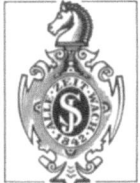

Maschallah Nadjmi (Editor)

Imaging of
Brain Metabolism
Spine and Cord
Interventional Neuroradiology
Free Communications

XVth Congress of the
European Society of Neuroradiology
Würzburg, September 13th - 17th, 1988

With 330 Figurers

Springer-Verlag Berlin Heidelberg New York
London Paris Tokyo Hong Kong

Prof. Dr. med. Maschallah Nadjmi
Abteilung für Neuroradiologie
Kopfklinik der Universität Würzburg
Joseph-Schneider-Straße 11
8700 Würzburg
FRG

ISBN-13: 978-3-642-74339-9   e-ISBN-13: 978-3-642-74337-5
DOI: 10.1007/978-3-642-74337-5

Offsetprinting: Saladruck, Berlin; Bookbinding: B. Helm, Berlin
2121/3020-543210 – Printed on acid-free paper

Preface

This volume contains papers given at the recent 15th Congress of the European Society of Neuroradiology, Würzburg.

The book consists of four main parts. The first three deal with new methods for imaging of brain metabolism (PET and MR spectroscopy), the spine and spinal cord, and interventional neuroradiology, while the fourth includes contributions on various topics including multiple sclerosis, AIDS, and the hypophysis.

Where manuscripts for papers given at the Congress were not available, short summaries based on abstracts submitted before the conference have been included.

We are very much obliged to Schering (Berlin) for their cooperation and for supporting this book. We also thank Springer-Verlag, especially B. Lewerich and M. Botsch, for the competent preparation and good design of this volume.

M. Nadjmi
President of the 15th Congress
of the European Society of
Neuroradiology

Table of Contents

Spine

X

Interventional Neuroradiology

XIV

Miscellaneous

PET and MR Spectroscopy

In Vivo Characterization of Pituitary Adenomas Using Positron Emission Tomography

K. Bergström, C. Muhr, M. Bergström, P. O. Lundberg, P. Lundin
and B. Långström

INTRODUCTION

Positron emission tomography (PET) is a technique which enables characterization of a large number of functional and biochemical parameters in vivo and thus vastly expands the diagnostic potentials of present neuroradiology.

We have used PET for the last 6 years with the aim of characterizing pituitary adenomas in order to establish the role of PET in the diagnosis of these tumors as a complement to radiological techniques such as MRI and CT.

MATERIALS AND METHODS

Altogether we have examined 81 patients with a pituitary adenoma. Most of these tumors were large with extra-sellar tumor extension, selected on the basis of possibility to perform a PET-study. Most of the cases were patients with a prolactinoma or a non-secreting pituitary adenoma, but a few cases with GH-, TSH- and ACTH-secreting adenomas were also included.

The patients were examined with PET using a brain scanner with 3 slices and 8 mm resolution. In the study of amino acid metabolism the patient was given an i.v. injection of ^{11}C-labelled L-methionine. For the investigation of dopamine D_2-receptor binding two studies were performed using ^{11}C-labelled dopamine D_2-antagonists, Raclopride or N-methylspiperone. Before the second study the patient was given Haloperidol in order to block the receptor binding, thereby indicating the non-specific binding. Subtraction of the second study from the first gives images of the specific receptor binding.

RESULTS

Pituitary adenomas are characterized by high amino acid metabolism (Muhr et al. 1984; Muhr et al. 1986b; Bergström et al. 1987a) which makes PET an ideal tool in the visualization of the adenomas. Of even greater importance is the high sensitivity of PET in recording treatment effects (Fig. 1). Thus, already within a few hours, the metabolism of prolactinomas is reduced by 30-50 % after the i.m. injection of bromocriptine (Bergström et al. 1987b). This early metabolic effect is later, within several weeks or months, accompanied by a significant tumor shrinkage (Muhr et al. 1988a; Muhr et al. 1988b).

The prolactinomas and some of the GH-secreting adenomas have high amounts of dopamine D_2-receptors as visualized with PET (Muhr et al. 1986a; Muhr et al. 1986b; Muhr et al. 1988c). The non-secreting adenomas demonstrate low or minimal receptor binding (Fig. 2). The potential of PET to determine the D_2-receptor status is of therapeutic importance in the selection of patients for bromocriptine treatment since a high amount of receptors is a prerequisite for good effect of dopamine agonist treatment.

4

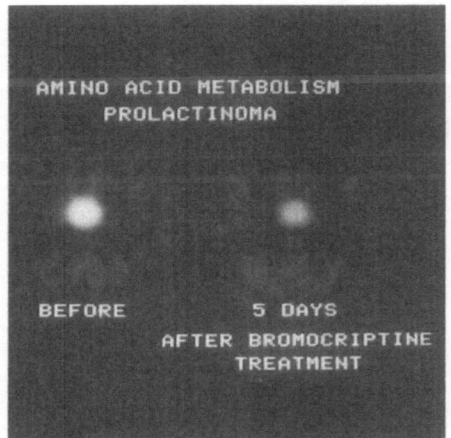

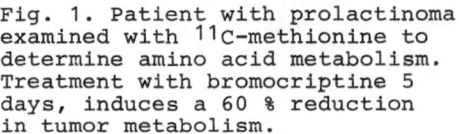

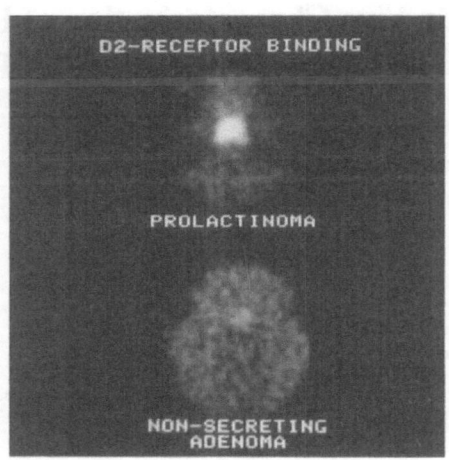

Fig. 1. Patient with prolactinoma
examined with ^{11}C-methionine to
determine amino acid metabolism.
Treatment with bromocriptine 5
days, induces a 60 % reduction
in tumor metabolism.

Fig. 2. Patient with prolactinoma
(upper image) and patient with non-
secreting adenoma (lower) examined
with the ^{11}C-labelled dopamine anta-
gonist Raclopride demonstrates the
significant differences in receptor
binding in the two types of adenomas.

DISCUSSION

With the use of the two different tracers we have been able to demonstrate
a role of PET in the diagnosis and treatment follow-up of pituitary adenomas with impacts on the clinical handling of the patients. The information obtained could not be deduced from other radiological techniques.
The relatively low resolution of present PET scanners still necessitate
complementary studies with CT and MRI.

With the rapid evolution of fast techniques for synthesis of ^{11}C-lab-
elled substances we foresee an increased role of PET in clinical routine and research in pituitary adenomas as well as in other tumors and
neurological disorders.

REFERENCES

Bergström M, Muhr C, Lundberg P O, Bergström K, Lundqvist H, Antoni G,
    Fasth K-G, Långström B (1987a) In vivo study of amino acid distribu-
    tion and metabolism in pituitary adenomas using positron emission
    tomography with ^{11}C-D-methionine and ^{11}C-L-methionine. J Comput Ass
    Tomogr 11:384-389
Bergström M, Muhr C, Lundberg P O, Bergström K, Gee AD, Fasth K-G,
    Långström B (1987b) Rapid decrease in amino acid metabolism in pro-
    lactin-secreting pituitary adenomas after bromocriptine treatment -
    in vivo study with positron emission tomography. J Comput Ass Tomogr
    11:815-819
Lundberg P O, Muhr C, Bergström K, Thuomas K-Å, Hartvig P, Lundqvist H,
    Antoni G, Långström B (1986) PET and NMR in diagnosis of pituitary
    adenomas. In: Battistin L, Gerstenbrand F (eds) PET and NMR: New per-
    spectives in neuroimaging and in clinical neurochemistry, Alan R.
    Liss, New York, pp. 407-424
Muhr C, Lundberg P O, Antoni G, Bergström K, Hartvig P, Lundqvist H,
    Långström B, Stålnacke C-G (1984) The uptake of ^{11}C-labelled bromo-
    criptine and methionine in pituitary tumors studied by positron emis-

sion tomography (PET). In: Lamberts SWJ, Tilders FJH, van Der Veen EA, Assies J (eds) Trends in diagnosis and treatment of pituitary adenomas, Free University Press, Amsterdam, pp. 151-155

Muhr C, Bergström M, Lundberg P O, Bergström K, Hartvig P, Lundqvist H, Antoni G, Långström B (1986a) Dopamine receptors in pituitary adenomas: PET visualization with C-11-N-methylspiperone. J Comp Ass Tomogr 10:175-180

Muhr C, Bergström M, Lundberg P O, Bergström K, Thuomas K-Å, Långström B (1986b) Dopamine receptors in pituitary adenomas and effect of bromocriptine treatment - evaluation with PET and MRI. Proceeding from the 14th International Cancer Congress, Budapest

Muhr C, Bergström M, Lundberg P O, Hartman M, Bergström K, Pellettieri L, Långström B (1988a) Malignant prolactinoma with multiple intra-cranial metastases studied with positron emission tomography. Neuro-surgery 22:374-379

Muhr C, Bergström M, Lundberg P O, Bergström K, Långström B (1988b) Positron emission tomography for the in vivo characterization and follow up of treatment in pituitary adenomas. In: Landolt AM, Hetz PU, Zapf J, Girard J, del Pozo E (eds) Advances in pituitary adeno-ma research, Advances in biosciences, vol 69, Pergamon Press, Oxford, pp. 163-170

Muhr C, Bergström M, Lundberg P O, Långström B, Bergström K (1988c) Pituitary imaging with positron emission tomography. Proceeding from 8th International Congress of Endocrinology, Kyoto

Early Changes in Regional Cerebral Metabolic Rates for Glucose and Oxygen and in Regional Cerebral Blood Flow of Malignant Gliomas After Intraarterial Chemotherapy with ACNU: Positron Emission Tomography Studies in 14 Patients

N. Roosen, K.-J. Langen, T. Kuwert, J. C. W. Kiwit, T. Kahn, H. Herzog, E. Rota, W. J. Bock, and L. E. Feinendegen

The prognosis of malignant gliomas remains grave despite surgery, radiotherapy and various kinds of adjuvant therapy, including chemotherapy. At our institution these tumors are treated with a combination of postoperative radiotherapy and intra-arterial (i.a.) chemotherapy with ACNU (iaACNU) as is reported elsewhere in the Proceedings of the XVth Congress of the European Society of Neuroradiology, Würzburg 1988. Because only some of these neoplasms respond to chemotherapy, a number of patients are treated unnecessarily with i.a. chemotherapy, which may have serious side effects. The measurement of early metabolic effects of iaACNU may provide important information to distinguish responders from non-responders. Previously published reports concerning the metabolic effects of chemotherapy in malignant gliomas dealt with longterm changes observed after completion of chemotherapy or after at least several cycles of radiochemotherapy. The present study reports on early effects of iaACNU in patients with malignant gliomas as measured with the use of positron emission tomography (PET).

POSITRON EMISSION TOMOGRAPHY: TECHNIQUE AND METHODS

The regional cerebral metabolic rate for glucose (rCMRglc) was determined using the $[^{18}F]$-2-fluoro-2-deoxy-D-glucose (FDG) method according to Phelps et al (1979). As suggested by others, the kinetic rate constants and the lumped constant of normal brain tissue were used (Di Chiro et al 1984; Hawkins et al 1986; Mineura et al 1987). rCMRglc was expressed in µmol/100g/min. These PET studies were performed with a *Scanditronix PC-4096* 8-ring PET scanner having a spatial resolution of 5mm. The regional cerebral metabolic rate for oxygen (rCMRO$_2$), the regional oxygen extraction ratio (rOER), and the regional cerebral blood flow (rCBF) were determined with the ^{15}O-steady-state inhalation method (Frackowiak et al 1980). Because of some errors in the absolute quantification of rCBF the data were analyzed as tumor-to-cortex ratios. These observations were obtained using an *ORTEC II* 1-ring PET scanner with a spatial resolution of 16mm.

INTRA-ARTERIAL CHEMOTHERAPY WITH ACNU: MANAGEMENT PROTOCOL

All patients having histopathologically proven malignant glioma of WHO grade IV or III, were treated with a combined management protocol involving cranial irradiation and iaACNU. ACNU is a relatively hydrophilic nitrosurea (Mori et al 1979; Hori et al 1987). ACNU was administered via the internal carotid artery ipsilaterally to the tumor. The first 100mg iaACNU course was given within 10 days after surgery. Subsequently 60Gy of irradiation was administered. Upon completion of radiotherapy 100mg ACNU were infused i.a. for

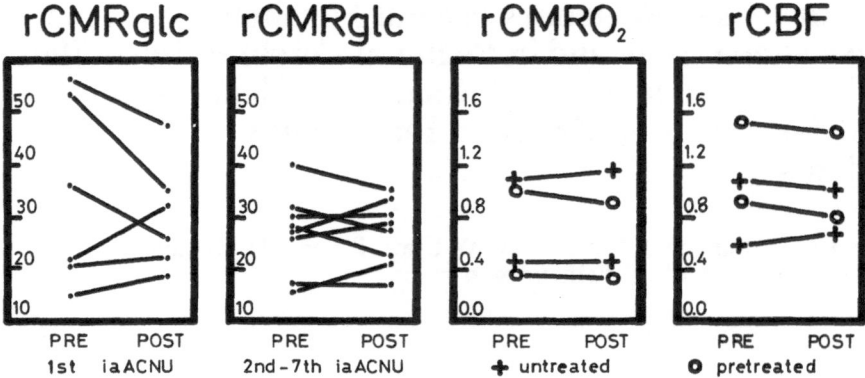

Fig. 1. rCMRglc, rCMRO$_2$, and rCBF of malignant gliomas, that were pretreated (i.e. 2nd-7th iaACNU) or untreated (i.e. 1st iaACNU). rCMRglc is given in µmol/100g/min, and rCMRO$_2$ as well as rCBF are expressed as tumor-to-cortex ratios.

the second time, and this procedure was repeated every 6-8 weeks up to a total of 7 i.a. infusions. Out of this group 14 subjects with partially extirpated or stereotactically diagnosed tumors were selected for PET studies. PET was performed within 3 days before iaACNU and within 6 days after iaACNU. Some patients were investigated during several iaACNU cycles. Ten patients were studied for rCMRglc. Six of them had not received any adjuvant therapy at the time of their first PET examination, whereas 4 were pretreated with radio- and chemotherapy. rCMRO$_2$, rOER, and rCBF were investigated in 4 more cases. Two were not pretreated, and 2 were pretreated with radio- and chemotherapy at their first PET study.

RESULTS (Fig. 1)

In untreated gliomas rCMRglc levels were heterogeneous: 2 tumors had an elevated rCMRglc (>50µmol/100g/min) and the remaining neoplasms in this group showed rather low rCMRglc. After iaACNU both tumors with elevated rCMRglc demonstrated an obvious decrease in glucose consumption (18 and 18%). The tumors of the untreated group with low rCMRglc revealed no change (5%) or an increase in rCMRglc (30, 31, and 57%). Of these 6 patients 2 died relatively early, due to systemic mycosis in one case and without known reason in the second case. Two of the four remaining patients had progressive disease, one remained stable, and one showed good tumor response to therapy. The two patients with progressive disease had either an increase in rCMRglc after iaACNU or no change of rCMRglc after iaACNU. The patient with stable disease had also no change in rCMRglc after iaACNU. The one patient with a good tumor response and a marked reduction in tumor size had shown an important reduction of rCMRglc after the first chemotherapy with iaACNU. In pretreated there was no case with high glucose consumption, almost all values being less than 30µmol/100g/min, and there were no significant changes after iaACNU.

The rCBF tumor-to-cortex ratios showed considerable differences between these tumors: the ratios ranged from 0.6 to 1.5 without obvious change after iaACNU. The same was true for rCMRO$_2$ and consequently for rOER. Pretreatment of gliomas did not seem to have any influence on rCBF, rOER, or rCMRO$_2$.

DISCUSSION

PET has been used to examine various physiological and biochemical parameters such as glucose consumption, amino acid uptake, oxygen metabolism, and blood flow in malignant gliomas (Brooks et al 1986). rCBF and rCMRO$_2$ are known to vary considerably from patient to patient without any significant correlation to malignancy (Leenders et al 1985). In the present study no effects of chemotherapy on rCBF and rCMRO$_2$ were observed which is in agreement with previous reports (Mineura et al 1987).

Contrary to rCBF and rCMRO$_2$ glucose consumption is supposed to correlate with malignancy and prognosis of malignant gliomas (Di Chiro et al 1982; Patronas et al 1982). These investigators observed variable rCMRglc in gliomas of different patients which is consistent with our own results. Mineura et al (1987) studied rCMRglc using PET in eight patients before and several weeks after radiochemotherapy with ACNU and N-(2-tetrahydrofuryl)-5-fluorouracil. In that study seven from eight patients showed a decrease of rCMRglc after radiochemotherapy and a reduction in tumor size while one patient with an increase in rCMRglc had progressive disease. Thus, a positive correlation between changes in rCMRglc in tumor tissue after chemotherapy and clinical outcome seems probable. Mineura et al (1987), however, reported only late effects of radiochemotherapy, which was completed at the time of the second PET scan; the results of the PET studies could not have an impact on continuation, interruption or modification of ongoing radiochemotherapy.

The present study investigated early effects of chemotherapy in order to get parameters for modification of individual therapy. The preliminary data reported herein indicate that in pretreated patients rCMRglc in tumors does not change after chemotherapy while in untreated patients the observed changes in rCMRglc appeared to correlate with clinical outcome. Similar results have been reported measuring the early effect of chemotherapy on amino acid uptake (Derlon et al 1987).

The relationship between the cytotoxic effects of nitrosoureas and the metabolic reaction as studied with PET remains unclear. Probably, one of the critical features of the metabolic effects of nitrosourea chemotherapy is the degree of cellular repair activity and its efficacity (Kohn et al 1981). The reduction of rCMRglc after chemotherapy may be caused by cytotoxic cell necrosis or by metabolic inhibition. An increase of rCMRglc may reflect an activation of reparative processes.

The measurement of early effects on rCMRglc at the first cycle of our management protocol with adjuvant iaACNU after surgery appears to be useful to monitor therapeutic effectiveness in order to optimize individual tumor therapy.

REFERENCES

Brooks DJ, Beaney RP, Thomas DGT (1986) The role of positron emission tomography in the study of cerebral tumors. Semin Oncol 13:83-93

Derlon JM, Bourdet C, Chatel M, et al (1987) Study of ^{11}C-L-methionine uptake in brain gliomas by positron emission tomography: metabolic grading, and effects of radiotherapy and intra-arterial chemotherapy. In: Chatel M, Darcel F, Pecker J (eds) Brain oncology. Biology, diagnosis and therapy, pp 179-184. Martinus Nijhoff Publ, Dordrecht, Boston

Di Chiro G, Brooks RA, Patronas NJ, et al (1984) Issues in the *in vivo* measurement of glucose metabolism of human central nervous system tumors. Ann Neurol 15 (Suppl):S138-S146

Di Chiro G, De La Paz RL, Brooks RA, et al (1982) Glucose utilization of cerebral gliomas measured by $[^{18}F]$fluorodeoxyglucose and positron emission tomography. Neurology 32:1323-1329

Frackowiak RSJ, Lenzi GL, Jones T, Heather JD (1980) Quantitative measurement of regional cerebral blood flow and oxygen metabolism in man using ^{15}O and positron emisssion tomography: theory, procedure, and normal values. J Comput Assist Tomogr 4:727-736

Hawkins RA, Phelps ME, Huang SC (1986) Effects of temporal sampling, glucose metabolic rates, and disruptions of the blood-brain barrier on the FDG model with and without a vascular compartment: studies in human brain tumors with PET. J Cereb Blood Flow Metab 6:170-183

Hori T, Muraoka K, Saito Y, et al (1987) Influence of modes of ACNU administration on tissue and blood concentration in malignant brain tumors. J Neurosurg 66:372-378

Kohn KW, Erickson LC, Laurent G, et al (1981) DNA crosslinking and the origin of sensitivity to chloroethylnitrosureas. In: Prestayko AW, Baker LH, Crooke ST, et al (eds) Nitrosoureas. Current status and new developments, pp 69-83. Academic Press, New York, London

Leenders KL, Thomas DGT, Beaney RP, Brooks DJ (1985) Cerebral gliomas studied with positron emission tomography. In: Voth D, Krauseneck P (eds) Chemotherapy of gliomas. Basic research, experiences and results, pp 101-109. Walter de Gruyter, Berlin, New York

Mineura K, Yasuda T, Kowada M, et al (1987) Positron emission tomographic evaluation of radiochemotherapeutic effect on regional cerebral hemocirculation and metabolism in patients with gliomas. J Neuro-Oncol 5:277-285

Mori T, Mineura K, Katakura R (1979) A consideration on pharmacokinetics of a new water-soluble anti-tumor nitrosourea, ACNU, in patients with malignant brain tumor. No To Shinkei 31:601-606 (Jpn)

Patronas NJ, Di Chiro G, Brooks RA, et al (1982) Work in progress: $[^{18}F]$-Fluorodeoxyglucose and positron emission tomography in the evaluation of radiation necrosis in the brain. Radiology 144:885-889

Phelps ME, Huang SC, Hoffman EJ, et al (1978) Tomographic measurement of local cerebral glucose metabolic rate in humans with (F-18)2-fluoro-2-deoxy-D-glucose: validation of method. Ann Neurol 6:371-388

ACKNOWLEDGEMENT

The authors are indebted to Ms. Dr. H. Hüttmann, ASTA-Degussa Pharma, D-6000 Frankfurt/Main, for continuous support of brain tumor research at the University of Düsseldorf.

PET in the Differential Diagnosis and Evaluation of Treatment in Dementias

W.-D. Heiss, K. Herholz, G. Pawlik, B. Szelies, and K. Wienhard

INTRODUCTION

Under normal conditions, function, metabolism and blood flow of the central nervous system are closely interlinked. Therefore, the cerebral structures involved in different activities can be demonstrated by studying these physiological parameters. Since disturbances of cerebral function are followed by changes in metabolism and blood flow, and pathological impairments of blood supply and energy metabolism themselves lead to functional deficits, in many diseases of the CNS these parameters are measurably altered without it being possible to draw conclusions with respect to aetiology. Dementias, which are clinically manifested primarily as non-localizable disturbances of cerebral function, can hardly be diagnosed in the early stages by conventional supplementary neurological investigations, which detect mainly localized morphologic lesions. Since glucose is the most important substrate of cerebral energy metabolism, studies of glucose metabolism are currently the best method of detecting and quantifying functional disturbances of the brain. The glucose metabolic rate can be determined regionally and three-dimensionally in the brain by means of positron emission tomography.

Glucose metabolism in healthy subjects
The different rates of glucose metabolism in various regions of the brain depending on their functional activity have been determined in a number of studies (review by Heiss et al. 1984). In our studies the mean glucose turnover rate of 42 normal subjects (age 43 + 19.1 years, 14 women, 28 men) was 34.6 + 3.83 µmol/100 g cerebral tissue/min. Highly significant regional differences with values between 40 and 50 µmol/100 g/min were detected in the striatum, upper limbic system, insula, frontal cortex and primary visual cortex, between 35 and 40 µmol/100 g/min in the other grey structures of the hemispheres, between 30 and 35 µmol/100 g/min in the cerebellum and hippocampal structures and below 20 µmol/100 g/min in the medullary layer. The findings of different PET laboratories as regards the age-dependence of cerebral glucose metabolism are contradictory. Our own studies confirm the existence of a certain age dependency: the global rate of cerebral glucose metabolism showed a decline with advancing age which, although statistically significant (p < 0.05) represented less than 2 % per decade. A detailed analysis revealed that the individual brain regions were affected symmetrically but to rather differing degrees (p < 0.0001).

Primary degenerative dementias
Primary degenerative dementias of the Alzheimer type (AD) which are accompanied by a loss of cortical neurons disturbances of various transmitter systems but also by selective reduction of specific projection systems (especially the cholinergic system, Coyle et al. 1983) and also by typical pathological changes (plaques and fibrils), account for more than 50 % of all dementia disorders. Patients with AD show a reduction of cerebral glucose metabolism proportional to the severity of the dementia, in which the reduced metabolism is detectable before the occurrence of atrophic changes in CT and shows significant regional differences: the bilateral local reductions are especially pronounced in the parieto-temporal and frontal cortex and do not affect the primary visual and sensorimotor cortex or the subcortical structures and the cerebellum (Kuhl et al. 1983, Friedland et al. 1983, Duara et al. 1986). In studies which compared results of PET and neuropsychological tests, it was possible to demonstrate a relationship between leading symptoms and the localization of especially reduced glucose metabolism: when an aphasic disorder was predominant, glucose metabolic disturbance was more pronounced in the left than in the right parietal lobe, when

apraxic symptoms predominated this parameter was disturbed more on the right than the left, while on predominance of amnestic deficits no asymmetry was present (Foster et al. 1983).

In the second, but much rarer form of primary degenerative dementia, Pick's disease, the first and most marked metabolic changes - in analogy to the primary localization of pathological changes - are seen in the frontal and temporal lobe (Szelies and Karenberg 1986). This distinctly different pattern of damage allows Pick's disease to be differentiated from AD; in moderate cases it is often not possible to make this distinction on the basis of clinical findings alone.

The pattern of metabolic disturbance is also characteristic in Huntington's chorea which in addition to the extrapyramidal-hyperkinetic syndrome is always accompanied by dementia disorders. The glucose turnover rate in the neostriatum is already significantly reduced in the early stages of this disease and as the severity and duration of the disease increases, metabolism is seen to be reduced in the nucleus caudatus and putamen, and later (according to the degree of severity of dementia) also the cerebral cortex (Kuhl et al. 1984). Since the metabolic disturbances precede the clinical manifestations of the disease, PET studies may possibly help to identify persons at risks in chorea families, and these studies as well as genetic investigations can be used to establish a prognosis for the subsequent appearance of the disease (Hayden et al. 1987, Mazziotta et al. 1987).

Vascular dementias

Focal cerebral lesions caused by blood flow disturbances can induce dementia syndromes through two mechanisms in particular: multiple lesions in mostly neurologically silent, frequently subcortical regions impair cerebral function in the form of dementia (multi-infarct dementia) when they exceed a total volume that cannot be precisely defined (80-150 cm^3). In rare cases, relatively small infarcts of critical localization can cause dementia syndromes in addition to the focally dependent neurological symptoms.

Multi-infarct dementias (MID) together with the AD-MID mixed forms account for about 30 % of all dementia syndromes. A clinical differentiation on the basis of rating scales (Hachinski et al. 1975) is often difficult, and diagnostic classification is often easier on the basis of morphological lesions demonstrated by CT or MRT. In MID patients, PET can clearly differentiate mostly multilocular metabolic reductions from the pattern typical of AD (Kuhl et al. 1983). Detection of ischemic lesions in the medullary layer in MID and Binswanger's disease can be performed with great sensitivity by means of T_2-weighted MRT (Heiss et al. 1986), and the regions of reduced metabolism then correspond to the superjacent deafferentated cortical areas.

Infarctions in the cerebral regions which are particularly important for the integrity of the personality lead to disturbances of behaviour, affect, mood and intellectual performance. This is especially true of infarcts in the area supplied by the anterior cerebral artery, after which the mental changes often outlast the focal neurological symptoms. Small localized infarcts in strategically important regions, for example unilaterally in the anterior centre of the thalamus or bilaterally in the median thalamus lead to permanent cognitive and amnestic losses.

Dementias of other aetiology

Inflammatory diseases of the brain may affect regions important for overall performance and thereby lead to dementia, or extensive inflammatory changes may cause diffuse cell losses and thereby impair higher cerebral functions. The typical example of localized inflammatory destruction of tissue is herpes simplex encephalitis, because its site of predilection is the lower temporal lobe frequently with bilateral involvement. When the inflammatory changes are limited to mesial temporal structures, pure amnestic syndromes may occur. Further extended bilateral lesions additionally cause cognitive and behavioural disturbances resembling the Klüver-Bucy syndrome described for monkeys after experimental bilateral temporal lobotomy and amygdala ablation. Creutzfeld-Jakob disease, a subacute spongiform encephalitis caused by slow virus infection, leads to progressive dementia, pyramidal, extrapyramidal and cerebellar disturbances and myoclonus with early fatal outcome. Glucose metabolism was patchily reduced in such patients (Horowitz et al. 1982). In HIV encephalitis, which often appears as the initial disease manifestation but may also develop later on in the course of HIV disease, regional reductions of glucose metabolism were detected, but these were not significantly correlated with test results (Navia et al. 1987). In patients with progressive paralysis glucose metabolism was globally reduced and the most pronounced disturbances affected the lower and mesial temporal lobe and the insula bilaterally and slight hypometabolism was detectable in superior intraparietal, pre- and mid-frontal locations. This metabolic pattern could in turn explain the characteristic symptoms of progressive paralysis.

Severe craniocerebral traumata which leave behind extensive cerebral damage sometimes cause permanent impairments of cognitive and affective cerebral function. In PET the globally reduced cerebral glucose metabolism is particularly pronounced bilaterally in the orbitofrontal, parietal and lower temporal cortex. In normal hydrocephalus the clinical picture is characterized by a decrease in cognitive function, disturbances of gait and incontinence. Glucose metabolism is reduced especially in cortical areas at the level of the ventricles (32 % reduction compared to control group, Jagust et al. 1985). This study could help in delineating this disorder from other forms of dementia (particularly AD) and in selecting patients for shunt operations.

Korsakoff's syndrome is an example of a relatively selective memory disturbance. The most frequent cause is thiamine deficiency in chronic alcohol abuse, although several other diseases may also cause similar memory impairments. Metabolism was diffusely moderately reduced and was disturbed especially bilaterally in the hippocampus, hypothalamus and thalamus.

It is often difficult to differentiate the affective disorders with impairment of drive and psychomotoricity seen in depressions from similar symptoms in the early stages of dementia. The metabolic patterns observed in depressed patients are not comparable to the characteristic changes seen in dementias, particularly in AD. When the overall metabolic level is in relation to the mood (Baxter et al. 1987) there are sometimes regional differences of varying distribution; a pattern typical of depression or correlations between the metabolic values of certain regions with the severity of specific symptoms or function deficits have not so far been described.

Evaluation of drug effects
Because the functional activity in Alzheimer dementias is reflected in metabolic values, measurements of this kind may be valuable in assessing the effects of drugs. Metabolic investigations could then also be useful in providing objective evidence of therapeutic results within a relatively short time, when clinical improvements or a slowing of the progression of the deficits would not yet be apparent.

Therapeutic concepts developed in the last few years include measures for substitution of cholinergic function. Some therapeutic approaches centering on the cholinergic activity - inhibition of cholinesterase with physostigmine or administration of tetrahydroaminoacridine (Summers et al. 1986) - have reportedly brought about improvements in the memory disturbances typical of AD.

The use of PET to objectivize the effects of drugs is still rare and has so far been limited to small groups of patients. Glucose metabolism was monitored for six to twelve weeks in eight patients with AD of differing severity undergoing therapy with a muscarinic choline agonist (Szelies et al. 1986). Over this period the global metabolic rate decreased under therapy, but there was a compensation of the heterogeneous metabolic pattern typical of AD. This effect was especially pronounced in patients who became clinically stabilized on this therapy and showed improved performance in several functions; this group which profited from the therapy originally showed regional glucose metabolic rates diverging relatively little from the norm and were also those whose AD was less severe.

Another study (Heiss et al. 1988) examined whether piracetam, which improves memory performance when administered in combination with precursors of acetylcholine (Ferris et al. 1982, Smith et al. 1984) has metabolic effects in AD. Of 16 patients with dementia syndrome nine fulfilled the criteria for AD (McKhann et al. 1984) and the remaining seven were graded as MID or unclassifiable and used as a control group. Under piracetam treatment (6 g piracetam b.i.d. (Nootrop, UCB Chemie) for 14 days as a short infusion) the glucose metabolism values in the AD group increased in the frontal, central, parieto-occipital, visual, auditory and cingulate cortex, basal ganglia and thalamus whereas no significant changes were detected in the non-AD group. The differences in the effects of treatment between AD and non-AD groups were statistically significant (ANOVA $p < 0.02$ for interactions between regions, treatment and group). These results were supported by improvements in five AD patients during the short therapy phase with respect to their clinical deficits and their performance in tests, but controlled clinical studies will be needed in order to justify the large-scale clinical use of piracetam in AD.

REFERENCES

Baxter LR, Phelps ME, Mazziotta JC et al (1987) Arch Gen Psychiat 44: 211-218
Coyle JT, Price DL, Delong MR (1983) Science 219: 1184-1190
Duara R, Grady C, Haxby J et al (1986) Neurology 36: 879-887
Ferris SH, Reisberg B, Crook T et al (1982) In: Corkin S et al (eds) Alzheimer's Disease: A Report of Progress. Raven Press, New York, pp 475-481
Foster NL, Chase TN, Fedio P et al (1983) Neurology (Cleveland) 33: 961-965
Friedland RP, Budinger TF, Ganz E et al (1983) J Comput Assist Tomogr 7: 590-598
Hachinski VC, Iliff LD, Zilkha E et al (1975) Arch Neurol 32: 632-637
Hayden MR, Hewitt J, Stoessl AJ et al (1987) Neurology 37: 1441-1447
Heiss WD, Hebold I, Klinkhammer P et al (1988) J Cereb Blood Flow Metab 8: 613-617
Heiss WD, Herholz K, Böcher-Schwarz HG et al (1986) J Comput Assist Tomogr 10: 903-911
Heiss WD, Pawlik G, Herholz K et al (1984) J Cereb Blood Flow Metab 4: 212-223
Horowitz S, Benson DF, Kuhl DE, Cummings JL (1982) Neurology 32: A167
Jagust WJ, Friedland RP, Budinger TF (1985) J Neurol Neurosurg Psychiat 48: 1091-1096
Kuhl DE, Metter EJ, Riege WH, Markham CH (1984) Ann Neurol 15 (Suppl): S119-S125
Kuhl DE, Metter EJ, Riege WH et al (1983) J Cereb Blood Flow Metab 3 (Suppl 1) S494-S495
Mazziotta JC, Phelps ME, Pahl JJ et al (1987) New Engl J Med 316: 357-362
Navia B, Sidtis JJ, Moeller JR et al (1987) J Cereb Blood Flow Metab 7 (Suppl 1): S388
Smith RC, Vroulis G, Johnson R, Morgan R (1984) Psychopharmacol Bull 20: 542-545
Summers WK, Majovski LV, Marsh GM et al (1986) New Engl J Med 315: 1241-1245
Szelies B, Herholz K, Pawlik G et al (1986) Fortschr Neurol Psychiat 54: 364-373
Szelies B, Karenberg A (1986) Fortschr Neurol Psychiat 54: 393-397

Image-Guided Localized ^{31}P NMR Spectroscopy of the Human Brain: Preliminary Clinical Results

W. Heindel, J. Bunke, and G. Friedmann

Introduction

For biomedical research, the application of phosphorus-31 NMR spectroscopy (^{31}P MRS) to living tissues and organisms is of particular interest. The phosphorus-containing compounds in the human body play an important role in cellular metabolism, in the supply and utilization of chemical energy, and are present in sufficient concentration to permit detection by MR spectroscopy. This study was designed to evaluate the diagnostic usefulness of a combination of hydrogen-1 MR imaging (^{1}H-MRI) and ^{31}P-MRS in diseases of the human brain. A great number of patients suffering from intracranial tumors was examined, whereas our experiences with ischemic brain lesions and degenerative brain lesions are still limited.

Materials and Methods

A 1.5 T whole body MR system (Gyroscan S15, Philips) operating at 64 MHz for ^{1}H and 25.9 MHz for ^{31}P MR was used. For a combined examination - imaging and spectroscopy - of the brain, a ^{31}P head coil was inserted into the standard ^{1}H head coil. ^{1}H MRI preceded spectroscopy in order to judge the pathologic tissue changes macroscopically and to define the volume of interest (VOI) within the lesion. For spatial assignment of the acquired ^{31}P spectra a modification (Luyten et al. 1986) of the "Image-Selected in Vivo Spectroscopy (ISIS)"-technique (Ordidge et al. 1986) was applied.

For a VOI of at least 35 x 35 x 35 mm 512 FIDs were accumulated using an interpulse delay of 3 seconds. With this procedure, the duration of a combined examination with imaging and spectroscopy lay between 60 and 90 minutes. The spectra were uniformly post-processed by multiplication with a Lorentz-Gauss filter function, a convolution difference filter and linear phase correction. Tissue pH was determined from the PCr-P$_i$ chemical shift difference using the formula proposed by Petroff et al. in 1985.

Up to now, more than 60 patients suffering from large brain tumors were examined according to this protocol (Heindel et al. 1988). Four patients with inoperable brain tumors were treated with radio- and/or chemotherapy. Tumor response to this treatment was monitored spectroscopically by follow-up studies. Three patients with symptoms of cerebral ischemia were studied.

Results and Discussion

Compared to normal brain tissue, spectra from meningiomas demonstrated the most obvious differences:

The phosphocreatine peak decreased markedly, typically below the level of ATP. Additionally, the phosphodiester peak was reduced, whereas the phosphomonoesters showed an increase in several cases. Calculation of tissue pH resulted in normal values or values shifted to the alkaline range. In contrast to ischemic infarction no tissue acidosis could be observed in tumors.

The study of intrinsinc tumors revealed less distinct spectral changes:

In malignant gliomas a reduced and sometimes splitted signal from phosphodiesters was observed. This was the only pathological finding in some cases of intraaxial tumors. In several gliomas the resonance of PCr was decreased as well, but not below the level of ATP. Fig. 1 shows a glioblastoma of the temporo-parietal region as an example.

In four cases of low-grade astrocytomas the ^{31}P spectrum could not be differentiated from a comparative measurement in normal brain tissue. This result demonstrates the difficulties of interpreting ^{31}P MR spectra without the information from imaging.

In spite of a sufficiently large measuring volume, no regular spectrum could be measured within two epidermoid cysts. Accordingly, difficulties were encountered in the evaluation of cystic tumors due to their much lower signal intensity.

In follow-up studies of inoperable tumors undergoing treatment by radio- and/or chemotherapy ^{31}P MRS demonstrated metabolic changes in two patients at a time, when imaging methods did not detect any change of tumor size or structure. Above all a recovery of the phosphocreatine peak could be observed. Further investigations have to be done in order to evaluate the usefulnes of ^{31}P MRS for detecting therapeutic response.

Our experiences with ischemic brain lesions are still very limited. A study of a transient ischemic attack as well as of a PRIND - in each case 24 hours after subsidence of clinical symptoms - revealed no spectroscopic changes. This was different in a patient with a hemorrhagic infarct: The intracellular pH was calculated as 6.75, thus indicating tissue acidosis.

Conclusions

The procedure for a combined imaging and spectroscopic examination of the brain on a clinical MR system is established. Volume-selective spectroscopy, which provides data on regional tissue function and pathophysiologic alterations, extends the morphologic information obtained from imaging.

Examination of different intracranial tumors showed characteristic spectral patterns. An increased number of cases and quantification will demonstrate whether the observed spectral changes can be correlated to histology. Moreover, ^{31}P MRS might emerge as a potentially valuable tool for detecting therapeutic response in tumors after radio- or chemotherapy, before any changes are evident by imaging modalities.

References

Heindel W, Bunke J, Glathe S, Steinbrich W, Mollevanger L (1988)
    Combined ^{1}H MR Imaging and Localized ^{31}P MR Spectroscopy of Intracranial Tumors in 43 Patients. J Comput Assist Tomogr, in press

Luyten PR, Groen JP, Arnold DA, Balériaux D, den Hollander JA (1986) ^{31}P Localized Spectroscopy of the Human Brain in Situ at 1.5 Tesla. SMRM, 5th Annual Meeting - Book of Abstracts 1083

Ordidge RJ, Conelly A, Lohmann JAB (1986) Image-selected in Vivo Spectroscopy (ISIS). A New Technique for Spatially Selective NMR Spectroscopy. J Magn Res 66: 283-294

Petroff OAC, Prichard JW, Behar KL, Alger JR, den Hollander JA, Shulman RG (1985) Cerebral Intracellular pH by ^{31}P Nuclear Magnetic Resonance Spectroscopy. Neurology 35: 781-788

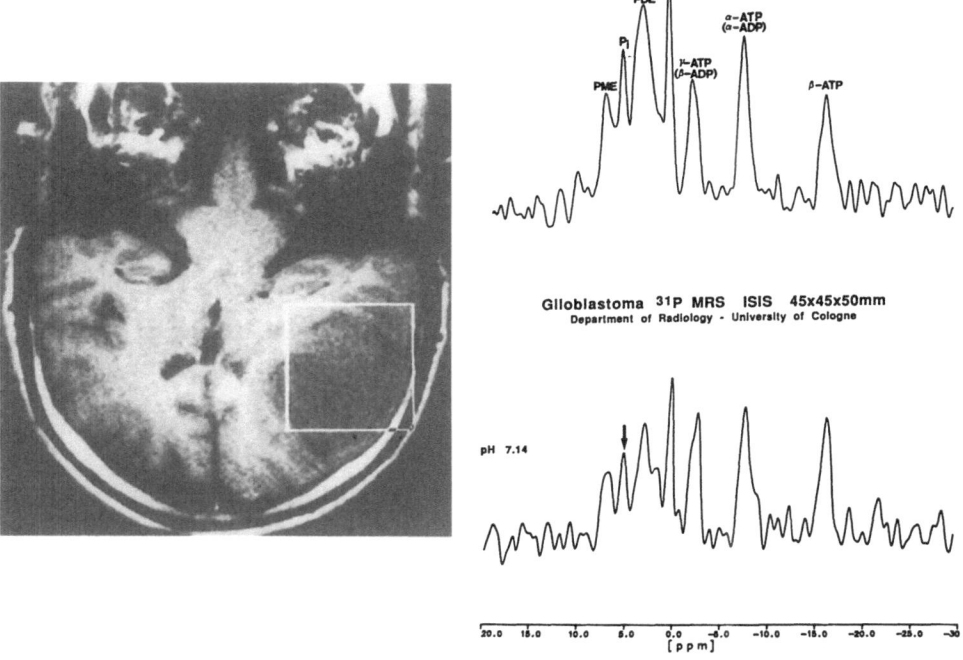

Figure 1. Image-guided localized ^{31}P MRS in a glioblastoma.

- Proton image (SE 250/30). The volume of interest is localized in the tumor tissue.
- ^{31}P spectra of normal brain (top), and a glioblastoma (bottom) with a decrease of phosphodiesters (PDE) and phosphocreatine (PCr). The chemical shift of the inorganic phosphate peak (P$_i$) indicates intracellular alkalosis.

Potentials of Magnetic Resonance Spectroscopy in Neuroradiology

S. Felber, R. Sauter, and W. Löffler

Introduction

Magnetic resonance refers to the ability of nuclei with a nonzero spin to undergo processing proportional to an external magnetic field. Two different applications of this physical phenomenon exist: magnetic resonance imaging (MRI) and magnetic resonance spectroscopy (MRS). In MRI, differences of the resonance frequency reflect mainly the position of the atoms in space, depending on the use of magnetic gradients, as experimentally demonstrated by Lauterbur in 1973. The hydrogen atom, by far the most common atom in living organisms, permits MRI with high spatial resolution and excellent soft-tissue contrast. Proton MRI has been developed into a routine diagnostic modality in neuroradiology with high sensitivity, but it still has limited specificity. Much interest is therefore now directed to MRS which, on the basis of experimental results in animal studies and human muscle disorders (Radda 1986), promises the introduction of biochemical information into clinical neuroradiology.

In Vivo Magnetic Resonance Spectroscopy

Since the initial experiments in 1946 by Bloch and Purcell, MRS has been used in chemistry and biochemistry. In contrast to MRI, the differences in resonance frequency do not encode the location but the molecular constitution of a given nucleus (chemical shift). Therefore, MRS requires high homogeneity of the magnetic field and high field strength, because the chemical shift is proportional to the magnetic field. Recent technical developments allow both MRI and MRS in whole-body systems (den Hollander and Luyten 1986).

Application of MRS in vivo carries the problem of localizing the MR signal of diseased tissues. The use of surface coils has been successful in disorders near the surface of the object, but focal disease in the depth of the organism requires more sophisticated techniques (Aue 1986). Lack of sensitivity is the other problem of in vivo MRS. Table 1 shows the sensitivity of biologically important nuclei relative to hydrogen. ^{19}F exhibits the highest relative sensitivity but normally is not detected by MRS within the organism. One possible application is the use of ^{19}F-labeled drugs (Wolf et al. 1987). Also ^{13}C, due to its natural abundance of 1.1% increases the necessity for labeled substances. Sodium has a quadrupolar nucleus and is suited for MRI. However, the biexponential T2 decay complicates the differentiation of intra- from extracellular compounds (Perman et al. 1986). Future applications may offer insights into brain edema and tumors as well as tissue osmolality.

The most promising data are available on ^{1}H and ^{31}P spectroscopy, and these will be discussed in detail.

Table 1. Sensitivity of biologically important nuclei relative to hydrogen

Atom	Relative sensitivity (%)	Natural abundance (%)	Resonance frequency at 1.5 T (MHz)	Spin
^{1}H	100	99.9	63.8	1/2
^{19}F	83	100	60	1/2
^{23}Na	9.2	100	16.8	3/2
^{31}P	6.9	100	25.8	1/2
^{13}C	1.5	1.1	16.6	1/2

Localized ^{31}P Spectroscopy

The particular interest directed to ^{31}P spectroscopy depends on the central role of phosphate compounds in the bioenergetics of living cells. MRS resolves the resonances of adenosine triphosphate (ATP), phospohcreatine (PCr), and inorganic phosphate (Pi). Phosphorous spectra of the brain also contain the broad resonances of phosphordiesters (PD) and phosphormonoesters (PM). The chemical shift between Pi and PCr can be used to calculate tissue pH. ^{31}P spectroscopy has already contributed to the understanding of muscle disorders, especially in mitochondrial myopathies (Argov et al. 1987). Application of ^{31}P MRS to brain asphyxia in newborns showed significant reduction of PCr/Pi ratios (Hope et al. 1984). Surface-coil ^{31}P MRS at 1.5 T in chronic infarction of four adults (Bottomley et al. 1986) did not exhibit differences in the ratios of energy-phosphate metabolities, but a decrease in the total MRS signal in the infarcted area was noted. Using surface coils with slice-selective saturation (FROGS; Sauter et al. 1987), we compared the healthy with the affected hemisphere in two patients with chronic middle cerebral artery infarction and obtained similar results. One explanation is that there are still metabolically active glial cells within the infarcted area, but there was also evidence of partial-volume averaging with normal brain tissue in our patients. Therefore a crossed Helmholtz coil was used in the further studies (Requard et al. 1988), which allowed ^{1}H imaging and ^{31}P MRS without repositioning of the patient and ubiquitous positioning of the VOI.

Subsequently a series of patients with gliomas (n = 6) and meningiomas (n = 3) has been examined following a standardized protocol. Only tumors with an extension of more than 4×4 cm in plane and 4 cm in the orthogonal plane and with a homogeneous consistution on MRI were selected. The patients were positioned within the crossed Helmholtz coil. Shimming was performed using the linear gradients. In all patients, a water-proton line width of less than 0.5 ppm, usually 20-22 Hz, was achieved within 10 min. After the shimming procedure FLASH images in

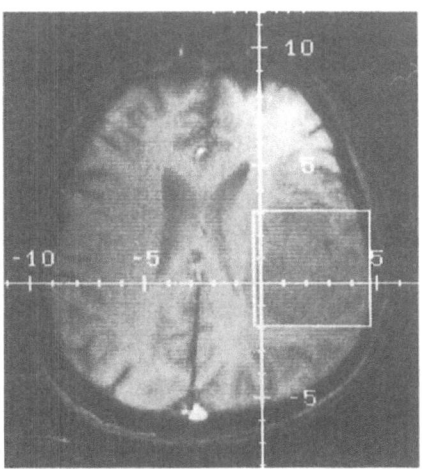

Fig.1. Axial FLASH image. The selected VOI is positioned over a surgically proven meningoma

orthogonal orientations for rapid VOI selection were performed. Using image-selected in vivo spectroscopy (ISI; Aue 1986), a 125-ml VOI was positioned over the tumor region (Fig.1). Eight free induction decays (FIDs) are accumulated with the ISIS sequence. The first ISIS FID is measured without gradients and reflects the ^{31}P spectrum of the whole brain. The following FIDs are acquired in the presence of magnetic gradients, and an addition/subtraction algorithm calculates the ^{31}P signal originating from the VOI. TR of the ISIS sequence was 3-4 s, and 32 acquisitions were taken, resulting in an examination time of 15 min. The ^{31}P spectrum of the tumor voxel was compared either to the first ISIS spectrum or a second VOI placed within the normal hemisphere.

No significant changes in the PCr/ATP ratio and tissue pH were observed from the tumors. This may reflect our selection of homogeneously appearing tumors without evidence of tumor necrosis or hemorrhage. The meningioma spectra were characterized by an elevated phosphormonoester level, probably due to phosphoethanolamine (Fig.2). This result is in accord with the findings of Segebarth et al. (1987).

In the glioma group all tumors were low-grade astrocytomas. The low-grade astrocytomas exhibited no consistant abnormality of the ^{31}P spectra. In two cases the PM level appeared to be even lower than that of the normal brain.

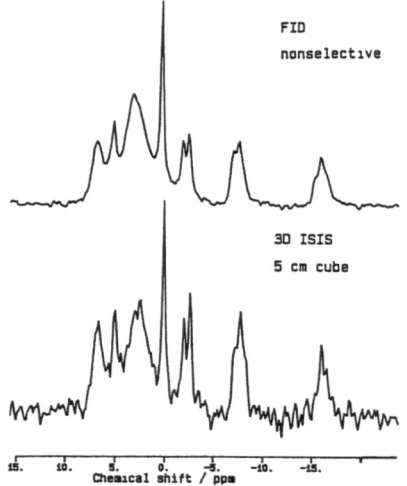

FID
nonselective

3D ISIS
5 cm cube

Chemical shift / ppm
15.   10.   5.   0.   -5.   -10.   -15.

Fig.2. ^{31}P signals. Upper spectrum, signal of the whole brain. The resonances are assigned to PM, Pi, PD, PCr, γ-ATP, α-ATP, β-ATP (left to right). Lower spectrum, from the meningioma: elevated PM level

Localized ^{1}H MRS

The ^{1}H FID of the brain is characterized by the dominant water-proton
resonance. Within the brain, access to the biochemically important
metabolities (lactic acid, creatine, and neurotransmitters) requires
sufficient suppression of the H_2O resonance (Tanaka et al. 1986).
Additional to water suppression, selection of a VOI is necessary for
evaluation of focal brain disease and must be implemented in a clinical
MR imager (Luyten and den Hollander 1986).

Recently the STEAM spectroscopy sequence, proposed by Frahm et al.
(1988), has been employed in our system. This sequence allows single-
step localization by exciting three intersecting planes of a VOI
smaller than 30 ml. Shimming is performed on the localized volume.
Then a chemical shift-selective radiofrequency pulse, preceding the
sequence, is used to suppress the water resonance. After successfully
suppressing the H_2O resonance, N-acetylaspartate, choline, and creatine can be assigned, as shown in a 27-ml VOI in the frontal white
matter of a normal volunteer (Fig.3).

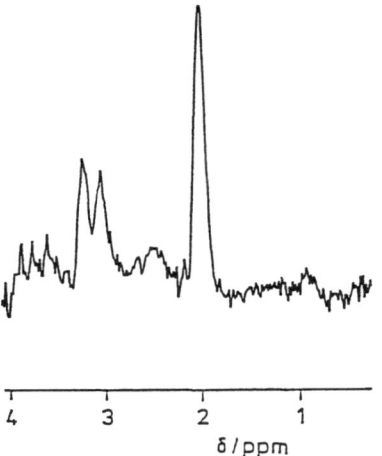

δ/ppm

Fig.3. ^{1}H spectrum obtained from a 27-ml VOI placed within the frontal
white matter of a normal volunteer. TR = 1.5 s; TE = 270 ms; AC = 512.
From left to right, the resonances of choline, creatine, and N-acetylaspartate are resolved

Discussion

Magnetic resonance imaging has developed into a routine imaging
modality in neuroradiology. Diagnosis of pathology depends predominantly on anatomical display and proton T1 and T2 relaxation parameters. MRS is now available in 1.5-T imaging systems and allows biochemical assessment of human pathology. However, human MRS does not
reach the sensitivity observed in animal studies, and the spatial resolution is limited. Further clinical experience is necessary to assess the potential of ^{31}P MRS in the differential diagnosis of intracranial tumors. The information of cellular energy metabolism obtained
by ^{31}P MRS promises to be important in monitoring of neoplastic
brain disease. It has already been demonstrated that MRS detects
metabolic response of extremity neoplasms to chemotherapy earlier
than tumor regression is visible in MRI (Semmler et al. 1986). The
first clinical applications of ^{31}P MRS to brain tumor treatment
indicate that ^{31}P MRS improves the clinical and therapeutic management of patients (Segebarth et al. 1987). Water-suppressed ^{1}H MRS
allows the definition of smaller VOIs than ^{31}P MRS. First results
in intracranial disorders (Bruhn et al. 1988) indicate not only the
differentiation of tumors by ^{1}H MRS but also a more sensitive approach to ischemic brain lesions. Further clinical application may
improve our understanding of demyelinating and degenerative diseases.

In conclusion, proton and phosphorus spectroscopy can now be performed in a clinical setting with routine 1.5-T imaging magnets. MRS
has a great potential in neuroradiology, but further controlled
studies are necessary to assess the diagnostic, prognostic, and
therapeutic impact of combined MRI and multinuclear MRS in clinical
routine.

Acknowledgement. We thank S. Fuchs for help in manuscript preparation.

References

[1]   Argov Z, Bank WJ, Maris J, Peterson P, Chance B (1987) Bio-
      energetic heterogeneity of human mitochondrial myopathies:
      phosphorus magnetic resonance study. Neurology 37: 257-262
[2]   Aue WP (1986) Localisation methods for in vivo nuclear magnetic
      resonance spectroscopy. Rev Magn Reson Med 1: 12-72
[3]   Bottomley PA, Drayer BP, Smith LS (1986) Chronic adult cere-
      bral infarction studied by phosphorus NMR spectroscopy. Ra-
      diology 160: 763-766
[4]   Bruhn H, Frahm J, Gyngell ML, Merboldt KD, Hänicke W,
      Sauter R (1988) Localized proton spectroscopy of tumours in

vivo: patients with primary and secondary cerebral tumours.
In: Abstracts of 7th annual meeting, Society of Magnetic Resonance in Medicine 1: 253

[5] Frahm J, Bruhn H, Gyngell ML, Merboldt KD, Hänicke W.
     Sauter R (1988) Localized high resolution proton NMR spectros-
     copy using stimulated echoes. Initial application to human
     brain in vivo. Magn Reson Med (submitted)

[6] Hollander JA den, Luyten PR (1986) ^{31}P and ^{1}H spectroscopy on
     a whole body MR scanner. Medicamundi 31 (2): 64-67

[7] Hope PL, Costello AM, Cady EB et al. (1984) Cerebral energy
     metabolism studied with phosphor NMR spectroscopy in normal
     and birth asphyxiated infants. Lancet 2: 366-370

[8] Lanterbur PC (1973) Image formation by induced local inter-
     actions: examples employing nuclear magnetic resonance. Na-
     ture 242: 190-191

[9] Luyten PR, den Hollander JA (1986) Observation of metaboli-
     ties in the human brain by MR spectroscopy. Radiology 161:
     795-798

[10] Perman WH, Turski PA, Houston LW, Glover GH, Hayes CE (1986)
     Methodology of in vivo human sodium MR imaging at 1.5 T.
     Radiology 160: 811-820

[11] Radda GK (1986) The use of NMR spectroscopy for the under-
     standing of disease. Science 233: 640-645

[12] Requard H, Offermann J, Sauter R (1988) Radiology (submitted)

[13] Sauter R, Mueller S, Weber H (1987) Localisation in in vivo
     ^{31}P NMR spectroscopy by combining surface coils and slice-
     selective saturation. J Magn Reson 75 (1): 167-173

[14] Segebarth CM, Baleriaux DF, Arnold DL, Luyten PR, Hollander
     JA den (1987) MR-image-guided ^{31}P MR spectroscopy in the
     evaluation of brain tumor treatment. Radiology 165: 215-219

[15] Semmler W, Gademann G, Kaick G v, Zabel HJ, Lorenz WJ (1986)
     In vivo ^{31}P spectroscopy of human tumors and their response
     to therapy using a 1.5 T whole body scanner. In: Abstracts
     of 5th annual meeting, Society of Magnetic Resonance in
     Medicine 1: 39

[16] Tanaka C, Naruse S, Horikawa Y, Hirakawa K, Yoshizaki K,
     Nishikawa H (1986) Proton nuclear magnetic resonance spectra
     of brain tumors. Magn Reson Imaging 4: 503-508

[17] Wolf W, Albright J, Silver MS, Weber H, Reichardt U, Sauer R
     (1987) Fluorine 19 NMR spectroscopic studies of the metabo-
     lism of 5-fluorouracil in the liver of patients undergoing
     chemotherapy. Magn Reson Imaging 5: 165-169

Brain Infarction: SPECT Examination of Regional Cerebral Blood Flow (RCBF) and Volume (RCBV) Compared with Gadolinium (Gd)-DTPA-Enhanced MRI

M. Cordes, H. Henkes, H. Eichstädt, C. Lefebre, N. Hosten, M. Langer, and R. Felix

Introduction

In the course of ischemic brain infarctions hemodynamic changes and impairment of cellular integrity are well recognized phenomena. Highly developed imaging modalities (eg. SPECT and MRI) are able to detect correlates of pathphysiologic mechanisms as:
- edema, to be depicted on T2 weighted images (WI),
- disruption of blood-brain-barrier (BBB), to be shown as contrast enhancement of Gd-DTPA on T1WI (1),
- vasoparalysis, resulting in increased rCBV and
- collateral formation, causing increased rCBF.
Besides other metabolic factors may contribute to the complex pathphysiology of cerebral infarctions.
Purpose of this investigation was to compare the hemodynamic changes (rCBF and rCBV) measured by SPECT with those changes (edema and BBB disruption) detected by MRI in the course of cerebral infarctions.

Patients and methods

28 patients, 17 males and 11 females, aged 35 to 84 years were examined. The patients were categorized in two groups with respect to the age of the brain infarction.
Group 1: subacute infarctions. 20 patients with 22 lesions, 4 through 45 days after clinical onset.
Group 2: chronic infarctions. 8 patients with 8 lesions, more than 180 days after clinical onset.
All infarctions were prooven by clinical data and CT examinations. SPECT examinations were carried out after i.v. application of 555 MBq 99mTc-HM-PAO (rCBF) and in vivo labeling of red blood cells with 740 MBq 99mTc-O4 (rCBV) (Tab. 1). Semiquantititative evaluation of all SPECT examinations was done by calculating regional indices (RI).

Tab. 1. Acquisition parameters of SPECT examinations

acquisition time:	20 sec/frame
rotation angle:	360 degrees
matrix size:	64 x 64 pixels
prereconstruction filter:	Wiener (damp 1, FWHM 10mm)
rCBF:	555 MBq 99mTc-HM-PAO, IV
rCBV:	740 MBq 99mTcO4 labeled red blood cells

MRI examinations were performed on a .5T Magnetom. All patients had plain T1WI and T2WI as well as Gd-DTPA enhanced T1WI (Tab. 2). The signal intensity (SI) of edema and contrast enhancement was graded 0 (none), 1 (mild), 2 (moderate) or 3 (marked). Time between MRI, rCBF and rCBV examinations was 3 days or less.

Tab. 2. Acquisition parameters of MRI examinations

T2WI: spin echo mode, TR 1600 ms, TE 30, 70 ms
T1WI: FLASH, TR 315 ms, TE 14 ms
contrast media: Gd-DTPA, 0.1mmol/kg BW

Results

Group 1: subacute infarctions
All 22 lesions detected by CT appeared on T2-weighted MR images as hyperintense lesions. Edema ranged from grade 1 to grade 3. 17/22 lesions showed contrast enhancement of Gd-DTPA, graded 1 to 3. All 22 lesions showed increased rCBV (mean RI: 1.24 , range: 1.08 to 2.48). The rCBF was increased in 7/22 lesions (mean RI: 1.38, range: 1.05 to 1.75), normal in 3/22 lesions (mean RI: 1.0, range 0.96 to 1.04) and decreased in 12/22 lesions (mean RI: 0.78, range: 0.38 to 0.95) (Tab. 3).

Group 2: chronic infarctions
All 8 lesions detected by CT were identified as lesions with increased SI on T2WI. None of the lesions showed contrast enhancement on T1WI. The rCBV was decreased in 6/8 lesions (mean RI: 0.81, range: 0.65 to 0.91) or normal in 2/8 lesions (mean RI:1.0). The rCBF was decreased in 8/8 lesions (mean RI: 0.78, range: 0.36 to 0.92 (Tab. 4).

Tab. 3: MRI and SPECT findings in subacute infarctions, n = 22

SI on T2WI↑   :   22/22. Grade 1 to 3.
SI on T1WI↑   :   17/22. Grade 1 to 3.
 (after Gd-DTPA)

rCBV increased :   22/22. Mean RI: 1.24, range: 1.08 - 2.48
     normal   :   0/22.
     decreased :   0/22.

rCBF increased :   7/22. Mean RI: 1.38, range: 1.05 - 1.75
     normal   :   3/22. Mean RI: 1.0, range: 0.96 - 1.04
     decreased :   12/22. Mean RI: 0.78, range: 0.38 - 0.95

Tab. 4: MRI and SPECT findings in chronic infarctions.
        n = 8

```
SI on T2WI↑        :      8/8
SI on T1WI↑        :      0/8
 after Gd-DTPA)

rCBV increased:    0/8
     normal   :    2/8. Mean RI: 1.0.
     decraesed:    6/8. Mean RI: 0.81, range: 0.65 - 0.91

rCBF increased:    0/8
     normal   :    0/8
     decreased:    8/8. Mean RI: 0.78, range: 0.36 - 0.92
```

Discussion

Our prelimanary results show that all lesions detected by CT could be demonstrated as lesions with increased SI on T2WI. Contrast enhancement was found in 17/22 of subacute lesions. Contrast enhancement could be first recognized in a lesion 4 days after clinical onset of stroke. The contrast enhancement on MRI examination was more marked than on CT examination at the same time. Since CT examinations with contrast media were carried out only in a few cases we were not able to compare MRI with CT findings systematically.
Interestingly all subacute lesions showed an increased rCBV, which may be caused by vasoparalysis in the infarcted territory. Pathologically this phenomenon is recognized as red veins in pale infarctions. The rCBV may be still increased 45 days after the clinical onset of infarction.It may be inhomogeneous in the infarcted area. As well defined pattern we observed a markedly increased rCBV of the margin of the infarcted area while it was gradually reduced in the center. Subacute infarctions in our series showed either an increased, normal or decreased rCBF, which may depend on the hemodynamic support by collateral formation or by reopening of occluded vessels. Hyperperfusion was commonly seen until 20 days after clinical onset, however in one case we found an increased rCBF 36 days after clinical onset.
In chronic brain infarctions we could not find any contrast enhancement on T1WI. This may be due to complete scar formation in the infarcted area. This correlates with reduced rCBV and rCBF. In some cases the rCBV was slightly increased in the margins of the infarctions. These sites probably represent ischemic areas with compensatory increased rCBV (2).

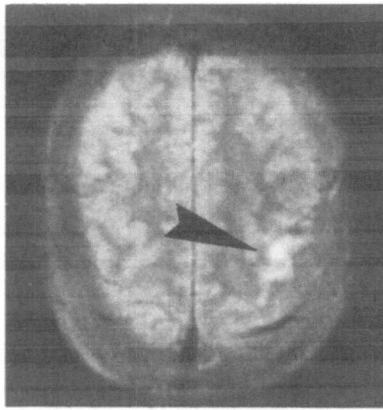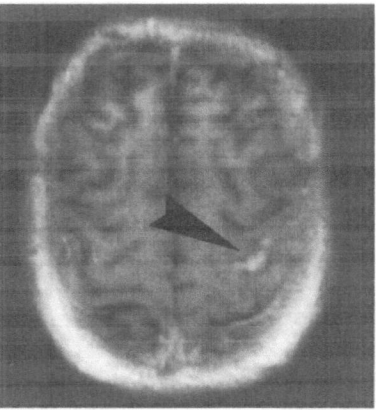

Fig. 1. MRI in a patient with left parietal infarction
a) T2WI showing increased SI in the infarcted region
b) T1WI demonstrates contrast enhancement after i.v.
application of Gd-DTPA

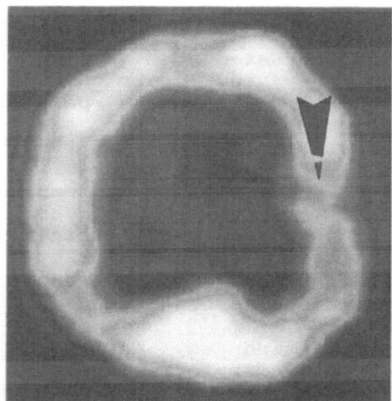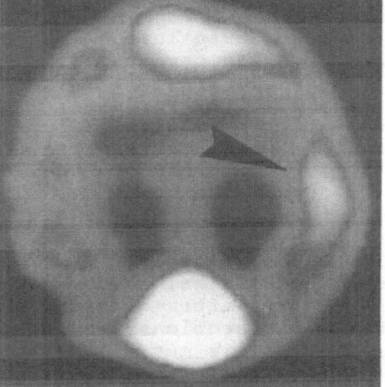

Fig. 2:. SPECT images of the same patient as in fig.1
a) rCBF is decreased, while the
b) rCBV is increased in the infarcted area.

References

(1) Runge VM, Price AC, Wehr CJ, Atkinson JB, Tweedle MF (1985):
Contrast enhanced MRI: evaluation of a canine model of osmotic BBB
disruption.
Invest Radiol 8: 830-844

(2) Ter-Pogossian MM, Herscovitch P (1985): Radioactive oxygen-15
in the study of cerebral blood flow, blood volume and
oxygen metabolism.
Sem Nucl Med 15: 377-394

Emerging Clinical Application of Phosphorous Chemical Shift Imaging of Neoplastic Disease

H. C. Charles, H. D. Sostman, M. Dewhirst, K. A. Leopold,
M. Baker, and J. A. Tucker (Durham, NC, USA)

The purpose of this study is the evaluation of clinical utility of phosphorous chemical shift imaging (31P CSI) of neoplastic disease. The current role of 31P CSI can be considered twofold, the differentiation of tumor from non-tumor in diagnosis and the evaluation of neoplastic therapy by serial monitoring of localized 31P information from neoplastic lesions.

Hydrogen images and spectroscopy studies were obtained at 1.5 Tesla on a clinical magnetic resonance spectrometer (SIGNA) using pulse sequences supplied by the manufacturer or written by one of the authors using pulse programming software provided by the manufacturer. A 6 cm home-built transmit/receive surface coil was used for acquisition of the spectroscopy data. The spectroscopic data is stored and transferred to an off-time system for processing and curve deconvolution. Data analysis (area ratios, height ratios, pH and other parameters) using a spreadsheet and statistical analysis program is performed on a personal computer. Biopsy and pathologic findings are used as the standard for these studies.

Results of monotoring resonances from PME, Pi, PDE, PCr and nTP show that differentiation of fibrosis/other lesions from tumor is facilitated with 31P CSI when conventional imaging is non-conclusive and that neoplastic therapy may be monitored using 31P CSI indicating the response of the tumor to treatment providing information not available from conventional hydrogen imaging.

31P CSI can be carried out in a clinical environment in conjunction with conventional imaging yielding clinically useful and pathologically confirmed information about neoplastic disease.

The PET Revolution in the Neurosciences

H. N. Wagner Jr. (Baltimore, USA)

Positron emission tomography (PET) has the potential of revolu-
tionizing clinical neurosciences, by making it possible for the
first time to measure in vivo chemistry in the living human
brain, expressing the results in absolute units of meters, kilo-
grams, and seconds (the MKS system). When we can measure the rate
of a chemical process in a region of the brain, there is the possibility of at least two diseases, one in which the rate of the chemical process is abnormally slow, and another in which the process
is abnormally fast. PET studies of brain chemistry fall into two
categories: substrate metabolism and information transfer. Advances in the use of simple probe detector systems are being used
to monitor the response of a given patient to drug treatment, and
to reduce the incidence of untoward side effects. PET can at times
detect abnormalities before anatomical changes have occurred, for
example, in epilepsy, Huntington's disease or cerebrovascular disease. In patients with epilepsy and brain tumors, PET scanning
provides information useful in the planning and monitoring of surgical treatment. PET can be used to determine whether there is an
epileptic focus, or in patients with tumor, to assess the effectiveness of surgery, radiation and chemotherapy. PET scanning can document the extent of tumors, and progression or regression with different forms of treatment. Up to now, treatment has been based primarily on histopathological examination of biopsies; biochemical
characterization may be an even better way to classify tumors.
Studies of patients with stroke indicate that metabolic abnormalities seen on PET frequently are more extensive than the corresponding
CT findings, and the pattern of metabolic abnormalities in PET correlates with the clinical syndrome and with the degree of eventual recovery. Abnormal D_2 dopamine receptor concentrations have been found
in the caudate and putamen of many patients with psychotic depression. PET studies have brought about a whole new approach to biological psychatry.

PET in the Evaluation of Response to Treatment of Brain Tumours

K. Ericson (Stockholm, Sweden)

Positron emission tomography (PET) with ^{11}C-methionine has been shown to be of value in the delineation and assessment of brain tumours in a majority of the cases. With the application of a kinetic model, the transport of the tracer from the blood and the accumulation in the tumour may be quantified. Such an analysis was performed in a small series of patients with astrocytomas and oligo-astrocytomas before and about two years after treatment with open surgery, conventional radiotherapy or stereotactic precision irradiation. In a majority of the patients, tumours with a pathologically increased methionine accumulation showed a significant normalization after treatment. However, exceptions were noted. There were a few patients with radiation necrosis and also patients with progression of the tumours to more malignant forms. The results were consistant with the findings of computed tomography (CT), but the changes were usually better visualized with PET.

Astrocytomas grade II are slowly growing tumours and a follow-up period of two years is too short for definite conclusions to be drawn as to the long-term effects of the treatment. However, PET seems to provide an effective means for monitoring the response to treatment and for detection of tumour recurrency. Difficulties may arise in the differentiation between radiation reaction and tumour regression, and in such cases PET with glucose or deoxyglucose may be superior.

PET in Brain Gliomas – Biological and Morphological Aspects

A. Lilja

Imaging of cerebral gliomas by CT, MRI and angiography provides valuable diagnostic information, which however can be used to predict tumour biology only in an indirect and empirical way. An increasing number of tracers developed for positron emission tomography (PET) can give more direct, and in many cases more specific, information about tumour biology. They may also aid in evaluating the effects of therapy on the tumor and on the surrounding brain.

In the table below, some of the radiopharmaceutical tools that have been used to characterize pathophysiological events in gliomas and in brain are listed. For some, like labeled carbonmonoxide and carbondioxide for blood volume and flow calculation, or ^{18}F-deoxyglucose (^{18}FDG), validated models for the interpretation of tracer kinetics exist, and quantitation of flow or glucose consumption is possible, at least in non-tumorous brain. In the case of ^{18}FDG, estimates of tumor glucose comsumption are used clinically, although some debate is continuing about details in tracer kinetic modeling in neoplastic tissue. For other substances, like some labeled amino acids, tracer kinetic models are not generally accepted, and the results with such substances are thus qualitative rather than quantitative, but may nevertheless be of great value.

SOME APPLICATIONS IN CEREBRAL GLIOMAS OF TRACERS USED IN PET

REGIONAL BLOOD VOLUME	$C^{15}O$ labeled erythrocytes
REGIONAL BLOOD FLOW	$C^{15}O_2$ - $H_2^{15}O$
BLOOD-BRAIN BARRIER FUNCTION	^{68}Ga-EDTA; ^{82}Rb
REGIONAL OXYGEN UTILIZATION AND EXTRACTION	$^{15}O_2$
REGIONAL GLUCOSE METABOLISM	^{18}FDG
-"- -"- TRANSPORT	^{11}C-methylglucose
REGIONAL pH	^{11}C-DMO
AMINO ACID TRANSPORT (PROTEIN SYNTHESIS)	L- or D-methyl-^{11}C-methionine, ^{11}C-L-leucine, ^{11}C-valine, ^{11}C-tryptophan
REGIONAL PHARMACOKINETICS/DRUG DISTRIBUTION	^{57}Co-bleomycin, ^{11}C-BCNU, ^{18}F-5-fluorouracil

A number of the physiological features of high-grade gliomas have been explored with PET (Beaney 1984). The normal coupling between blood volume and flow, provided by autoregulation, is disrupted in the neo-vasculature of high-grade tumors, a fact which emphasizes that identification of tumor vessels by angiography does not permit an adequate prediction of blood flow . Oxygen consumption in tumor tissue is frequently low, despite adequate supply of oxygenated blood. In contrast to this, glucose utilization is usually locally increased in malignant tumours. This means that anaerobic glycolysis is taking place (Rhodes et al 1983). Tyler et al (1987), using ^{11}C-DMO, have reported local pH in gliomas to consistently be more alkalotic than in brain.

As most high-grade gliomas display areas of increased glucose consumption, this property has been used to differentiate them from low-grade tumors, which generally have a glucose consumption lower than or equal to normal brain (Di Chiro et al 1987 a). Di Chiro et al have found grading of gliomas to be more accurate with ^{18}FDG PET than with CT. This group also found that an increase of tumor glucose utilization by a factor 1.4 or more, compared with contralateral brain, means a poor prognosis for patients treated by surgery and radiotherapy or chemotherapy. These results have been reproduced by several (Mineura et al 1986), but questioned by occasional other investigators (Tyler et al 1987).

Since 1982, in the groups working in Uppsala and Karolinska hospitals, we have used methionine, labeled with ^{11}C in the methyl position, in examinations of gliomas. Virtually all high-grade gliomas examined by us have shown markedly increased ^{11}C-methionine uptakes in comparison with contralateral brain (Lilja et al 1985; Mosskin et al 1987). The high tracer accumulation is mediated by increased transport via the vascular barrier (BBB). Provided the BBB is not grossly disrupted, this transport can be modified by competition with other amino acids, and is stereospecific, as in normal brain (Bergström et al 1987 a,b). The increased uptake also reflects enhanced protein synthesis, and additionally, to a lesser extent, metabolism or increased amino acid pools, as indicated in recent laboratory studies (Bustany et al 1986; Ishiwata et al 1988). In most high-grade gliomas, and in the majority of low-grade gliomas PET with ^{11}C-methionine delinates tumor tissue more accurately than CT or routine spin echo MRI (Mosskin et al 1987, Tovi et al 1986). There is a rough correlation between the magnitude of amino acid accumulation and malignancy grade, with a 2.5-fold increase of methionine accumulation in viable glioma tissue strongly suggestive of a high tumor grade (Mosskin et al 1987, Lilja et al 1985).

In gliomas treated by irradiation a gradual further depression of oxygen consumption, and a decrease in tumor blood volume and flow has beeen reported (Beaney 1984). The partial cell loss occuring in irradiated normal brain did not appear to be caused by ischemia secondary to the vascular damage, as has been assumed. In patients examined early after irradiation acute decreases in glucose consumption in tumor and brain have been found (Di Chiro et al 1987 b, Ogawa et al 1988). We found methionine transport to be unchanged during and soon after radiation therapy (Bergström et al 1988). In a preceding presentation Ericson et al (this issue) have described the long term results of irradiation on low-grade gliomas, with reductions of the ^{11}C-methionine accumulation in some cases. Cortico-steroid medication seems to lower cortical blood volume and flow (Beaney 1984). We have found steroids to have a greater effect on methionine transport in tumor tissue than in brain (Bergström et al 1988). Both findings could indicate an effect of the medication on the vasculature.

With increasing aggressiveness of therapy for gliomas, it becomes increasingly important to measure effects and side effects on tumor and brain. CT offers little help in this respect, due to its rather low sensitivity and to the fact that density alterations are often non-specific. With PET, a differentiation betweeen tumor recurrence and brain lesions induced by radiation or intraarterial chemotherapy can be made using for instance ^{18}F-deoxyglucose (Di Chiro et al 1987 b). ^{11}C-methionine seems to aid in differentiating between tumor and edema even in aggressively treated cases (Lilja et al 1988).

The future importance and perspectives of PET in brain tumor disease may to some extent be in the characterization of brain tumors, by defining possible differencies in metabolism, protein synthesis, growth rate, or receptor structures. Such efforts could be especially valuable in predicting the susceptibility to more specific treatment, to ameliorate the present shortcomings of surgical and radiological therapy of gliomas and might actively aid in formulating new therapy. The interest shown in the effects of current therapy for gliomas on tumor and brain with PET provides a good basis for evaluation of possible new therapeutic modalities. Studies of the pharmacokinetics of chemotherapeutic agents have already been made using PET (Beaney 1984). Further investigations of secondary effects of brain tumors, like the studies of distant effects by tumors on glucose metabolism (Di Ciro et al 1987 a), e. g. of mechanisms in the formation of peritumoral edema, would also be valuable.

REFERENCES

Beaney R P (1984) Positron emission tomography in the study of human tumors. Semin Nucl Med 16:324-341

Bergström M et al (1987 a) PET study of methionine accumulation in glioma and normal brain tissue: competition with branched chain amino acids. J Comput Assist Tomogr 11:208-213

Bergström M et al (1987 b) Comparison of the accumulation kinetics of L-methyl-^{11}C-methionine and D-methyl-^{11}C-methionine in brain tumours studied with positron emission tomography. Acta Radiol 28:225-229

Bergström M et al (1988) Effect of radiation therapy and cortisone treatment on amino acid transport in glioma and normal brain tissue. Submitted

Bustany P et al (1986) Brain tumor protein synthesis and histological grades: a study by positron emission tomography (PET) with C11-L-methionine. J Neuro-Oncol 3:397-404

Di Chiro G (1987 a) Positron emission tomograpy using (^{18}F)fluoro-deoxyglucose in brain tumors. Invest Radiol 22:360-371

Di Chiro G et al (1987 b) Cerebral necrosis after radiotherapy and/or chemotherapy for brain tumors. AJNR 8:1083-1091

Ishiwata K et al (1988) Comparison of L-(1-^{11}C)methionine and L-methyl-(^{11}C)methionine for measuring in vivo protein synthesis rates with PET. J Nucl Med 29:1419-1427

Lilja A et al (1985) Dynamic study of supratentorial gliomas with L-methyl-^{11}C-methiomine and positron emission tomography. AJNR 6:505-514

Lilja A et al (1988) Positron emission tomography and CT in
    differential diagnosis between recurrent or residual glioma and
    treatment induced brain lesions. Accepted for publication
Mineura et al (1986) Positron emission tomographic evaluation of
    histological malignancy in gliomas using oxygen-15 and
    fluorine-18-fluorodeoxyglucose. Neurol Res 8:164-168
Mosskin M et al (1987) Positron emission tomography with [11]C-
    methionine and computed tomography of intracranial tumours
    compared with histopathologic examination of multiple biopsies.
    Acta Radiol 28:673-681
Ogawa T et al (1988) Changes of cerbral blood flow, and oxygen
    and glucose metabolism following radiochemotherapy of gliomas:
    a PET study. J Comput Assist Tomogr 12:290-297
Rhodes C G et al (1983) In vivo disturbance of the oxidative
    metabolism of glucose in human cerebral gliomas. Ann Neurol
    14:614-626
Tovi M et al (1986) Tumour delineation with magnetic resonance
    imaging in gliomas. Acta Radiol Suppl 369:161-163
Tyler J L et al (1987) Metabolic and hemodynamic evaluation of
    gliomas using positron emission tomography. J Nucl Med 28:
    1123-1133

PET Studies in Cerebro-Vascular Disorders

J. C. Baron (Orsay, France)

Positron emission tomography (PET) allows to measure locally in humans not only the cerebral blood flow but also the rates of oxygen consumption and glucose utilization and the intracellular pH, permitting an assessment of energy metabolism-perfusion interrelationships.

In acute cerebrovascular occlusions, the earlier the PET study the more frequent the demonstration of parenchymal ischemia (in the form of "poverty perfusion"), but some degree of ischemia-oligemia can be occasionnally observed up to the 4th day; in the remaining cases, PET studies demonstrate the spontaneous return of circulation (in the form of "luxury-perfusion"), which can occur within hours of stroke onset.

A depression of energy metabolism in brain areas distant from the lesioned area is frequently documented, affecting for example the contralateral cerebellar cortex or the ipsilateral cerebral cortex in cases of supratentorial brain damage or thalamic stroke, respectively: these sometimes transitory effects of deafferentation ("diaschisis") may underlie part of the clinical expression of, as well as of the functional recovery subsequent to, stroke in humans. PET studies have also allowed to characterize the long-term circulatory and metabolic cerebral consequences of carotid-artery obstructions, and have demonstrated the hemodynamic nature of some cerebrovascular events.

Spine

MR Anatomy of the Spine and Spinal Cord

M. Gado, M. Vannier, and G. Conroy

TECHNICAL CONSIDERATIONS

The spinal cord has a small diameter, it lies within a rigid bony canal and it contains important neural elements. Therefore, relatively small lesions within the parenchyma or in the extraaxial space often present with serious neurologic deficits. For these reasons, imaging of the spine and spinal cord is demanding in terms of spatial resolution and contrast discrimination. Amongst non-invasive methods, MRI has the highest capability for imaging of the spinal cord (Figs. 1 & 2). Paradoxically, MR imaging of the spine is challenging in

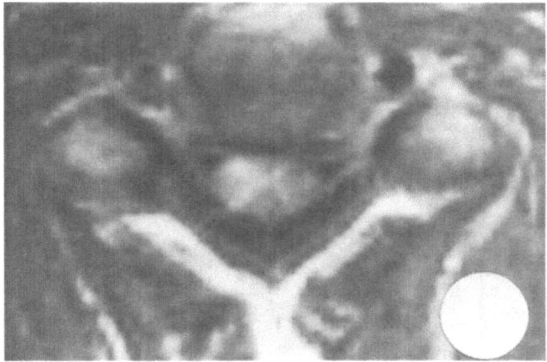

Fig. 1: Normal spinal cord. Axial MRI, 1.5 T. T1-WI (TR 500 msec, TE 21 msec) at the level of a cervical intervertebral foramen. The spinal cord, the ventral and dorsal nerve roots are contrasted against the dark CSF.

view of the numerous sources of "errors" of measurement and processing of measured data. These result in serious artifacts which should be discussed.

1. Chemical shift effects cause edge artifacts on MRI (Babcock et al. 1985). Fat in bone marrow of the vertebral bodies and appendages creates a chemical shift artifact when the interface between fat-containing tissue and water containing tissue is across the frequency encoding (readout) gradient. The artifact is most noticeable on T1-weighted images and is more obvious in high field imaging (Fig. 3). It appears as a band of signal loss when fat lies on the side of the lower frequency and vice versa. Rotating the gradients may eliminate the artifact at the lower or upper border of the vertebra but will create a new artifact at the posterior or anterior border. A similar artifact may be seen between the dorsal aspect of the dural sac and the epidural fat between the laminae of thoracic vertebrae.

2. Truncation artifact is another interface phenomenon caused by the fourier transform of measured data in processing of images (Lufkin et al. 1986; Czervionke et al. 1988). The artifact originates when a high contrast interface lies across the phase encoding gradient. Therefore in a sagittal or axial image of the cord the artifact will arise if the phase encoding gradient is oriented from front to back of the patient. The artifact appears as a

44

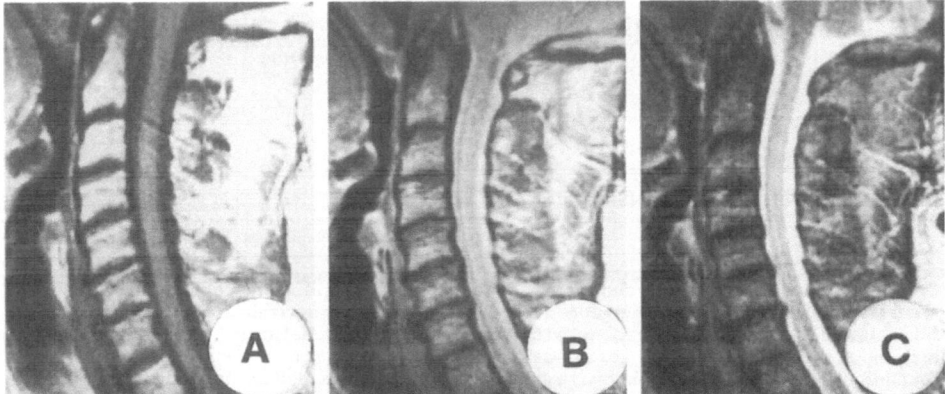

Fig. 2: Normal spinal cord. Same case as Fig. 1. Sagittal MRI 1.5 T. A: T1-WI (TR 500 msec, TE 21 msec). B: Bal-I (TR 2200 msec, TE 35 msec). C: T2-WI (TR 2200 msec, TE 90 msec. Contrast of the spinal cord and CSF is noted best in T1-WI and to a less extent at T2-WI. There is poor contrast of spinal cord and CSF in Bal-WI.

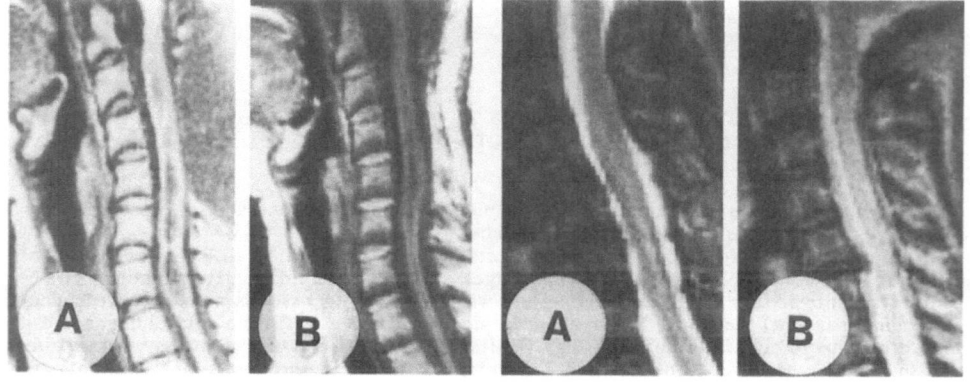

Fig. 3   Fig. 4

Fig. 3: Effect of field strength on appearance of chemical shift artifact. Patient with syringohydromyelia. A: Sagittal MRI, .5 T, T1-WI. The chemical shift artifact is not obvious. B: Same case, sagittal MRI, 1.5 T, T1-WI. The chemical shift is obvious; signal loss at the lower border of the vertebral body. The readout gradient is in the up-down direction.

Fig. 4: Two manifestations of truncation artifact in two different patients. Sagittal MRI, 1.5 T, T2-WI. A: A high intensity streak in the center of the cord resembles a cavity filled with fluid. B: Edge enhancement at the interface between the anterior border of the spinal cord and CSF results in "sculptured" appearance.

central strand of low signal in T1-weighted images and high signal in T2-weighted images (Fig. 4A). The artifact thus resembles the central canal or central gray matter of the spinal cord. It may be misinterpreted as a small cavity in the cord. The same principle is responsible for the artifactual edge enhancement at high contrast interfaces, such as sculptured appearance (Fig. 4B).

3. CSF motion is a source of several problems in MRI of the spinal cord: a. Ghosts of abnormal signal intensity appear as streaks propogated along the phase encoding axis. b. Loss of signal of CSF in T2-weighted images may also result from CSF motion. The signal loss is variable and unpredictable and therefore interferes with interpretation. Artifacts due to CSF motion can be reduced by cardiac gating (Enzman et al. 1987) and/or pulse sequences with motion compensation (Haacke and Lenz 1987). c. Even with these provisions, motion of CSF may result in curvilinear streaks of signal void resembling arteriovenous malformations.

4. Surface coil receivers are essential for MRI of the spine (Modic et al 1986). When single planar loops are used as surface receiver coils, there is signal drop-off the further the tissues are from the receiver coil. This may interfere with correct interpretation of normal or abnormal signal intensities.

ANATOMIC-RADIOLOGIC STUDY

Three fresh cadavers were scanned by MRI in the 3 orthogonal planes, using 1.5 Tesla Magnetom imager (Siemens, Islin). Two spin echo sequences were performed in each plane to generate three images of each anatomic level; T1-weighted image (T1-WI): TR = 750 msec, TE = 17 msec; balanced image (Bal-I): TR = 2500 msec, TE = 28 msec; T2-weighted image (T2-WI): TR = 2500 msec, TE = 90 msec. The cadavers were then frozen, the cervical spine removed and sectioned using a ban saw. The specimens were sectioned one each, in the sagittal, axial and coronal planes. Photographs of the anatomic sections were compared with the corresponding MR images.

RESULTS

1. Sagittal Series
a. In the Midsagittal plane (Fig. 5), the odontoid process lies in front of the myelomedullary

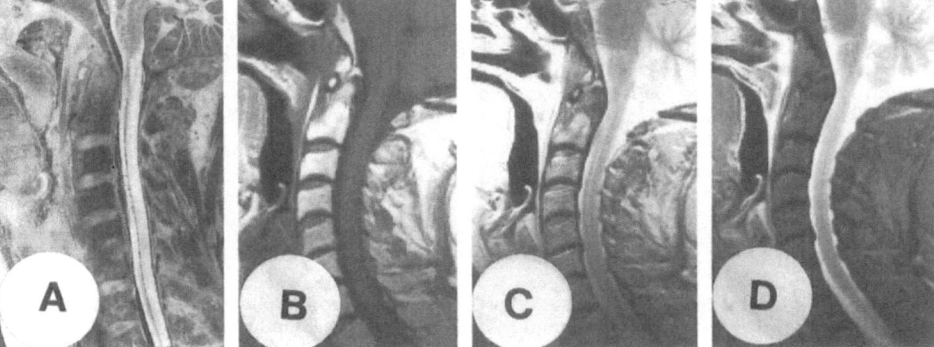

Fig. 5: Anatomic radiologic correlation, cadaver #1. A: Mid-sagittal anatomic section. B-D: Sagittal MRI 1.5 T of the same cadaver before sectioning at same plane as A. B: T1-WI. C: Bal-I. D: T2-WI.

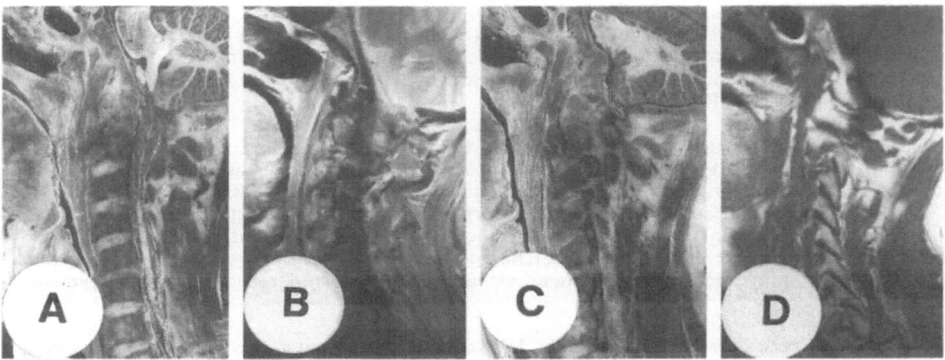

Fig. 6: Anatomical radiologic study cadaver #1. A: Anatomic sagittal section at 12 mm to the right of the midline. B: Sagittal MRI, 1.5 T, Bal-I of the same cadaver before sectioning at a level corresponding to A. C: Sagittal anatomic section at 18 mm to the right of the midline. D: Sagittal MRI, 1.5 T, Bal-I of the same cadaver before sectioning, at a level corresponding to C.

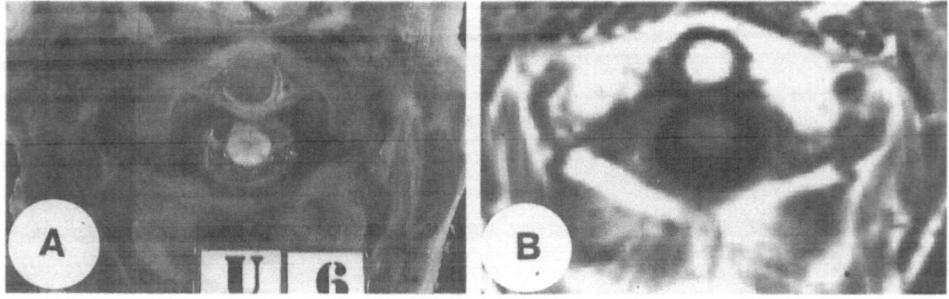

Fig. 7: Anatomic radiologic study, cadaver #2. A: Axial anatomic section at the level of the articulation between the odontoid process and the anterior arch of the atlas. The ligamentum transversarum is well seen on the posterior aspect of the odontoid process. B: Axial MRI of the same cadaver before sectioning. 1.5 T, T1-WI. The ligamentum transversarum is clearly demonstrated.

junction. The synovial bursa on the dorsal surface of the odontoid process is identified. The dura, the transverse and cruciate ligaments of the atlas are indistinguishable from one another and appear as one linear strand of signal void extending from the lower end of the clivus, behind the synovial bursa and blends with the posterior surface of the body of the axis. In the Bal-I, the central gray matter of the spinal cord is distinguishable from the white matter by its higher signal intensity. It appears as a thin strip and lies closer to the anterior surface of the cord than the posterior surface. b. In the sagittal section through the lateral part of the bony spinal canal (Fig. 6A,B), the ventral and dorsal nerve roots were clearly seen in the anatomic section but not on the corresponding MRI. This part of the spinal canal was best evaluated in axial sections (see below). c. Further laterally, the anatomic section ran through the lateral masses of the vertebrae and the intervertebral foramina (Fig. 6C,D). The corresponding MRI showed clearly the atlanto-occipital joints lying parallel to the transverse plane. The spinal nerve C1 appeared directly posterior to the atlanto-occipital joint in front of the vertebral artery on the superior aspect of the posterior arch of the atlas. The cervical root C2 lies immediately below the posterioir arch of the atlas and directly posterior to the atlanto-axial joint. From the level of C2 downwards the four joints are oriented in an oblique direction (approximately 45°). The nerves exit at the <u>anterior</u> aspect of the corresponding joint. While there are no exit foramina for spinal nerves C1 and C2, the nerves below C2 exit through intervertebral foramina. But, in sagittal MRI sections the bony anterior border of the intervertebral foramen is absent due to the angled orientation of the foramina. Therefore the vertebral artery or a para-vertebral muscle lies directly in front of the exiting nerve, unless oblique imaging is used (Yenerich and Haughton 1986).

2. Axial Series.
Axial MR sections at the level of the articulation between the odontoid process and anterior arch of the atlas show clearly the ligamentum transversarum in its extent from side to side (Fig. 7). The nerve roots in the lateral parts of the spinal canal are well shown in axial plane; hence the need to include axial images in MRI protocols of the spine. The epidural space in the cervical region is occupied by a venous plexus rather than fat (Fig. 8 & 9). The veins showed high signal in the Bal-1 and T2-WI of the cadaver. High signal of the venous structures may also be seen in T1-weighted images in life due to flow-related enhancement. The epidural space is widest at the level of C1 and becomes smaller at lower levels. The spinal nerves exit in the foramina anterior to the facet joints.

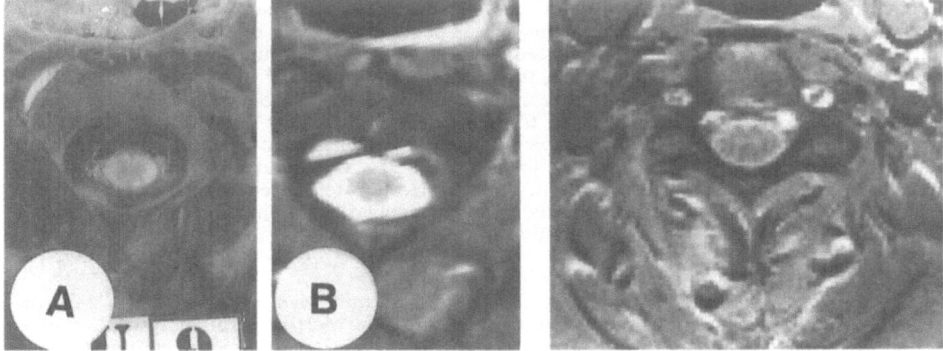

Fig. 8   Fig. 9

Figure 8: Anatomic radiologic study cadaver #2. A: Axial anatomic section at the level of the lateral masses of the axis. B: axial MRI of the same cadaver before sectioning, at the same plane as A. 1.5 T, T2-WI. The epidural space is filled with a venous plexus rather than fat. This is responsible for the high signal in the epidural space in T2-WI.

Figure 9: Cadaver #1 axial MRI, 1.5 T, Bal-I. The inner structure of the spinal cord is depicted. The gray matter with its characteristic H-configuration stands out in contrast to lower signal of white matter.

48

3. Coronal Series.
The vertebral bodies, lateral masses and the unique orientation of the atlanto-occipital and atlanto-axial articulations are demonstrated in MR images corresponding to the anterior coronal sections (Fig. 10). The anterior atlanto-occipital membrane may also be shown in one of these sections. More posteriorly, the myelomedullary junction is displayed and further posteriorly, the dorsal elements of the vertebrae and the surrounding muscles. At the craniocervical junction, the lower cranial nerves exit at the internal auditory canals, jugular foramina and hypoglossal canals.

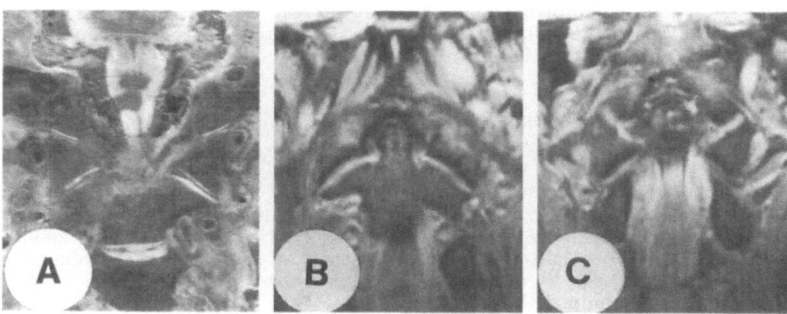

Fig. 10: Anatomic radiologic study, cadaver #3. A: Coronal anatomic section through the atlanto-occipital and atlanto-axial articulations. B & C: Coronal MRI of the same cadaver before sectioning. 1.5 T, Bal-I. The orientation of the anatomic sections was at a slightly different angle from the MR images. The corresponding structures, however, can be identified.

4. Signal Intensities.
The signal intensities seen in this study reflected the known magnetic characteristics of parenchyma and CSF with a few differences. In the fresh specimen, the contrast of gray and white matter in the T1-weighted image was poor, presumably due to decrease in blood volume. In the balanced and T2-weighted images, however, the higher signal intensity of gray matter was obvious. Furthermore, the signal intensity of CSF was much higher than is usually seen in life. This is probably related to the absence of CSF motion in the cadaver and is therefore more representative of the true effect of the long T2 of CSF on the signal. The inner structure of the spinal cord was also clearly demonstrated in the balanced images, both in the sagittal (Fig. 5) and axial images (Fig. 9). Gray matter shows higher signal intensity. This contrast pattern is usually lost in life due to degredation of images by the effect of motion. These observations indicate the amount of the inherent information lost and could be captured by better correcting for motion effects.

5. Multispectral Enhancement and Color Display.
The three spin echo images obtained for each anatomic level display signal patterns reflecting varying degrees of predominance of T1 and T2. Multispectral analysis allows the combination of these different patterns in one display. For this purpose, we entered the three spin echo images of the same anatomic level into a digital image processing system (model 75 and system/600 software from International Imaging Systems, Inc. of Milpitall, CA). These data were scaled to 8 bits per channel and pseudocolored by displaying each gray scale spin echo image as red, green and blue respectively. A simple color composite image was produced by displaying the three images simultaneously in full registration of the pixels (Fig. 11).

There was strong longitudinal non-uniformity in the original gray scale image. To improve the image contrast and gray scale uniformity, a Wallis imager enhancement operator was applied to the color composite image. The Wallis enhancement, performed on a VAX-11/750 computer improved the subjective quality and overall uniformity of contrast in the color image. The image enhancement operation used in conjunction with color display was helpful in comparing and combining the results of the three spin echo images for the study of individual components of the scene, i.e. brain, spinal cord, bone, muscle, ligaments, fat, etc.

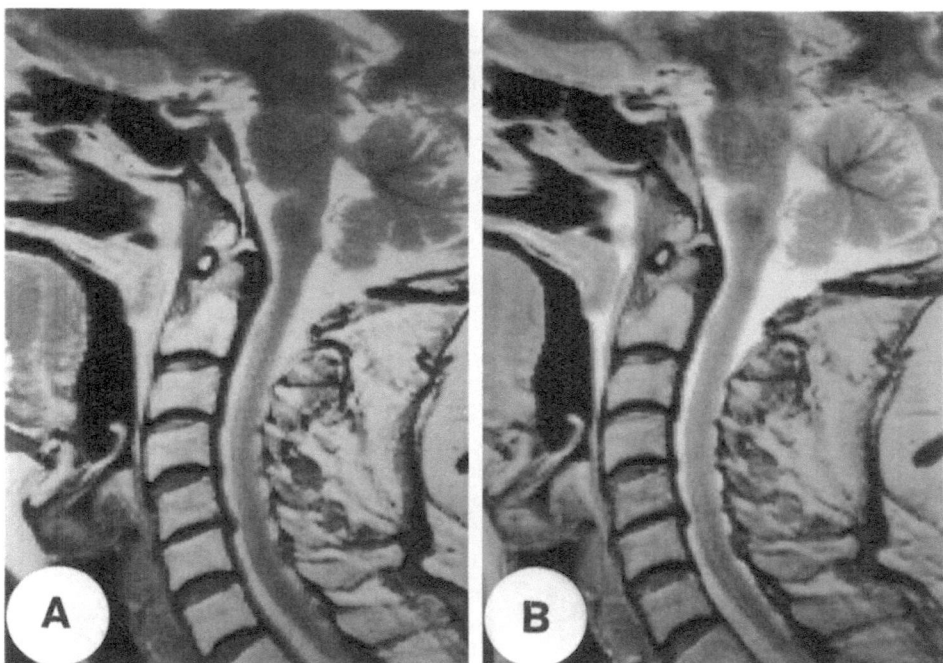

Fig. 11: Multispectral analysis. Two composite images created from the midsagittal MRI images shown in Fig. 5B-D. The resultant color of the individual structures on the composite image depends on the color assignments to the three images of the original data set. A & B show examples of different color assignments of the same data set.

REFERENCES

Babcock EE, Brateman L, Weinreb et al (1985) Edge artefacts in MR images: chemical shift effect. JCAT 9:252

Czervionke LF, Czervionke JM, Daniels DL et al (1988) Characteristic features of MR truncation artifacts AJNR 9:815

Enzman DR, Rubin JB, Wright A (1987) Use of cerebrospinal fluid gating to improve T2-weighted images. Radiology 162:763

Haacke EM, Lenz GW (1987) Improving MR image quality in the presence of motion by using rephasing gradients. AJR 148:251

Lufkin RB, Pusey E, Stark DD et al (1986) Boundary artifact due to truncation errors in MR imaging. AJR 147:1283

Modic MT, Masaryk TJ, Paushter DM (1986) Magnetic resonance imaging of the spine. Radiol Clin North Am 24:229

Yenerich DO, Haughton VM (1986) Oblique plane MR imaging of the cervical spine. JCAT 10:823

Craniocervical Junction: MR Study of Normal Paravertebral Soft Tissues and Bony Structures

C. Faubert, J. L. Dietemann, H. Sick, M. Vouge, and A. Wackenheim

INTRODUCTION

MRI provides simultaneous display of soft tissues, bony structures, and vasculonervous structures. In this study, we intend to correlate the in-vivo 3-D tomographic tissular visualization MRI provides with macro- but essentially micro-anatomic (histological) sections of the craniocervical junction.

SUBJECTS AND METHOD

This study is based on our own experience covering a two year period, involving over 200 patients. We used a GE-CGR Magniscan 5000 (0.5 T) and standard head coil. T1- weighted images were obtained using standard gradient echo (TR 400-600/ TE 16-18) and spin echo (TR 500-700/ TE 26-28) sequences with 4 excitations. Sagittal +++, Frontal ++, Axial +, 5mm thick slices were obtained.

RESULTS AND DISCUSSION

Analysis of T1- weighted sections allows precise visualization of prevertebral ligaments which appear as low intensity areas. Anteriorly, because of the presence of high intensity contrasting preodontoid fat, the anterior longitudinal ligament, the anterior atlanto-occipital membrane, the anterior atlanto-axial membrane, the anterior and posterior parts of the medial atlanto-axial joint, the lateral atlanto-axial joints, the apical ligament of dens, the cruciform ligament (transverse ligament, superior longitudinal band, inferior longitudinal band) and its relationship with the alar ligaments, the membrana tectoria and the posterior longitudinal ligament are discussed.

Posteriorly the posterior atlanto-occipital membrane and ligamentum nuchae are quickly presented. The interspinous ligaments are not developped in this region.

Non ligamentous non vasculonervous structures in front include the hypersignal pharyngeal tonsils (composed of lymphoid tissue and mucus glands) with its ondulated aspect, the pharyngeal bursae (a median recess), the pharyngobasilar fascia (isointense) at the level of opening the auditory tubes. The superior pharyngeal constrictor muscle (isointense) is readily visualized on sagittal sections extending up to the anterior arch of the atlas.

52

NMR scans are less informative than CT or polytomograms for bony structures. However most anatomical landmarks are easily recognized. As on polytomograms the odontoid process and the anterior arch of the atlas appear heterogeneous in relation with variable distribution of cortical (hypointense) and cancellous bone (isointense). Remains of Bergman's ossiculum terminale is often seen on frontal sections as a low intensity triangular area. The remains of the synchrondrosis between the dens and body of the axis (fusion normally occurs between the ages of 5-12) are often responsible for a hypersignal in this area.

Anterior and posterior muscles (which appear isointense) are well demonstrated on MR scans: in front of the craniocervical junction it is possible to identify the rectus capitis anterior , the rectus capitis lateralis , and the longus capitis. Suboccipital muscles (rectus capitis posterior, obliquus capitis superior and inferior, semispinalis capitis and splenius capitis) and the suboccipital triangle may be identified in many cases.

REFERENCES

Brand-Zawadzki M., Norman D. (1987) MRI of the CNS. Raven Press,
Cabanis E.A., Doyon D., Halimi Ph. et al. (1988) Atlas d'IRM del'encephale et de la moelle. Masson.
Daniels D.L., Haughton V.M., Naidich T.P.(1987) Cranial and Spinal MRI:An atlas and guide. Raven Press.
Dietemann J.L., Doyon D., Aubin M.L., Manelfe C.(1988) Chapter 19:Jonction cervico-occipitale normale et pathologique in "TDM et IRM du Rachis". Eds:C.Manelfe, Vigot, Paris. (in print).
Koritke J.G., Sick H. (1983) An atlas of sectional human anatomy. Index 1:Head, Neck, Thorax. Urban & Schwarzenberg.
Stark D.D., Bradley W.G. (1988) Magnetic Resonance Imaging. Mosby, St.Louis.
Wackenheim A. (1974) Roentgen diagnosis of the cranio-vertebral region. Springer Verlag, Berlin.
Williams P., Warwick (1980) R.Gray's Anatomy, 36 th Edition, Churchill Livingstone.

Spinal CSF Pulsations

G. Schroth, U. Klose, and W. Grodd

Knowledge of CSF production, distribution and absorption has gradually accumulated since the introduction of radionuclide scanning (Di Chiro 1966) and X-ray contrast cisternography (Du Boulay 1966). But the present understanding of cerebrospinal (CSF) flow is still incomplete and hampered by the fact that lumbar punction of the closed system of ths CSF spaces may disturb observations of physiological CSF movement.

With Magnetic Resonance imaging (MRI) normal and disturbed CSF circulation can be visualized and quantified noninvasively and a mapping of the flow pattern can be achieved in a variety of pathological conditions.

METHODS:

Our investigations were performed on a 1.5 Tesla Magnetom (Siemens Corp., Erlangen, FRG). Using ECG gated FLASH sequences (Fig.2) CSF flow was measured during the cardiac cycle in 120 normal volunteers and patients. With a time resolution of normally 75 ms, the CSF movement was calculated by flow induced signal enhancement on magnitude images and by analysis of the velocity-dependent phase of the protons on phase images. To obtain high contrast between flowing and stationary structures, a large flip angle of 90 degree was applied (Klose 1987, Schroth 1987). To monitor the dependency of CSF flow during respiration, RACE-real time acquisition of flow was performed by a special projection technique (Müller 1988). In addition a variety of phantom experiments and computer simulations was performed to quantify both methods.

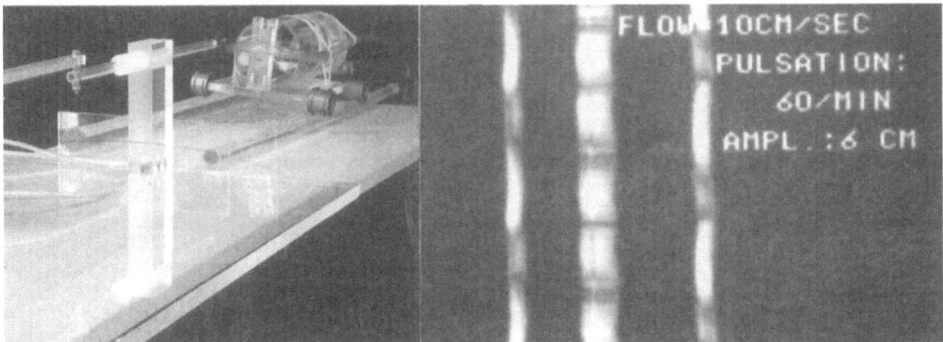

FIG.1. Left side: Flow phantom to simulate oscillation and continous laminar motion: Concentric acrylic tubes, perfused with water (passively driven by gravity acting on the difference in the water level in reservoirs at each end) are fixed on a waggon, and moved sinusoidal through the magnetic field. By variations of the amplitude and frequency of the waggons motion and the flow velocity inside the tubes any kind of combination of flow and superimposed oscillating motions (as expected in the spinal canal) can be performed.
Right side: Race-real time phantom experiment (FLASH, TR=50ms, TE=10ms, flip angle = 90 degrees, without phase encoding gradient; the horizontal direction shows one dimensional fourier transformation in readout direction; the vertical axis represents the time of measurement (3,5sec from the top to the bottom). The middle column (a closed tube) indicates oscillation of the waggon. Comparable to the CSF pulsations in the canals of the cervical spine, the intensity peaks in the lateral tubes are shifted against one another by half a cycle of the waggons oscillation (frequency: 60/min, amplitude: 6cm) due to the opposite directed flow in both lateral tubes (10 cm/sec).

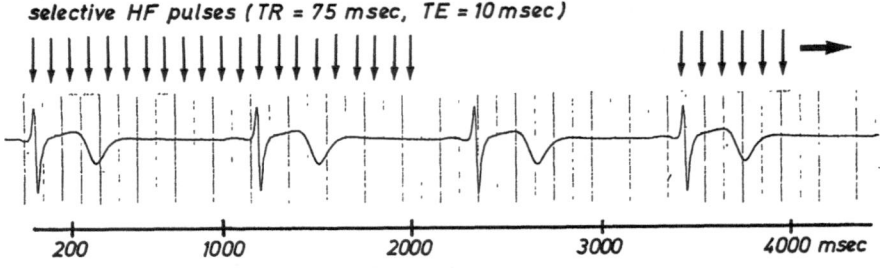

selective HF pulses (TR = 75 msec, TE = 10 msec)

200   1000   2000   3000   4000 msec

Fig.2: ECG gated FLASH sequence for detection of signal changes within the cardiac cycle. Starting every second or third R-wave of the ECG, the same slice is excited 20 or 40 times in an orientation perpendicular to the expected flow.

RESULTS AND DISCUSSION

A striking feature of FLASH images is the high-intensity appearance of flowing structures, especially for motion perpendicular to the imaging plane. The mechanism for this signal enhancement is a wash in of fully relaxed spins between subsequent radio frequences, whereas the signal intensity of stationary structures is decreased by saturation effects (Fig.3 and 4).

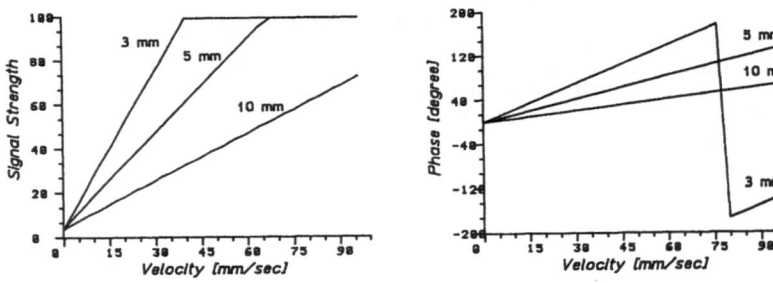

Fig.3: Diagram of computer simulated changes in magnitude and phase of spins for an increasing flow perpendicular to slices of 3, 5 and 10mm thickness.

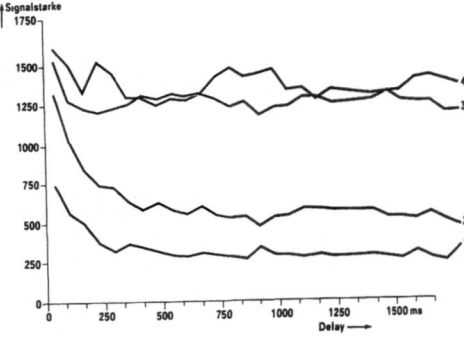

Fig.4: Plot of signal intensity versus time for 20 FLASH excitations, starting with the R-wave of the ECG until the delay time of 1500ms. Whereas the signal intensities of the spinal cord (1) and muscle tissue (2) decreases, due to saturation effects, the intensities of blood vessels remain high. The intensity peaks of the jugular vein (4) are caused by acceleration of the veinous blood flow during the cardiac diastole. Continous blood flow in the internal vertebral veinous plexus (3).

Related to time and direction we found simultaneous pulsatile CSF-flow in both the foramina of Monro and the cerebral aqueduct.

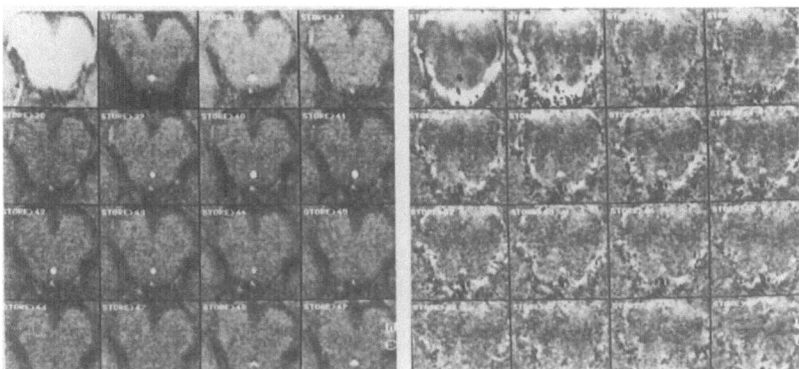

Fig.5: ECG gated axial FLASH-images through the midbrain (inferior colliculus of the tectum mesencephali) starting simultaneously with the R-wave of the ECG and follow up with a time delay of 75 msec. The magnitude images *(left side)* show the change of signal intensities of the aqueduct, whereas the signal of the adjacent dorsal vein (superior cerebellar vein) demonstrates constant blood flow during the cardiac cycle. *Right side:* corresponding phase images. Flow downwards is encoded as a decrease, upwards as an increase of signal intensity.

Fig.6: Plot of signal strength and phase of normal CSF flow within the cerebral aqueduct during the cardiac cycle as a function of R-wave delay. The flow induced signal enhancement of the CSF protons follows the phase of the hydrogen nuclei with some time delay which is typical for an oscillating motion. The CSF flow from the third to the fourth ventricle normally

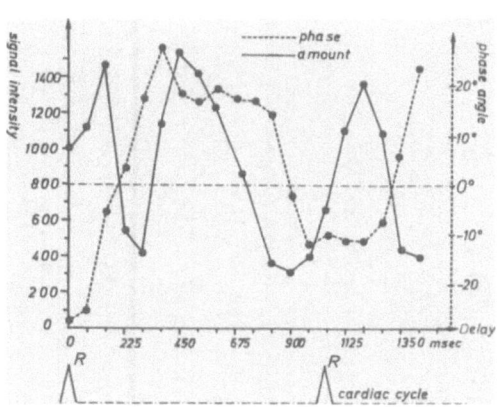

-    starts 150 to 300 ms after the R-wave of the ECG;
-    simulates an arterial pulse pattern (peak and shoulder);
-    lasts for 55-60% of the cardiac cycle;
-    is followed by a backflow from the fourth to the third ventricle, with a slower velocity and which takes a shorter time.

In contrast to the two peaks of signal strength, within the aqueduct, only one peak occurs in the frontal and lateral cervical subarachnoidal spaces (SAS) during the cardiac cycle (Fig.7).

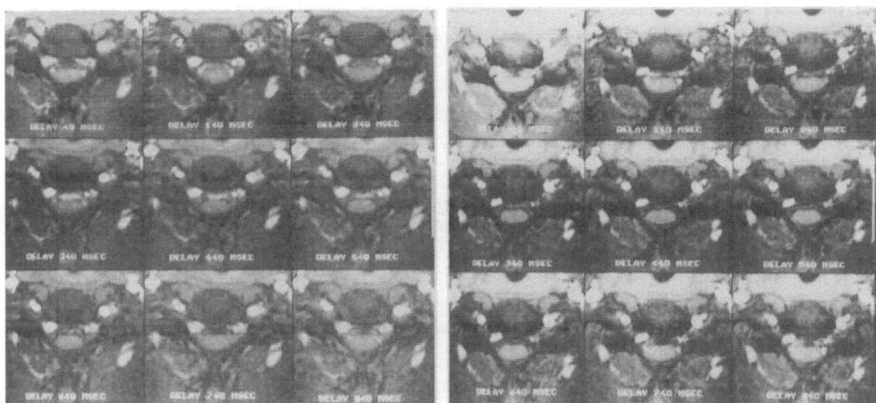

Fig.7: Signal intensities of the cervical spinal canal during the cardiac cycle on axial FLASH images *(left)*. After saturation of a distant slice above *(right)* the signal increase in the frontal SAS (300 - 400 ms after the R-wave of the ECG) is diminished.

The phase (Fig.8) demonstrates synchroneous oscillating motion of both, frontal and lateral SAS, with a negative shift in the lateral SAS, indicating an additional flow upwards. On the magnitude images, the resulting intensity peak is increased, when oscillating and directed flow move into the same direction and the signal is reduced when oscillation and directed flow are opposed.

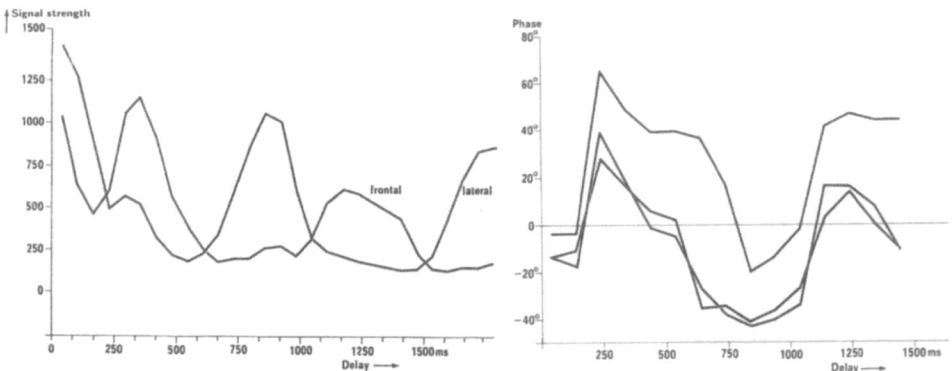

Fig.8: Plot of phase and signal strength of CSF in the frontal and lateral cervical SAS as a function of R-wave delay of the ECG.

This MRI-analysis of phase and magnitude images of CSF protons shows, that the cardiac related CSF pulsations are superimposed by a continous flow, moving downwards in the frontal and upwards in the lateral subarachnoidal canals.
To confirm this findings additional saturation pulses were used. After saturation of a plane situated cranially to the examined slice the signal peak resulting from flow downwards will be missed, as demonstrated in Fig.7 on the right side.

The results are summarized in Fig.9. After application of a saturation pulse above the frontal flow is reduced and the signal increase of the lateral SAS disappeares after saturation of a slice below.

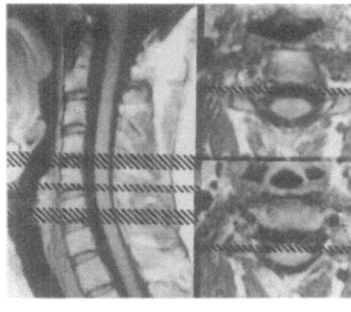

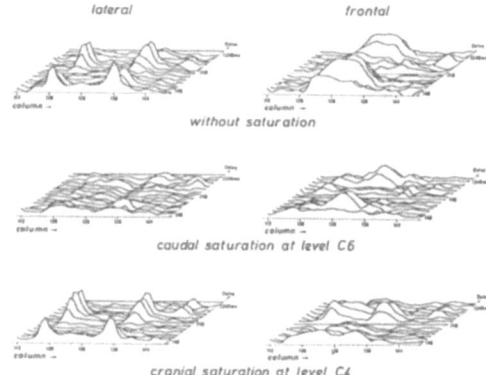

lateral   *frontal*

without saturation

caudal saturation at level C6

cranial saturation at level C4

Fig.9: Plot of the change of signal intensity of two lines through the lateral and frontal cervical SAS, as shown on the left side, before and after saturation of additinal slices above and below.

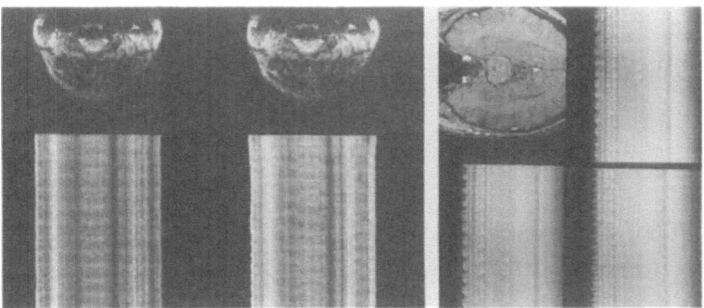

Fig.10: RACE-real time mesurement of CSF-flow in the aquaeduct and spinal canal (after saturation of the structures surrounding the spinal canal). *Left side:* de- and increase of the spinal CSF pulsation during normal respiration (left). Marked increase of the spinal CSF flow immediately after the beginning of respiration (right).
Right side: de- and increase of aqueductal CSF-flow during normal respiration (top, right side). Increase of the aqueductal CSF flow 2-3 heart beats after the beginning of inspiration (bottom, left). Reduction of aqueductal CSF flow during exspiration (bottom, right).

During thoracical inspiration the venous backflow to the heart is increased. Thus the volume of the spinal epidural veins is decreased, which is immediately followed by an increase of CSF flow downwards (Fig. 10, left side). During the following heart beats, this increased blood volume passes the pulmonary circulation and arrives at the intracranial cavity 2 or 3 heart beats later, resulting in a delay between start of inspiration and the increase of aqueductal CSF pulsation (Fig.10, right side).

REFERENCES:
Bergstrand G et al. (1985) J Comput Assist Tomogr 9(6): 1003-1006.
Di Chiro O (1966) Acta Radiol Diagn (Stockh) 5: 988-1002.
Du Boulay GH (1966) Br J Radiol 39: 255-262.
Du Boulay GH et al.(1972) Acta Radiol Diagn (Stockh) 13: 496-523.
Klose U et al. (1987) Fortschr Röntgenstr 147: 313-319.
Müller E et al. (1988) Abstracts SMRM VII, (San Franzisko) p. 729.
Schroth G et al. (1987) Abstracts SMRM VI, (New York) p. 119.

CSF Pulsations in the Cervical Region Studied by MRI

J. T. Wilmink, E. L. Mooyaart, R. L. Kamman, and D. J. Zeilstra

Introduction

Cine MR is a new technique using a movie loop of sequential gradient reversal echo images obtained during various points of the cardiac cycle, thus allowing cinegraphic display of structures and substances demonstrating movements related to cardiac function. Although the application of the method has until recently focused on cardiovascular studies, pulsatile movements synchronous with the arterial pulse have been described and studied by fluoroscopic filming and videodensitometry of movements of contrast media introduced into the CSF spaces [1,2].

In cerebral MRI the flow void sign produced by the movement of CSF through the aqueduct is a well-known phenomenon. Cine-MR can be used to demonstrate the intermittent nature of this CSF movement related to the arterial pulse, and also to highlight similar pulsatile CSF movements in other regions where such movement effects are not so readily noticeable by "conventional" MRI.

In the cervical region complete obstruction of contrast medium ("myelographic block") is known to stop all CSF pulsation distal to it, while pulsation persists on the cranial side though usually diminished. The presence of a myelographic block is universally regarded as conclusive evidence that spinal cord compression of some kind is present. MRI provides a good image of the cord and the surrounding CSF when the spinal canal is of normal width.

In cases with degenerative spinal narrowing however the cord is often difficult to delineate and in marginal situations it is difficult to differentiate between a cord which is compressed and one which has just escaped compression. Using CT myelography, criteria have been developed based upon measurement of cross-sectional cord area in order to ascertain a symptomatic degree of cord involvement [3], but such cross-sectional cord measurements by MRI at present are not fully reliable under the conditions mentioned above.

The present study aims by means of cine MR imaging to study the CSF pulsations in the cervical region in normal individuals and those with cord compression, with a view to reproducing the phenomenon of myelographic block.

Material and Method

Five normal individuals were studied, as well as nine patients with clinical and radiological signs of cervical cord compression. In two of these cases an intraspinal neoplasm (meningeoma and metastasis respectively) was involved. The seven other cases were suffering from cervical myelopathy due to degenerative spinal narrowing. Myelograms were available for scrutiny in six of these, and showed a complete block in cervical spinal extension in four and an incomplete block in two.

Cine MR (multiphase imaging) by means of gradient reversal echo imaging using a small flip angle, was performed in a 1.5 Tesla system (Philips Gyroscan). Sagittal T_1 weighted images (spin-echo, TR 650 msec, TE 30 msec) 5 mm thick were acquired, and the most appropriate section was selected for the cine-loop sequence. Depending on the cardiac frequency 11 to 16 images were acquired during the cardiac cycle, starting 15 msec after the R-wave. The cine study was obtained using gradient echoes and a 10° pulse angle. The echo time was 20 msec and the interval between images 33 msec. Four measurements were made, the field of view was 300 mm with matrix of 180 x 256. Flexion-extension studies were performed in six of the cases with degenerative spinal narrowing.

Results

In the normal individuals pulse-related CSF movements were seen as rythmically-appearing areas of signal loss in varying degrees in all cases. The least movement was seen in those with large CSF spaces around the cord while pulsatile movements appeared especially noticeable in those with a less roomy spinal canal. In some individuals a wave front of CSF movement could be observed passing dorsal and ventral to the cervical cord.

The two tumor cases demonstrated a virtually complete block to CSF movements at the level of the lesion, with small jets of CSF being forced past the block with every heartbeat.

In the seven cases with degenerative spinal narrowing a complete block to CSF movements was seen in six. In three of these the MRI block could be reduced by flexion of the cervical spine; pulsatile movements could now be seen above and below the involved level. The myelogram showed an incomplete block in two of these. Three cases in whom the MRI block could not be reduced by flexion demonstrated a complete myelographic block.

In the seventh case cine MR showed an incomplete block and myelography a complete block, but MRI was performed with the cervical spine in the mid-position and a flexion extension study was not done in this case.

Discussion

Intracranial pressure variations synchronous with the arterial pulse have been said to constitute a CSF pump forcing the fluid from the cranium in systole into the spinal dural sac which is elastic and surrounded by an easily compressible valveless epidural venous system. Pulsatile CSF movements in the cervical region resulting from this have been previously studied by observing the movements of contrast media introduced into the cervical arachnoid space [1,2].

Lane and Kricheff reported mean deflections in the upper cervical region of 9.6 mm (range 3-30 mm), with a caudal movement occurring in cardiac systole and a cranial movement in diastole. Going from cervical flexion to extension the mean amplitude of the pulsations increased somewhat in normals, and one may speculate whether this is due to narrowing of the CSF space around the cord which always occurs in cervical extension. It is our impression that in normal individuals CSF movements studied by cine MR are more pronounced in those with a relatively narrow spinal canal, as was also described by du Boulay, but precise quantification is not possible with this technique and the number of normal studies is small.

In patients with spondylotic spinal cord compression Lane and Kricheff observed decreased pulsation amplitudes above and below the block, and this was also noted by du Boulay. In three of our seven cases with spinal narrowing CSF pulsations were abolished in cervical flexion as well as in extension and there was a complete myelographic block.

In three other cases the CSF movements, absent in extension, could be restored by cervical flexion and in these cases the myelogram showed an incomplete block. It might seem that cine MR is more sensitive to obstruction of CSF flow than myelography, but difference in posture of the cervical spine between the two examinations appears a more likely explanation. The same may apply to the seventh case, in whom myelography performed in cervical extension showed a complete block and cine MR in the mid-position an incomplete block.

In conclusion, cine MR is a non-invasive easily performed method of studying CSF dynamics. The present study indicates that the obliteration of the CSF space around the cervical cord may be reliable demonstrated by this technique, so that the phenomenon of myelographic block may be reproduced without the disadvantages of myelography.

References

1. du Boulay GH (1966) Pulsatile movements in the CSF pathways.
   Br.J.Radiol. 39: 255-262

2. Lane B, Kricheff II (1974) CSF pulsations at myelography: a video-densitometric study. Radiology 110: 579-587

3. Penning L, Wilmink JT, van Woerden HH, Knol E (1986) CT myelographic findings in degenerative disorders of the cervical spine: clinical significance. AJNR 7: 119-127

DOPE – A Fast Method to Measure CSF Motion

D. Ott and J. Hennig

Introduction

The physiology of CSF circulation is not yet fully understood. Various invasive methods and recently some noninvasive MR methods have been used to study bulk motion and local CSF pulsations. DOPE (double phase encoding) is a new MR method (Hennig 1988) that allows one to measure quantitatively the CSF flow over a wide region within seconds during routine examinations. The flow patterns in normal volunteers and in patients with suspected disturbed CSF circulation will be discussed.

Material and Method

All examinations were performed with a low field (0.23 T) iron shielded resistive system (Tomikon, Bruker Medizintechnik). A total of 45 examinations of the head and craniocervical junction, 19 of the cervical spine, 47 of the thoracic spine, and 23 of the lumbar spine were performed, with 2 to 10 scans each.

The DOPE method derives from RARE myelography. Two myelography datasets are made to interfere with the result of a myelographic image with an overlying linear pattern. Slow flow within a fluid space will produce a curvilinear deformation on the interference pattern. The acquisition time (19 s) is much longer than the cardiac cycle, and thus the fast systolic-diastolic pulsations are not depicted. The smallest velocity detectable is 0.8 mm/s/pixel, the upper limit being given by the flow void of the RARE signal (Hennig 1988).

Results

Physiological Flow Patterns

The flow patterns in normal volunteers and patients with unrelated pathology are not uniform. Although there is mostly CSF flow within the fourth ventricle (1 to 4 pixels upwards, equaling 0.8 to 3.6 mm/s), some normal individuals do not display flow within the fourth ven-

tricle. Rather consistent upward flow is detected in the prepontine
and premedullary cistern. The flow velocity in the aqueduct cannot be
measured in healthy people for the physiological invisibility in myelograms due to partial volume and flow-void phenomenon. The physiological
bulk movement of CSF from the lateral ventricles through the foramina
Monroi can only rarely be seen with maximal 0.8 mm/s. The lateral ventricles seem otherwise static. The CSF flow within the spinal canal is
summarized in Fig.1. The cervical region consistently displayed flow
in a caudad direction (maximal 3.6 mm/s) ventrally. In a few cases we
detected bilaterally in the ventrolateral cervical aspect slow upward
CSF flow corresponding to the suspected CSF flow channels. The main
flow in the thoracic region, with the cord primarily lying anterior,
is directed downwards in the dorsal aspect. Laterally we find an upward motion of CSF also in the thoracic area, more or less pronounced
and not always symmetrical. CSF flow is usually detectable down to
the conus medullaris. The lumbar region itself never shows any greater
physiological CSF motion with this method.

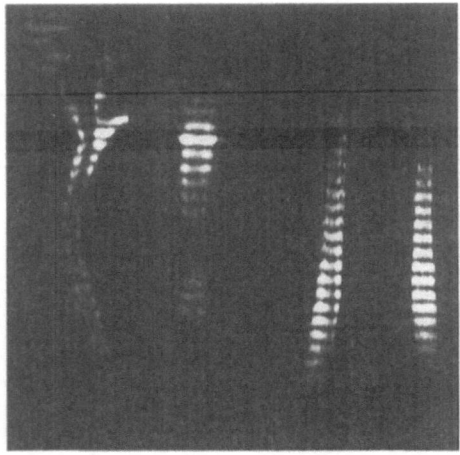

Fig.1. Normal flow pattern in the cervical and thoracic spinal canal

Pathological Flow Patterns

From the hydrocephalic patient group we measured quantitatively five
patients with NPH, two of which seemd to be in a compensated chronic
state, with only little change in the flow pattern (no or normal upward movement in the fourth ventricle, no movement in the third ventricle, and only slight forward movement in one lateral ventricle).

The apparently more typical pattern is a "reflux pattern" with upward
flow through the foramina Montroi and forward and backward motion within the lateral ventricles, together with higher velocities in the
third ventricle with mixed directions (max. > 4 mm/s) (Fig.2).

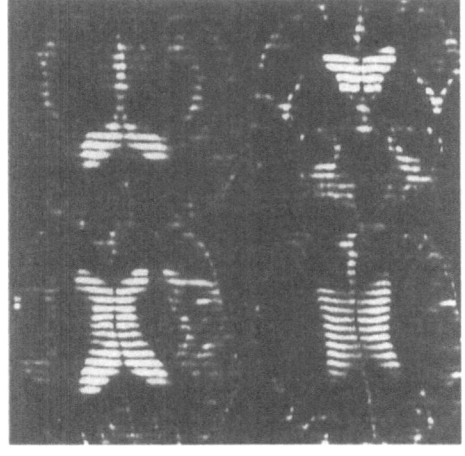

Fig.2. Abnormal flow pattern in NPH

Aqueductal stenosis leads to the expected change in flow pattern, as
illustrated in an example of almost total stenosis without any flow
within the fourth ventricle and caudal part of the third, accompanied
by high bidirectional flow in the suprasellar cister/anterior third
ventricle (Fig.3).

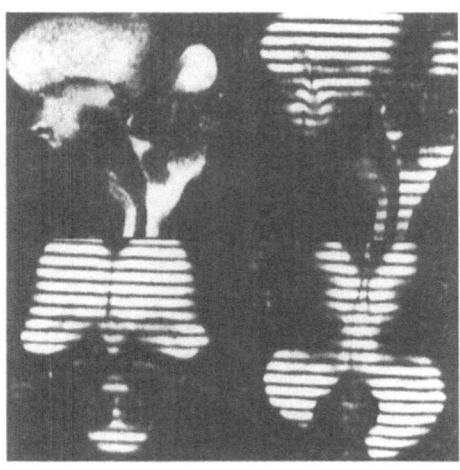

Fig.3. Aqueductal stenosis

Among the space-occupying intracranial lesions one case of unilateral blockage of the foramen Monroi was demonstrated with this method. Subarachnoid cysts that do not communicate are found to be static, unlike the surrounding CSF, verified in four cerebral, two spinal subarachnoid cysts, and in one root sleeve avulsion. Spinal canal stenosis and spinal tumors were found to inhibit CSF motion when complete compression occurred with otherwise rather normal flow patterns. Only one patient with syringomyelia was examined with a cervical cyst: there was discrete motion within the cyst and reduced flow in the surrounding CSF space. Two patients with basilar impression without syrinx show cephalic CSF flow anteriorly at the cranio cervical junction, diminished by head extension.

The iatrogenic disturbance of CSF flow after insertion of a ventricular shunt was tested in three patients. All show abnormal flow within the lateral ventricles, asymmetrically in a unilateral shunt. The comparison of the preshunt images with two postshunt images demonstrates the increased flow towards the shunt immediately after its insertion, with less velocity after some days accompanied by reduction of ventricular size (Fig.4).

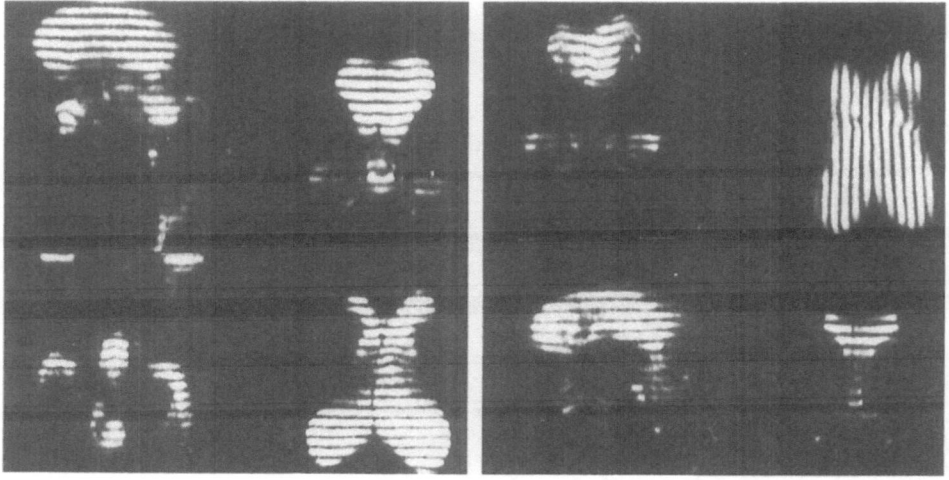

__Fig.4.__ Hydrocephalus occlusus. a: Before shunting. b: After shunting. Increased flow velocities, decreasing after efficient reduction of ventricular size (__lower__ __right__)

Discussion

The qualitative analysis of the flow-void phenomenon does not seem accurate enough to study the CSF circulation. The existing quantitative MR methods (Feinberg and Mark 1988) are time consuming and require postprocessing of the data. DOPE is a newly developed method that directly visualizes CSF flow velocity and direction over a rather large area (e.g., head, cervical and thoracic spinal cord in one image). The time resolution does not allow one to examine the cardiac cycle in terms of pulsations, yet the results prove that the slower motions yield important information. The physiological variability is highest in the spinal cord, with some variations of cerebral flow patterns confirming reports in the literature (Rubin and Enzmann, 1987; Shermann and Citrin, 1986). The clinical value of the method lies in the additional functional information that can be obtained in the routine examination setting. Especially the still difficult differentiation between NPH requiring a shunting procedure and compensated or atrophic ventriculomegaly may be helped by DOPE studies. In our first cases NPH was associated with higher flow velocities than usual and with what can be interpreted as a "reflux pattern." A higher incidence of void sign and quantitative measurements of reduced compliance in these patients are in agreement with these preliminary findings (Bradley et al. 1986).

Other valuable applications are the demonstration of communication versus noncommunication of cysts; this might be important for differentiating neoplastic from nonneoplastic cysts, reported on spinal cysts by Enzmann et al. (1987). The question of whether or not a compression is functionally complete can rarely be answered by MRI; DOPE, however, shows a complete blockage when there is no flow distal to the lesion in a physiologically nonstatic CSF compartment.

A possible role in the functional testing of ventricular shunts has to be clinically confirmed after these promising results.

Apart from intensive studies of physiological flow patterns that will be continued with Valsalva's maneuver and other provocative tests, the clinical application will be tested in larger series in patients with hydrocephalus and other disorders of the CSF circulation - especially the effect of craniocervical anomalies that might help to understand the pathogenesis of syringomyelia.

References

[1] Bradley WG, Kortman KE, Burgoyne B, Eng D (1986) Flowing
    cerebrospinal fluid in normal and hydrocephalic states:
    appearance on MR images. Radiology 159: 611-616
[2] Enzmann DR, O Donohue J, Rubin JB, Shuer L, Cogen P,
    Silverberg G (1987) CSF pulsations within nonneoplastic spinal
    cord cysts. AJR 149: 149-157
[3] Feinberg DA, Mark AS (1987) Human brain motion and cerebro-
    spinal fluid circulation demonstrated with MR velocity imaging.
    Radiology 163: 793-799
[4] Hennig J (1988) Generalised MR interferography. Proceedings
    SMRM 1988, San Francisco
[5] Mark AS, Feinberg DA, Brant-Zawadzki MN (1987) Changes in size
    and magnetic resonance signal intensity of the cerebral CSF
    spaces during the cardiac cycle as studies by gated, high
    resolution magnetic resonance imaging. Invest Radiol 22:
    290-297
[6] Rubin JB, Enzmann DR (1987) Imaging of spinal CSF pulsation
    by 2DFT MR: significance during clinical imaging. AJNR 8:
    297-306
[7] Sherman JL, Citrin CM (1986) Magnetic resonance demonstration
    of normal CSF flow. AJNR 7: 3-6

Analysis of Spinal CSF-Flow Phenomena with an MR Cine Mode Using Fast Sequences. Demonstration by MR-Movie

G. Schuierer, J. Grebmeier, and W. J. Huk

Spinal CSF flow had formerly been difficult to analyse. It is pulsatile, highly dependent on the heart cycle, changes direction and magnitude rapidly and it could only be studied invasively (duBoulay 1966). The ability of MR imaging in demonstrating flow phenomena is well known. Gradient echo imaging provides a new MRI method for the noninvasive study of fast, pulsatile flow, since data acquisition can be triggered by the R-wave and is very fast (Frahm et al. 1987), providing a time resolution down to less than 30 msec (MR-cine mode).

We studied spinal CSF flow by MR imaging in 16 patients, 8 normal and 8 with spinal pathology including spinal stenosis, disc hernias and cord atrophy. Three patients had syringomyelia, two of them were also examined after surgery. Altogether 20 studies, mainly of the cervical spine, were performed in axial and/or sagittal orientation with surface coils.

For imaging of the spinal CSF flow we used the FISP sequence (Oppelt et al. 1987) with R-wave triggering, since in the study of cerebral CSF flow it had proven to render the highest signal intensity variations. Further imaging data are shown below.

Imaging data for the FISP sequence

field strength	1.5T	matrix	256x256
flip angle	50°	TE	10 msec
TR (eff)	30-60 msec	(dependent on heart rate)	
slice thickness	6 mm	FOV	28 cm
images/series	19	averages	4

Experience showed, that triggering on every second R-wave improved image quality, so each series needed about 9-10 minutes, depending on the heart rate. During each recorded R-R-intervall 19 data acquisitions were done, so each of the final 19 images represents a different phase within the heart cycle.

Besides visual evaluation, the image series can be analysed with a standard software, which creates curves of relative signal intensity versus time within a region of interest.

A more vivid visual impression of spinal CSF flow, especially of its pulsatile character, is gained by displaying images of a series in a closed loop, which we call a MR movie. One has to be aware that this is a composite and not a real-time movie.

Using gradient echo sequences, signal intensity depends mainly on the inflow of unsaturated protons into the plane of scanning. Therefore, up to a threshold value, higher intensity represents higher flow. Turbulences cause signal loss due to dephasing. The sequence used gave no information about the direction of flow.

Analysis of the axial images of the normal patients and some of
those with spinal pathology showed quite a similar pattern: areas
of maximum flow were found laterally on both sides and in the
midline ventral or dorsal to the cord. These areas showed the
highest variations of signal intensity, in some phases of the
heart cycle separated by low signal regions. As already published
by others (Schroth et al. 1987), the flow maxima are asynchronous
(Fig 1a). But we also had studies with synchronous peaks of flow.
We attribute this to the variations of anatomy and the different
levels of scanning.
The plots of most of the signal intensities showed two more or
less pronounced peaks with a variable delay in between. Although
strongly dependent on arterial pulsations, no constant correlation
of peak CSF flow and arterial or venous flow maximas was found.
In sagittal scans absolute changes of pixel intensity were less
pronounced, the curves showing only small variations. Nevertheless
the sagittal MR movies of normal patients made these flow
phenomena, which were oscillating up and down in front of the cord
and in the upper cervical spine also dorsally, quite obvious. The
pattern gave the impression of an oscillating wave, but as yet we
do not have enough experience to prove this.

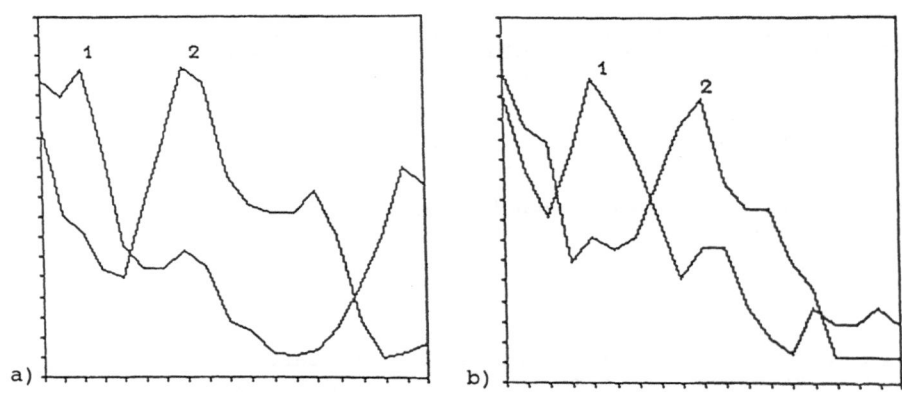

Fig 1. Plots of relative signal intensities (not normalised)
    versus time (50 msec/unit).
a) normal pattern with asynchronous CSF-flow lateral (1) and
    ventral (2) to the cord.
b) asynchronous peaks of CSF-flow within the syrinx (1) and the
    spinal canal (2).

Of special interest were the studies in a 62-year old female with
a large cervicothoracic syringomyelia, which after shunting of the
syrinx showed a considerable collapse of the cavity. The axial and
sagittal study before surgery demonstrated only small regions of
definite flow outside the cord in the lateral recesses. Within the
two syrinx cavities strong pulsations were observed, in sagittal
orientation oscillating up and down.

After shunting the flow pattern changed dramatically. Outside the collapsed cord the flow phenomena observed in normals with frontal and lateral maxima were found. Inside the two cavities pulsatile flow was still present, which was asynchronous with CSF flow in the spinal canal (Fig 1b).

Based on the limited number of studies we can summarize our experiences as follows:

1. Gradient echo imaging with ECG triggerung facilitates the demonstration of spinal CSF flow phenomena with very good image quality and high time resolution.

2. There seem to exist normal flow patterns in the sagittal and axial planes. But final conclusions cannot as yet be drawn, especially if one considers the various factors which can influence spinal CSF flow.These are e.g. absolute and relative size and shape of the spinal canal and cord, arterial and venous blood pressure, the systolic-diastolic pressure gradient, breathing, the level of scanning and also spinal pathology.

3. Display of the image series as a movie makes spinal CSF-flow phenomena more obvious and easier to perceive visually. It may help also in the differentiation of low intensity tumors from cysts or artefacts.

4. Although our experience is limited, we think that this method will aid in the understanding of CSF dynamics in syringomyelia.

References

duBoulay GH (1966) Pulsatile movements in the CSF pathways.
  Br J Radiol 39:255-262
Frahm J, Haase A, Matthaei D (1986) Rapid MR imaging of dynamic
  processes using the Flash technique. Magn Resonan Med 3:312-327
Oppelt A, Graumann R (1986) FISP:eine neue schnelle Pulssequenz
  fr die Kernspintomographie. Electromedica 54:15-20
Schroth G, Klose U, Gawehn J, Petersen D, Varallyay G (1987)
  ECG-related pulsations of the CSF. SMRM book of abstracts 1:119

Comparison of Strategies for CSF and Blood Flow Motion Artifacts Suppression in T2-Weighted Spin-Echo MR Imaging of the Spine

M. Citrin, J. L. Sherman, and R. Gangarosa

INTRODUCTION

The cerebrospinal fluid flow void sign has previously been described (Sherman and Citrin 1986). This sign is related to the pulsatile and turbulent flow of cerebrospinal fluid through narrow areas of the ventricular system. When this occurs, CSF is visualized as a zone of hypointensity due to time of flight and spin dephasing effects. However, in evaluation of the spine, this sign tends to obscure interfaces between the discs and the thecal sac, as well as between the thecal sac and the spinal elements residing within the thecal sac. Reduction of the cerebrospinal fluid flow void sign can be affected by acquiring data in a fashion that is synchronized to the R-R interval of the heart or by the application of special gradients which reduce these moments of motion. We evaluated these two techniques in order to determine the most efficient way to perform T2-weighted imaging of the spinal canal.

MATERIALS AND METHODS

Seven volunteers were examined on a 0.5 Tesla MR imager. Either the lumbar or cervical spine was examined employing T2-weighted imaging sequences (TR 2000 TE 80) and using a combination of techniques to reduce motion artifacts secondary to cerebrospinal fluid motion. Patients were scanned employing 4 different techniques (1) no motion suppression, (2) cardiac gating only, (3) MAST (motion artifact suppression technique), (4) a combination of cardiac gating and MAST. Comparison between the results of these various techniques was performed in a blinded fashion and evaluated for:

1. The prominence of abnormalities within the spinal canal,
2. Appearance of signal arising from zones of CSF flow, and
3. Conspicuity of anatomical detail.

RESULTS

MAST and MAST-gated images were superior to the non-MAST techniques in all image criteria in all subjects. Artifacts on the non-gated, non-MAST axial images and gated non-MAST axial images simulated lesions in 2 subjects and obscured abnormalities that were present. MAST and MAST-gated images were equal for visualization of abnormalities that were incidentally found in these volunteers. MAST-gated images were slightly superior to MAST axial and sagittal cervical spine images and lumbar sagittal images. MAST images were judged to be superior to MAST-gated axial images in the lumbar area.

Setup time was significantly longer for cardiac gated images. In addition, the TR was determined by the cardiac R-R interval and was therefore variable and not under operator control.

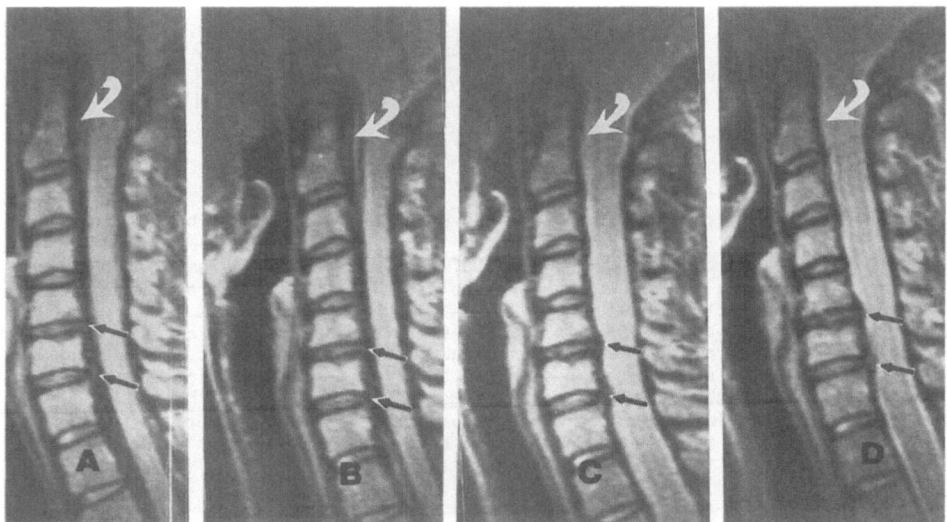

Figure 1.   T2-weighted midline sagittal images obtained at 0.5T. TE=80 msec, non-gated TR=1800 msec, gated TR=1866 msec, section thickness = 5mm. (A) Non-gated image without MAST (B) Gated image without MAST (C) Non-gated image with MAST and (D) Gated image with MAST.   Note hypointense CSF on images A & B, especially at the C1 level (curved white arrows).   Minor discogenic disease is much better visualized on MAST images C & D (black arrows).

DISCUSSION

The application of MAST was more successful than utilizing cardiac gated data acquisition alone. The slight improvement in the MAST images by combining this technique with cardiac gating was not considered significant when considering the added time of setup and lack of control of the TR. The non-MAST images appeared less sharp and were less bright. Unusual artifacts were identified in 2 non-MAST images (including a gated image) that could be misinterpreted as pathological lesions.

MAST requires no setup time or increase in acquisition time. MAST employs specially shaped read and slice select gradient wave forms which null the various temporal moments of motion preventing their propagation as phase errors. This results in reduced motion artifact secondary to CSF pulsation. The suppression occurs within view motion (during data collection) but does not suppress view to w motion (between data acquisitions). MAST compensates for velocity of flow, eleration of flow, and turbulence of flow. There is some inherent reduction in ge sharpness with MAST, but this is compensated for by the reduction in CSF w artifact. This is particularly well seen in sagittal scans (Figs. 1A-D) but also apparent on axial images.

ERENCES

rman JL, Citrin CM: Magnetic resonance demonstration of normal CSF flow. AJNR 7:3-6, 1986.
rman JL, Citrin CM, Gangarosa, RE, et al: The MR appearance of CSF pulsations in the spinal canal. AJNR 7:879-884, 1987.

Gadolinium DTPA in Magnetic Resonance Imaging of Spinal Tumours and Angiomas

I. Isherwood, J. M. Hawnaur, and J. P. R. Jenkins

The value of Gadolinium DTPA (Gd-DTPA) in Magnetic Resonance Imaging (MRI) of intracranial pathology is well established (Stack et al. 1985). The usefulness of Gd-DTPA in MRI of the spine is the subject of recent studies (Baleriaux et al. 1987; Bydder et al. 1985; Slasky et al. 1987; Sze, Abramson et al. 1988; Sze, Krol et al. 1988). This report concerns our experience of spinal tumours encountered in one hundred and four patients with spinal disorders examined by MRI and Gd-DTPA.

METHOD

104 patients, aged between 16 and 75 years (56 male and 48 female), presenting with various spinal disorders have been studied with MRI using Gd-DTPA (Schering-AG). Patients with neurological dysfunction were selected on the basis of a clinical and radiological diagnosis of underlying spinal disease. The majority had undergone myelography and/or Computed Tomography (CT) and/or CT myelography of the spine. A minority in appropriate clinical circumstances also had spinal angiography. All MRI (MR) scans were performed on a 0.26 Tesla Picker International Superconducting magnet system, using a surface coil and a 30cm field of view. Contiguous multi-section images of 7mm slice thickness were obtained in the sagittal plane, supplemented in most cases by transverse or coronal sections. T1- and T2-weighted Spin Echo (SE) sequences (TR = 560-3000, TE = 26-120ms) and a Partial Saturation Recovery (PSR) gradient echo sequence (TR = 500, TE = 18ms) were obtained at the relevant spinal levels. The T1-weighted SE and PSR gradient echo sequences were repeated following intravenous injection of Gd-DTPA in a dose of 0.2mmol/kg body weight. Scanning was continued up to one hour, depending on the clinical problem. Image reconstruction was by a two-dimensional Fourier transform technique.

RESULTS AND DISCUSSION

Table 1: Diagnoses in 104 patients undergoing MRI with Gd-DTPA

INTRAMEDULLARY	Tumour	20
	Syringomyelia	15
	Angioma	2
	Trauma	3
	Multiple sclerosis	1
	Radiotherapy change	1
	Infarction	1

Table 1: Diagnoses in 104 patients undergoing MRI with Gd-DTPA (Continued)

EXTRAMEDULLARY			
	Intradural	Tumour	11
		Dermoid cyst	1
		Arachnoid cyst	1
			13
	Extradural	Epidural fibrosis & disc	11
		Fibrosis alone	7
		Disc alone	9
		Tumour	5
		Osteomyelitis	2
		Trauma	2
		Rheumatoid arthritis	1
		Vertebral haemangioma	1
		AVM	1
			39
		Angiomas	6
NORMAL			3

SPINAL TUMOURS

Table 2: Diagnoses in 47 patients with spinal tumour or angioma

INTRAMEDULLARY	Ependymoma	6
	Astrocytoma	5
	Glioma - no biopsy	6
	Metastases	3
		20
INTRADURAL	Neurofibroma	1
	Meningioma	1
	Haemangioblastoma	3
	Angiolipoma	1
	Metastases	3
	Dermoid cyst	1
	Arachnoid cyst	1
	Leukaemic deposits	1
	Lymphoma	1
		13
EXTRADURAL	Lymphoma	3
	Neurofibroma	1
	Liposarcoma	1
	AVM	1
		6
ANGIOMAS	Intramedullary	2
	Extramedullary	6

INTRAMEDULLARY TUMOURS

Most primary intramedullary tumours were detected on pre-contrast sequences by virtue of irregular expansion of the spinal cord with heterogenous abnormal signal (long T1/long T2). It was not always possible, however, to differentiate a cystic glioma from syringomyelia or post-operative/post-radiotherapy change from residual tumour without Gd-DTPA.

All intramedullary tumours enhanced to varying degrees, independent of histological type or grade of malignancy. Cystic gliomas of the cord showed early cyst wall enhancement concomitant with enhancement of the more solid component of the tumour. On delayed scans (i.e. after approximately 20 minutes) there was a measurable increase of signal intensity within tumour cysts, suggesting gradual accumulation of Gd-DTPA (Fig. 1). No enhancement of syrinx cavities or surrounding cord occurred in idiopathic or post-traumatic syringomyelia, even in those patients in whom abnormal signal (long T2) was present in the adjacent cord on pre-contrast scans. Residual or recurrent intramedullary tumour showed obvious enhancement on both T1-weighted SE and PSR gradient echo sequences obtained immediately after injection of Gd-DTPA whereas post-radiation necrosis gave rise only to subtle patchy enhancement within myelomalacic areas on delayed scans. Areas of cord containing post-operative haemorrhage or oedema showed no evidence of enhancement.

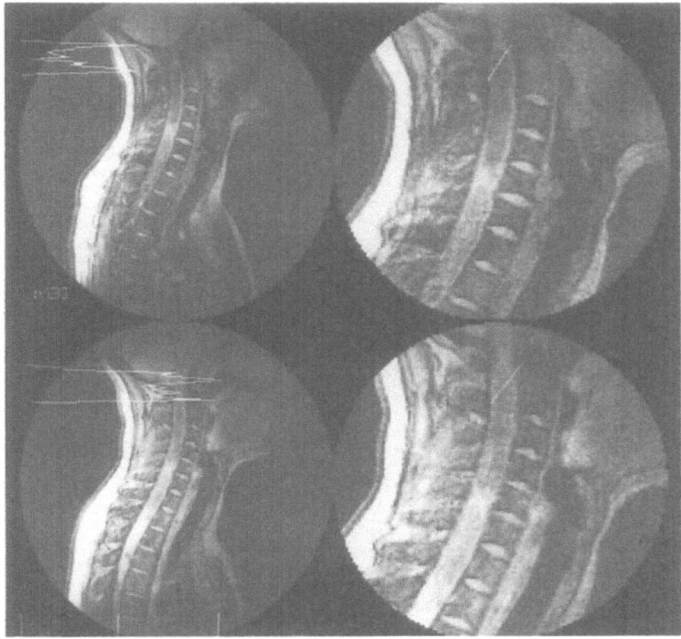

Fig. 1. Cystic ependymoma on sagittal PSR gradient echo 500/18 scans (a) & (b) pre- and (c) & (d) 45 minutes post Gd-DTPA. Enhancement of tumour cyst wall and cyst contents are indicated by a change in the signal intensity profiles

Intramedullary metastases were manifest as one or more ill-defined areas of increased signal on T2-weighted SE and PSR gradient echo sequences, with little or no morphological change in the spinal cord. Conspicuity of metastases was increased after Gd-DTPA, the lesions showing ill-defined enhancement on both T1-weighted SE and PSR gradient echo sequences. Similar multifocal, ill-defined areas of enhancement occurred in two cases of extensive angioma. Solitary lesions showing similar signal characteristics on both pre- and post-Gd-DTPA sequences were considered on clinical grounds to be areas of cord infarction.

INTRADURAL TUMOURS

Multiple intradural tumours from 5-30mm in diameter were demonstrated in von Hippel-Lindau's disease, neurofibromatosis and metastatic carcinoma. Although discrete areas of signal abnormality were detectable within the subarachnoid space on pre-contrast scans, the smaller lesions in particular were relatively inconspicuous, and delineation was significantly improved by the enhancement after Gd-DTPA.

En plaque intradural disease due to leukaemic or lymphomatous infiltration and angioblastic meningioma was detected as non-specific diffuse enlargement of the cauda equina and spinal cord, respectively, with enhancement following Gd-DTPA (Fig. 2).

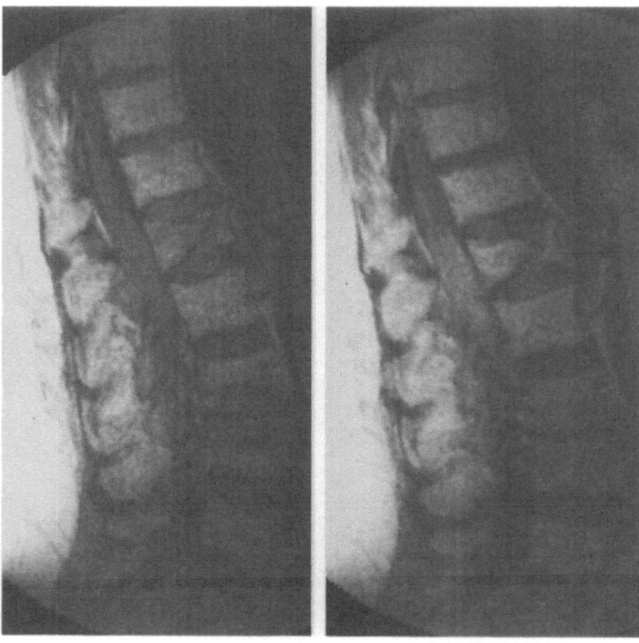

Fig. 2. Intradural lymphoma on sagittal SE 700/40 scans (a) pre- and (b) post-Gd-DTPA showing moderate enhancement of an enlarged conus. The partially collapsed L1 vertebral body is also enhanced due to lymphomatous infiltration

An increase in cerebrospinal fluid signal intensity on T2-weighted
and PSR gradient echo sequences may be observed in the presence of a
very high concentration of CSF protein.

One patient with an intradural dermoid tumour presented with acute
low back pain and sciatica together with signs of meningism. MRI of
the dorso-lumbar region demonstrated a lobulated intradural mass
compressing and infiltrating the conus with heterogenous areas of
short and long T1, and long T2 consistent with both fatty and cystic
components. Peripheral enhancement of the tumour occurred after Gd-
DTPA. Intraventricular and subarachnoid fat globules in the cranial
cavity were demonstrated by both MRI and CT (Fig. 3).

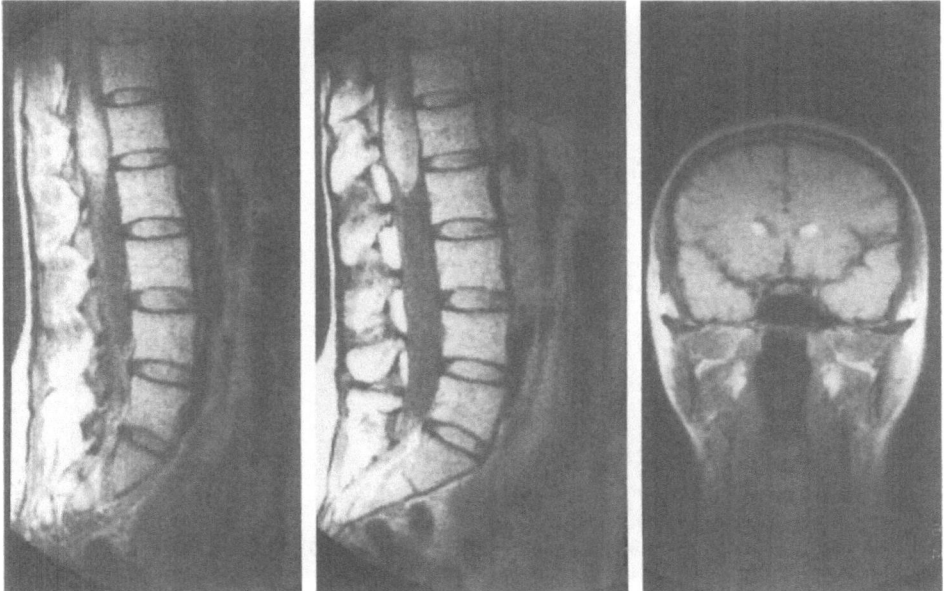

Fig. 3. a) Intradural dermoid cyst of the conus on contiguous
sagittal SE 1000/40 pre Gd-DTPA scans
        b) Coronal SE 820/26 brain scans showing high signal fat
deposits in the frontal horns of the lateral ventricles, and in the
subarachnoid space

The signal intensity of an arachnoid cyst was similar to CSF on all
sequences and no enhancement occurred after Gd-DTPA.

EXTRADURAL TUMOURS

Extradural tumours were detected in 3 patients with lymphoma and in
one each with neurofibroma and liposarcoma. The bony and soft
tissue tumour components both enhanced following Gd-DTPA. Soft
tissue tumour was particularly well seen contrasted against

paravertebral and extradural tissue on all sequences following Gd-DTPA. Enhancement of bony deposits, however, only served to reduce contrast between tumour and fatty marrow on T1-weighted SE sequences, particularly following radiotherapy. Gd-DTPA PSR gradient echo scans were of value in highlighting both the extradural and extraspinal extent of soft tissue tumour and increasing the conspicuity of bony involvement (Fig. 4).

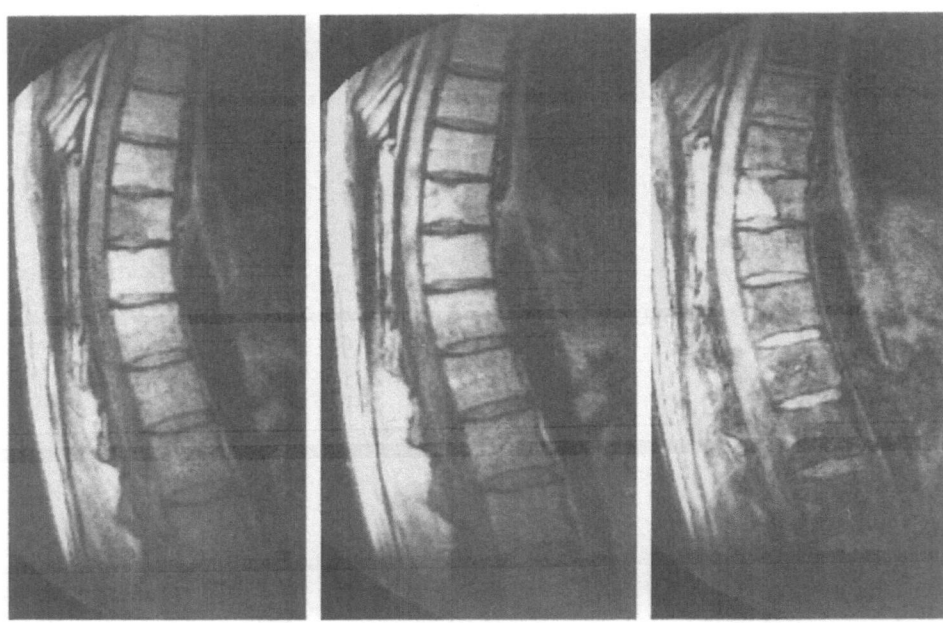

Fig. 4. Enhancing intramedullary and vertebral metastases following laminectomy and palliative radiotherapy on sagittal post-Gd-DTPA scans a) & B) SE 1000/40 Pre- and post-Gd-DTPA and c) PSR gradient echo 500/18 post-Gd-DTPA. Intramedullary lesions are well shown in both sequences but the bony component is rendered more conspicuous on the post-Gd-DTPA PSR gradient echo scans

ANGIOMAS

8 of the 9 patients with angiomas had enlarged intradural vessels demonstrated by myelography or angiography. In the remaining patient, with a predominantly extraspinal arterio-venous malformation, myelography demonstrated thecal displacement by an extradural mass.

Serpiginous linear and punctate low signal areas representing intradural vessels could be detected in all cases, optimally contrasted against CSF and cord on T2-weighted SE sequences. Two patients presented acutely with back pain and meningism clinically diagnosed as subarachnoid haemorrhage. Both, on MRI, showed focal expansion of the lower dorsal cord, with a central "nidus" of small well-defined low signal areas representing intramedullary vessels. In one, abnormal signals (long T1/long T2) in the adjacent cord were interpreted as oedema. Some of the low signal vessels within the intramedullary "nidus" increased in signal intensity following Gd-DTPA but there was no enhancement of surrounding cord (Fig. 5).

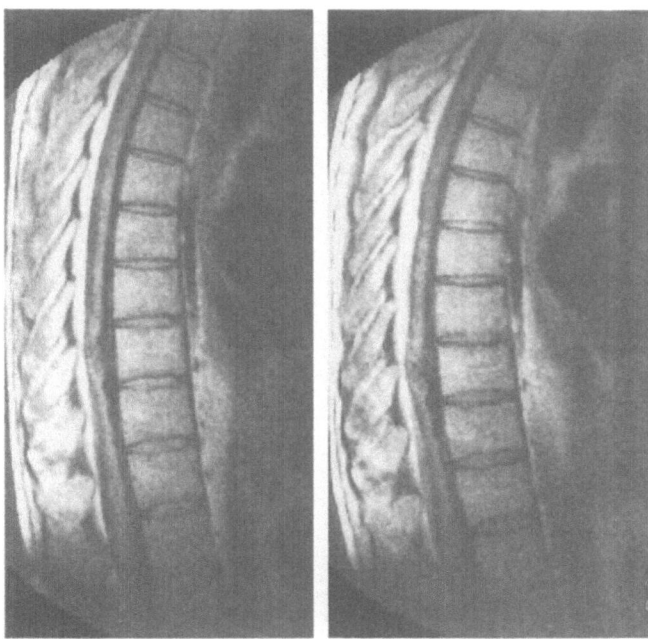

Fig. 5. Intramedullary angioma on sagittal SE 700/40 scans (a) pre- and (b) post-Gd-DTPA. Part of the intramedullary "nidus" at D9 shows increased signal intensity following Gd-DTPA but there is no enhancement in adjacent cord

Extramedullary angiomas had a variable appearance on MRI. In four patients no intramedullary abnormality was demonstrated either before or after Gd-DTPA. In one of these patients, the arterio-venous malformation was predominantly extraspinal (Fig. 6). In two patients, spinal MRI demonstrated diffuse enlargement of the lower dorsal cord and conus with heterogenous signal abnormality (long T1/long T2) pre-contrast together with prominent intradural vessels. Following Gd-DTPA the expanded portion of the cord showed diffuse homogenous enhancement more intense on delayed scans (i.e. after approximately 30 minutes) than on immediate post-contrast scans (approximately 5 minutes) (Fig. 7). These patients presented with chronic symptoms of progressive gait disturbance and impaired sphincter control.

In two patients (one of whom also had an intradural angiolipoma) discrete multifocal areas of enhancement occurred after Gd-DTPA, the corresponding areas of spinal cord appearing normal on pre-contrastsequences. In one of these patients an area of short T1/long T2 identified in the cord pre-contrast was attributed to haemorrhagic infarction secondary to venous thrombosis. These patients presented with acute paraplegia which subsequently partially improved.

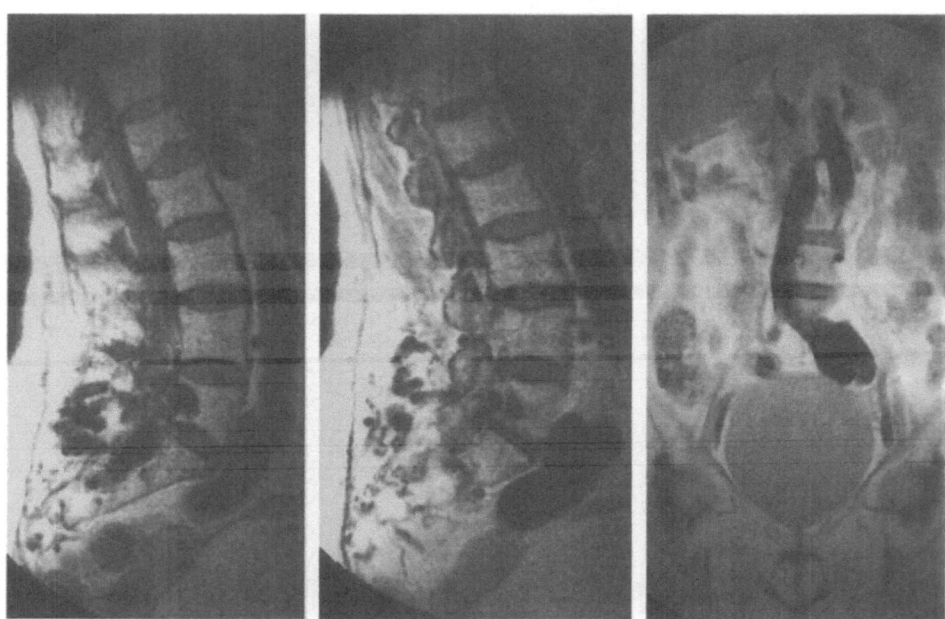

Fig. 6. a) & b) Large extraspinal arterio-venous malformation (AVM) on contiguous sagittal pre-Gd-DTPA SE 700/40 scans of the lumbosacral spine. There is erosion of the bony sacrum with extension of venous drainage into the spinal canal
        c) Coronal post-Gd-DTPA SE 1000/40 scan demonstrating aneurysmal diltation of the left iliac and ascending lumbar veins involved in the AVM

It is difficult to correlate the various MRI signal abnormalities and enhancement characteristics of spinal angiomas with pathology without detailed operative or histological evidence. The results here presented support the postulate that compression of the coronal venous plexus by large arterialised veins draining an extramedullary angioma results in venous congestion of the cord (Aminoff et al. 1974; Kendall et al. 1977; Dormont et al. 1987). This is manifest on MRI as diffuse swelling and signal change consistent with an increased water content. Enhancement within the affected cord seems likely to be due to accumulation of Gd-DTPA in the extravascular compartment of the cord secondary to raised venous pressure, by the same mechanism as oedema formation. An alternative hypothesis might be that an altered arteriovenous pressure gradient results in reduced arterial flow into the cord with consequent ischaemic hypoxia. Fluid and/or Gd-DTPA accumulation might then occur secondary to diffuse malfunction of the spinal "blood-brain barrier". Rapid resolution of cord enlargement and signal abnormality, together with symptomatic improvement has been reported after surgical closure of such dural spinal arteriovenous fistulae (Assouline et al. 1988; Mazaryck et al. 1987). Angiomas having an intramedullary "nidus" are thought to drain away from the spinal cord, perhaps directly into epidural veins, with no significant obstruction to the normal draining veins. Disappearance of dilated intradural veins and the intramedullary "nidus" on MR has been reported following embolisation of an intramedullary angioma (Doppman et al. 1987).

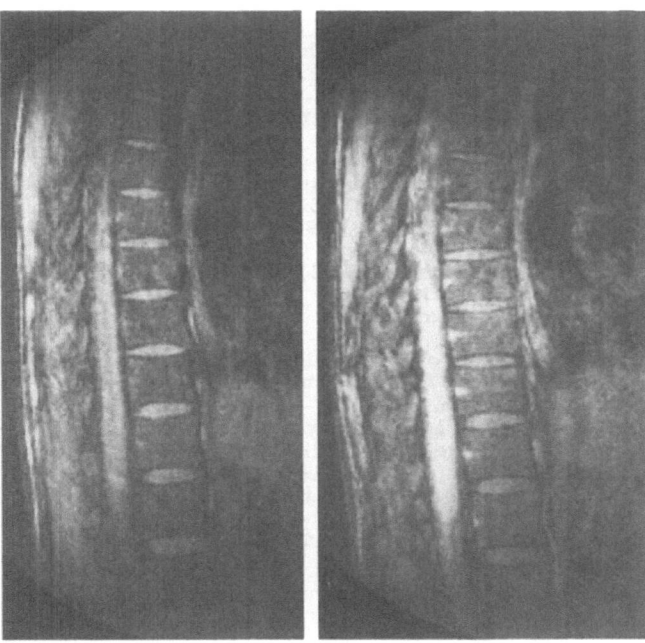

Fig. 7. Extramedullary angioma on sagittal PSR gradient echo PSR 500/18 scans (a) pre- and (b) 30 minutes post-Gd-DTPA. Note enlarged intradural vessels surrounding expanded cord which shows marked delayed enhancement following Gd-DTPA

In two patients clinical symptoms and signs were consistent with cord infarction and ill-defined foci of enhancement were observed following Gd-DTPA. it is possible that thrombosis or compression of normal spinal veins may predispose to venous infarction in the cord. Alternatively, such foci or enhancement may represent intramedullary angiomas with an abnormal vascular network at capilliary level.

SUMMARY

Gd-DTPA in a dose of 0.2mmol/kg has proved to be a safe contrast medium with no significant side-effects and a high degree of patient acceptibility. The conspicuity and detailed delineation of lesions was improved by the administration of Gd-DTPA. In some patients enhancement resulted in detection of lesions not visible on pre-contrast MRI scans. Enhancement following Gd-DTPA was not specific for tumour and consideration of the pattern of enhancement together with the clinical history and examination is necessary in order to provide more specific diagnoses. It is suggested that the variable enhancement of spinal cord in the presence of extramedullary angiomas is related to the degree of intramedullary venous congestion and may therefore prove of value in pathophysiological studies of spinal vascular malformations.

REFERENCES

Aminoff MJ, Barnard RO, Valentine L (1974) The pathophysiology of spinal vascular malformations. J Neuro Sci 23:255-263

Assouline E, Gelbert F, Dormont D, Reizine D, Merland JJ (1988) MRI Study of Dural Arteriovenous fistulae draining into the external spinal veins. J Neuroradiol 15: 1-12

Baleriaux D, Parizel PM, Niendorf HP, Rodesch GL, Segebarth C (1987) Value of intravenous Gd-DTPA Contrast Injection in the MR evaluation of spinal tumours. AJNR 8 (5): 952

Bydder GM, Brown J, Niendorf HP, Young IR (1985) Enhancement of cervical intraspinal tumours in MR imaging with intravenous Gadolinium-DTPA. J Comput Assist Tomogr 9 (5): 847-851

Doppmann JL, Di Chiro G, Dwyer AJ, Frank JL, Oldfield EH (1987) Magnetic resonance imaging of spinal arteriovenous malformations. J Neurosurg 66: 830-834

Dormont D, Assouline E, Gelbert F, Helias A, Halimi P, Chiras J, Bories J, Doyon D, Merland JJ (1987) MRI Study of Arteriovenous malformations. J Neuroradiol 14: 351-364

Kendall BE, Logue V (1977) Spinal epidural angiomatous malformations draining into intrathecal veins. Neuroradiology 13: 181-189

Mazaryck TJ, Ross JS, Modic MT, Ruff RL, Selman WR, Ratcheson RA (1987) Radiculomeningeal vascular malformations of the spine: MR imaging. Radiology 164: 845-849

Slasky BS, Bydder GM, Niendorf HP, Young IR (1987) MR Imaging with Gadolinium-DTPA in the Differentiation of Tumour, Syrinx and Cyst of the Spinal Cord. J Comput Assist Tomogr 11 (5): 845-850

Stack JP, Antoun NM, Jenkins JPR, Metcalfe R, Isherwood I (1988a) Gadolinium DTPA as a contrast agent in magnetic resonance imaging of the brain. Neuroradiology 30: 145-154

Sze G, Abramson A, Krol G, Liu D, Amster J, Zimmerman RD, Deck MDF (1988) Gadolinium-DTPA in the evaluation of intradural extramedullary spinal disease. AJNR 9: 153-163

Sze G, Krol G, Zimmerman RD, Deck MDF (1988) Malignant extradural spinal tumours: MR imaging with Gd-DTPA. Radiology 167: 217-223

MR in Craniocervical Malformation

C. F. Andreula, M. Resta, M. A. Gentile, and A. Carella

Introduction

MR imaging represents the first choice examination for craniocervical malformations, with superb contemporary evaluation of the different structures of the region.

Material and Method

The MR study was performed on patients with standard radiographic evidence of osseous craniocervical malformation. We utilized the MR Max superconductive system by GE, operating at 0.5 T. The pulse sequences used were spin-echo with TR 500-600 ms and TE 30 ms, for T1-weighted images good for accurate morphologic evaluation, and TR 2000 ms and TE 28-100 ms for proton density, and T2-weighted images and fast scanning with partial flip angle of 15°, TR 200 ms and TE 20 ms.

Discussion

The relatively high incidence of the association of bone and nervous craniocervical malformations, whatever the gravity of osseous malformation, is an argument for the utilization of the neuroimaging technique.

The results yielded by the protocol used in recent years - initial X-ray examination followed by CT and possibly myelo-CT - were good but sometimes not exhaustive. Nowadays, MR imaging discloses the multicompartmental system of the craniocervical junction, with unsuspected time saving and less discomfort for the patient.

Conclusions

MR plays a fundamental role in the study of craniocervical malformations. Such a technique must not be reserved for major anomalies, but is also suggested in symptomatic minor ones. It sometimes shows a more important malformational pathology of the vascular and nervous system of the region (Fig.1-5).

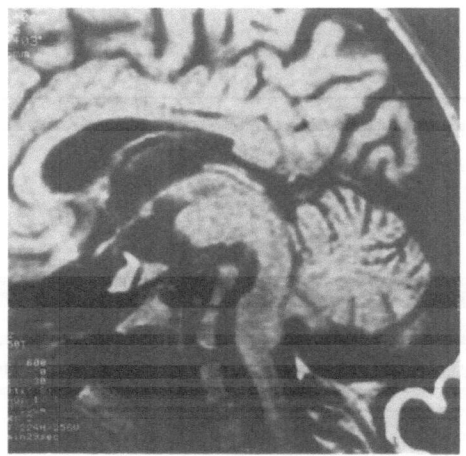

Fig.1. MR T1-weighted image. Very important basilar impression. The bone anomaly causes compression on the midbrain

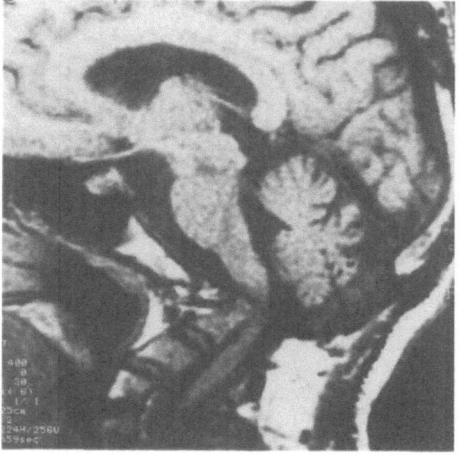

Fig.2. MR T1-weighted image. Important distortion of the upper spinal cord with anterior compression by malformed C1 and C2, dislocated upwards and backwards

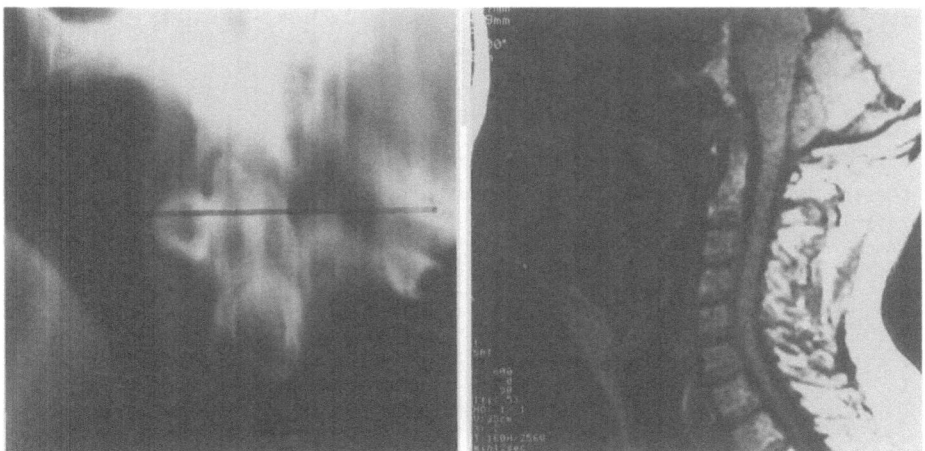

Fig.3. a: Moderate basilar impression and dysplasia of the dens.
b: T1-weighted image of same case, with normal nervous structures

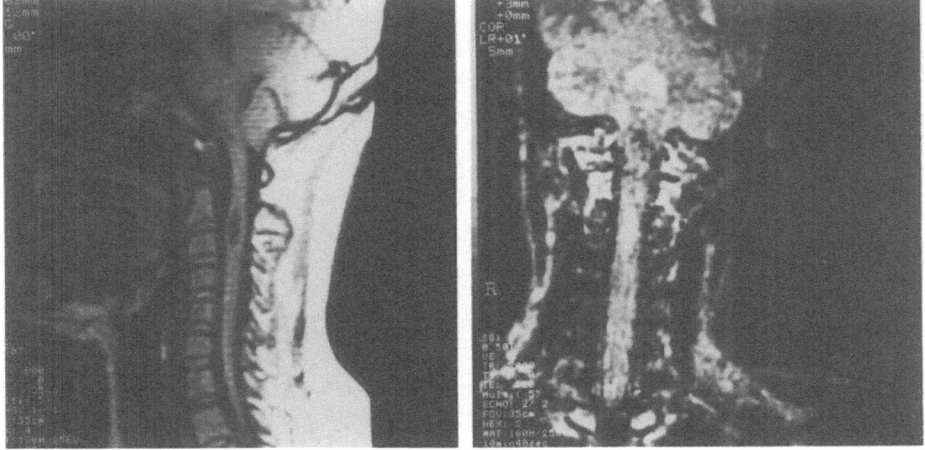

Fig.4. a: T1-weighted images. No osseous craniocervical malformations
but small hydrosyringomelic cyst. b: T2-weighted image of same case

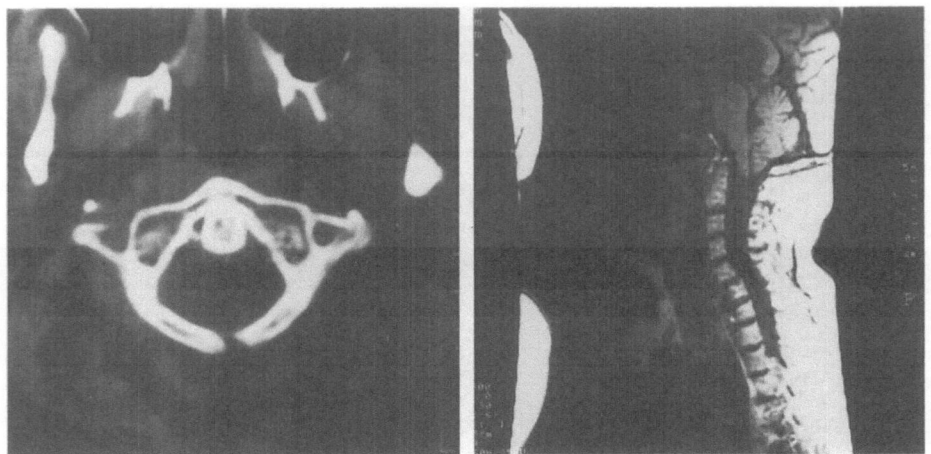

Fig.5. a: CT image. Slight cleft of the posterior arch of the atlas.
b: T1-weighted image. Wide cervicodorsal syringomyelia

Bibliography

[1] Hawkes RC. Holland GN, Moore WS (1983) Craniovertebral junction
    pathology: assessment by NMR. AJNR 4: 232-233
[2] Modic MT, Weistein MA, Pavliceck Z, Boumphrey F, Steines P,
    Duchesneau PM (1983) Magnetic resonance imaging of the cervical
    spine. Techniques and clinical observations. AJR 141: 1129-1136
[3] Newton TH, Potts DG (1983) Advanced imaging techniques. Clavadel,
    San Francisco, pp 159-186 (Modern neuroradiology. Vol 2)

Normal Postnatal Maturation of the Spine

Th. P. Naidich (Miami, FL, USA)

To date, scant normative data define the maturation of the vertebral body, intervertebral disc, basivertebral venous plexus, epidural fat, dura, subarachnoid space, cord, roots, laminae, facet joints, ligamentum flavum, spinous processes, interspinous ligament and paravertebral musculature from birth to adulthood. This presentation addresses the results available thus far from an ongoing evaluation of the postnatal development of these structures, in both imaging and necropsy material.

Vascular Anatomy and Microangiography of the Spinal Cord

A. K. Thron (Aachen, FRG)

We present a radio-anatomical study on the angioarchitecture of the spinal cord in man. Normal findings of in vivo angiography are compaired with those of postmortally injected specimens.

The demonstration of radicular feeders, of the longitudinal arterial trunks, the anastomotic circles and networks and of the superficial drainage routes is supplemented by a three-dimensional reproduction of intrinsic spinal arteries and veins using microradiographical techniques.

Even though the main arterial trunks may exhibit narrow segments or even interruptions, it can be shown that the network is supplemented by other longitudinal anastomoses such as connections between central arteries at the anterior median fissure. The gross regional variability of arterial supply conditions and of the intrinsic territories correspond to locally variable blood requirements. In contrast to the pattern of arterial supply with a dominance of the anterior and central (centrifugal) system, the intrinsic drainage pattern of the spinal cord parenchyma can be characterised as a radially symmetric, largely horizontally oriented system. The superficial blood collecting venous trunks in anterior and posterior midline location are connected by numerous transmedullary anastomoses of large caliber. Physiological and pathophysiological aspects of anatomical findings are illustrated by appropriate examples.

Brain Stem Anatomy and MRI

G. De Chambenois, T. N. Jee, N. Girard, J. Sedat,
and G. Salamon (Marseille, France)

The authors have studied brain stem MRI and show that at any level
the external aspect of the slice, the configuration and the shape
of the fourth ventricle correspond to different nuclei of the brain
stem.

The value of this work is confirmed by comparison with myelin stain
sections for anatomy and by verified tumors studied with MRI for pathology.

Craniocervical Juncture: MRI vs CT in Congenital and Acquired Diseases

R. A. Zimmerman (Philadelphia, PA, USA)

The purpose of this study was to demonstrate the benefits and limitations of MR in demonstrating and understanding disease processes
affecting the craniocervical region.

One hundred and thirty-four patients, 70 adults and 64 children,
were evaluated with high field (1.5 Tesla) MR utilizing one of 2 GE
Signa MR systems. Fifty-five patients had congenital malformations,
48 had neoplasms, while 31 others had a wide spectrum of diseases.
The MR results were compared to those obtained with CT and to operative and post-mortem findings (where available).

Location and alignment of vertebral and CNS structures, compression
and cavitation of cord and brain stem, and tumor encasement of, or
extension within, cord or involvement of cervical soft tissues were
all demonstrated in a superior fashion by MR. CT retains an important
role in interpreting the nature of intrinsic bone disease. Recent
application of MR flow and motion compensation schemes, 3D acquisition gradient echo-contiguous thin sections (1.5 mm) with T1 or T2
weighting, and the use of an intravenous paramagnetic contrast agent
(Magnevist) now provide greater sensitivity in demonstrating disease
processes in the craniocervical region.

Lesions Involving the Foramen Magnum: Diagnostic Management

E. Schindler, R. Stiglbauer, and A. Neuhold

The value and significance of MRI in assessing lesions involving the
foramen magnum are well established. This has been shown in tumors,
syringobulbia, hematomas in the medulla oblongata, Chiari malformations, and rheumatoid arthritis involving the craniocervical junction
(Lee et al. 1985; Spinos et al. 1985; Biller et al. 1986; Friedburg
et al. 1986; Sherman et al. 1987; Pettersson et al. 1988). Since all
these lesions are excellently visualized with MRI, the question is
raised whether conventional neuroradiological examinations and CT can
be omitted today in patients whose signs and symptoms point to a
foramen magnum lesion. The diagnostic management should imply therapeutic considerations, particularly surgical planning (Perneczky 1987)
- the neuroradiologist has to decide the imaging method in order to
demonstrate as exactly as possible the pathology that the neurosurgeon
will encounter during operation. In respect of this fact we have evaluated the neuroradiological findings in our patients with lesions involving the foramen magnum.

MATERIAL AND METHODS

Neuroradiological examinations were carried out in 28 patients with
various foramen magnum lesions (Table 1). All space occupying lesions
were histologically (resp. surgically) verified. All patients had plain
film radiography and were examined with CT and MRI. MRI was performed
on an 0.5T or on an 1.5T superconductive magnet, using the spin-echo
sequences to get T1- and T2-weighted sagittal images; in 14 cases additional axial, and in 5 cases additional coronal slices were made;
slice thickness was 5 resp. 3 mm; gadolinium-DTPA was administered in
7 cases. Conventional tomography of the craniocervical junction was
carried out in 7 patients. 13 patients had (mostly bilateral) vertebral
angiography. The findings of all these examinations were evaluated,
particularly in regard to their contribution to neurosurgical planning.

RESULTS

Plain film radiograms were normal in all lesions situated in the medulla
oblongata and in most of the extramedullary space occupying lesions involving the foramen magnum. In all cases of skeletal malformation, however, plain radiography revealed abnormal findings. In these cases, conventional tomography was very helpful to assess extent and degree of the
malformation. Moreover, the pathologic tomograms contributed consider-

ably to radiation therapy planning in one case of breast cancer metastasis (Fig. 1). MRI has proved to be most informative since it was
conclusive in all space occupying lesions, as it demonstrated both
their topography and the condition of the medulla (Fig. 2). For operation planning, T1-weighted sagittal images turned out to be of greatest
value; additional axial or coronal slices, however, supplied useful
information in many cases (Fig. 3). MRI with gadolinium did not essentially contribute to therapy planning - in all our cases the lesion
was already discernible on the plain MR images, and in none of our
cases it was detected only after gadolinium administration. Although
the CT findings were abnormal in many cases, CT did not supply definite information concerning the site and size of the lesion and the
involvement of the adjacent structures. Angiography revealed shifting
of one or both vertebral arteries in many space occupying lesions involving the foramen magnum. Strikingly, none of the meningiomas in
our series showed a distinct tumor stain.

Table 1. Lesions involving the foramen magnum, pathology (28 cases)

Tumors:		13
low grade astrocytomas	3	
ependymomas	2	
neurinoma (accessory nerve)	1	
meningiomas	4	
osteoma (atlas, posterior arch)	1	
metastases	2	
Non-tumorous lesions:		9
aneurysm (vertebral artery)	1	
arachnoidal cyst	1	
syringomyelia-syringobulbia	2	
Chiari I malformation	2	
osteomyelitis (from mastoiditis)	1	
rheumatoid arthritis	2	
Skeletal malformations:		6

DISCUSSION

The evaluation of the neuroradiological findings in our series has
proved that MRI is the most informative examination method for diagnosing foramen magnum lesions. Other examinations, however, have not
lost their value since MRI is available. Nevertheless, plain radiography should remain the first diagnostic step if signs and symptoms
indicate such a lesion. Even though plain radiography does not yield
abnormal findings in most tumor cases, skeletal malformations can be
ascertained with this examination. If plain radiograms point to such
a malformation, conventional tomography will be very valuable to demonstrate the condition of the skull base, the topography of the atlantooccipital joints and the position of the dens.

MRI has to be carried out whenever a lesion involving the foramen
magnum is surmised, no matter what the plain films have shown. For
therapy and prognosis, it is of decisive significance whether the
lesion is an intramedullary or an extramedullary one. There is no
other diagnostic method to definitely answer this crucial question
than MRI. If an operation on the foramen magnum is planned, we think
that T1-weighted images provide with more information on the patho-

logic condition of this region than T2-weighted images. In our opinion, T1-weighted sagittal and additional T1-weighted axial or coronal images are more useful than T1- and T2-weighted images in one plane only. MRI with paramagnetic agents does not appear to be helpful for neurosurgical strategy, but may contribute to differential diagnosis in some cases.

CT can be omitted in lesions involving the foramen magnum (if MRI is available), because it does not yield sufficient information on the location of such lesions and does not clearly answer whether the adjacent structures are involved or not. Angiography, however, is indispensable, particularly in all neurosurgical cases. Information on the position of the vertebral arteries and on their topographic relation to the lesion is essential for planning the approach to the foramen magnum.

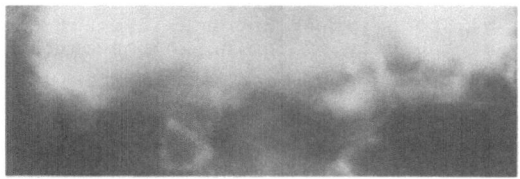

Fig. 1. Osteolytic lesion involving the atlantooccipital articulation and the jugular foramen on the right. Breast cancer metastasis

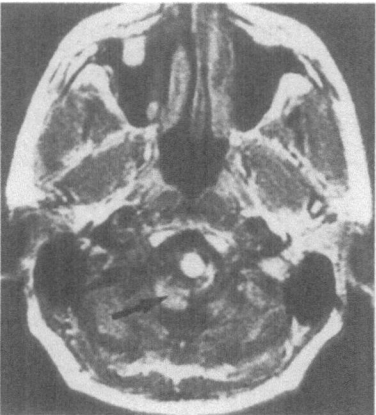

Fig. 2. Hyperintense lesion that displaces the medulla oblongata (arrow) to the right. Thrombosed aneurysm of the left vertebral artery. SE, TR 400/ TE 30

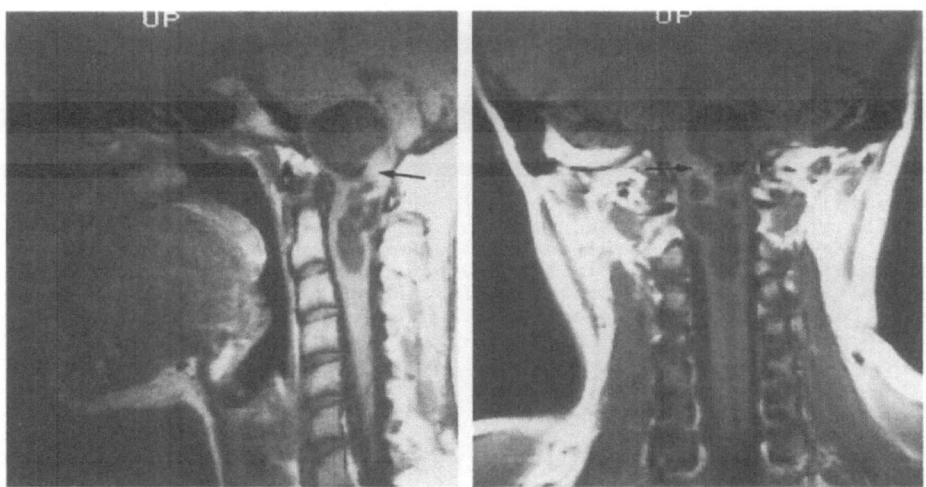

Fig. 3. MRI with Gd-DTPA, a sagittal, b coronal image. Intramedullary tumor with cystic components that indents the 4th ventricle from below and occludes its outlets. There is some Gd-enhancement (arrows), but this supplies no further information on the tumor type. Histological diagnosis: ependymoma

REFERENCES

Biller J, Gentry LR, Adams HP Jr, Morris DC (1986) Spontaneous hemorrhage in the medulla oblongata: clinical MR correlations. Case report. J Comput Assist Tomogr 10:303-306
Friedburg H, Schumacher M, Hennig J (1986) Pathologie des kraniozervikalen Übergangs in der magnetischen Resonanztomographie. 68 Fälle. ROFO 145:315-320
Lee BCP, Deck MDF, Kneeland JB, Cahill PT (1985) MR imaging of the craniocervical junction. AJNR 6:209-213
Perneczky A (1987) The posterolateral approach to the foramen magnum. In: Samii M (ed) Surgery in and around the brain stem and the third ventricle. Anatomy, pathology, neurophysiology, diagnosis, treatment. Springer, Berlin
Pettersson H, Larsson EM, Holtås S, Cronqvist S, Egund N, Zygmunt S, Brattström H (1988) MR imaging of the cervical spine in rheumatoid arthritis. AJNR 9:573-577
Sherman JL, Citrin CM, Barkovich AJ (1987) MR imaging of syringobulbia. J Comput Assist Tomogr 11:407-411
Spinos E, Laster DW, Moody DM, Ball MR, Witcofski RL, Kelly DL Jr (1985) MR evaluation of Chiari I malformations at 0.15 T. AJNR 6:203-208

Tumors of the Craniocervical Junction: Experiences with Conventional and Special MRI Techniques

E. Hofmann, H. Friedburg, D. Ott, and H. Bertalanffy

MRI has become the most sensitive and accurate imaging technique in patients with spinal diseases. Absence of beam hardening artifacts and a high intrinsic tissue contrast permit a reliable and noninvasive demonstration and diagnosis of tumors involving the craniocervical junction (Epstein and Wisoff 1987, Friedburg et al. 1986).

Materials and Methods

From 1984 to 1988 we examined a total of 21 patients with tumors at the craniocervical junction.
All MRI scans were performed on a low-field resistive iron-shielded system (BRUKER Tomikon BMT 1100, 0.23 T) with extended head coils. Routinely at the beginning of every examination a MR-myelography (RARE "liquorgraphy") was done as a pilot scan.
RARE (Rapid Acquisition with Relaxation Enhancement) is based on the principles of echo imaging with long echo trains, each of the echoes being differently phase encoded for spatial coordinates. The resulting image contrast is dominated by the transverse relaxation time T2. Suppression of all signals representing a T2 < 500 ms results in images that are specific for aqueous fluids. So, within a short acquisition time of less than 10 seconds, nontomographic myelography-like images can be obtained without the intrathecal application of a contrast medium.
A paramagetic contrast medium (Gd-DTPA) was applied i.v. in 5 patients in order to get a more precise information about tumor extent and location.

Results

Among the 21 tumors (Table 1) few were originating from the craniocervical junction and restricted to it. In the majority of cases this region was involved secondarily by tumors of the cervical spine or the skull and brain.

Table 1. Tumors involving the craniocervical junction (n=21)

Intramedullary:		Extramedullary:	
Astrocytoma	n=5	Metastasis	n=3
(Sub-)Ependymoma	n=4	Meningioma	n=3
Hemangioblastoma	n=1	Chordoma	n=1
Medulloblastoma	n=1	Neurinoma	n=1
		Lipoma	n=1
		Inflammat. Pseudotumor	n=1

RARE-myelography played an essential role in patient positioning and in planning the subsequent T1 and T2-weighted imaging sequences. Applying conventional myelography criteria, usually a distinction betwen intra- and extramdullary tumors could already be made according to the "liquorgraphy". The use of Gadolinium proved essential in intramedullary neoplasias where nonenhanced scans failed to tell the tumor from the surrounding reactive changes.

Discussion

Intramedullary neoplasms involving the craniocervical junction are very effectively displayed by MR. The tumor can be distinguished as an area of abnormal signal intensity. Apart from lipomas and hemangioblatomas, however, the tumors have nonspecific findings (Scotti et al. 1987). Even after application of Gadolinium DTPA, a differentiation between ependymomas and astrocytomas, the most common intramedullary tumors, is impossible. Gadolinium proves beneficial in telling tumor from surrounding reactive changes (edema, cyst formation) and therefore has a direct impact on the operative approach (Bydder et al. 1985) (Fig. 1).

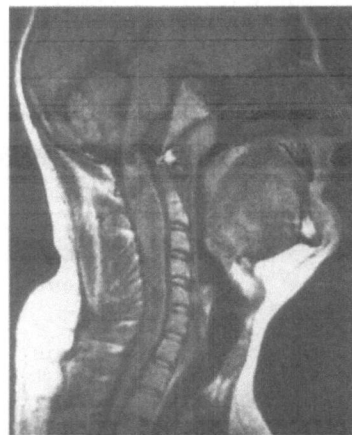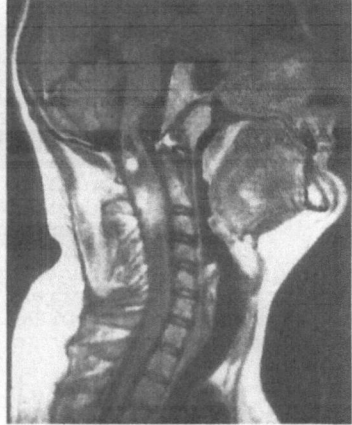

Fig. 1. Pilocytic astrocytoma of the craniocervical junction. On the conventional T1-weighted series (left) the tumor cannot be distinguished from reactive changes. After Gd-DTPA enhancement (right) the tumor blushes at the C2-level. At surgery it proved to be well-circumscribed.

In one of our patients, the use of Gadolinium was vital to depict the solid nodule of a hemangioblastoma which had been otherwise undetected. However, the correlation between enhancement and tumor extent still remains an unsolved problem as tumor cells can be found some distance away from enhancing areas (Earnest et al. 1988).
Among the extramedullary tumors, especially meningiomas are prone to be overlooked on unenhanced T1-weighted scans. Gd-DTPA not only makes the tumor blush but also demonstrates the infiltration

of adjacent dura mater and bone (Schroth et al. 1987) thus allowing a relatively specific diagnosis.

In patients with craniocervical tumors, lumbar or subatlantal
puncture to perform a convential myelography may be hazardous.
RARE-myelography, on the other hand, is a quick noninvasive
method to obtain nontomographic heavily T2-weighted images comparable to myelograms (Hennig 1984, Hennig 1986a,b). We found RARE
imaging an indispensible tool for exact patient positioning.
Beyond that, it visualizes tumor cysts and shows the extent and
location of spinal space occupying lesions (Friedburg et al.
1987) (Fig. 2).

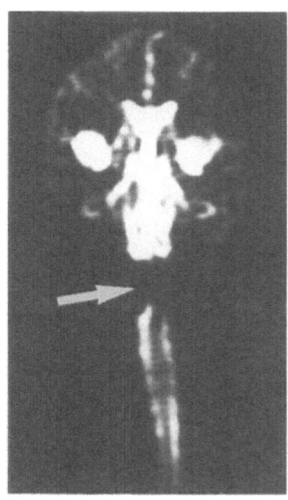

Fig. 2. RARE myelogram of a craniocervical meningioma clearly
indicating the extraaxial nature of the tumor (arrow) with displacement of the spinal cord.

References

Bydder GM, Brown J, Niendorf HP, Young IR (1985) Enhancement of
    Cervical Intraspinal Tumors in MR Imaging with Intravenous
    Gadolinium-DTPA. JCAT 9,5:847-851
Earnest F, Kelly PJ, Scheithauer BW, Kall BA, Cascino TL, Ehman
    RL,   Forbes GS, Axley PL (1988) Cerebral Astrocytomas:
    Histologic Correlation of MR and CT Contrast Enhancement with
    Stereotactic Biopsy. Radiology 166:823-827
Epstein F, Wisoff J (1987) Intra-axial tumors of the cervicome-
    dullary junction. J Neurosurg 67:483-487
Friedburg H, Schumacher M, Hennig J (1986) Pathologie des
    kraniozervikalen Übergangs in der magnetischen Resonanztomo-
    graphie. Fortschr Röntgenstr 145,3:315-320
Friedburg H, Hennig J, Schumacher M (1987) RARE-Myelographie in
    der klinischen Routine. Fortschr Röntgenstr 146,5:584-590
Hennig J, Nauerth A, Friedburg H, Ratzel D (1984) Ein neues
    Schnellbildverfahren für die Kernspintomographie. Radiologe
    24:579-580

Hennig J, Nauerth A, Friedburg H (1986) RARE Imaging: A Fast
    Imaging Method for Clinical MR. Magnetic Resonance in Medicine
    3:823-833
Hennig J, Friedburg H, Ströbel B (1986) Rapid Nontomographic
    Approach to MR Myelography Without Contrast Agents. JCAT
    10,3:375-380
Schroth G, Thron A, Guhl L, Voigt K, Niendorf HP, Garces LRN
    (1987) Magnetic Resonance Imaging of Spinal Meningiomas and
    Neurinomas. J Neurosurg 66:695-700
Scotti G, Scialfa G, Colombo N, Landoni L (1987) Magnetic
    Resonance Diagnosis of Intramedullary Tumors of the Spinal
    Cord. Neuroradiology 29:130-135

Value of Paramagnetic Contrast Agents in the Evaluation of the Craniocervical Junction by MRI

F. E. Zanella, G. Friedmann, and W. Heindel

INTRODUCTION

Magnetic resonance imaging (MRI) is the modality of choice in imaging the craniocervical junction (2,3,5). Therefore there is no need to demonstrate obvious findings, but rather an interest in documenting the sensitivity for small or unsuspected findings. We want to demonstrate the possibilities of MRI for imaging the craniocervical junction and emphasize the value of paramagnetic contrast agents.

ANATOMY

There is no conclusive *definition of the craniocervical junction*; therefore the nomenclature of the anatomists will be used (4,6). The craniocervical junction is defined by the osseous structures of the base of the occipital bone including the foramen magnum and the first and second vertebra of the cervical spine. All structures located within these bony borders also belong to the craniocervical junction. These structures are pons, medulla oblongata, upper cervical spinal cord, vertebral artery and cranial nerves XI and XII.

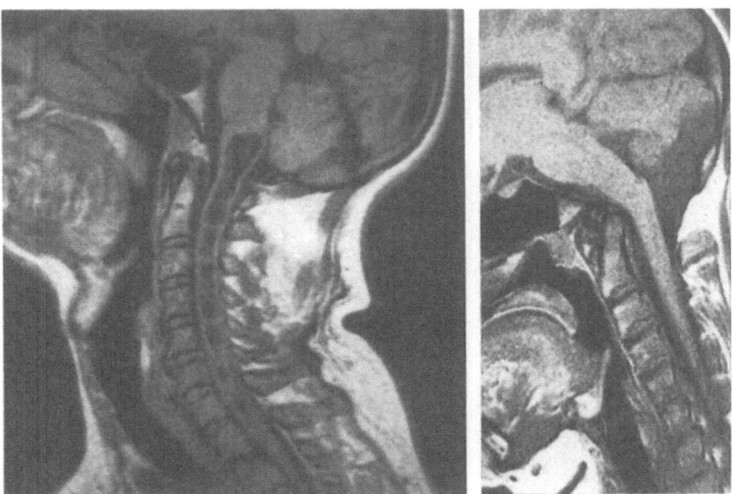

Fig. 1 a,b; Abnormalities of the craniocervical junction: Syringomyelia with cavities in the cervical spinal cord and the brainstem (syringobulbia). There is no need for Gadolinium DTPA (Fig. 1a). Basilar invagination with demonstration of the compression of the brainstem without administration of Gadolinium DTPA (Fig. 1b).

RESULTS

The changes regarding the craniocervical junction can be divided into three groups:

1:    no need for Gadolinium DTPA;
2:    Gadolinium DTPA facilitates diagnosis, although the changes are already seen without it;
3:    Gadolinium DTPA is required to find the correct diagnosis.

No Gadolinium DTPA is necessary in abnormalities of the craniocervical junction (2,3,5) such as basilar invagination (Fig. 1a), Arnold Chiari syndrome or proven syringomyelia or syringobulbia (Fig. 1b).

Gadolinium DTPA often facilitates diagnosis of pathologic changes, although the lesion is already seen without it. The real extent of a tumor and the relationship to the neighbouring structures are better demonstrated after Gadolinium DTPA (1,2,7). A remarkable enhancement of a lesion after Gadolinium DTPA does not only show the tumor better, but also facilitates the histological diagnosis (Fig. 2 a,b). The most common enhancing tumors will be meningioma and ependymoma. Inflammation can also cause a considerable enhancement.

In all these cases T2-weighted images render the correct diagnosis more difficult, because they produce a similar high signalintensity between tumor and surrounding cerebrospinal fluid. Additionally, T2-weighted images take a long time; therefore there may be a lot of motion artifacts that reduce the quality of imaging and therefore the diagnostic potential.

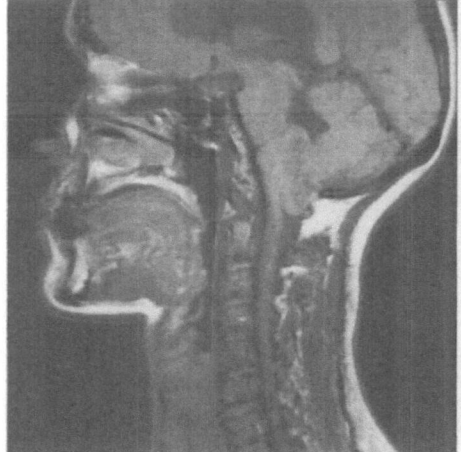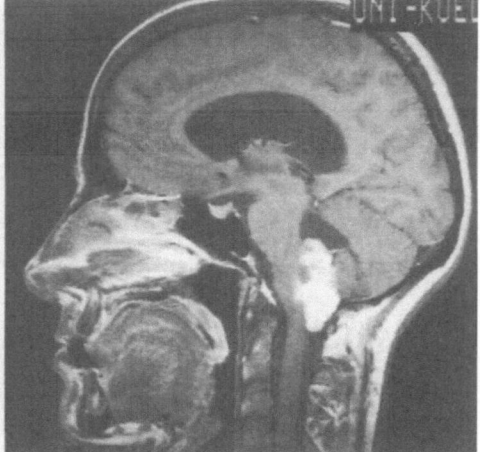

Fig. 2a,b ; Ependymoma at the bottom of the fourth ventricle. The image without Gadolinium demonstrates the tumor at the bottom of the fourth ventricle (Fig. 2a). After Gadolinium DTPA there is a remarkable enhancement of this lesion (Abb. 2b). The real extent of the tumor and the relationship to the neighbouring structures are better demonstrated after Gadolinium DTPA.

Most important are those cases, where *Gadolinium DTPA is imperative* to establish the correct diagnosis. This is especially true in all kinds of intramedullary tumors (1,2,7). In these cases T2-weighted images demonstrate a large region of high signal intensity; but this high signalintensity is produced by the intramedullary neoplasm as well as by the reactive edema. The real extent of the tumor is demonstrated after Gadolinium DTPA.

We also administer Gadolinium DTPA "on principle", if there is suspicion of multiple tumors. A typical example for this group is the neurofibromatosis von Recklinghausen. After Gadolinium DTPA in some cases multiple extramedullary nodes were seen as an expression of this multifocal disease (Fig 3 a,b). Even more, in one case Gadolinium DTPA revealed an intramedullary tumor in the lower cervical cord, additionally.

Inflammatory disease of the brain stem and upper cervical cord often reveals on T1-weighted images no changes and on T2-weighted images sometimes only a slight increase of signalintensity. In case of activity of the inflammation the images after Gadolinium show a remarkable enhancement.

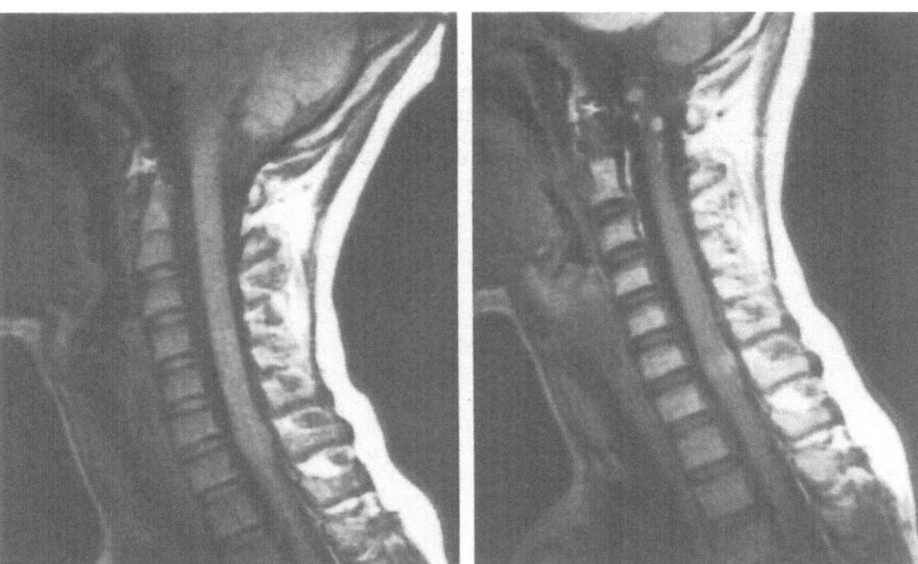

Fig. 3 a,b; Neurofibromatosis in a 8 year old boy: Before Gadolinium DTPA there is only a suspicious finding in the region of the craniocervical junction (Fig. 3a). After administration of Gadolinium DTPA there are found multiple nodes with considerable enhancement as an expression of this multifocal disease (fig. 3b).

CONCLUSIONS

* The sensitivity and specificity af magnetic resonance imaging of the craniocervical junction can be inmcreased by use of Gadolinium DTPA.
* Paramagnetic substances are not necessary in congenital or acquired abnormalities of the craniocervical junction.

* Paramagnetic substances may be helpful in a many, where the lesion is already seen before administration of Gadolinium DTPA. In these cases Gadolinium DTPA facilitates diagnosis by enhancing the tumor. There is often a better demarcation from surrounding structures.
* Paramagnetic substances should be administered in all intramedullary neoplasms and if there is suspicion of multifocal disease. Paramagnetic substances should be administered in all cases, when clinical symptoms are present and magnetic resonance imaging reveals no pathologic finding.

REFERENCES

1. Bydder GM, Brown J, Niendorf HP, Young IR (1985) Enhancement of cervical intraspinal tumors in MR imaging with intravenous Gadolinium DTPA. J Comput Assist Tomogr 9:847-851
2. Friedburg H, Schumacher M, Hennig J (1986) Pathologie des kraniozervikalen Überganges in der magnetischen Resonanztomographie. Fortschr Röntgenstr 145:315-320
3. Han JS, Benson JE, Yoon YS (1984) Magnetic resonance imaging in the spinal column and craniovertebral junction. Radiol Clin North Am 22:805-827
4. Lanz T, Wachsmuth W (1982) Praktische Anatomie. Springer, Berlin Heidelberg New York
5. Lee BCP, Deck MDF, Kneeland JR, Cahill PT (1985) MR imaging of the craniovertebral junction. AJNR 6:209-213
6. Pernkopf E (1980) Atlas der topographischen und angewandten Anatomie des Menschen. Urban und Schwarzenberg, München
7. Scotti G, Scialfa G, Colombo N, Landoni L (1985) MR imaging of intradural extramedullary tumors of the cervical spine. J Comput Assist Tomogr 9:1037-1041

The Craniocervical Junction in Skeletal Dysplasia: MRI in Flexion and Extension

J. L. Sherman, S. E. Kopits, and C. M. Citrin

Congenital dysplasia of the craniocervical junction is a serious cause of morbidity in patients with skeletal dysplasia. Compression or restriction of normal mobility of the medulla or cervical spinal cord can lead to chronic myelopathy of variable severity. The compressive effects are due to enchondral bone hypoplasia in achondroplasia (ACP). Patients with Morquio's syndrome, spondyloepiphyseal dysplasia congenita, and other miscellaneous skeletal dysplasias are prone to the development of cervicomedullary compression due to odontoid dysplasia and atlantoaxial instability. MR imaging offers the ability to visualize noninvasively the effects of the dysplasia on medulla and spinal cord. When combined with flexion and extension positioning, MR provides dynamic information which more accurately reflects the severity of the dysplasia.

In this paper we review the findings we have obtained with MR imaging of the craniocervical junction in 52 patients with skeletal dysplasia.

MATERIALS AND PATIENTS

Fifty-two patients with skeletal dysplasia were evaluated with MR. There were 19 with Morquio syndrome (MPS IV) (Fig. 1); 11 with spondyloepiphyseal dysplasia congenita (SEDc) (Fig. 2); 14 with achondroplasia (ACP) (Fig. 3); 2 with diastrophic dwarfism (DD) (Fig. 4A); 2 with Conradi-Hunerman (CH); 2 with Kneist dysplasia (KD) (Fig. 4B); 1 with metatropic dwarfism (MD); and 1 with spondylometaphyseal dysplasia (SMD). Thirty-five were evaluated on a 0.6 T imager and 17 on a 1.5 T imager. A variety of pulse sequences was employed. All patients had sagittal flexion and extension images.

RESULTS

Instability was found in 20/52 patients: MPS-IV (7), SEDc (7), DD (2), CD (2), KD (1), SMD (1). This included 15 patients with C1-2 instability and 5 patients with C2-3 instability. Cord deformity (myelopathy) was found in 34 patients: MPS-IV (13), SEDc (8), ACP (9), DD (1), KD (1), CH (1), SMD (1). Flexion/extension images showed more cord deformity than neutral images in 14 patients: MPS-IV (5), SEDc (6), ACP (1), DD (1), CH (1). This included 4 patients in whom the deformity was not apparent on neutral images. Foramen magnum stenosis was present in 13/14 with ACP and, to a lesser degree, in 9 with MPS-IV. Dysplastic vertebrae and intervertebral discs, spinal stenosis, disc herniation, and abnormal spinal curvatures were also identified.

DISCUSSION

The main indication for MRI of the cervical spine and craniocervical junction in patients with skeletal dysplasia is to evaluate suspected myelopathy. The signs and symptoms of myelopathy are variable and may be obscured by complicated expressions of the skeletal dysplasia in other body systems. Myelopathy leading to paraplegia is frequent in patients with MPS-IV and SEDc (Stevenson 1979). Myelopathy, if present, may be reversible or irreversible. It may be caused by bony impingement, ligamentous impingement, craniocervical instability, disc herniation, or a combination of these findings. Subluxation or instability may occur if there is excessive ligamentous laxity or anomalous odontoid development. Not all patients with odontoid dysplasia are unstable, and not all patients with instability develop a myelopathy (Lipson 1977; Kopits et al. 1972). MR with flexion and extension imaging is able to reveal dynamically the relationships of the bony, cartilaginous, ligamentous, and neural structures of the craniocervical junction. It is advocated as an ideal screening procedure since it is non-invasive. Together with the clinical findings it helps determine which patients will benefit from surgical procedures (fusion, suboccipital craniectomy, laminec-tomy, etc.) and the timing of such procedures.

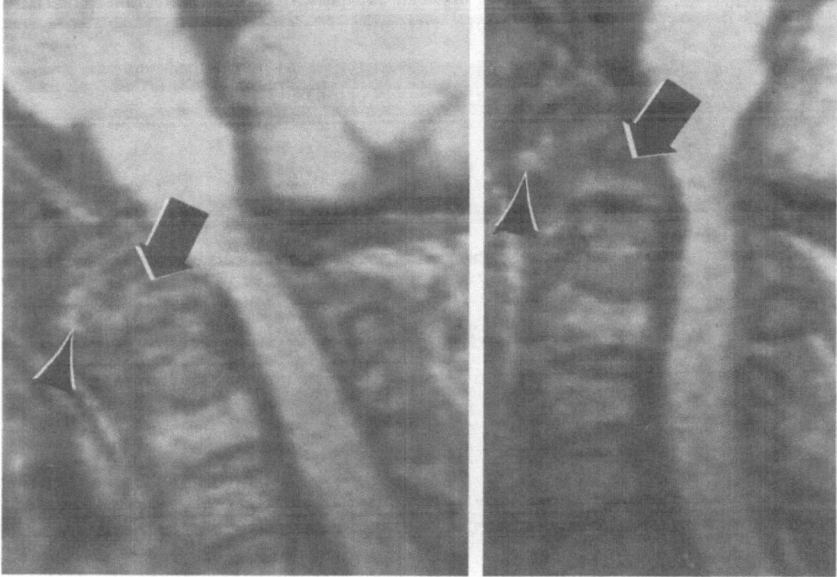

Fig. 1. 17-year-old female with MPS-IV. Flexion and extension sagittal images. There is odontoid dysplasia (arrows) and C1-2 subluxation (arrowheads). Note narrowing of upper cervical canal, craniocervical junction, and deformity of spinal cord.

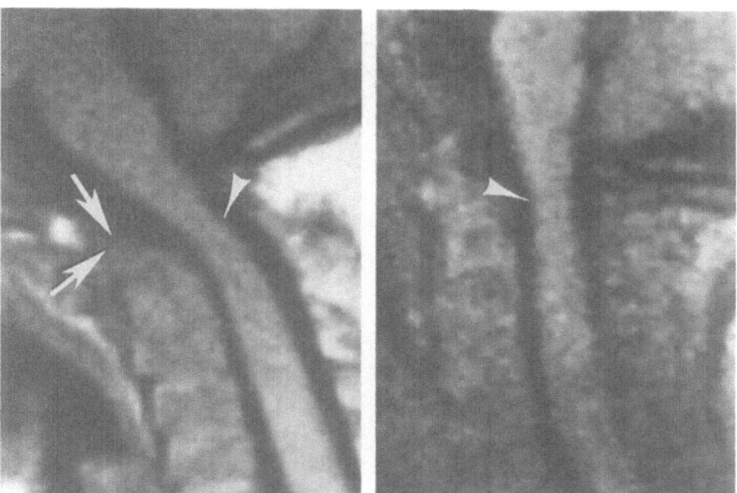

Fig. 2. 8-year-old female with SEDc. Flexion and extension images reveal hypoplastic dysplastic odontoid (arrows), C1-2 subluxation, and cord deformity which is most marked in flexion (arrowheads).

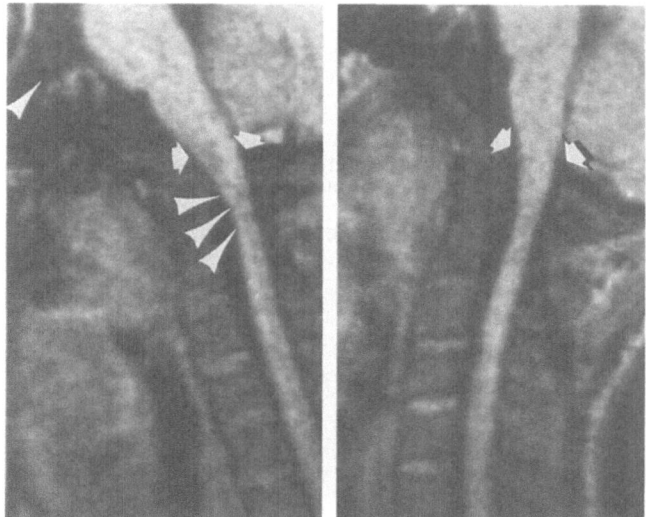

Fig. 3. 18-year-old female with achondroplasia (ACP). Flexion and extension images. The odontoid is well formed. There is foramen magnum stenosis (arrows) and deformity of the spinal cord which is more pronounced in flexion (arrowheads).

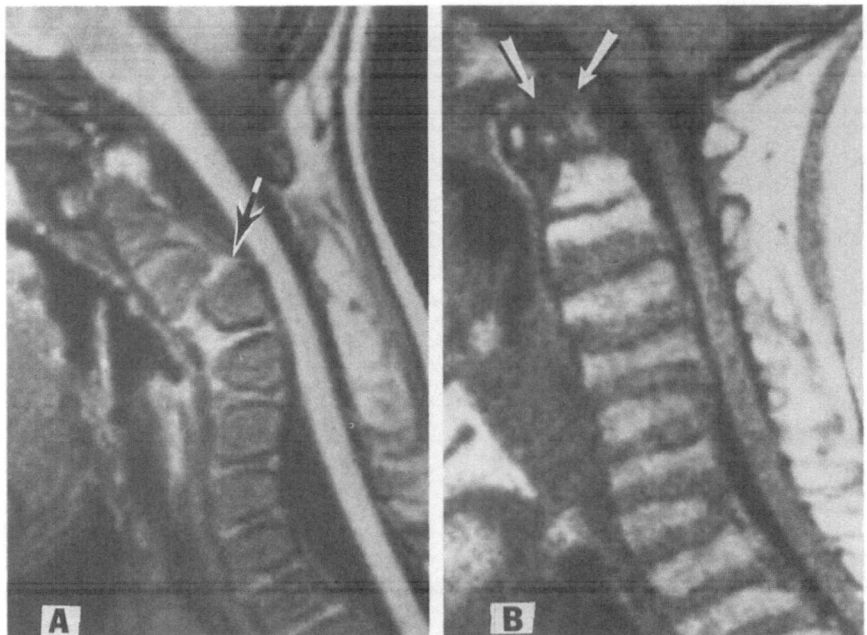

Fig. 4. (A) Diastrophic dysplasia (DD). 4-year-old female. Flexion image reveals typical deformity of C3 to C6 with subluxation at C2-3 (arrows).

Fig. 4. (B) Kneist dysplasia (KD). 8-year-old male. Note dysplasic vertebrae and odontoid process (arrows). There is non-fusion of the odontoid with C1-2 subluxation. Canal stenosis is present between C2 and C5.

REFERENCES

Kopits SE, Perovic MN, McKusick V, Robinson RA, Bailey JA (1972) Congenital atlantoaxial dislocations in various forms of dwarfism. JBJS 54A:1349-1350
Lipson SJ (1977) Dysplasia of the odontoid process in Morquio's syndrome causing quadriparesis. JBJS 59A:340-344
Stevenson RE (1979) Mucopolysaccharidosis IV. In: Bergsma D (ed) Birth defects compendium, second edition, syndrome identification, original article series. Liss, New York, p 732

Diagnostic Concept of Spinal Tumours
Results of 235 Patients

B. Schuknecht, M. Nadjmi, M. Ratzka, and K. Eberhardt

Over a period of 5.5 years 235 patients were diagnosed to derive symptoms from a spinal tumour. Cases were selected on the basis of a positive MRI, CT or CT-Myelography finding. In all patients tissue diagnosis was supported by either histology or the presence of a primary neoplasm at a different site. Tumours associated with spinal dysraphism are not included. Primary diagnosis and follow-up examinations for spinal tumour comprise 6 % of CT-, 8.9 % of MRI-investigations. The frequency of the different tumours and their distribution with regard to location is depicted in table 1. Compared to the literature our figures are representative taken into account that greater series in the past were frequently published in the neurosurgical literature, where metastases are infrequently operated on.

Neurinomas in 28, neurofibromas in 11, ganglioneuromas in 4 and meningiomas in 26 patients constitute the majority of spinal tumours in the "strict" sense (3, 9). Meningiomas exhibit a unique thoracic predilection (69.2 %), commonly in dorso-lateral intradural location, may calcify and preferentially affect women in 84.6 %. Multiple meningiomas and neurofibromas (fig. 1) were associated with von Recklinghausen disease as was malignant tumour conversion in 2 cases. A dumb-bell appearance in 10 patients (23.2 %), the extradural growth and bone erosion was readily identified by CT. Delineation of the intradural component requires intrathecal enhancement.

High sensitivity of MRI provides excellent discrimination of CSF, myelon and tumour, even in locations where artifacts from adjacent bone or body parts outside the reconstruction circle degrade CT images (e.g. craniocervical and cervico-thoracic junction). Axial and coronal reconstructions are advisable (1, 4). By means of intravenous contrast enhancement intra- and extradural tumour extension is more readily appreciated (7).

This is also true for intrinsic spinal cord tumours present in 8.5 % of our patients, 20 % of intraspinal tumours respectively (table 2). Ependymomas outnumber astrocytomas by 2:1 in adult patients (6) and comprise 70 % of intramedullary lesions (table 2) typically extending over multiple levels in the cervical and thoraco-lumbar (ependymoma) and cervicothoracic region (astrocytoma). Ependymomas of the conus and filum terminale occasionally present with signs mimicking a herniated lumbar disc. Information provided by myelography and CT-myelography is frequently restricted to the contour of the cord. Albeit a delayed CT-myelography may demonstrate a contrast filled cyst (10).

MRI will distinguish between solid and cystic tumour portions (8, 14), which were found to be present in 38 % of astrocytomas and 46 % of ependymomas respectively in an autopsy study (11). Synechiae may lead to a segmented appearance (fig. 2). Cord expansion, lack of distinct lesion margins, signal inhomogeneity are MRI-criteria in favour of an intrinsic intramedullary tumour (13). Hemangioblastomas linked to the presence of von Hippel-Lindau disease in 33 %, were found to be associated with intramedullary cysts (2). Hemangioblastomas and cavernous angiomas were

present in 3 cases in our series respectively. Serpiginous filling defects encountered by Myelography pointed to the vascular nature, which
was defined by selective DSA (fig. 3).
Leukemias and lymphomas commonly presented as an epidural and/or paraspinal mass (5). Osseous involvement is uncommon (5) and was noticed in 1
patient with Hodgkin lymphoma. Dissemination into the subarachnoid space
had occured in 3 patients. Multiple filling defects demonstrated by
myelography, at autopsy proved to be subarachnoid patches and nodules of
Burkitt's lymphoma in 1 patient (fig. 4).

Due to superior spatial resolution CT readily defines the extent of
cortical bone erosion and cancellous bone infiltration caused by plasmo-
cytoma or metastatic neoplastic disease (12). CT myelography is mandatory
in cases where myelography reveals complete obstruction of CSF pathways
as was present in 33/56 (58.9 %) of patients examined for metastatic
disease. Frequently contrast material may trickle past the obstacle
allowing definition of the craniad end.

In MRI neoplastic infiltration of cancellous bone will lead to a relative
signal loss, reflecting prolongation of T1 (12). Sagittal T1 weighted
images are advantageous in patients where on the basis of plain film
findings multiple level involvement is suspected (8). In the majority of
patients MRI will offer advantages over myelography in the evaluation of
metastatic spinal disease.

Conclusion:
The CT, MRI and CT-myelography findings of 235 patients are presented who
were diagnosed to derive symptoms from a spinal tumour. The investigatory
modalities are described. Limitations are mentioned.

Though a tissue specific diagnosis frequently cannot be established, CT
and MRI, supplemented by DSA or intravenous contrast application, may
provide criteria which allow a high degree of tissue characterisation.

TABLE 1: DISTRIBUTION OF 235 SPINAL TUMOURS BY HISTOLOGY AND LOCATION

Type:	N Pat.		Cervical	Thoracic		Lumbosacral
Neurinoma, -fibroma	43	18.3 %	16	6		21
Meningioma	26	11.1 %	6	18		2
Ependymoma	12	5.1 %	4	8		-
Astrocytoma	8	3.4 %	3	5		-
Angioma	6	2.5 %	2	3		1
Lipoma	5	2.1 %	-	3		2
	100	42.5 %	31	35	8	26
Plasmocytoma	14	5.9 %	3	10		1
Leukemia/Lymphoma	16	6.8 %	1	11		4
Bone Tumour	15	6.4 %	2	4		9
Metastases and	78	38.3 %	18	53		20
Meningiosis	12		intradural dissemination			
	135	57.5 %				

TABLE 2: LOCALIZATION OF 235 SPINAL TUMOURS

intra-medullary		intradural		intra-extradural		extradural	
Astrocytoma	7	Meningioma	25	Neurinoma	6	Metastases	73
Ependymoma	6	Neurinoma	17	Meningiosis	2	Neurinoma	20
Angioma	2	Meningiosis	12	Meningioma	1	Bone tumour	15
Lipoma	2	Ependymoma	6	Angioma	1	Plasmocytoma	14
Metastases	2	Leukemia	4	Metastasis	1	Leukemia	12
Oligo-dendroglioma	1	Angioma	3			Lipoma	1
		Lipoma	2				
	20		69		11		135
	(8.5 %)		(29.4 %)		(4.7 %)		(57.4 %)

REFERENCES

1. Braun M, Cosnard G, Cabanis EA, Iba-Zizen MT, Pharaboz C, Jean-Bourquin D, Deroster C, Perfettini C, Tamraz JC, Bocquet M (1986) NMR imaging and neuromas. J Neuroradiology 13:209-225
2. Browne TR, Adams RD, Roberson GH (1976) Hemangioblastoma of the Spinal Cord. Arch Neurol 33:435-441
3. Dorwart RH, LaMasters DL, Watanabe TJ (1983) Computed Tomography of the Spine and Spinal Cord. Newton-Potts, San Anselmo, p. 155
4. Gawehn J, Schroth G, Thron A (1986) The value of paraxial slices in MR-imaging of spinal cord disease. Neuroradiology 28:347-350
5. Holtas SL, Kido DK, Simon JH (1986) MR Imaging of Spinal Lymphoma. J of Comp Ass Tomogr 10:111-115
6. Kopelson G, Linggood RM, Kleinman G, Doucette J, Wang CC (1980) Management of Intramedullars Spinal Cord Tumors. Radiology 135:437-439
7. Lapointe JS, Graeb DA, Nugent RA, Robertson WD (1985) Value of Intravenous Contrast Enhancement in the CT Evaluation of Intraspinal Tumors. AJNR 6:939-943
8. Norman D (1987) Magnetic Resonance Imaging of the Central Nervous System Brant-Zawadzki-Norman, New York, p 289
9. Salah S, Horcajada J, Pernecky A ((1975) Spinal Neurinomas - A comprehensive clinical and statistical study on 47 cases. Neurochirurgica 18:77-84
10. Scotti G, Scialfa G, Colombo N, Landoni L (1987) Magnetic resonance diagnosis of intramedullary tumors of the spinal cord. Neuroradiology 29:130-135
11. Sloof JL, Kernohan JW, MacCarty LS (1964) Primary intramedullary tumours of the spinal cord and fileum terminale. WB Saunders, Philadelphia
12. Weigert F, Reiser M, Pfändner K (1987) Die Darstellung neoplastischer Wirbelveränderungen durch die MR-Tomographie. Fortschr Röntgenstr 146: 123-130
13. Williams AL, Haughton VM, Pojunas KW, Daniels DL, Kilgore DP (1986) Differentiation of Intramedullary Neoplasms and Cysts by MR. AJR 149:159-164
14. Zanella FE, Steinbrich W, Friedmann G, Koulousakis A (1986) Magnetische Resonanztomographie (MR) bei spinalen Raumforderungen. Fortschr Röntgenstr 145:326-330

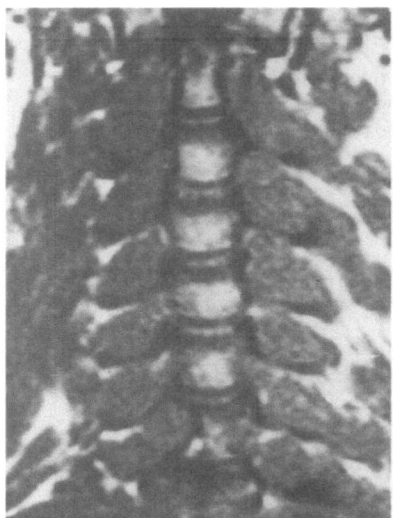 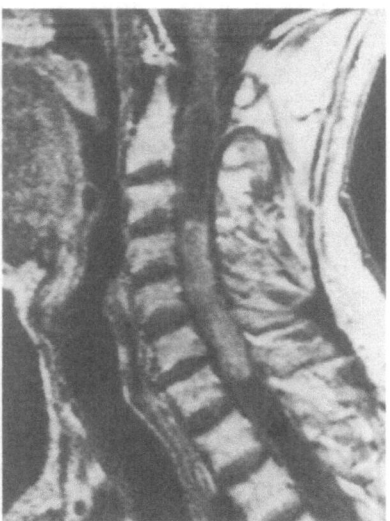

Fig. 1. Characteristic T1 weighted coronal MR image (TR 400 TE 20) in a young patient with neurofibromatosis. Multiple almost symmetrical spinal nerve root involvement is depicted.

Fig. 2. Sagittal spin echo image (TR 600 TE 20) shows inhomogenous increased signalintensity of a cervical ependymoma after intravenous administration of Gadolinium DTPA. The solid and cystic partially segmented components are readily identified.

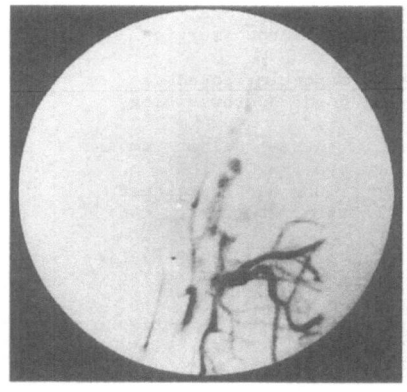 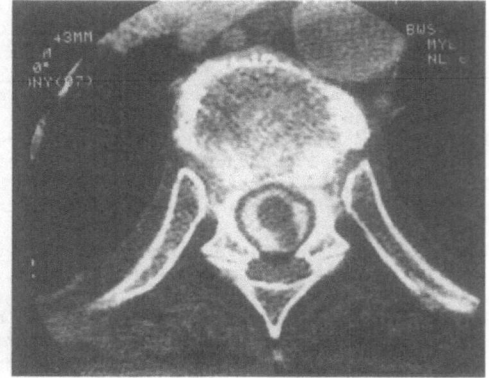

Fig. 3. Selective spinal DSA in a 25 year old patient with von Hippel-Lindau disease and a lumbar L1-L3 hemangioblastoma. Pathognomonic angiographic appearance with clusters of capillary vessels.

Fig. 4. CT-Myelogram in a patient with Burkitt's lymphoma. Focal subarachnoid deposit attached to the dorsal aspect of the thoracic cord.

Difficulties in Intubation For Cervical Surgery: Airway Assessment with Magnetic Resonance Imaging

M. Boukobza, D. Bouguet, M. Metzger, R. Roy-Camille, and P. Viars

Introduction

Cervical spine surgery may involve difficulties in intubation if the cervical spine is arthrotic or if the spinal cord is compressed by tumors or traumatic lesions (1). Magnetic resonance imaging (MRI) provides multidimensional imaging and is now widely performed before spinal surgery (2). For the cervical region, T1-weighted images in the sagittal plane offer anatomic visualization of airways, including soft tissues, from mouth to trachea (Fig.1). The purpose of this study was to evaluate the ability of MRI to predict difficult intubations.

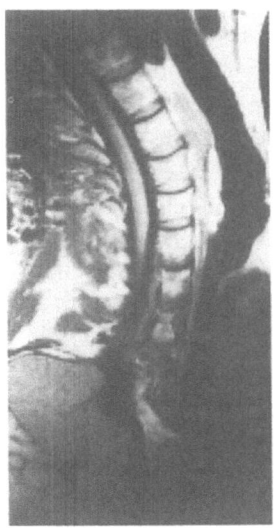

Fig.1. C4 metastasis, normal airways, uneventful intubation

Methods

From July 1986 to January 1988, 102 patients were scheduled to undergo cervical spine surgery (60 traumatic lesions, 40 tumors, 2 cervical myelopathies). Preoperatively, all underwent careful physical examina-

tion (3), cervical roentgenography and MRI. Awake endotracheal intubation was performed using topical anesthesia and neuroleptanalgesia.
Before February 1987, MRI data were not reviewed by the anesthesiologist prior to surgery (group I: n = 34 patients); following a case
where intubation was difficult, MRI data were systematically reviewed
(group II: n = 68 patients). MRI analysis was done by both the neuroradiologist and the anesthesiologist and included: alignment between
rhinopharynx and trachea (blind nasal intubation), angle and distance
between epiglottis and base of tongue (exposure of larynx during
laryngoscopy), size of trachea, and prevertebral hematomas (subglottic
obstacle).

Results

Group I. Intubation was difficult in five cases (15%), although difficulties had been clinically predicted in three. Retrospective analysis
of MRI was informative in all cases (hematoma = 1; angle of 90° between
epiglottis and base of tongue = 3; misalignment between rhinopharynx
and trachea = 1).

Group II: Intubation was difficult in nine cases (13%), all of which
had been predicted by preoperative review of MRI results (hematoma = 1;
angle of 90° between epiglottis and base of tongue = 8). Although only
six cases could have been predicted clinically, intubation techniques
were adapted to the nine patients according to MRI findings (Fig.2):
blind nasotracheal intubation for difficult exposure of the larynx
when there was good alignment between thinopharynx and trachea, smaller
internal diamter tube for hematomas, use of a flexible fibroptic bron-
choscope for nasal intubation when there was misalignment between the
trachea and thinopharynx.

Conclusion

Preoperative review of MRI results by the anesthesiologist can be helpful in predicting difficulties in intubation during cervical spine surgery. Direct assessment of the airways shows the cause of the difficulties and shows the anatomic solutions. Whenever this procedure is available, the anesthesiologist will benefit from careful preoperative MRI
analysis.

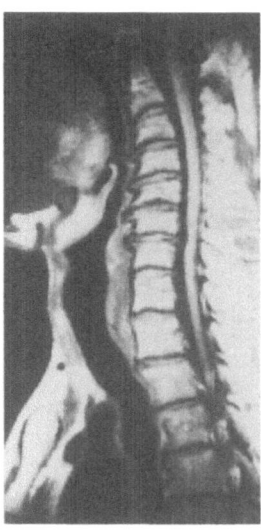

Fig.2. Cervical myelopathy. Angle of 90° between epiglottis and large base of tongue, narrow oropharynx. Difficult intubation

References

[1] Benzel E, Larson SJ (1987) Functional recovery after decompressive spine operation for cervical spine fracture. Neurosurgery 20: 742-746
[2] Modic M, Hardy W (1984) Nuclear magnetic resonance of the spine: clinical potential and limitation. Neurosurgery 15: 583-592
[3] Samsoon G, Young JR (1987) Difficult tracheal intubation, a retrospective study. Anaesthesia 1987, 42: 487-490

MR of the Spine in Breast Cancer

E. Touboul, M. Boukobza, J. Kardouss, G. Amiel, and J. Metzger (Paris, France)

Metastatic bone disease of the spine was evaluated in 20 consecutive patients at the time of the first metastasis of breast cancer. All patients presented other bone and visceral metastatic lesions and/or positive bone marrow biopsy. The serum CEA and CA 15-3 levels were always increased. The spine of patients was examined by anterior-posterior and lateral plain X-Ray films of the spine, bone scintigraphy after intravenous injection of Tc-99 m labeled methyldiphosphonate (Tc 90 m MDP) and MR using T1 spin echo sequence in the sagittal plane. The sensitivity of the three methods to detect bone vertebrae metastases was evaluated. The metastatic involvement of vertebral bodies was detected more often by MR than conventional radiography or bone scintigraphy. Early imminent impingement of the spinal cord can be observed, before neurologic symptoms.

MR in Lumbar Spondylolisthesis

S. Cronqvist, S. Holtås, M. Annertz, and B. Jönsson (Lund, Sweden)

MR examination was performed in 16 patients with lumbar spondylolisthesis and with progressive low back pain. In all, the shapes of the intervertebral foramina were altered due to vertebral displacement and to posteriorly and laterally extending disc protrusion. In addition, the MR findings permitted separation into three groups: (1) normal fat in the intervertebral foramina, nerve roots of normal shape; (2) reduced fat, compressed nerve roots; (3) no remaining fat, nerve roots not identifiable.

Eight patients with bilateral symptoms had bilateral changes. In seven with mainly unilateral symptoms, MR showed a more pronounced narrowing of the foramen on the affected side. A discrepancy was present in one case between the side with the symptoms and the side with the most severe changes. Images obtained in coronary projections demonstrated the nerves passing through the intervertebral foramina. In this projection it was possible to directly observe local dislocation and/or compression. MR thus makes it possible to demonstrate foraminal changes in two different projections, which has been of great importance in the operative management of these patients.

MRI of Postoperative Lumbar Spine after Surgery: Assessment of Recurrent Herniated Disk

C. Manelfe, I. Berry, C. Nomblot, J. Prère, Ph. Arrué and A. Bonafé

Failed back surgery syndrome is a rather frequent entity in the postoperative setting of herniated nucleus pulposus (HNP) removal. Various conditions may be involved in the recurrent pain; these include persistent or recurrent HNP and pathologic scarring, which must be differentiated as reoperation gives opposite results. Radiologic assessment of these patients is one of the most difficult problems in neuroradiology. To date, plain computed tomography (CT) followed by CT after IV injection of contrast material has been the most widespread modality, although a significant number of false diagnoses result (Braun et al. 1985). Some institutions perform diskography. Recently, magnetic resonance imaging (MRI) with injection of contrast material (Gd-DOTA) has been reported (Hueftle et al. 1988), giving great hope that the problem can be solved in higher proportion of patients. The aim of the study reported here is to further test the ability of MRI in this setting.

Methods

Thirty-one patients (8 female, 23 male) aged 33 to 73 years (mean 50 ± 9 years) were included in the study. They had undergone back surgery 3 weeks to 30 years previously (9 ± 16 years). Ten of them had had multiple operations. Levels of operation were as follows: L3-L4, 4 patients; L4-L5, 18 patients; L5-S1, 25 patients. Twenty-four patients had recently been examined by CT, although mostly in other institutions and somtimes without IV injection of contrast material. Sometimes only a report based on the CT was available.

MRI was performed at 0.5 T (Magniscan 5000/GE-CGR, France) with 5-mm sagittal and axial of slices. T1-weighted sequences were performed in all planes (gradient echo, TR 400, TE I4, 4 excitations). T2-weighted sequences were sometimes added (spin echo, TR 2000, TE 50-100, 2 excitations; or gradient echo, TR 400, TE 30, flip angle 15°).

Gadolinium-DOTA (Guerbet Labs, France) was injected at the usual
dose of 0.1 mmol/kg over 3 min and all T1-weighted sequences were
subsequently repeated. The agent could be injected into 18 of the
31 patients. This subpopulation included patients whose previous
surgery had been from 3 weeks to 26 years ago.

Results

Noncontrast MRI evaluation showed 14 possible cases of recurrent
HNP in the 31 patients. Seven of them were reoperated on, and a
herniated disk was confirmed in six. In only one patient who was
reoperated on was fibrosis found. CT evaluation of the same population suggested recurrent HNP in only 7/24 patients. This discrepancy not only reflects the smaller number of examinations performed, but also the lower sensitivity of the method as it was
used. Indeed, two cases of HNP were correctly assessed, as confirmed by surgery; four other suggested cases of HNP do not have
surgical confirmations, twice because surgery is pending, twice
because MRI did not confirm HNP and no surgery followed. The same
false positive as previously mentioned for MRI occurred. Therefore,
CT overdiagnosed three cases of HNP; on the other hand, in three
cases CT was negative for HNP while MRI indicated HNP (surgery is
pending in one case and confirmed HNP in the others two). In one
case, CT was inconclusive, while MRI favored a diagnosis of HNP,
confirmed surgically. Therefore, CT missed four cases of HNP.

Of the subpopulation who received Gd-DOTA intravenously, HNP was
suggested in four patients and fibrosis in five. Nine patients
showed other findings (spinal stenosis, arachnoiditis, etc.). Three
patients were reoperated on; HNP was confirmed in two, while the
third case corresponded to the same false positive as mentioned
previously (Fig.1). It is noted that no HNP was suggested by contrast MRI which was not suggested by noncontrast MRI. On the other
hand, of the seven patients in whom recurrent HNP was suggested on
the basis of noncontrast MRI and who have not been reoperated on,
two had different results of contrast MRI. Indeed, Gd-DOTA-enhanced
images showed evidence of fibrosis while plain images seemed to indicate HNP (Fig.2).

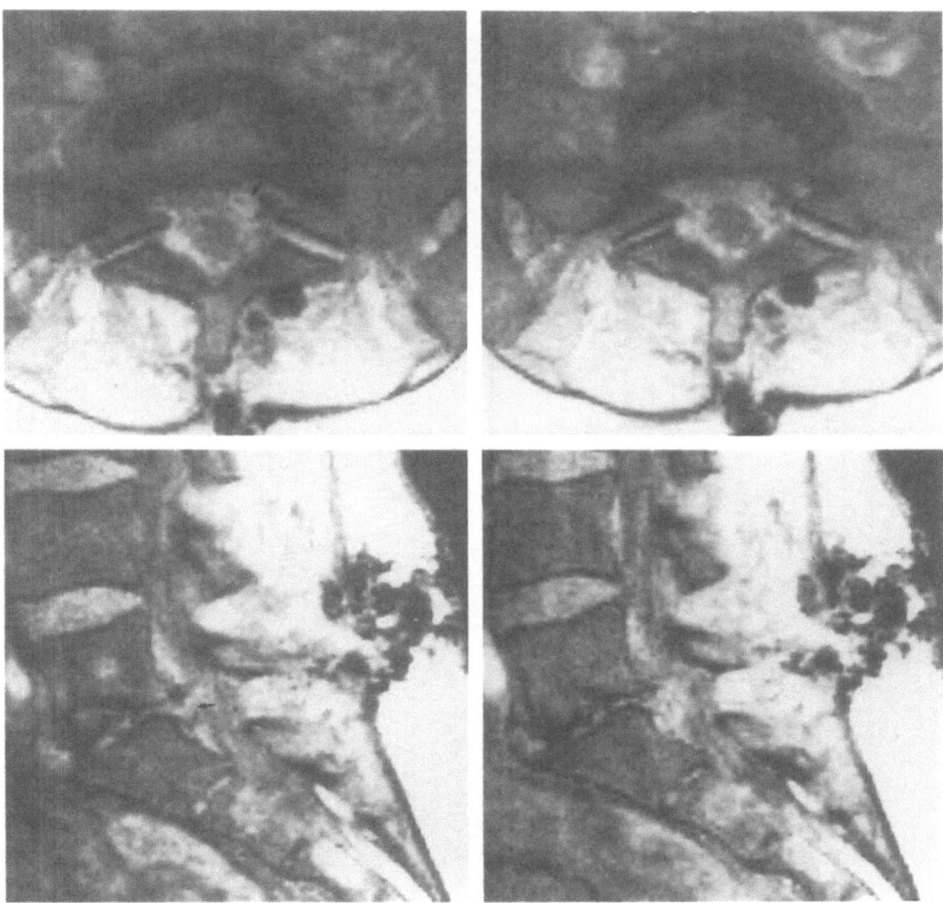

Fig.1. 47-year-old woman, operated on at the L5-S1 level 6 months
previously, with recurrent pain. Both CT and MRI (with and without
Gd-DOTA) suggested recurrent HNP. At surgery, only scar tissue was
found. a,b: Pre- and postcontrast T1-weighted axial images showing
abnormal tissue in the left lateral recess with partly rimmed high
signal intensity and partly very low signal intensity (arrow). After contrast injection there is hardly any enhancement. c,d: Pre-
and postcontrast T1-weighted left parasagittal images with impression of herniated material out of the L5-S1 interspace into the epidural space (arrow). After contrast injection, blurring of the
posterior margin could only with hindsight have suggested fibrosis

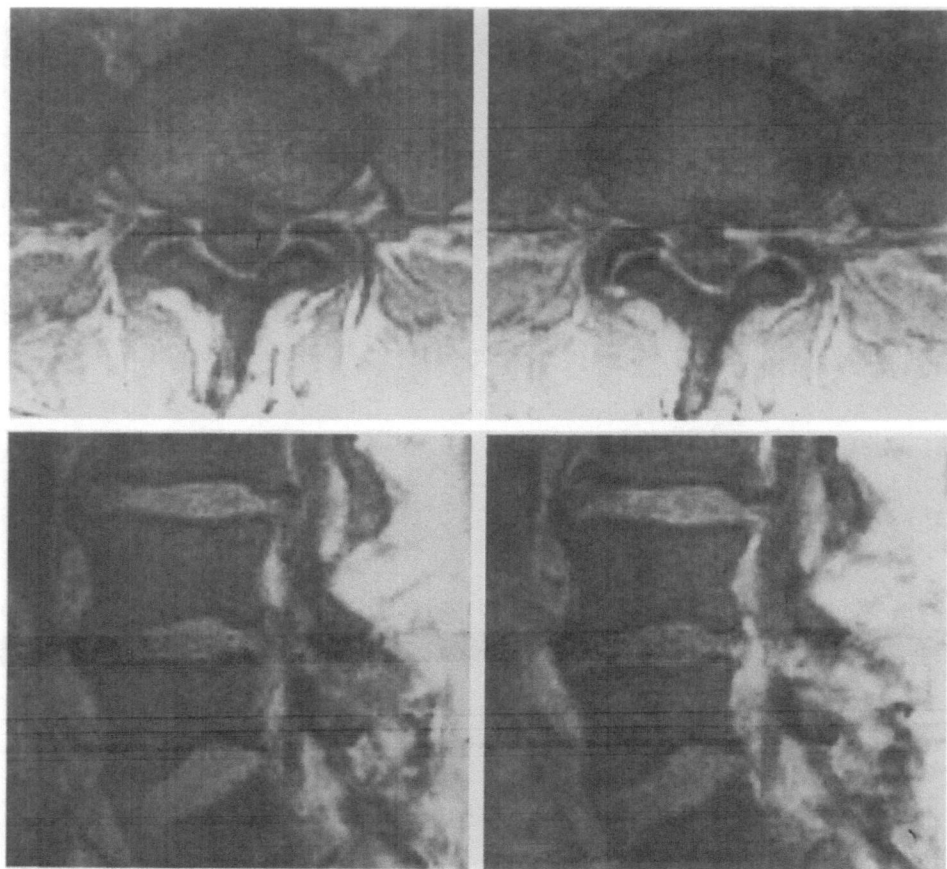

Fig.2. 61-year-old man who had undergone diskectomy 10 years before and had left L5 radiculopathy. Noncontrast MRI suggested recurrent HNP, while results after Gd-DOTA injection seem to rule out this possibility. No reoperation occurred. a,b: Axial pre- and postcontrast T1-weighted images. Precontrast image suggests a small lesion bulging in the left epidural space, with similar intensity to the disk (arrow). Postcontrast image shows homogeneous enhancement of the lesion. Note adhesive arachnoiditis with anterior displacement of the nerve roots of the cauda equina. c,d: Sagittal pre- and post-contrast T1-weighted images where posterior margin of the L4-L5 disk is better delineated by the enhancement of epidural tissue, ruling out bulging of the disk which was difficult to assess before

Discussion

MRI seems to be able to assess recurrent HNP with a sensitivity at least as good as that of CT. It seemed superior in this series, but our CT comparison was not optimal. Although on T1-weighted images scar tissue may have the same intensity as the disk, such similarity is not observed on T2-weighted images, in which fibrosis is of higher intensity than herniated disk.

The differentiation could be much better assessed using the Gd-DOTA, postinjection T1-weighted sequences; fibrosis was always enhanced while herniated disk was usually not. Scar enhancement occurred regardless of its age (up to 26 years) and became more homogeneous with time. Disk enhancement occurred occasionally, most often on delayed images, around the diskectomy bed.

In two cases Gd-DOTA enhancement of fibrosis helped delineate the posterior margin of a disk which, from the noncontrast image, was thought to be herniated, thus increasing the specificity of MRI. On the other hand, no example was found in which noncontrast, T1-weighted MRI did not indicate HNP which would have been seen with contrast MRI. Therefore, Gd-DOTA does not seem to increase sensitivity in this postoperative setting.

References

[1] Braun IF, Hoffman JC, Davis PC, Landman JA, Tindall GT (1985) Contrast enhancement in CT differentiation between recurrent disk herniation and postoperative scan: prospective study. AJNR 6: 607-612
[2] Hueftle MG, Modc MT, Ross JS, Masaryk TJ, Carter JR, Wilbert RG, Bohlman HH, Steinberg PM, Delamarker RB (1988) Lumbar spine: postoperative MR imaging with Gd-DTPA. Radiology 167: 817-824

MR Post-Diskectomy Imaging

M. Resta, F. Dicuonzo, A. Lorusso, and A. Carella

Introduction

The failed back surgery syndrome is a frequent condition. Burton [2] reported the incidence of the syndrome to be 10%-40%. This may involve disk herination (12%-16%), lateral spinal stenosis (58%), central spinal stenosis (7%-14%), arachnoiditis (6%-16%), or epidural fibrosis (6%-8%). The crucial problem is the distinction between epidural scar and recurrent disk herniation, because only reoperation on recurrent disk herniation leads to a good surgical result.

Contrast-enhanced CT scans are helpful [7]; confidence in the differential diagnosis between recurrent disk herniation and scar thereby improves, but its accuracy remains about 80% [1]: MR has been applied to the preoperative diagnosis of disk herniation, and with the development of surface-coil MR imaging [5,6] and with the use of gadolinium DTPA, major attention has been given to postoperative spinal MR imaging [1,3,4]. To investigate present diagnostic MR accuracy in operated lumbar disk herniations we undertook a prospective MR study (still in progress). We present some explicative cases here.

Materials and Methods

A total of 16 patients, operated for lumbar disk herniation with failed back surgery syndrome were examined with enhanced CT and unenhanced MR; in only four cases was gadolinium DTPA also injected. At present surgical correlations are not available. CT scans were obtained using a GE CT 9800; contrast material was a nonionic water-soluble contrast medium (Iopamiro, Bracco). MR studies were performed on the MR MAx GE 0.5 T superconductive magnet with surface coils. A complete study consists of seven spin echo acquisitions or nine acquisitions after gadolinium injection and 11 acquisitions for delayed enhancement:

1. Coronal (for patient positioning) TR 300, TE 30, matrix 128 × 128
   1 nex
2. Sagittal TR 500, TE 30 matrix 160 × 256 4 nex
3. Sagittal 15° partial flip angle TR 200 TE 20 matrix 160 × 256 8 nex
4. Sagittal 45° partial flip angle TR 500 TE 25-30 matrix 160 × 256
   4 nex
5. Axial TR 500 TE 30 matrix 160 × 256 4 nex
6. Axial TR 2000 TE 28 (proton density) matrix 160 × 256 2 nex
7. Axial TR 2000 TE 100 matrix 160 × 256 2 nex
8. Sagittal postgadolinium TR 500 TE 30 matrix 160 × 256 4 nex
9. Axial postgadolinium TR 500 TE 30 matrix 160 × 256 4 nex.

We repeat the last two images (numbers 8,9) after 30-45 min for delayed enhancement. The gadolinium dose was 0.1 mmol/kg.

Results and Discussion

Laminectomy-diskectomy and laminectomy-diskectomy-foraminotomy
were the most frequent types of surgery in our cases. In the CT
imaging we evaluated the morphologic aspects, location, mass effect,
and density of epidural soft tissue. In MR imaging we considered
bone signals, epidural soft tissue morphology, signal characteristics, mass effect, and disk morphology. "Abnormal epidural soft
tissue" (soft-tissue signal) refers to the edema in immediate
postoperative period and fibrosis or disk material in late postoperative period. Laminectomy is always recognized by loss of bone
signals and presence of soft tissue with an intermediate signal in
T1 weighted images (w.i.) and an isohyperintense homogeneous signal
in T2 w.i. The only finding in laminotomy is the absence of ligamentum flavum. The normal picture in diskectomy consists of linear-
ly decreased signal in T1 and T2 w.i., similar to that in preoperative anulus fibrosus. The presence of a soft-tissue hypoisointense
signal in T1 and T2 w.i. with parent anulus, contiguous to the intervertebral disk, with mass effect, indicates a recurrent disk herniation. The fragments may be hyperintense in T2 w.i. The findings
for scar diagnosis have been the following: aberrant soft tissue
unrelated to the disk space, no mass effect, intermediate signal in
T1 w.i., and hyperintense signal in T2 w.i. as regards anulus. When
the criteria for both recurrent disk herniation and scar are present,
we suggest the use of gadolinium DTPA.

Epidural soft tissue that is enhanced indicates disk material (Fig.1);
epidural soft tissue that is not enhanced indicates scar (Fig.2); a
central nonenhancing area with peripheral enhancement indicates a disk
wrapped with scar (Fig.3).

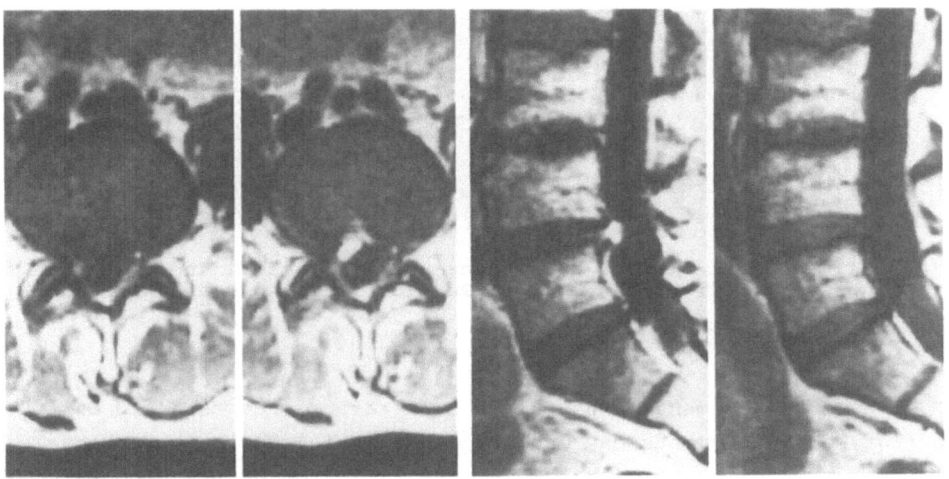

Fig.1. T1 Weighted images. a: Without and with gadolinium. Epidural
nodular scar. b: With and without gadolinium. Epidural nodular scar.

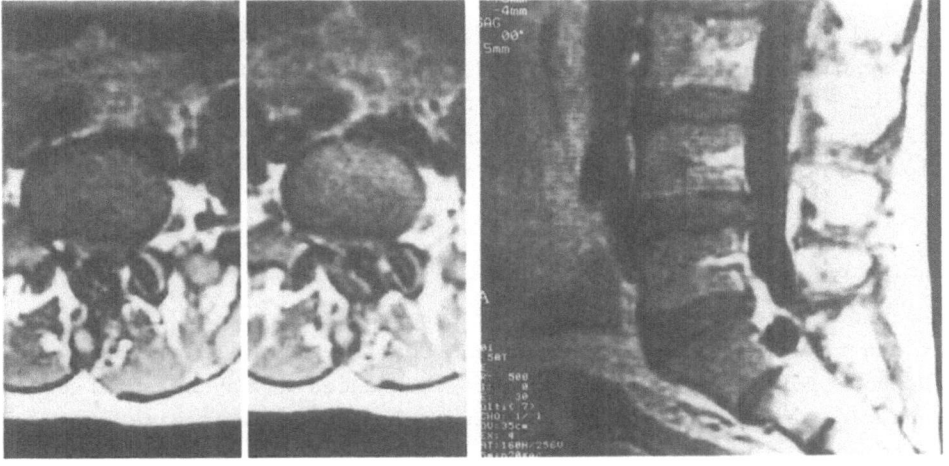

Fig.2. T1 Weighted images. a: Without and with gadolinium. Soft
tissue not enhanced indicates recurrent disk herniation at L4-L5
level. b: With gadolinium. Recurrent disk herniation at L4-L5 level
and epidural scar at L5-S1 level. Note the sacral radicular cyst

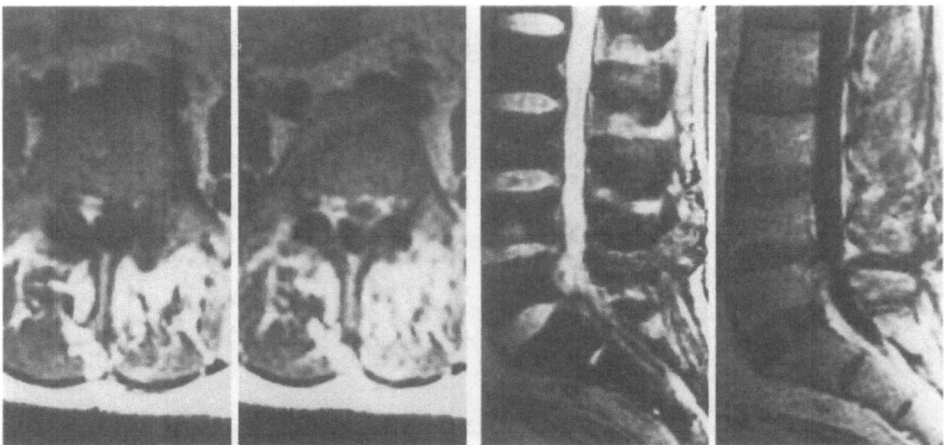

Fig.3. T1 Weighted images. a: Without and with gadolinium. Free disk fragment wrapped with scar. b: 45° Partial flip angle and with gadolinium

MR delayed enhancement is useful in small areas, not enhanced early. In fact, disk fragments may enhance in delayed images; nerve roots entrapped in scar never enhance. According to the literature, CT advantages are an accuracy of 80% (similar to MR) and analysis of vascular and bone changes, MR advantages are an accuracy of 80% (similar to CT), multidimensional imaging, and a larger area than with CT. CT disadvantages are single-plane imaging, radiation, and contrast material. MR disadvantages are difficult bone valuation, poorer spatial resolution (interslice gap), decreased signal to noise ratio, and cost. However, a high-resolution surface coil with appropriate pulse sequence (we suggest fast-scanning technique with adequate flip angles) and gadolinium MR can improve the accuracy of MR.

Conclusion

We can summarize our findings regarding the differential diagnosis between recurrent disk herniation and scar as follows: (a) unenhanced CT is never sufficient, (b) unenhanced MR may be sufficient, (c) enhanced MR or appropriate pulse sequence is always sufficient.

Regarding the other causes of failed back surgery syndrome, in bone changes and spondylolisthesis CT remains the best technique; in arachnoiditis we propose enhanced MR or myelography.

References

[1] Bundschuh CV, Modic MT, Ross JS (1988) Epidural fibrosis and re-
    current disk herniation in the lumbar spine: MR imaging assess-
    ment. AJNR 9: 169-178
[2] Burton CV, Kirkaldy-Willis WH (1981) Causes of failure of sur-
    gery on the lumbar spine. Clin Orthop 157: 191-199
[3] Hueftle MG, Modic MT, Ross JS (1988) Lumbar spine: postoperative
    MR imaging with Gd-DTPA. Radiology 167: 817-824
[4] Maravilla KR, Lesh P (1985) Magnetic resonance imaging of the
    lumbar spine with CT correlation. AJNR 6: 237-245
[5] Modic MT, Masaryk T (1986) Lumbar herniated disk disease and
    canal stenosis: prospective evaluation by surface coil MR, CT,
    and myelography. AJNR 7: 709-717
[6] Ross JS, Masaryk TJ, Modic MT (1987) Lumbar spine: postoperative
    assessment with surface-coil MR imaging. Radiology 164: 851-860
[7] Teplick JG, Haskin ME (1984) Intravenous contrast-enhanced CT of
    the postoperative lumbar spine: improved identification of re-
    current disk herniation, scar, arachnoiditis, and diskitis.
    AJNR 5: 373-383

Spinal Dysraphism – Assessment of the Role of MR Imaging

T. Jaspan, C. I. Rothwell, I. M. Holland, and B. S. Worthington

INTRODUCTION

The spinal dysraphisms represent a complex array of abnormalities related to disordered embryogenesis of the spine. Traditionally CT assisted myelography (CTM) has been employed in our institution to investigate patients with these lesions. The recent introduction of MRI has led us to undertake a comparative assessment of these two techniques in order to establish a rational approach to the investigation of this group of patients.

MATERIALS AND METHODS

87 patients were examined over a 30 month period. All patients underwent total spinal myelography. Subsequent CT examination, on a Picker 1200 SX Scanner, was performed 1 to 4 hours after myelography. Neuroleptanalgesia or general anaesthesia was employed for infants and children. Late scanning was performed on a Picker Vista 0.15T resistive unit with appropriate surface coils. Initially infants and children were examined under general anaesthesia. In the latter 2 years of the study this was replaced by oral sedation with chloral hydrate (50-70 mg/kg). Routine sagittal and axial T_1 weighted spin echo (TR=500 msec, TE=40 msec). Sequences were used in all cases with supplementary coronal views in the presence of scoliosis. A T_2 weighted sequence (TR=1600 msec, TE=80 msec) was used in selected cases for further tissue characterization. A 256 x 256 acquisition matrix was used with 7 mm slice thickness. All examinations were analysed in terms of (1) lesion definition (2) tissue characterization (3) demonstration of cord cavitation and (4) assessment of the craniocervical junction. The MR examination in each case was categorized as providing (1) superior (2) equivalent or (3) inferior detail or information in comparison with the corresponding CTM study.

RESULTS

29 male and 58 female patients were studied with an age range of 2 months to 51 years and an average age of 16.9 years. Table 1 displays the incidence of lesions found in all patients. Many patients exhibit more than one abnormality. The comparative analysis of the two investigative techniques and incidence of hydrosyringomyelia is also tabulated.

Table 1   Incidence of lesions, associated hydrosyringmyelia
                 and comparative assessment of MRI v CTM

Lesion Type	No of Lesions	MRI Superior	MRI=CTM	CTM Superior	Cord Cavities
Tethered cord/thick filum	56	15	20	21	12
Diastematomyelia	33	16	3	14	14
Lipoma/dermoid	21	10	9	2	4
Dermal sinus	10	7	2	1	1
Meningomyelocoele	11	9	2	0	5
Lipomyelomeningocoele	11	5	5	1	4
Meningocoele	11	9	2	0	1
Others*	6	4	2	0	0

* Chiari II malformation, intramedullary lipomatosis, neuroepithelial cyst,
   arachnoid cysts (3)

Detail of the filum terminale and other neural structures was better demonstrated
by CTM (Fig. 1) however MRI frequently provided important additional information,
often unsuspected on the CTM, such as focal cord cavitation, disc degeneration and
sacral meningcoeles.

Tissue characterization by MRI was superior especially in terms of clearly
differentiating lipomatous and neuro ectodermal tissues from normal cord and
assessing the nature of cystic lesions (Fig. 2).

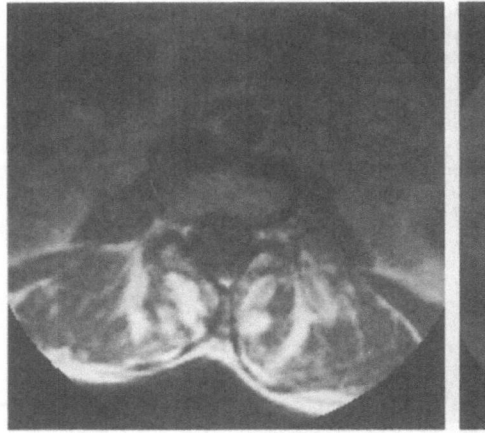
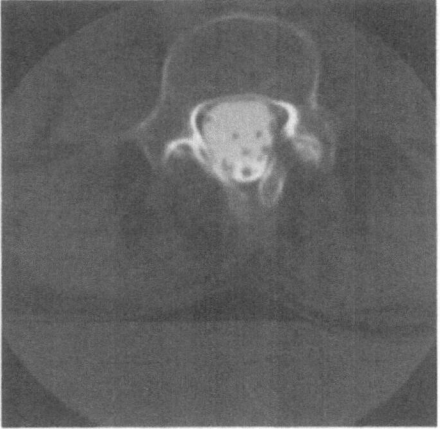

a.   b.

Fig. 1   31 year old female a. MRI b. CTM at same level. CTM shows superior
         delineation of the thick filum terminale.

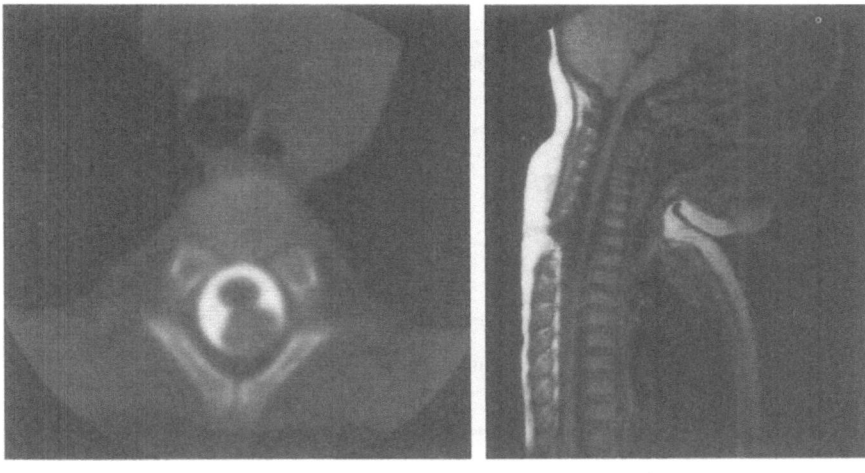

a.   b.

Fig. 2   6 year old female a.   CTM showed an intradural mass posterior to the cord at
T$_2$, closely related to a dermal sinus track.   Density measurements suggested
a solid mass   b.   MRI shows the dermal sinus track however the contents of
the canal at T$_2$ are of CSF signal intensity suggesting the mass was an
arachnoid cyst (confirmed at operation).

Cord cavitation was demonstrated in 41/87 (47.1%) of patients.   In 39/41 (95.1%)
cases the syrinx was found to be adjacent to a zone of cord tethering or in the
distal cord tethered by a thickened filum terminale.   MRI facilitated monitoring
of these patients (Fig. 3) enabling the surgeons to time their drainage procedures.

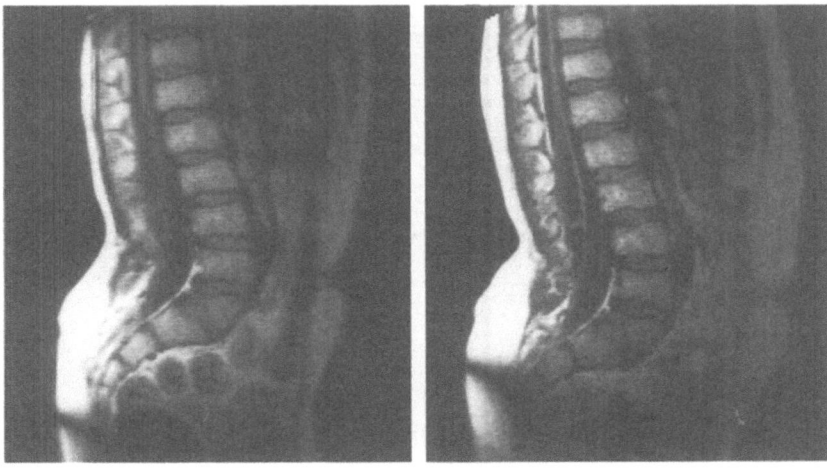

a.   b.

Fig. 3   9 year old boy.   Sequential MRI scans demonstrating enlargement of the
ventriculus terminalis.

In 5/41 cases the syrinx was demonstrated immediately above or contiguous with a myelo- or lipomyelomeningocoele. One patient with a repaired lumbar myelomeningocoele and a mild Chiari II abnormality had a syrinx occurring remotely in the upper thoracic region.

The anatomical relationships at the craniocervical junction were in all cases more precisely defined by MRI, Chiari II malformations being demonstrated in 10/11 of the patients with meningomyelocoeles. There was one case of a Chiari III malformation.

CONCLUSION

The essential requirement of the neurosurgeon in the assessment of spinal dysraphism is the clear definition of the lesion, presence of any associated lesions and their sequelae. In our study, spina bifida cystica lesions were generally better assessed by MRI in terms of more clearly demonstrating the various involved tissue elements, presence of cord cavitation and nature of any craniocervical abnormalities. CTM remains, however, more accurate for demonstrating the location and orientation of finer neural elements such as nerve roots, filum terminale and the arachnodural envelopes, fibrous bands and osseous spurs of diastematomyelia. Of greatest material importance to the surgeon is the ability to define the pathological filum terminale which, on a low field system, remains at present in the realms of CTM.

This study confirms our initial findings based on a smaller study (1) and lends further support to other groups (2,3) who propose the use of MRI as the primary investigation of suspected spinal dysraphism. CTM may still be required in selected cases for further definition of finer neural detail such as the state of the filum terminale. MRI has helped to underline the relatively high incidence of cord cavitation in dysraphism, which may reflect the sequela of focal damage either due to chronic ischaemia or repetitive minor traumatic episodes consequent upon cord tethering. Monitoring of this potentially serious complication should be undertaken by MRI scanning.

REFERENCES

Altman N R, Altman D H (1987) MR imaging of spinal dysraphism. AM J Neuroradiol 8: 533-538
Barnes P D, Lester P D, Yamanashi W S, Prince J R (1986) Magnetic resonance imaging in infants and children with spinal dysraphism. Am J Neuroradiol 7: 465-473
Jaspan T, Worthington B S, Holland I M (1988) A comparative study of magnetic resonance imaging and computed tomography-assisted myelography in spinal dysraphism. Br J Radiology 61: 445-453

ACKNOWLEDGEMENTS: We would like to thank the MRC and DHSS for financial support of the MRI project.

Diagnosis of Lumbar Dysraphias by CT Myelography and Nuclear Magnetic Resonance Imaging

M. Ratzka, N. Sörensen, M. Nadjmi, and B. Schuknecht

Clinical investigations aim at the least possible delay in cord tethering. Frequent conditions are lipomeningomyeloceles, tight filum, dermoid cysts, and retethering after early myelocele repair (Table 1). Less frequenlty, diastematomyelia occurs if the institution does not have a scoliosis center (Fitz and Harwood-Nash 1975). Dermoids and lipomeningoceles are usually presented for diagnosis in the first year of age. The tight filum, diastematomyelia, and retethering of early closed myeloceles at first develop symptoms or deteriorate during periods of rapid growth at about 5 years of age on average (Hall et al. 1988). This corresponds to our own observations in the past 8 years. Worsening dysraphic signs force one to check the whole CNS to exclude lesions at a higher level.

This report is based on experience with more than 130 operated cases of lumbar dysraphies since 1980 and is confined to the lumbar site.

Table 1. Incidence of lumbar dysraphias, 1980-1988

manifestation	n
Lipomeningo(myelo)celes	50
Conus tethering (mostly tight filum)	32
Dermal sinuses	25
Meningoceles	10
Diastematomyelia	10
Caudal regression syndromes	3

In the first 3 years diagnosis was established by plain films and conventional myelograms, sometimes supplemented by noncontrast CTs. Since 1983 high resolution with target scanning, 512 matrix, and high-contrast algorithms has provided very clear and precise results.

After a short initial period the method was optimally standardized. It allowed precise description of all conditions of dysraphia and tethering in close accordance with operative results (Figs.1-4).

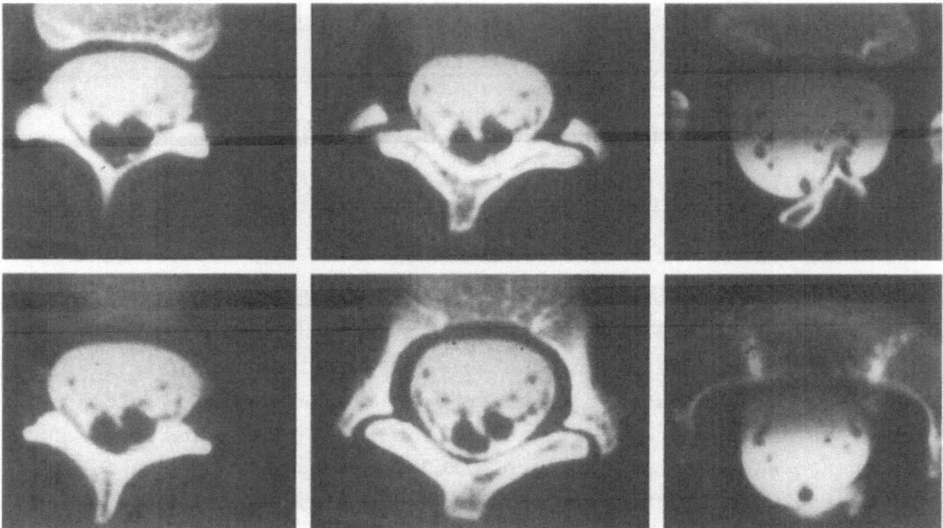

Fig.1. Tethering at the level of the 5th lumbar vertebra in a case of diastematomyelia. The partition of the cord, roots the rudimental dorsal spur, and tight filum are clearly distinguishable

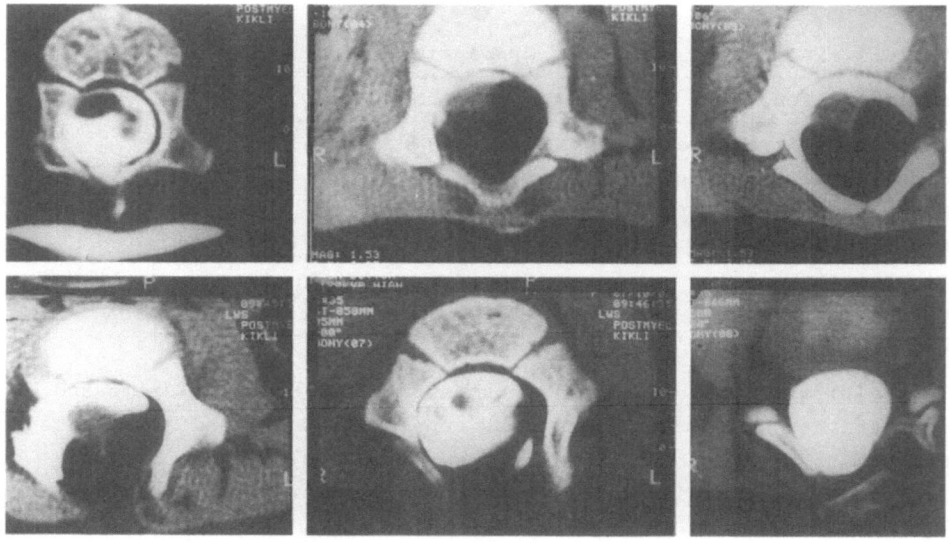

Fig.2. Tethering in a case of lipomeningocele with normally shaped conus and nerve root pattern

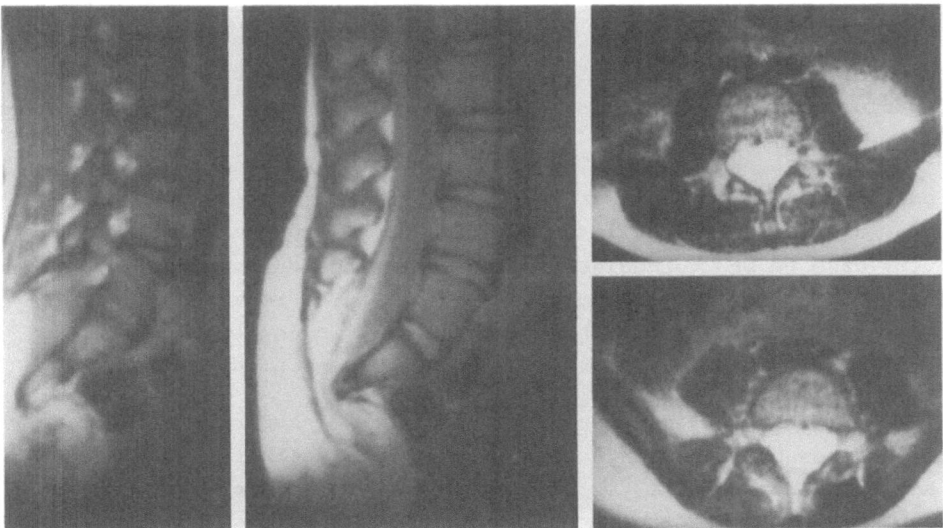

Fig.3. Early MRI pictures (0.35 T). While the sagittal slices are diagnostic, the transversal T2 sequence was not sufficient

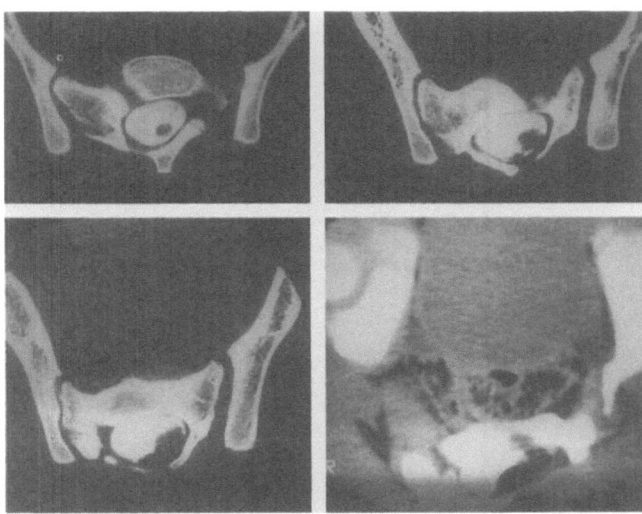

Fig.4. The corresponding CT myelography of the same case as in Fig.3 shows the very low tethering with a lipomeningomyelocele, roots, placode, lipoma, and suspected site of fixation

Although we would not emphasize any risk except in children with seizures or severe scoliosis, CT myelography remains invasive and is therefore restricted to inpatients. General anesthesia is preferable in infants as it is in MRI.

Since the introduction of MRI the situation has changed for us. Suddenly we had to deal with many external MRI pictures which has been made before the children came for special consultation. In every case we had to decide together with the neurosurgeon whether the MRI pictures indicated surgery or had to be repeated or supplemented by CT myelography. Sometimes we were in doubt, but in fact the frequency of CT myelographies has decreased significantly.

After initial problems, recent MRI pictures of superior quality have caused us to hesitate to follow up with another investigation only for minor details, especially if anesthesia was required. Undoubtedly, smaller details of the conus shape or the nerve roots, which might influence the postoperative prognosis, can be demonstrated much more clearly by CT myelography, as is shown in Figs.5 and 6. Problems with the diagnosis if only MRI is performed are reported by Hall et al. (1988). In only two of five cases a tight filum could be detected by MRI, a diagnosis which is very clear in CT myelography. The problem emerges if only T1-weighted sequences

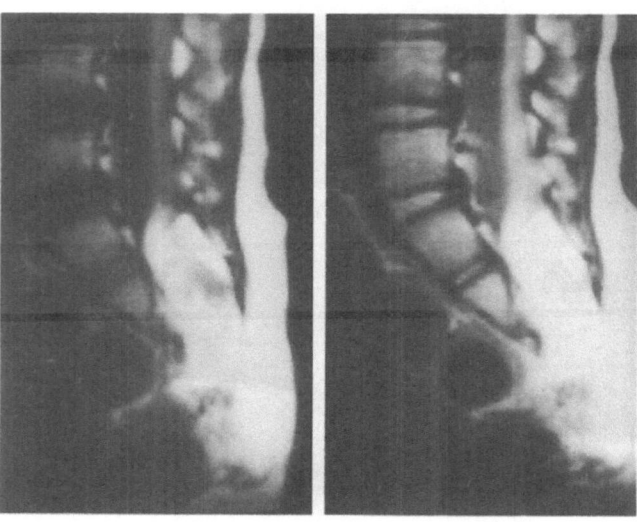

Fig.5. Lipomeningomyelocele in sagittal T1 and proton-density sequence

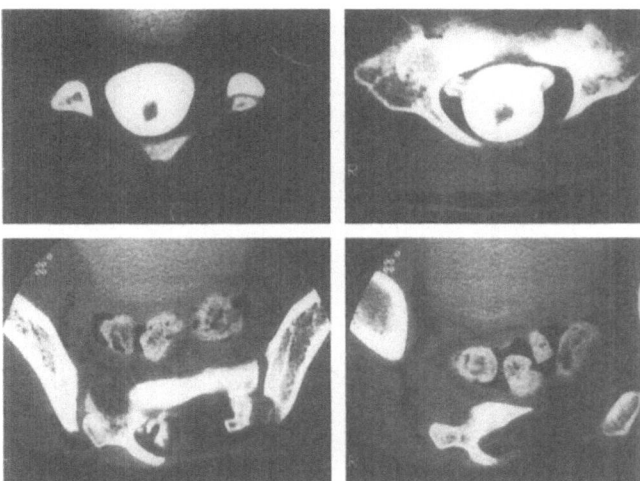

Fig.6. CT myelography of the same case as in Fig.5 which we would
not have performed if transverse slices had been available

are performed at lower caudal levels. New, improved MRI pictures
with more contrast and better tissue differentiation show details
much better (Figs.7,8).

Figure 9 shows high-frequency T1 sequences in a case of diastematomyelia. The same quality can also be gained with spin-echo sequences. Whereas the sagittal picture enables a first-glance diag-

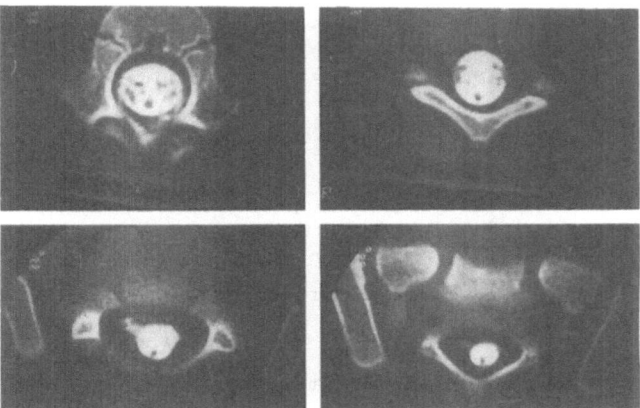

Fig.7. Classical aspect of the tight filum with its dorsally fixed
and therefore caudally opening circular structure

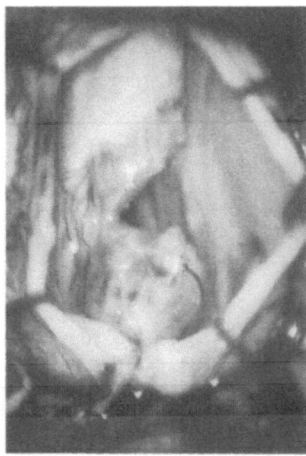

Fig.8. The corresponding site to that in Fig.7 during operation.
The filum is remarkably strong and has been partly cut already

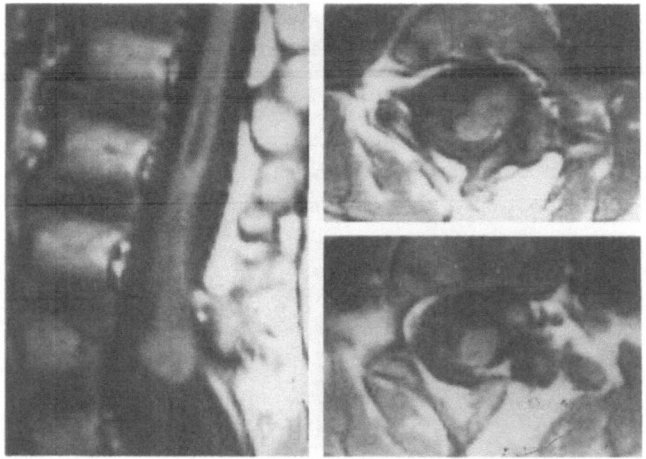

Fig.9. Diastematomyelia in high-frequency T1 sequences

nosis, the transverse one show the asymmetry of the cord partition
and details of the spinal roots.

If it seems necessary to obtain specific information from myelography in special cases, for example, in tight filum, asymmetrically
fixed lipoceles, or scoliosis, it is possible to simulate CT myelograms by strongly T2-weighted transverse sequences

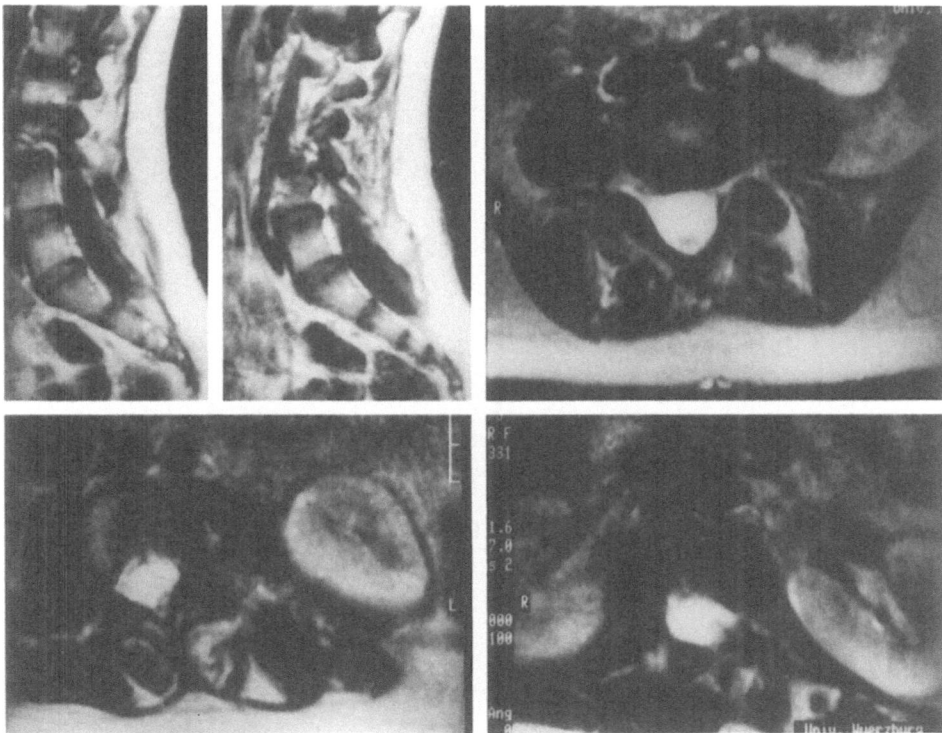

Fig.10. Lipomeningomyelocele with tethering demonstrated by MRI

Figure 10 demonstrates MRI findings of tethering in another case of lipomeningomyelocele. Due to scoliosis the sagittal pictures cannot give the topographic continuity; the result of a transverse sequence suffices as it clearly separates placode, roots, and the presumed zone of tethering.

We support the development of this technique of transverse, strongly T2-weighted sequences as we are convinced that their diagnostic value may soon reach that of CT myelography. Then CT could be reserved for cases with extended bone surgery (as an additional investigation without contrast, CT myelography could be available only for extremely difficult cases), or if MRI is not practicable for any reason.

References

[1] Fitz CR, Harwood-Nash DC (1975) The tethered conus. Am J Roentgenol Radium Ther Nucl Med 125: 515-523
[2] Hall WA, Albright AL, Brunberg JA (1988) Diagnosis of tethered cords by magnetic resonance imaging. Surg Neurol 30: 60-64

Lumbosacral Spinal Dysraphism – Examination with MRI Compared with Conventional Modalities: Management and Recommendations

E. Volle, J. Treisch, H. J. Kaufmann, J. P. Hedde, D. Köhler, and T. Michael

INTRODUCTION

Optimal planning of the diagnostic procedure is essential for an exact diagnosis and for the subsequent neurosurgical intervention in dysraphic myelodysplasias. A definitive diagnosis of the existing lesion and its ventral, dorsal and intraspinal extent is the least required of the imaging diagnostician. Previously, the invasive methods of myelography and CT-myelography produced the greatest possible yield of information (3, 4, 5).

Magnetic resonance imaging (MRI) now allows adequate differentiation of intraspinal and perispinal structures while avoiding stress on the infantile organism from ionising rays and obviating intrathecal contrast administration (1, 2). Our study compares the diagnostic yield and the respective value of the individual examination modalities.

MATERIAL AND METHODS

Nineteen patients (11 male and 8 female; aged: newborn to 39 years) presenting with the clinical symptoms of lumbosacral spinal dysraphism were examined initially by the diagnostic procedures as shown in Fig. 1.

In all 19 cases, sagittal, axial, T1- and T2-weighted MRI sequences were compared with the conventional X-ray films and with 12 high-resolution CT scans, 2 studies having been performed after contrast enhancement. Lumbar myelograms were available for 8 patients, post-myelographic CT studies in 6, and 2 newborns had been examined by ultrasound. The results of all examinations were compared with each other.

Eighteen of the 19 patients underwent lumbar surgery. The single exception was a patient with a suspected clinical diagnosis of lumbar spina bifida occulta and a confirmed cervical meningocele. Patients with diastematomyelia, syringomyelia and other purely intramedullary lesions were not included in this study.

Tab. 1. Summary of cases with lumbosacral spinal dysraphism

SPINA BIFIDA OCCULTA	n=14
with tethered cord n=6	
Dorsal Neurodermal Sinus	2
in combination with	
Lipomyeloschisis	5
Lipoma(extraspinal)	3
Currarino Trias	2
Dermoid	1
Megacauda	1
SPINA BIFIDA APERTA (CYSTICA)	n=5
dorsal Myelomeningocele	3
dorsal Lipomyelomeningocele	2

RESULTS

The repartition of the study population into 14 cases of occult
dysraphia and 5 of spina bifida cystica is shown in Tab. 1. The
diagnosis was confirmed at surgery in 18 cases (1 patient with a
megacauda did not undergo lumbar surgery). The findings on conventional X-ray studies were confirmed by MRI as follows: An increased
lumbosacral interpeduncular distance was demonstrated in 9 out of 15
cases (= 60 %). Incomplete closure of the arch was recognized in 12
out of 18 cases (= 67 %). An osseous defect (agenesis or dysgenesis)
was seen at MRI in 7 out of 9 cases (= 78 %). MRI demonstrated
locatable pathology in 11 out of 12 patients (= 92 %) with skin
changes (appendages, local tuft of hair).

In 42 % of patients with CT (including contrast enhancement studies)
and with myelography and post-myelographic CT scans, this combination
of examinations was superior to MRI in the differential diagnosis of
soft-tissue masses. With myelography/myelo-CT it was possible to
demarcate intraspinal calcifications, septa, cavity formations and
their communication with adjacent structures, particularly with the
subarachnoid space. In 5 out of 8 cases, myelography and myelo-CT
provided guiding information additional beyond that obtained with
MRI. Confirmation or exclusion of tissue components with CSF communication ventrally of the vertebral column or the demonstration of
a descended abscess cavity presacrally was possible only by myelography (in 2 cases) and by contrast-enhanced CT (in 1 case). In
addition, a rectal contrast enema provided the necessary information
for a correct preoperative diagnosis in Currarino's triad (n = 2
cases).

MRI and myelography were equal as regards determination of the craniocaudal extent of the lesions. CT is inappropriate because of the high radiation exposure (gonadal dose) in the individual scanning levels. CT furthermore provided no unequivocal information as regards the evaluation of a prolapsed medullary cone and/or a megacauda. Myelography/myelo-CT, on the other hand, displayed distinct advantages in respect of the demarcation of the terminal filament and individual nerve roots and their sacs (n = 8 = 100 %). The recognizable details of a lesion provided by sagittal, coronal and axial MRI projections demonstrate the superiority of this modality over myelography and the secondary reconstruction techniques of the post-myelographic examination. In 5 out of 19 cases (= 26 %), the guiding signs were seen only at myelography and myelo-CT and contrast-enhanced CT. A correct preoperative diagnosis was made with MRI in 14 of the 19 cases (= 74 %).

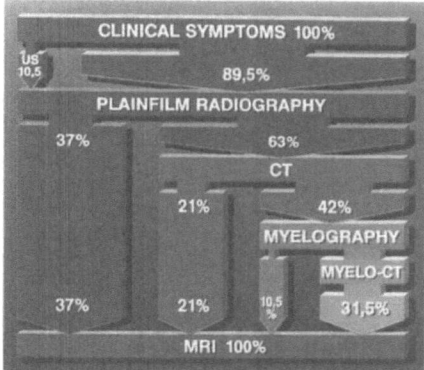

Fig. 1. Diagram shows the sequence of diagnostic procedures in chronological order

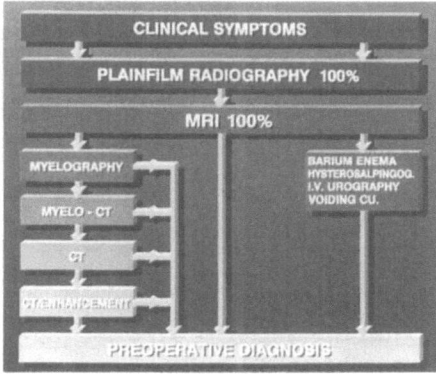

Fig. 2. Diagram listing our recommendation for the diagnostic work-up in lumbo-sacral spinal dysraphism

DISCUSSION

MRI is increasingly being recommended as a screening technique for spinal dysraphism with myelodysplasia (1, 2). We agree with these authors as regards the clinical picture of spina bifida cystica, but not as regards occult spinal dysraphism or more complex osseous malformation syndromes, since our study revealed a need for supplementary procedures (Fig. 2). In the case of osseous lesions, differential diagnosis has improved as experience with plain X-ray diagnosis and the different CT techniques have grown. Direct comparison of MRI and myelography shows that myelography is the more informative procedure when the aim is to demonstrate individual nerve sheaths, nerves, nerve root sacs and the terminal filament as a whole. Myelography and myelo-CT are the only examination procedures which supply unequivocal findings in the diagnosis of cystic cavities and their possible communication with the CSF system.

The advantage of magnetic resonance imaging lies in the avoidance of ionising radiation, the multidirectional scanning planes and the very exact recognisability of details of extradural soft-tissue components - particularly in T2-weighted scans. T1-weighted scans produce good images of neural structures comparable with those obtained with the standard procedures. In addition, a possible communication with the CSF system may be suspected in the presence of cystic lesions which display the same signal intensity pattern as the CSF.

For the preoperative diagnosis of myelodysplasia it is advisable to perform plain radiography (sonography in neonates) followed by MRI. This procedure is also to be recommended in occult spinal dysraphism and malformation syndromes of the vertebral column with pronounced osseous changes. Where necessary, myelography, myelo-CT or contrast-enhanced CT can then be performed as indicated.

SUMMARY

Magnetic resonance imaging is now the method of choice for the diagnosis of myelodysplasia - dysraphism - of the lumbar spine. Myelography followed by myelo-CT is required for the differentiation of perispinal lesions.

REFERENCES

Altman NR, Altman DH (1987) MR imaging of spinal dysraphism. AJNR 8:533-538
Barnes PD, Lester PD, Yamanashi WS, Prince JR (1986) Magnetic resonance imaging in infants and children with spinal dysraphism. AJNR 7:465-472
Naidich TP, Harwood-Nash DC, McLone DG (1983) Radiology of spinal dysraphism. Clin Neurosurg 30:341-365
Naidich TP, McLone DG, Mutluer S (1983) A new understanding of dorsal dysraphism with lipoma (lipomyelochisis): radiologic evaluation and surgical correction. AJNR 4:103-116
Sarwar M, Virapongse C, Ghimani S (1984) Primary tethered cord syndrom: a new hypothesis of its origin. AJNR 5:235-242

The Anatomic Basis of Vertebrogenic Pain in Lumbar Disc Extrusion: A Retrospective MR Study

J. R. Jinkins, A. R. Whittemore, and W. G. Bradley

Huntington Medical Research Institutes
10 Pico Street

INTRODUCTION

Extruded lumbar intervertebral discs have traditionally been categorized as posterior or postero-lateral in location (PDE), although occasional reports have addressed extrusions extending anteriorly (ADE) and centrally (CDE). the clinical state of neurogenic radiating pain accompanying posterior extrusions with somatic nerve root compression is well defined, however the uncomplicated ADE and CDE may also be associated with a definite clinical syndrome, which includes both local and referred symptoms with much the same somatic distribution as that observed in true sciatica.

METHODS

A detailed retrospective review of 250 MR examinations of the lumbar spine was performed in the axial and sagittal planes utilizing single and dual spin echoes respectively, on mid- and high field imagers. Extrusive abnormalities were sought along the periphery of the disc, anteriorly (ADE) or posteriorly (PDE) utilizing the lateral margin of the neural foramen as the boundary. A third category of central disc extrusion (CDE) was incorporated which indicated a herniation into or through the vertebral body itself to include Schmorl's nodes and limbus vertebrae.

RESULTS

Out of the total of 250 examinations, 236 extrusions were identified in all directions at all lumbar levels in 145 subjects, leaving 105 negative studies (42%). Of these 236 extrusions, 69 (29%) were ADE's, 34 (14.5%) were CDE's, and 133 (56.5%) were PDE's (Fig. 1).

DISCUSSION

The anatomic basis for the mediation of pain generated within the disc and paradiscal structures rests with afferent fibers from the two primary sources: 1) postero-lateral neural branches emanating from the ventral ramus of the somatic spinal root, and 2) neural rami projecting directly to the paravertebral autonomic neural plexus (Fig. 2). Thus, the conscious perception of pain originating in the vertebral column, although complex, has definite pathways represented in this dual peripheral innervation associated with closely related central ramifications.

Major clinical manifestations of this anatomic configuration include a tripartite syndrome of pain associated with vertebral pathology which involves varying superimposed combinations of:

1) well circumscribed local _somatic_ spinal pain;

2) centrifugally _referred_ pain to the low back, pelvic structures, and buttocks/lower extremities; and lastly,

3) centrifugally _radiating_ pain to cutaneous dermatomes if, and only if, the somatic spinal root is intimately involved with the pathologic process.

The first two elements of the above comprise _vertebrogenic_ pain, while the third represents _neurogenic_ (radicular/sciatic) pain.

CONCLUSION

The directional differentiation of lumbar disc extrusions utilizing MR, together with a clarification and appreciation of the accompanying clinical syndromes should contribute to the further elucidation of the specific causes of local somatic and referred vertebrogenic pain as well as the radiating neurogenic pain engendered by these distinct organic lesions.

REFERENCES

Brodal A (1981) The autonomic nervous system. In: Neurological Anatomy. Oxford University, New York, pp 698-787

Edgar MA, Ghadially JA (1976) Innervation of the lumbar spine. Clinical Orthopaedics and Related Research 115:35-41

Hirsch C, Ingelmark BE, and Miller M (1963) The anatomical basis for low back pain. Acta Orthop Scand 33:1-17

Hochaday JM, Whitty CWM (1967) Patterns of referred pain in the normal subject. Brain 90:482-496

Jackson HC, Winkelman RK, Bickel WH (1983) Nerve endings in the human lumbar spinal column and related structures. J Bone Joint Surg 48-A:1272-1281

Stilwell DR (1956) The nerve supply of the vertebral column and its associated structures in the monkey. Anatomical Record 125:139-169

Wiberg G (1949) Back pain in relation to the nerve supply of the intervertebral disc. Acta Orthop 19:211-221

Wyke B (1987) The neurology of low back pain. In: Jayson MIV (ed) The Lumbar Spine and Back Pain. New York:Churchill Livingstone, pp 56-99

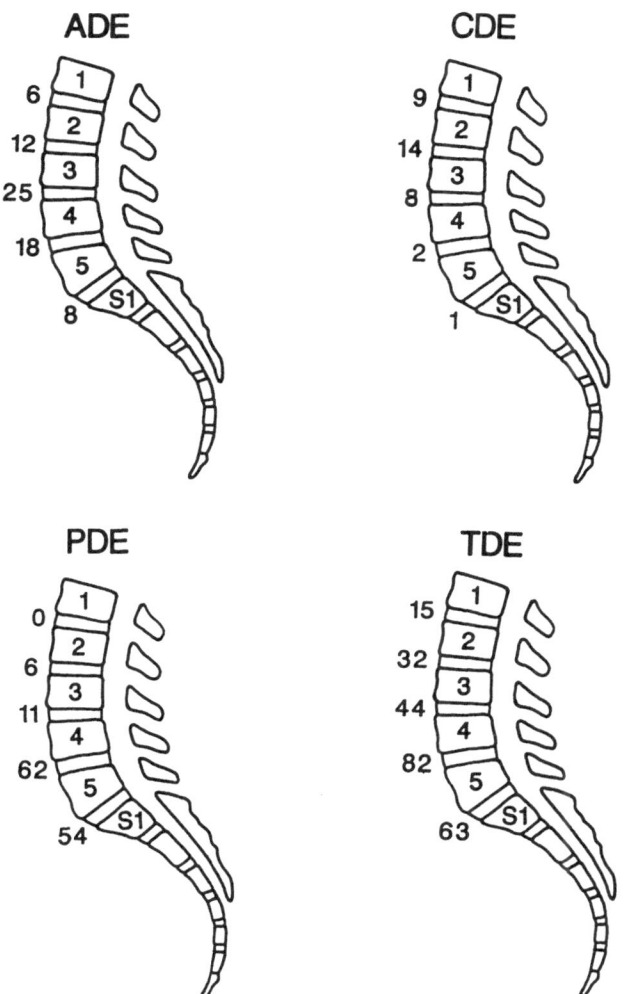

Fig. 1. Distribution of 236 total disc extrusions in 145 subjects with positive MR examinations:

ADE: Anterior disc extrusions (anterior to lateral border of neural foramen),
CDE: Central disc extrusions (Schmorl's nodes and limbus vertebrae),
PDE: Posterior disc extrusions (posterior to lateral border of neural foramen),
TDE: Total disc extrusions.

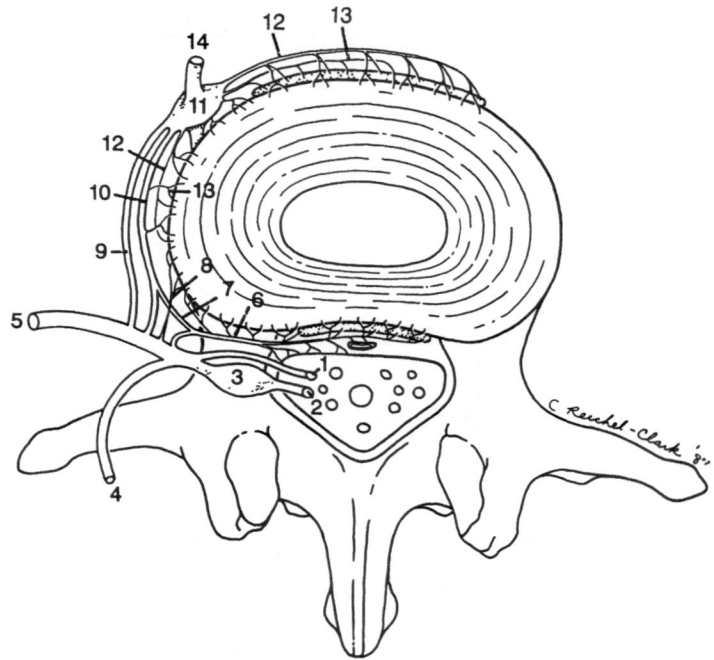

Fig. 2. Schematic diagram of the innervation of the anterior spinal canal and structures of the anterior aspect of the spinal column (1: ventral root, 2: dorsal root, 3: dorsal root ganglion, 4: dorsal ramus of spinal nerve root, 5: ventral ramus of spinal nerve root, 6: recurrent meningeal nerve (RMN: sinuvertebral nerve of Luschka), 7: autonomic afferent/efferent branch to RMN, 8: direct somatic afferent branch from ventral ramus to lateral disc, 9: white ramus communicans (not found caudal to L-2), 10: gray ramus communicans (multilevel irregular lumbosacral distribution), 11: paraspinal sympathetic ganglion, 12: anterior and lateral autonomic afferent sensory branches, 13: anterior and lateral autonomic efferent branches, 14: paraspinal sympathetic chain).

MRI in Degenerative Disease of the Lumbosacral Disc

P. Piazza, R. Menozzi, F. Cusmano, E. Ferri, M. Imberti, and P. Bassi

Introduction

Many papers have shown the ability of CT (Mall and Kaiser 1984; Dorwart 1984; Williams et al. 1982; Lutman 1987; Di Guglielmo et al. 1982) and especially of magnetic resonance (MR) (Edelman et al. 1985; Modic et al. 1986; Masaryk et al. 1988) to demonstrate with great detail the anatomical structures of the lumbosacral spine involved in degenerative disease, in particular the disc unit, made up of a nucleus and an anulus, the vertebral end plates, and the posterior longitudinal ligament, in order to differentiate between a contained and a noncontained disc herniation.

The aim of our investigation was to further evaluate the ability of MR in making such an important differentiation for conservative or surgical management of leg and low back pain.

Subjects and Methods

During a 6-month period, 55 patients (30 men, 25 women; 19-75 years old) with neurologic evidence of a degenerative disease of the lumbosacral discs were examined at our institution with a 1.5 T superconducting magnet (Philips Gyroscan S15) and a 10 × 50 cm rectangular surface coil.

Our examination consists of four different images (Table 1). The first is a coronal multiple-slice scout view, followed by a sagittal and then an axial multiple-slice sequence. The examination ends with a multiple-echo T2-weighted slice in the sagittal median or paramedian plane, depending upon vectors of herniated nucleus pulposus. All the sequences are performed with a 256 × 256 matrix and are cardiac gated; the examination lasts about 40 min. In the evaluation of degenerative disease of the lumbosacral disc we have considered four main situations: (a) bulging anulus, associated or not with spondylotic spurring of the vertebral body margins (Fig.1); (b) prolapsed disc (Masaryk et al. 1988) or subanular herniation

(Dorwart 1984), which we usually call discal protrusion (Fig.2);
(c) extruded herniation (Fig.3); (d) free-fragment of sequestered
disc (Fig.4).

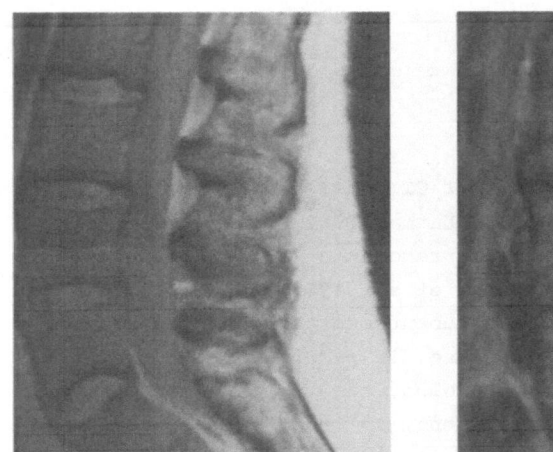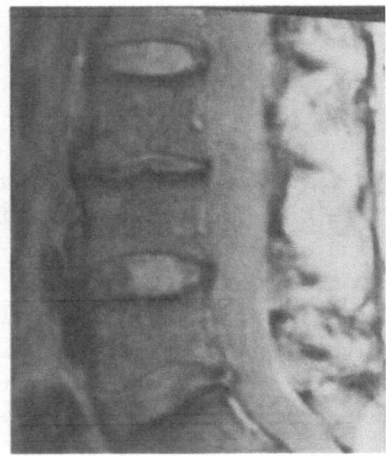

Fig.1. Bulging anuli at L3-4 and L4-5 level, characterized by a
generalized extension of disc margins beyond vertebral body end
plates

Fig.2. Subanular herniation appearing as focal extension of disc
margin, bounded by low signal intensity of outer anular fibers

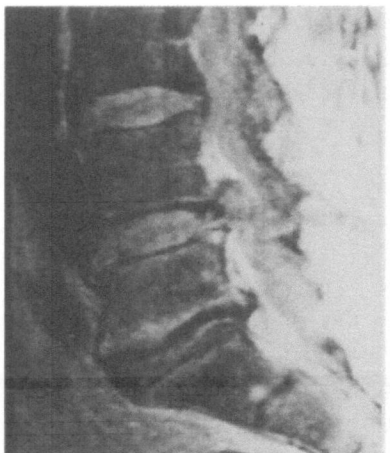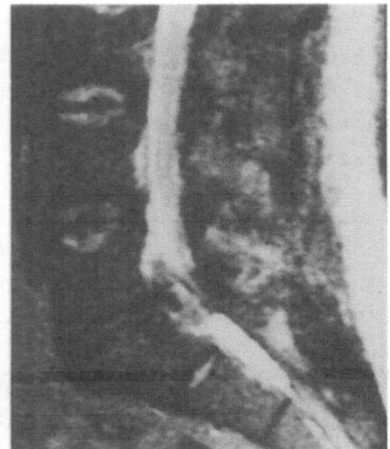

Fig.3. Extruded disc, no longer bounded by outer anular fibers

Fig.4. Free fragment or herniation of nuclear material no longer
attached to remaining disc

Table 1. Technical parameters

Plane	TR	TE	Slice thickness	Gap	Nex
1. Coronal	500	30	6 mm	10 mm	1
2. Sagittal	1100	30-60	5 mm	0.5 mm	2
3. Axial	1000	30-60	5 mm	0.5 mm	2-4
4. Sagittal	2100	30-60- ... -180	5 mm		2

Results

In our series the affected spaces demonstrated slight reduction in signal intensity on intermediate (TR = 1100) and proton-density weighted images and loss of signal on T2-weighted images. In our series (Table 2) sagittal images, especially proton-density weighted ones, were able to establish the integrity of outer anular fibers in subanular herniations, in extruded herniations, both sagittal and axial images showed very well the defects in posterior discs margin. T2-weighted images were superior in showing free fragments.

Table 2. Distribution of cases by type and location of disorder

	L2-3	L3-4	L4-5	L5-S1
Bulging anulus	2	2	1	6
Subanular herniation	3	2	7	5
Extruded herniation	2		9	5
Free fragment			1	1

MR findings were confirmed in 14 out of 16 extruded herniations which underwent surgical intervention at our institution. Extruded herniations with free fragment were also surgically confirmed.

Discussion

A long time has passed since many surgeons operated for herniated lumbar disc disease solely on the basis of their clinical impression. Nowadays, radiological evaluation of the lumbosacral spine plays an important role in determination of the discal origin of leg and low back pain.

While the present paper does not make a systematic comparisoon between MR and other investigative modalities, our results confirm other authors' findings (Masaryk et al. 1988; Modic et al. 1986) which demonstrate the superiority of MR over other techniques.

About strategies for efficient imaging of degenerative disease of the lumbosacral disc, a great number of parameters have been · utilized (Kios and Norman 1987). Our initial experience with T1-weighted images has been discouraging because of difficulties in distinguishing between the posterior disk margin and the thecal sac; therefore, we now prefer an intermediate TR = 1100-1200 ms which offers better contrast resolution and facilitates distinction between subanular and extruded herniations.

Conclusions

In conclusion, we would like to recall some advantages of MR such as: absence of ionizing radiations, which represents an important risk in CT examination (Grobovschek et al. 1987); an examined area which extends from the lumbosacral level to the conus medullaries; absence of contrast media; multiplanar examination, which facilitates distinction between contained discs (Figs.1,2) and noncontained ones (Figs.3,4), making easier the therapeutic choice between conservative, percutaneous, and conventional surgical procedures.

References

[1]   Di Guglielmo L, Vadalà G, Garbagna GP, Dorè R. Failoni S,
      Di Giulio G (1982) Valore della tomografia computerizzata nella
      diagnosi di ernia del disco lombare. Radiol Med 68: 51-56
[2]   Dorwart RH (1984) Fundamentals of computed tomographic evalua-
      tion of lumbar disc disease. In: Genant HK (ed) Spine update.
      San Francisco
[3]   Edelman RR, Shoukimas GM, Stark DD, Davis KR, New PFJ, Saini S,
      Rosenthal DI, Wismer GL, Brady TJ (1985) High resolution sur-
      face-coil imaging of lumbar disc disease. AJNR 6: 479-485
[4]   Grobouschek M, Hoffman W, Rahim H, Dinkhauser L (1987) Lumbo-
      sacral CT versus myelography-dosimetry, indications in compa-
      rison also with MR. In: Calabrò A, Leonardi M (eds) Computer
      aided neuroradiology. XIV Congress of the European Society of
      Neuroradiology, Udine, 1987
[5]   Kios BO, Norman D (1987) Strategies for efficient imaging of the
      lumbar spine. In: Brant-Zawadzki M, Norman D (eds) MRI of the
      CNS. Raven, New York
[6]   Lutman M (1987) La tomografia computerizzata nella sciatica
      lombare. Edizioni Libreria Cortina, Verona
[7]   Mall JC, Kaiser JA (1984) Critical evaluation of computed
      tomography versus myelography in assessing low back pain. In:
      Genant HK (ed) Spine update. San Francisco
[8]   Masaryk TJ, Ross JS, Modic MT, Boumphrey F, Bohlman H, Wilber G
      (1988) High-resolution MR imaging of sequestered lumbar inter-
      vertebral disks. AJNR 9: 351-358

[9]   Modic MT, Masarik T, Boumphrey F, Goormastic M, Bell G (1986)
      Lumbar herniated disk disease and canal stenosis: prospective
      evaluation by surface coil MR, CT, and myelography. AJNR 7:
      709-717

[10] Williams AL, Haughton VM, Meyer GA, Ho KC (1982) Computed tomo-
      graphy appearance of the bulging anulus. Radiology 142: 403-408

MRI in Spinal Dysraphism – Findings in 90 Children and Adolescents

M. Just (Mainz, FRG)

The spinal cord in 90 children and adolescents was examined by magnetic resonance imaging (MRI) many years after neonatal surgery of a meningomyelocele (average 12 years). In a high percentage of cases (88%) a diagnosis of tethered or retethered cord could be made. Associated anomalies like syringomyelia, lipoma, or dermoid could be found in 26% of the patients. Typical MRI features of tethered cord and associated anomalies are presented. In 30 cases additional head scans were done demonstrating complex cerebral malformations like ACM I and II, anomalies of the corpus callosum, absence of the falx, and low placed tentorium.

Since only few of our patients showed unequivocal progression of their neurological deficits, the high percentage of tethered cords is surprising. Obviously in most cases this finding is clinically asymptomatic or masked by preexisting neurological deficits. Instead associated anomalies like syringomyelia must be considered the reason for clinical deterioration in most cases.

As a result MRI proved to be a safe and highly effective modality for evaluating children with dysraphic myelodysplasia.

3D Gradient Echo Sequences in Examinations of the Spine

N. Obletter, H. Kett, and A. Breit (Passau, FRG)

Recent progress in MR imaging allows one to acquire an entire volume using 3D Fourier processing, resulting in a homogenous spatial resolution with a voxel-size of about one cubic millimeter. Acquisition time for a matrix of 256 × 256 × 128 amounts to less than 15 minutes, if gradient echo sequences are applied (FLASH/FISP).

The information contained in such a huge amount of data is retrieved with the aid of a special rapid data processing system.

Up to now about 100 3D data sets have been acquired from spines. The advantages of these processing techniques in comparison with the conventional spin echo sequences are discussed: the spatial resolution of 3D GE sequences with a slice thickness of 1.2 to 1.5 mm is significantly superior to that obtained with SE sequences.

This allows one to distinguish details such as vessels, small masses and nerve roots. Furthermore, the signal-to-noise ratio of 3D sequences is higher than in multi-slice technique. A decisive advantage is that it is possible to compute curved planes by postprocessing of the 3D data sets.

In single computed planes that follow the curvature of the spine or of other anatomical borders, it is possible to visualize intraspinal tumors and syringomyelias in their full extension.

Another practical advantage is the possibility of reconstructing from the 3D data sets any view desired by the surgeon.

Clinical Use of Three-Dimensional Spinal Computer Tomograpy

H. Becker

CT slices yield two-dimensional (2-D) representations of the human body. Secondary reconstructions, for example coronal or sagittal images, facilitate the conceptual spatial allocation of anatomical structures. Three-dimensional (3-D) imaging in CT has become possible through the development of special software. An experimental 3-D software programme has been available to us since 1985 on the GE 9800 CT-scanner. For a short time we have been using a very fast version, the "Quick 3-D" software programme, routinely. The object of our investigations was to test the use of the 3-D image procedures with CT and to determine its applicability for the imaging of the spinal region and also its clinical significance for neuroradiological diagnosis.

The 3-D image aquisition sequence is not very different from routine scanning. Usually we are using 3 or 5 mm axial continuous slices of the region of interest for 3-D reconstructions. The impression of a 3-D image develops through a range of grey tones. Structures which are more distant from the observer are imaged in dark shades, whilst structures facing towards the observer are imaged in light shades. The calculated bodies can rotate about all axes of the space. Full 360° rotation capability is provided at all orientations. Up to 360 static 3-D images may be produced in one full rotation with 1 degree angular intervalls. These images may be viewed sequentially like a movie to enhance the 3-D perception.

3-D reconstructions of the spine were calculated on the basis of the data from 50 CT-investigations. This method has been used especially for patients with a trauma of the spine. A comparison was made with conventional x-rays, axial CT scans and sagittal and coronal 2-D CT reformations.

In cases of C 1 fracture axial CT is superior to cervical spine x-rays. 2-D CT reformations are inaffectual in C 1 fractures. 3-D imaging with rotation around the x axis shows the traumatic changes clearly, especially the relation to C 2.

A fracture of the odontoid process can be precisely diagnosed with x rays, if necessary with additional conventional tomography. Axial CT are often not of diagnostic value. A sagittal 2-D CT reformation can be more helpful. 3-D imaging is problematic. For demonstration of the fracture of the odontoid process it is necessary to cut away the vertebral arch. For hidden structures with overlying details the section can be selected in such a way that a clear view is obtained of the region of interest.

In cases of complex C 2 fracture axial CT is better than conventional x ray. 3-D CT provides more informative images than 2-D CT reformations but without new diagnostic results.

The C 2-isthmus fracture can be seen more easily with axial CT than
with conventional radiographs, 2-D CT reformations are without any
diagnostic value in these cases. 3-D CT is able to show the fractures
of the vertebral arch very clearly, especially in cases with distinct
dislocation.

Fractures in the range of C 3 - C 7 can be usually demonstrated more
exactly in axial CT than in cervical spine x rays. 2-D CT reformations
have different diagnostic value, but in general 3-D CT were more
informative.

In cases of burst fractures the evidence of an intraspinal osseous
fragment is very important, because of the danger of fatal neurological complications. Axial CT and sagittal 2-D reformation are indicated. 3-D CT provides this information only if the spinal canal is
cut laterally (Fig. 1,2).

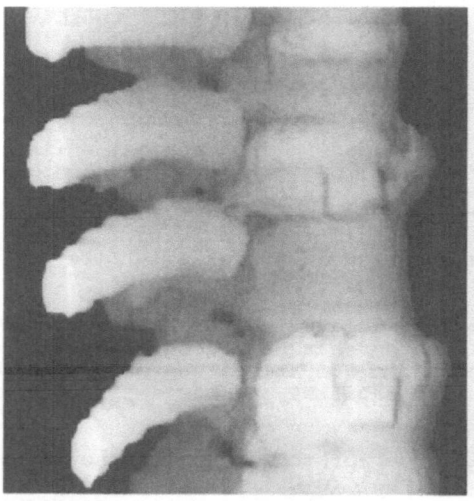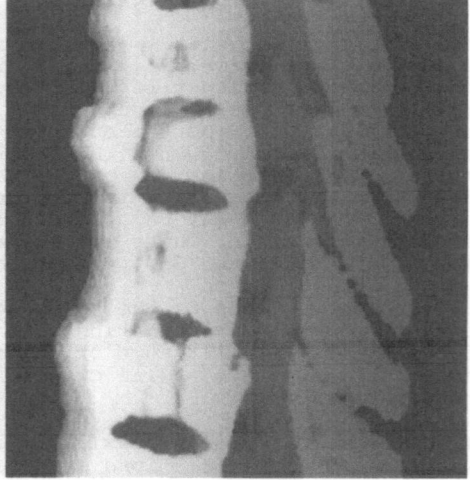

Fig. 1 and 2: 3-D CT of a burst fracture of Th 7 and 9

In patients with translation injuries of the spine with rotation and
luxation 3-D CT is most important. The complexity of the anatomical
relations can be shown by rotation of the vertebrae about the different axes.

There is a regulated relation between the plain of the course of the
fracture and the choice of the best reformation. If the fracture goes
in the sagittal plain, a 3-D CT is indicated with rotation around
the x axis. If the fracture is located in the coronal plain, then a
rotation around the x axis is preferable for the assessment of a
fracture within a single vertebra. A rotation around the z axis can
delinate altered intervertebral relations of several vertebral. A
sagittal or coronal 2-D CT reformation is sufficient in cases with
a fracture in the axial plane. Clearly visible dislocations of bony

fragments are basic requirements for a successful 3-D CT as the spatial resolution of 3-D images is inferior when compared to conventional radiographs and CT scans. In many cases it is more useful to generate a 3-D reformation than sagittal or coronal 2-D reformations.

Where tumours have caused the destruction of the vertebrae, the extent of the bone destruction and the altered position of the vertebrae in relation to each other can be made visible by 3-D CT. Generally the simultaneous display of soft tissue and bone is possible with a double density mode but the results remain unsatisfactory due to the poor distinctness and decreased differentiation of the reproduced structures. In cases with a strong enhancement of the tumour after intravenous injection of contrast medium or calcified tumours a 3-D CT can be done easily. When the tumour is located into the spinal canal the overlying arches of the vertebrae have to be cut away in the prescription of the 3-D image or the spinal canal must be cut laterally (Fig. 3 - 6).

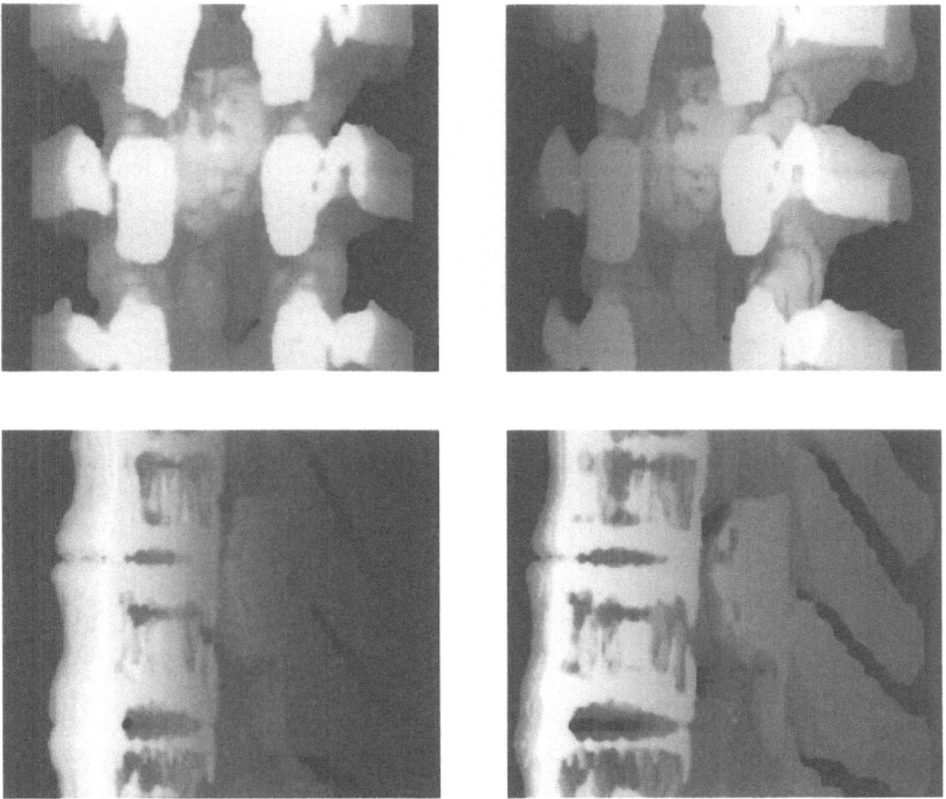

Fig. 3 - 6: Calcified meningioma at the level of Th 10/11

From our experience the 3-D CT does not result in any fundamentally new aspects in the diagnostical point of view. The clinically relevant information can already be obtained from the conventional 2-D images. However, a clearer understanding of the topography of the pathological findings can be obtained. Above all, a better spatial concept of the spine is conveyed using 3-D CT. This simplifies the communication between the neuroradiologist and the attending physician. For surgeons in particular, the preoperative planning can be improved.

REFERENCES

Becker H (1988) Dreidimensionale kraniale und spinale Computertomographie. Radiologe 28:239-242
Lang PH, Genant HK, Steiger P, Chafetz N, Morris JM (1988) Dreidimensionale Computertomographie und multiplanare CT-Reformationen bei lumbalen Spondylodesen. Fortschr. Röntgenstr. 148:524-529
Sartorius D (1986) 3-D display of CT data: new aid to preop surgical planning. Diagn Imag Intern 2:26-32

Significance of Modern Imaging Techniques in Patients with Friedreich's Ataxia

W. Müller-Forell, G. Schroth, and K. Wessel

Introduction

Friedreich's ataxia is an autosomal recessive hereditary disease with onset in childhood. As a prototype of afferent ataxia in its early stages primarily the posterior column and spinal cerebellar tracks are affected and only later the cerebellum itself. The neurological feature includes slowly progressing ataxia of gait and posture instability, deep tendon arreflexia, progressive muscle weakness in the lower extremities, dysarthria and decrease of vibration sensibility of the lower limbs (Geoffroy et al. 1976, Lamarche et al. 1984, Diener et al. 1986, Wessel and Diener 1987).

The diagnosis of FA is made clinically, the CT examination only shows minimal changes, especially in early stages (Claus and Aschoff 1982, Diener et al. 1986). The advantage of MRI is imaging nearly without artefacts, especially in the posterior fossa. Therefore we expected an exact definition of the structural lesions, in correlation to the neuropathological changes of FA.

Patients and methods

10 patients in the age of 18-30 years ($\female$: $\male$ = 8 : 2) were examined with CT and MRI. All met the clinical diagnostic criteria of FA. Using the disability scale of Kurtzke (1965) for multiple sclerosis, the score of our patients reached from 2 to 7.

CT scans were performed with a high resolution SOMATOM DRH-Scanner in a slice thickness of 4 mm, cerebellar atrophy was graduated in: 0 = normal, 1 = enlargement of at least one cerebellar or vermal sulcus, 2 = additional to enlarged basal cisterns, 3 = enlargement of at least 3 sulci and enlarged basal cisterns.

MRI was performed using a 1.5 Tesla-MAGNETOM (Siemens Co.). In medio-sagittal planes of T_1-weighted (SE 400/30) images the diameter of the IVth ventricle, of the pons, of the medulla oblongata cranial and caudal to the level of oliva an of the spinal cord at the level of Foramen magnum C_2 and C_3 were measured (Fig. 1). Further the ratio of the sagittal diameters of the pons and the medulla oblongata at the level of the Foramen magnum was built (Koehler et al. 1985). All values were analysed statistically and compared with those of a group of 15 healthy subjects.

Results

On CT only in patients suffering from a severe Friedreich's ataxia a markable or pronounced cerebellar atrophy with enlargement of the IVth ventricle was seen, without any correlation to the clinical score (Fig. 2). With MRI only the diameter of the medulla oblongata caudal to the oliva and the diameter of the spinal cord at the level

of the foramen magnum, C_2 and C_3 were reduced significantly in
patients suffering from Friedreich's ataxia (p <0,001) (Fig. 3, 4).
Especially the comparison of the ratios of the diameters of pons and
foramen magnum showed a pronounced significance (p = 0,000), but no
correlation to the clinical score could be assessed (Table 1).

Discussion

The clinical findings correlate closely with patho-anatomical and
histological lesions found at necropsy examination (Greenfield 1954,
Oppenheimer 1979, Lamarche et al. 1984). These changes do not reflect
very good on CT, partly because of the artefacts, partly because of
the fact that the only little reduction of the volume in a mild
atrophy is not visible on CT (Claus and Aschoff 1982, Diener et al.
1986). MRI has the possibility of a non-invasive evaluation of the
structures of the upper spinal cord and the brain stem, nearly
without artefacts (Flannigan et al. 1985, Gawehn et al. 1986). Our
results indicate that even in patients with a not very advanced
disease a significant atrophy of the caudal medulla oblongata and the
upper spinal cord can be demonstrated at the location of the autoptic
proven lesion, especially the ratio of the sagittal diameter of the
pons and medulla at the level of the foramen magnum is impressive.
But there is only poor correlation of the morphological changes,
shown in MRI, with the clinical score of the disease.

Our examinations may be recommended as a diagnostic marker, even in
cases with beginning Friedreich's ataxia.

References

Claus D, Aschoff JC (1982) Evaluation of infratentorial atrophy
    by CT. J Neurol Neurosurg Psychiatry 45:979-983
Diener HC, Müller A, Thron H, Poremba M, Dichgans J, Rapp H (1986)
    Correlation of clinical signs with CT findings in patients with
    cerebellar disease. J Neurol 233:5-12
Flannigan, MD, Bradley WG, Mazziota JC, Rauschning W, Bentson JR,
    Lufkin RB, Hieshima GB (1985) Magnetic resonance imaging of the
    brainstem: Normal structure and basic functional anatomy.
    Radiology 154:375-383
Gawehn J, Schroth G., Thron A (1986) The value of paraxial slices
    in MR-imaging of spinal cord disease. Neuroradiology 28:347-350
Geoffroy G, Barbeau A, Breton G, Lemieux B, Aube M, Leger C,
    Bouchard JP (1976) Clinical description and roentgenologic
    evaluations of patients with Friedreich's ataxia.
    Can J Neurol Sci 3:279-286
Greenfield, JG (1954) The spinocerebellar degenerations.
    Blackwell Scientific Publications Oxford
Koehler PR, Haughton VM, Daniels DL, Williams AL, Yetkin Z,
    Charles HC, Shutts D (1985) MR-measurements of normal and
    pathological brainsteim diameters. AJNR 6:425-427
Kurtzke JF (1965) Further notes on disability evaluation
    in multiple sclerosis with scale modifications.
    Neurology 15:   654-661
Lamarche JB, Lemieux B, Lieu HB (1984) The neuropathology
    of "typical" FRIEDREICH's ataxia in Quebec.
    Can J Neurol Sci 11:592-600
Oppenheimer DR (1979) Brain lesions in FRIEDREICH's ataxia.
    Can J Neurol Sci 6:173-176
Wessel K, Diener HC (1987) Degenerative Kleinhirnerkrankungen
    In: Brandt Th, Dichgans J, Diener HC (eds) Therapie und
    Verlauf neurologischer Krankheiten. Kohlhammer Stuttgart,
    685-696

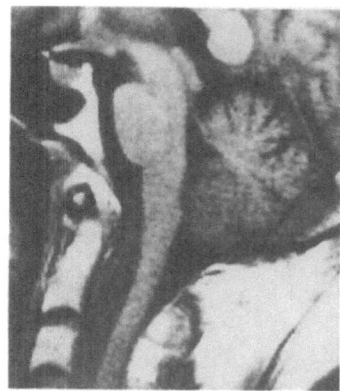 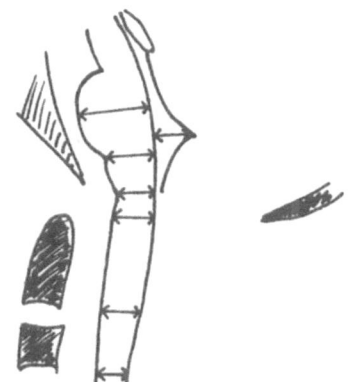

Fig. 1   a) Normal sagittal   b) Scheme of the
            slice of the cranio-   measurements
            cervicak region   (see text)
            (SE 400/30)

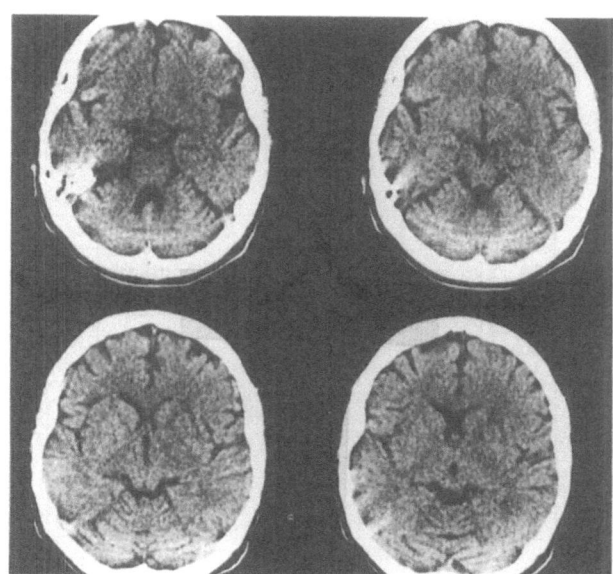

Fig. 2:
CT of a 24 year old
female suffering
from FA, cerebellar
and supratentor.
atrophy.

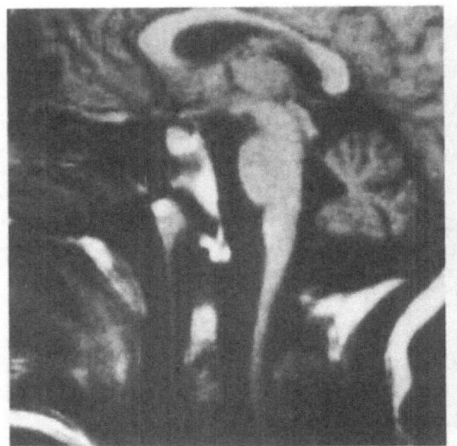 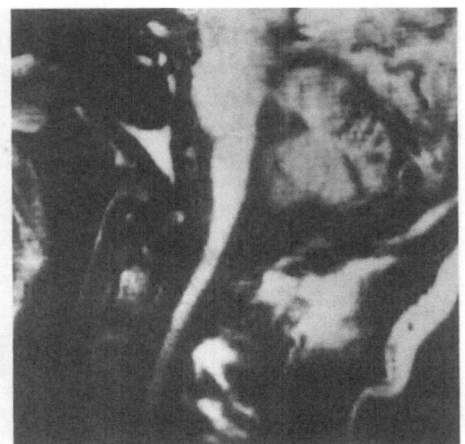

Fig. 3: 20 year old female   Fig. 4: 30 year old male

Both figures show the remarkable atrophy of the upper spinal cord and medulla oblongata.

Table 1· Clinical and neuroradiological results

Pat.-Nr.	age at beginning	examination	clinical score	CT Atrophy	KST IV. Ventr.	cranial of oliva	caudal of oliva	For. magnum	c_2	c_3	ratio
1	5	20	6	2	2,8	4,8	3,0	2,7	2,4	1,8	2,9
2	8	21	2	1	4,8	4,8	3,6	2,4	1,8	1,8	3,5
3	9	19	3	0	3,0	4,2	3,6	3,0	2,4	1,8	2,6
4	9	18	4	0	3,0	4,8	2,4	2,4	2,1	2,0	3,2
5	7	30	6	3	6,0	3,6	3,0	2,4	1,5	1,8	3
6	8	26	4	0	3,6	5,4	3,6	2,1	2,1	2,1	4
7	6	24	7	1	4,8	5,4	3,6	2,4	2,7	1,8	3,5
8	9	20	6	1	4,2	4,8	3,6	2,4	1,5	1,8	3,2
9	8	27	6	0	5,4	4,2	3,0	2,4	1,8	1,7	3,5
10	9	21	3	0	3,0	5,4	3,6	3,0	2,7	1,7	2,8
AM	7,8	22,6	4,7	0,8	4,06	4,74	3,3	2,52	2,1	1,83	3,22
S					1,15	0,6	0,42	0,3	0,45	,0,13	0,42
Control group (n = 15) AM					3,35	4,65	3,92	3,24	2,51	2,46	2,22
S					1,06	0,77	0,68	0,5	0,36	0,25	0,25
Significance					n.s.	n.s.	p<0,01	p<0,001	p<0,02	p<0,001	p=0,000

Table 1: Clinical and neuroradiological results.

Diagnosis of Vertebrospinal Vascular Malformations: 10 Years of Experience

J. Stojanović, A. Kamler, K. Čavka, A. Jušić, M. Šoštarko, N. Thaller, and A. Mandić

Introduction

Vertebrospinal AVMs are classified according to their clinical, topographic, pathoanatomic, and hemodynamic characteristics. Perman (1926), Töpfer (1928), Bailey and Bucy (1929), Junghanns (1932), Schmorl and Junghanns (1971), Djindjian et al. (1981), Stojanović et al. (1985), Laredo et al. (1986), Merland et al. (1987), Thron (1988), and many others gave descriptions of vertebral angioma based on standard rtg view radiographs, CT findings, and spinal angiography. Djindjan et al. (1981) classified vertebral angiomas into three types of vascular anomalies (A,B,C), mainly upon their angiographic appearance. Laredo et al. (1988) and Merland et al. (1987) divided vertebral angiomas into a group with and a group without symptoms. Extension into the spinal canal can be expected in the group with symptoms. Owing to the above-mentioned criteria, differentiation between clinically silent vertebral angiomas and those responsible for spinal cord compression is possible.

Recently, Kendall and Logue (1977), Merland et al. (1980, 1987), Bradač et al. (1984), Riche et al. (1984), Gueguen et al. (1987), Thron (1988), and others classified spinal AVMs into four groups of AV disturbances: intramedullar AVMs, perimedullar intradural AV fistulas, meningeal AV fistulas, and extradural AVMs. The first three at these groups of AV disturbances are drained via intradural perimedullar veins, the last one via extradural vessels only. Merland et al. (1987) classified perimedullar intradural AV fistulas according to their morphological and functional properties into three types, mainly considering AV shunt volume. In terms of these criteria for the classification of vertebrospinal AVMs, our patients over a 10-year period included 102 with vertebral angioma, 52 with spinal AVMs, 13 with complex vertebroparavertebral AVM, and 4 with spinal hemangioblastoma.

Patients and Methods

The study included 171 treated patients; their follow-up was performed in the Radiology Department, KBC University of Zagreb, and
SIT, Zagreb, in the period 1978-1988. The age of patients with vertebral angioma (65% women, 35% men) ranged from 18 to 72 years
(mean, 44.7). The age range of patients with spinal AVM (36.5%
women, 63.4% men) was 6-58 years (mean, 31.8).

Radiologic procedures included standard AP and lateral-view radiographs in all patients; myelography was performed in 101 patients
[we have recently been using Iohexol (Nycomed), for myelography
only]; CT was done in 97 and CT myelography in 75 patients. During
CT intravenous contrast application occurred in 62 cases, MRI was
performed in 2 patients, and spinal angiography in 141.

Results

Vertebral Angioma - Clinical Symptomatology. Angiomas were analyzed
according to regions and locations. In the cervical region angioma
was confirmed in 8, in the dorsal in 39, and in the lumbar in 55
patients. Their topographic distribution is presented in Table 1.

Table 1. Topographic distribution of
         116 angiomas in 102 cases

Cervical (n = 8)	Dorsal (n = 49)	Lumbar (n = 59)
C4 2	D3 2	L1 12
C5 2	D4 4	L1 17
C6 3	D5 4	L3 21
C7 1	D6 5	L4 6
	D7 3	L5 3
	D8 4	
	D9 6	
	D10 7	
	D11 6	
	D12 8	

The oligotopic location of vertebral angioma was most often in the
dorsal region. On the basis of clinical findings and results of
radiologic investigation we formed two groups of vertebral angiomas:

asymptomatic (64.7%) and symptomatic (35.3%). In the first group
these were inbedded in the vertebral spongiosa, mainly in the body,
and in the latter group prominence from the vertebral border was
observed. On the basis of angiographic and hemodynamic criteria,
four types of angioma were formed: type A in 28.8%, B in 40.8%,
C in 18.2%, and D in 12.2% of cases. A capillary-venous barrier
was the predominant angiographic finding in type D. In the group
of patients with vertebral angioma, spinal angiography was performed in 66. Origin in the Adamkiewicz arteries was established;
in five patients this was at the angioma level (7.5%), and three
had it on the neighboring level (4.5%).

Spinal AVMs - Clinical Symptomatology. All patients with spinal
AVM complained, for some time, of pain in the vertebral region
and/or in the lower limbs. Paraparesis with sensor and sphincter
disturbances (in some cases in three or four extremities) was confirmed in 37 (7.11%), paraplegia in 11 (21.1%) cases. Subarachnoid
hemorrhage was reported in 19 cases (36.5%).

Spinal AVMs - Neuroradiologic Findings. Neuroradiologic methods
confirmed intramedullar AVM in 8 patients, perimedullar intradural
AV fistula in 15, meningeal AV fistula in 22, extradural AVM in 6,
and solitary aneurysm in 1 patient. In the group with perimedullar
AV fistula, aneurysm was confirmed in 4 patients. Spinal AVMs and
hemangioblastomal topographic distribution is presented in Table 2.

Table 2. Topographic distribution: 52 AVMs and 4 hemangioblastomatas

	Cervical	Dorsal	Lumbar
AVM			
Intramedullar	3	5	0
Perimedullar	2	9	4
Meningeal	3	12	7
Extramedullar	1	3	2
Aneurysm	1	0	0
Hemangioblastoma	1	2	1

Vertebroparavertebral (complex) AVM was confirmed in 13 patients: in
the cervical region one, in cervicodorsal three, in dorsal three, in
dorsolumbar four, and in lumbosacral two.

Discussion

Classification was made according to neuroradiologic, pathogenetic,
and therapeutic results, mainly considering operative and histologic
findings. Besides clearly defined typical vertebrospinal AVMs (presented in "Results") co-called "mixed" or subtypes were evident in
almost every group of AV disturbances and mainly in the first three.
Rarely, a metameric form of malformation was found. In four cases
there were AVMs complicated with irrigating artery aneurysm (two
cass with two and two cases with one aneurysm). Also, in one case we
isolated a solitary aneurysm on the dorsal branch of the vertebral
artery (Table 2). In three cases we discovered a very rare meningeal
AV anomaly in the distal cervical territory. One was probably of
traumatic origin since it appeared after the posterior arcus atlas
fracture (dorsal meningeal AV fistula between C1 and C2). It was
not operatively treated. Three months after trauma spinal reangio-
graphy was normal. Also, spontaneous regression of clinical symptomatology was evident. The last two cases with anomalies were surgically verified and treated.

Conclusion

Accepted neuroradiologic criteria for the classification of vertebrospinal AVM enable the differentiation of various vertebral and
spinal AVMs on the basis of their location, morphology, hemodynamic
properties, and taking in consideration their "activity," mainly
that of the vertebral angioma.

References

[1] Bailey P, Bucy PC (1929) Cavernous hemangioma of the vertebrae.
     JAMA 92: 1748-1751
[2] Bradač GB, Pöll W, Merland JJ (1984) Extradurale Angiome mit
     venöser perimedullärer Drainage. Neurochirurgia 27: 136-140
[3] Djindjian R. Merland JJ, Djindjian M, Stoeter P (1981) Angio-
     graphy of spinal column and spinal cord tumors. Thieme, Stutt-
     gart
[4] Gueguen B, Merland JJ, Riche MC, Rey A (1987) Vascular malfor-
     mations of the spinal cord: intrathecal perimedullary arterio-
     venous fistulas fed by medullary arteries. Neurology 37: 969-979
[5] Junghanns H (1932) Über die Häufigkeit gutartiger Geschwülste
     in den Wirbelkörpern (Angiome, Lipome, Osteome). Arch Klin Chir
     169: 204-212
[6] Kendall BE, Lgue V (1977) Spinal epidural angiomatous malforma-
     tions draining into intrathecal veins. Neuroradiology 13:
     181-189
[7] Laredo JD, Reizine D, Bard M, Merland JJ (1986) Vertebral
     hemangiomas: radiologic evaluation. Radiology 161: 183-189

[8] Merland JJ, Riche MC, Chiras J (1980) Les fistules arterio-
     veineuses intra-canalaires, extra-medullaires a drainage
     veineux medullaire. J Neuroradiol 7: 271-320
[9] Merland JJ, Reizine D, Assouiine E et al. (1987) Le mal-
     formazioni vascolari vertebro-midollari. In: Pistolesi Gf,
     Bergamo Andreis IA (eds) L'imaging diagnostico del rachide,
     Edizioni Libreria Cortina, Verona, pp 522-562
[10] Perman F (1926) On hemangiomata in the spinal column. Acta
     Chir Scand 61: 91-105
[11] Riche MC, Melki JP, Merland JJ (1983) Embolization of spinal
     cord vascular malformations via the anterior spinal artery.
     AJNR 4: 378-381
[12] Riche MC, Reizine D, Melki JP, George B, Rey A, Merland JJ
     (1984) Treatment of vascular malformations of the spinal cord.
     Surg Rounds 60-75
[13] Schmorl G, Junghanns H (1971) The human spine in health and
     disease. Grune & Stratton, New York
[14] Stojanović J, Papa J, Buljat G, Tetičković E, Bradač GB (1985)
     Ein Beitrag der spinalen Angiographie zur Diagnostik eines
     Wirbelangiomas. Fortschr Röntgenstr 141: 348-350
[15] Thron AK (1988) Vascular anatomy of the spinal cord. Neuro-
     radiological investigations and clinical syndromes. Springer,
     Vienna New York
[16] Töpfer D (1928) Zur Kenntnis der Wirbelangiome. Frankfurt Z
     Pathol 36: 337-345

Pathophysiology of Spinal Dural Arteriovenous Fistula: A Hemodynamic Approach

W. Hassler, E. H. Grote, and A. Thron

Introduction

Dural arteriovenous fistulas (AVFs) are lesions with a meningo-radicular extraldural feeder. The fistula is located in the dural layer, and venous drainage is always intradural on the surface of the spinal cord. The special symptoms, such as slowly progressive myelopathy and mixed peripheral and central nervous disturbances, are said to be a cause of high venous pressure, with ischemia due to venous congestion and stagnation, with reduced arteriovenous pressure gradient and therefore reduced intramedullary blood flow. As no one had yet measured flow and pressure in these malformations, we have done these investigations.

Material and Methods

Among 25 operated cases we performed intraoperative measurements in eight cases. We measured venous pressure before and after fistula occlusion as well as flow velocity in fistula-feeding and -draining vessels. The flow velocity of spinal cord supplying arteries were measured before and after fistula occlusion, as was the CO_2 response of spinal cord arterioles. Flow velocity measurement was done with a mini-doppler probe (Microvascular Doppler ultrasonograph model MT 20, EME, Überlingen, FRG) with a diamter of 1 mm. The pressure measurements were done with a small needle (0.45×13 mm) in the proximal part of the draining vein; with an aneurysm clip the feeder was occluded so that stump pressure could be recorded.

Results

Feeders of fistulas had a high flow, but not as high as in cerebral angioma feeders. They often showed low end-diastolic flow velocities as a sign of an increased vascular resistance, even in the presence

of downstream AVF, thus proving disturbed venous outflow from the
spinal canal. Flow velocity increased at the location of fistulas
and decreased in the draining vein with its wide diameter. The flow
in the draining vein decreased with distance to fistulas (Fig.1).

Flow velocity in the small spinal cord supplying artery was low.
The venous flow was typically breathing dependent. After occlusion
of the fistula, flow velocity in the feeder was zero, and in the
draining vein flow velocity was very low, in most cases also zero.
In a special case, one radiculomeningeal feeder originated from
the fistula, and at the same level there also originated a spinal
cord supplying artery. These arteries are so small in diameter that
they cannot be seen on angiography. In embolization procedures they
may also be occluded. After fistula occlusion flow velocities rose
in spinal cord supplying arteries and veins.

Pressure in the draining vein of a spinal dural AVF was high, about
61%-87% of systemic arterial pressure. After fistula occlusion,
pressure dropped markedly, with a rest pressure of 16%-60% of the
former fistula vein pressure (Table 1).

Some examples show the typical changes: In the first case the mean
pressure of the draining vein was 81 mmHg. After clip occlusion of
the distal part of the vein, stump pressure rose to 107 mmHg. Removing
the clip, the pressure dropped to the former value of 81 mmHg. After
occlusion of the fistula, the fistula vein pressure dropped to
23 mmHg. In a second case the fistula vein pressure was 54 mmHg;
after clip occlusion of the fistula it dropped to 9 mmHg. And in a
final case the pressure in the vein was 78 mmHg, 86% of systemic
arterial pressure. After occlusion of the fistula, the pressure
dropped to 35 mmHg. With clipping of the feeder the measurement
could be repeated with the same results (Fig.1).

In summary, we can conclude that the pressure drop after occlusion
of a high-flow fistula is more pronounced than that of low-flow
fistulas (Table 1).

We were very lucky to operate a case in which the fistula was near
the main spinal cord supplying the artery of Adamkiewicz. The dural
fistula lay at the level of the L1 segment of the right side, and
the artery of Adamkiewicz enters at the level of T12 on the left side.

The diastolic flow velocity of Adamkiewicz's artery was low, whereas
the diastolic flow velocity in dural feeders and drainers was high

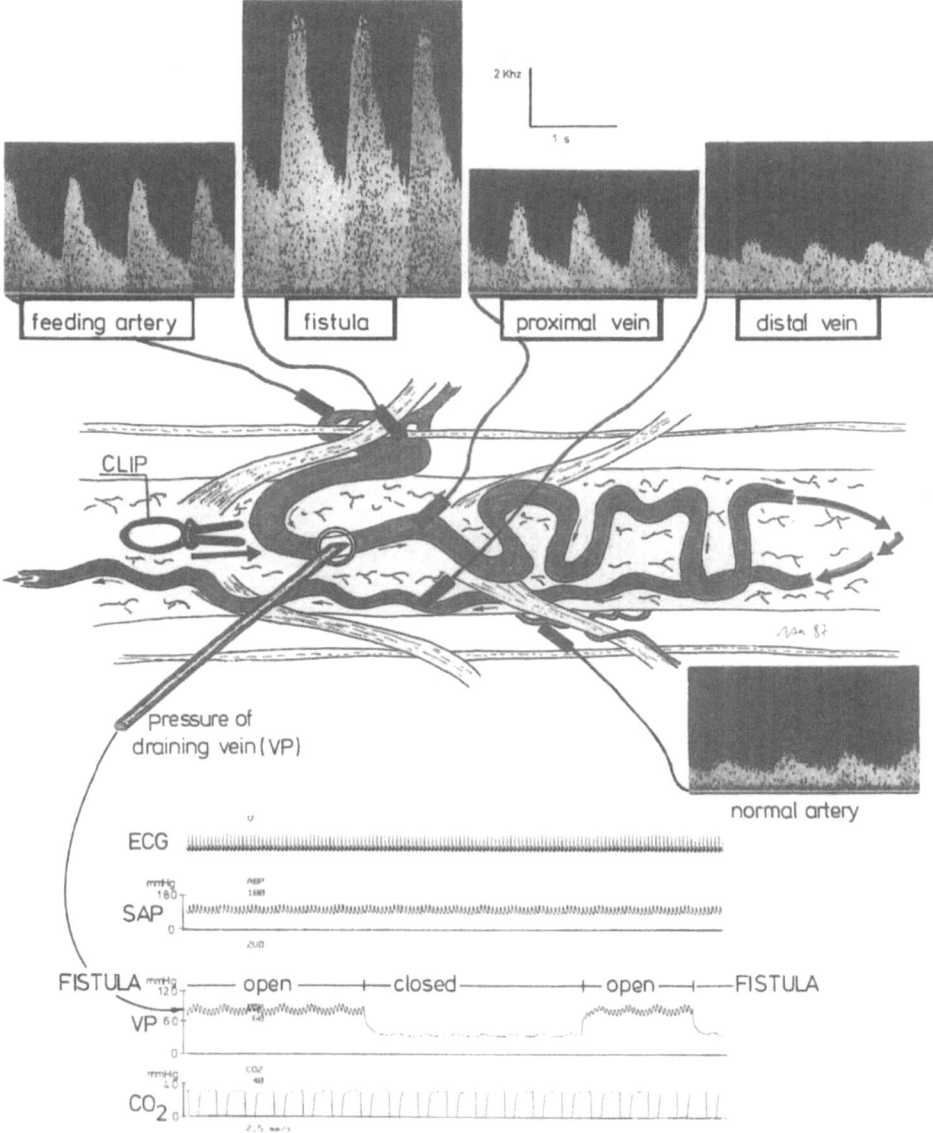

FLOW VELOCITIES AND PRESSURE IN DURAL ARTERIOVENOUS FISTULA

feeding artery   fistula   proximal vein   distal vein

CLIP

pressure of
draining vein (VP)

normal artery

ECG

SAP

FISTULA ——— open ——— closed ——— open —— FISTULA
VP

CO₂

Fig.1. Flow velocities and pressure in moderate-flow fistula system
and in normal spinal cord supplying vessels: at the site of maximal
pressure drop (fistula) the flow velocity is very high; in the draining vein with large diameter the flow velocity is low. With distance
to fistula the flow velocity in draining veins decreases. Small radicular spinal cord supplying arteries show a typical flow spectrum.
After occlusion of the fistula pressure in the draining vein drops
from 78 mmHg to mmHg (mean pressure)

Table 1. Venous pressures before and after removal of spinal dural AVF in relation to SAP and estimated shunt volume

Cases (name, sex, age)	Location of fistulas	Estimated shunt volume from angiography	SAP mmHg (mean)	Pressure in proximal part of draining vein			
				before removal mmHg (mean)	% of SAP	after removal mmHg (mean)	% of former vein pressure
W.A., F, 62	Th12/Li r	High	90	54	60	9	16.7
Q.E., M, 53	L2/Le l	High	90	55	61.1	9	16.4
R.E., M, 76	L1/L2 r	High	105	72	68.6	20	27.8
K.G., M, 62	Th6/7 r	Moderate	92	78	84.8	35	44.9
S.G., F, 67	Th10/11 l	Moderate	91	56	61.5	24	42.8
K.S., M, 52	Th8/9 r	Low	80	70	87.5	45	64.3
H.J., M, 72	Th12/L1 r	Low	90	70	77.8	37	52.8
S.E., F, 63	Th7/8 l	Low	67	54	80.6	22	40.7

(high flow lesion). After occlusion of the fistula flow velocity in Adamkiewicz's artery increased, and the flow output of the small venous vessels on the surface of the spinal cord also increased, as a sign of improved circulation.

In some cases we have done CO_2 reactivity tests of the flow velocity of spinal cord supplying arteries before and after fistula occlusion.

Before fistula occlusion the CO_2 response of the spinal cord supplying artery is good. After elevating CO_2 concentration to 60 mmHg, the flow velocity in Adamkiewicz's artery increased due to arteriolar dilatation. By hyperventilation and diminishing the concentration of CO_2 to 20 mmHg, the flow velocity decreased markedly as a sign of constriction of arterioles in the nervous tissue. After excision of the fistula the CO_2 reactivity did not change. This means that the vasomotoric response was not disturbed.

Conclusion

Our findings can be summarized as follows:

1. The venous pressure in a dural AVF is about 60%-90% of the systemic arterial pressure.
2. The fistula vein pressure changes with the systemic arterial pressure.
3. The pressure drop in high-volume or high-flow fistulas is higher than in low-flow fistulas after removal of the AVF.
4. After occlusion of the fistula no further flow is detectable in most cases in the draining veins, but after incision of the former draining vein a small retrograde bleeding is usually visible as a sign of venous drainage of the spinal cord in the fistula-draining veins.
5. The flow velocities in dural AVF-feeding and -draining veins are different and correlate with the angiographically estimated amount of shunt volume.
6. After occlusion of the fistula, flow velocity of the spinal cord supplying arteries rises, indicating improvement in circulation.
7. The CO_2 reactivity before and after AVF removal in spinal cord supplying arteries is normal, which means that the vasomotoric response (autoregulation) seems to be undisturbed.
8. The flow velocity in spinal cord supplying arteries is quite normal, so that proposed steal phenomena can be excluded.

Bibliography

[1] Aminoff MJ, Barnard RO, Logue V (1974) The pathophysiology of spinal vascular malformations. J Neurol Sci 23: 255-263
[2] Di Chrio G, Doppman JL, Ommaya AK (1971) Radiology of spinal cord arteriovenous malformations. Prog Neurol Surg 4: 329-354
[3] Hassler W (1986) Hemodynamic aspects of cerebral angiomas. Springer, Vienna New York
[4] Hassler W, Thron A, Grote E (1988) Hemodynamics of spinal dural arteriovenous fistulas. An intraoperative study. J Neurosurg
[5] Merland JJ, Riche MC, Chiras J (1980) Intraspinal extramedullary arteriovenous fistulas draining into the medullary veins. J Neuroradiol 7: 271-320
[6] Symon L, Kuyama H, Kendall B (1984) Dural arteriovenous malformations of the spine. Clinical features and surgical results in 55 cases. J Neurosurg 60: 238-247
[7] Thron A (1988) Vascular anatomy of the spinal cord. Neuroradiological investigations and clinical syndromes. Springer, Vienna New York

Cystic Necrosis in Compressive Cervical Myelopathy: A Comparison of Myelo CT and MRI

J. H. Faiss, G. Schroth, W. Grodd, B. Will, and E. Koenig

INTRODUCTION

Spondylotic stenosis of the spinal canal is a frequent phenomenon in elderly patients. Jeffreys (1986) reports that 75% of people over 65 years old show a narrowing of the cervical spinal canal. But only a minority of patients suffer from cervical myelopathy due to cervical stenosis. The results of neurosurgical treatment are not uniform and depend on the operation technique. In general, however, surgery has disappointed with regard to an improvement of clinical symptoms.

MATERIAL AND METHODS

Within a period from january 1986 to april 1988 34 patients suffering from cervical myelopathy due to spondylotic stenosis confirmed by X rays and myelography were examined by delayed high-resolution CT about 6-10 hours after myelography.

After surgical intervention 19 of our patients were examined for neurological dysfunction including neurophysiologic tests like SEP and EMG. Posturography, magnetic stimulation and MRI were also performed. In MRI T1-weighted (SE=600/15msec) sagittal and axial as well as flowcompensated axial T2-weighted (SE=3000/22/90msec) images were made, completed in some cases by gradient-echo sequences.

RESULTS

12 of our 34 patients showed bilateral collections of contrast medium within the myelon, portraying a double-barreled shape, as it is demonstrated in figures 1 and 2. This enhancement mostly extends cephalad of the level of maximal compression, less often in the caudal direction (see table 1).

	N
Group I	
Patients with intramedullary contrast medium	12
Group II	
Patients without intramedullary contrast medium	22

Table 1: Preoperative findings in myelo CT and patient groups.

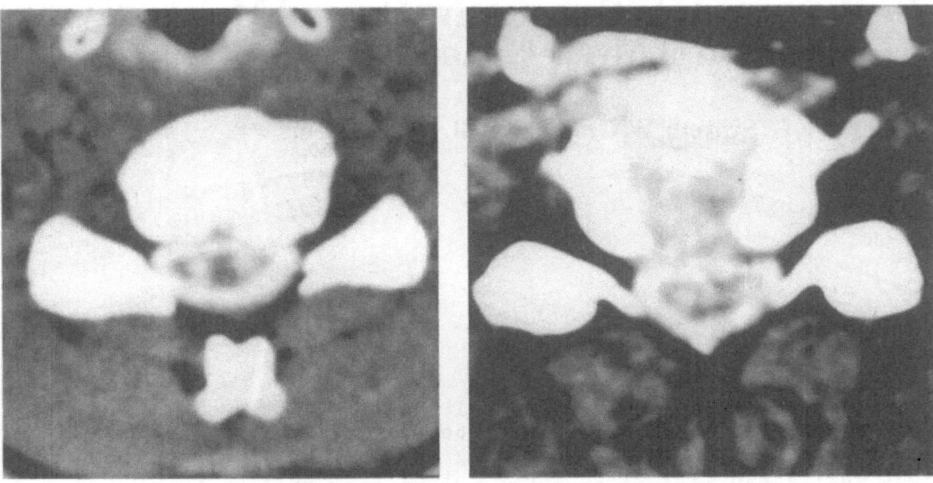

Fig.1 and 2: Intramedullary lesions demonstrated by myelo CT.

As in preoperative CT we were able to demonstrate the described
intramedullary lesions in postoperative MRI in 5 cases.
2 further patients which had no intramedullary lesions in preoperative CT, presented such lesion in postoperative MRI
(see table 2).

	With intramedul-lary lesions	No intramedul-lary lesions
Group I		
Patients with pre-operative intramedul-lary lesions (N=8)	5	3
Group II		
Patients without pre-operative intramedul-lary lesions (N=11)	2	9

Table 2: Postoperative findings in MRI

As a rule axial flowcompensated T2-weighted images displayed
the lesions as typical, bilateral, double-barreled regions of
increased signal intensity with a high degree of sensitivity
(see fig.3 and 4)

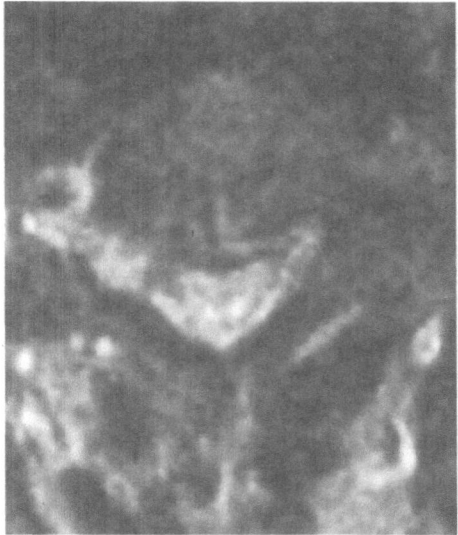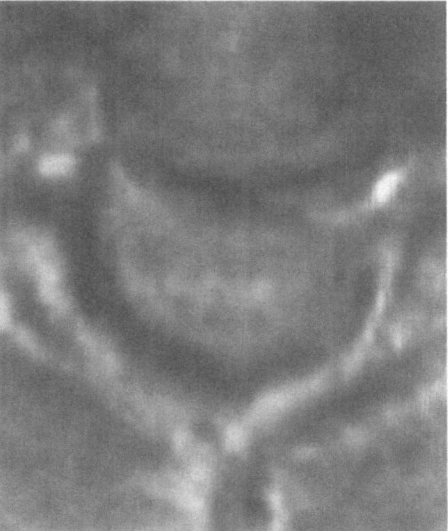

Fig.3 and 4: Intramedullary lesions demonstrated by MRI.

The postoperative clinical findings showed no significant
clinical improvement in most of the cases with intramedullary
lesions.

DISCUSSION

Delayed myelo CT has revealed intramedullary lesions developing
chronically near the level of compression from cervical
spondylosis (Jinkins et al. 1986, Al-Mefty et al. 1988, Mossman
and Jestico 1983). These lesions correlate with the cystic
necrosis present largely in the gray matter, as described by
pathologists (Stockdorph 1969).

We are now able to demonstrate these lesions in T2-weighted
MRI as regions of signal increase and as a low-intensity signal
in T1-weighted MRI (Macdonald et al. 1988, Al-Mefty et al.
1988, Quencer et al. 1986) with a high degree of sensitivity.

Central cystic necrosis of the spinal cord following trauma is
well-known. In the later stages of the disease a combination of
gliosis and edema can be found which finally may result in
syringomyelia due to progressive and regressive alterations. The
fact that our findings in patients with chronic compression of
the spinal cord resemble those of CT and MRI in syringomyelia
may suggest a similar pathogenesis of both conditions (Castillo
et al. 1988).

In studies on experimental canine cervical myelopathy, Hoff
(1977) demonstrated, that a combination of compression and
ischemia is cumulative in producing the severity of neurological deficits.Extreme compression first leads to a venous
compression and then to an occlusion of perforating arterioles
(Feldenzer et al. 1988, Kapadia 1984, Noble and Wrathall 1988).

Recently, Quencer et al. (1986), investigating the chronically inquired spinal cord, were optimistic regarding the ability of MRI to differentiate between myelomalacia and intramedullary cysts. They concluded that the difference in relaxation times between normal spinal cord tissue, myelomalacia and intramedullary cysts is the factor that allows MRI to be more accurate than delayed myelo CT in demonstrating the pathologic changes present in an injured cord.

Up to now, MRI and delayed myelo CT are complementary diagnostic method which may assist in determining the extent of spinal cord alterations and the prognosis for therapy in cases of spondylosis, spinal cord compression, spinal cord injuries and myelopathies of diverse etiologies.

REFERENCES

Al-Mefty O et al. (1988) Myelopathic cervical spondylotic lesions demonstrated by magnetic resonance imaging.
J Neurosurg 68: 217-222

Castillo M et al. (1988) Syringomyelia as a consequence of compressive extramedullary lesions: Postoperative clinical and radiological manifestations
AJR 150: 391-396

Feldenzer JA et al. (1988) The pathogenesis of spinal epidural abscess: Microangiographic studies in an experimental model
J Neurosurg 69: 110-114

Hoff JT et al (1977) The role of ischemia in the pathogenesis of cervical spondylotic myelopathy: a review and new micro-angiographic evidence.
Spine 2: 100-108

Jeffreys RV (1986) The surgical treatment of cervical myelopathy due to spondylosis and disc degeneration
Journal of Neurology, Neurosurgery and Psychiatry 49: 353-?

Jinkins JR et al. (1986) Cystic necrosis of the spinal cord in compressive cervical myelopathy: Demonstrating by Iopamidol CT-myelography
AJNR 7: 693-701

Kapadia SE (1984) Ultrastructural alterations in blood vessels of the white matter after experimental spinal cord trauma
J Neurosurg 61: 539-544

Macdonald RL et al. (1988) Microcystic spinal cord degeneration causing posttraumatic myelopathy: Report of two cases
J Neurosurg 68: 466-471

Mossman SS, Jestico JV (1983) Central cord lesions in cervical spondylotic myelopathy
J Neurol 230: 227-230

Noble LJ, Wrathhall JR (1988) Blood-spinal cord barrier disruption proximal to a spinal cord transection in the rat: Time course and pathways associated with protein leakage
Experimental Neurology 99: 567-578

Quencer RM et al. (1986) Magnetic resonance imaging of the chronically injured cervical spinal cord
AJNR 7: 457-464

Stockdorph O (1969) Pathologie des Rückenmarkes
In: Handbuch der Neurochirurgie Vol.7/1: 238-304.
Springer, Berlin, Heidelberg, New York

Contrast Enhanced MRI of Infectious Spondylitis

S. O. Rodiek, G. T. Werner, and G. Goede

INTRODUCTION

Unspecific infectious spondylitis is a potentially curable disease.In untreated cases it is frequently followed by a neurological deficit secondary to compression syndromes of spinal cord and nerve roots or severe axis deviation of vertebral column.Usually there is a rapid onset of symptoms including heavy dorsalgias,fever and an elevation of erythrocyte sedimentation rate.The disease was found to be responsible for low back pain in 0.4 % of 3000 patients,who consulted a medical rehabilitation department (Werner et al. 1988). In this paper typical MRI patterns of spondylitis before and after application of paramagnetic contrast agents are presented.Until now there have been only few communications on this topic (Reiser et al. 1986).

PATIENTS AND METHODS

MRI was performed in thirteen patients with infectious spondylitis and followed up in three cases.The studies were completed by plain films,spinal CT and radionuclide bone scans.MRI was performed with a superconductive 0.5 tesla MAGNETOM (SIEMENS AG, Erlangen).Typical examinations before contrast media administration were obtained from SE modes with TR 0.5/TE 30 and TR 1.6/TE 90. Gadolinium–DTPA enhanced images were applied in a TR 0.5/TE 30 SE mode. The administered dosage was 0.1 mmol/kg. After performance of TR/TE scans in sagittal plane for a topical orientation, inflamed spinal segments were examined with a surface coil in sagittal and axial slices.

RESULTS

On unenhanced T1–weighted scans acute spondylitis regularily exhibits a transdiscal signal decrease with a bivertebral extension,that does not exceed the contours of the distal endplates. On T1–weighted scans the affected segment is often found to be dilated in a barrel–shaped way due to a paravertebral subligamenteous spread of infection (Fig. 1a, 2a).The transdiscal signal void is a characteristic pattern of spondylitis.It is not noted in vertebral metastases,which also appear as areas of decreased signal intensity but typically spare the disc.Within the inflamed spinal region pathomorphological details like disc narrowing or bone destruction usually cannot be discriminated.
Additional information is supplied by T2–weighted images.In contrast to T1–weighted scans acute inflammation is recognized by a markedly increased signal intensity (Fig. 1b). At this stage a height reduction of disc,a simultaneous loss of contours of adjacent endplates and erosions of cancellous bone are observed.The intranuclear cleft of the intervertebral disc is no longer visualized. T2 signal intensity of normal discs in healthy individuals has a variable appearance which is influenced by the degree of hydration. With aging and in degenerated discs the loss of water content corresponds to a hypointense signal intensity as T2–weighting increases.

In these cases no interference with the bright signal caused by infected discs is noted. In younger patients,however,the normal disc hydration reveals a high signal intensity on T2-weighted images,which might interfere with the signal increase of inflamed discs (Fig. 2b).The diagnosis of discitis is then based alone on morpho-logical defects of postcontrast scans. Extravertebral spread of infection is a further common phenomenon,which is appreciated from a prevertebral and intraspinal bulging of the exudate with a displacement of hypointense anterior and posterior longitudinal ligaments. The detection of dural sac and cord compression on T2-weighted images might be obscured by isointensity of CSF and spinal cord with epi-dural exudate (Fig. 1b). Among a total number of thirteen patients the thoracic cord was found to be compressed in four,and the lumbar dural sac in seven cases. As could be seen from follow-up studies previous signal alterations fairly norma-lized with successful antibiotic therapy.

The IV administration of Gadolinium-DTPA was not followed by side effects.There is virtually no influence of paramagnetic contrast agents on the appearance of normal spine structures except a signal elevation of epidural veins,for instance within the basivertebral channel (Fig. 3b). In acute spine infection T1-weighted postcon-trast scans demonstrate a bright signal of involved spinal elements with a superior separation of anatomical details (Fig. 2c). Due to a low signal intensity of CSF an impingement of cord by exudate bulging is outlined more obviously than on T2-weighted scans (Fig. 1c). Concomitant inflammation of spinal muscles often concerns m. psoas. Myositic reactions present as muscular swelling and signal increase. Sclerotic bone reactions within the marrow are displayed as irregular borderlines of low intensity adjacent to the affected disc.This line is also obtained from T2-weighted scans but obscured on T1-weighted images (Fig. 1). At the subacute stage of spondylitis the application of contrast media effects only a mild signal increase.The normal bone marrow and diseased segments therefore will provide an isointense signal with a fogging effect on the infectious origin of the disease.

In conclusion the degree of highlightning following contrast agents application is a sensitive indicator of the activity of the inflammatory process. Residual lesions after spondylitis include collaps and fusion of vertebrae with hyperkyphosis of vertebral column or minor changes of cortical bone and discs which are all accurate-ly shown by MRI (Fig. 3).

DISCUSSION

In acute inflammatory processes the increased water content of tissue causes longer T1 and T2 relaxation times,which are proved highly sensitive by MRI (Stark and Bradley 1988).Infectious spondylitis is diagnosed from patterns of signal altera-tions and distribution of lesions,which are virtually characteristic and are not noted in neoplasms.This parallels experience of other authors (Brant-Zawadzki and Norman 1987). MRI turned out to be superior to other imaging techniques like plain films,CT or radionuclide studies (Modic et al. 1985) and was more definitive in the early detection of spinal abscesses (Angtuaco et al. 1987).MRI successfully docu-ments soft tissue involvement inside and outside the spine (Rodiek 1988). It also proves the activity of the disease,another important factor for therapy.The diag-nosis of acute spondylitis can already be made by using both,T1- and T2-weighted images.Contrast enhanced T1-weighted scans,however,turned out to display a more detailled pathology than without contrast.They also exhibit a better soft tissue resolution than T2-weighted scans with a better assessment of epidural exudate.In cases with normal disc hydration diagnosis of discitis is facilitated by postcon-trast scans.In the subacute forms of spondylitis the contrast agents might cause isointensity of inflamed and regular tissues,so that additional T1-weighted images are required to make the diagnosis.

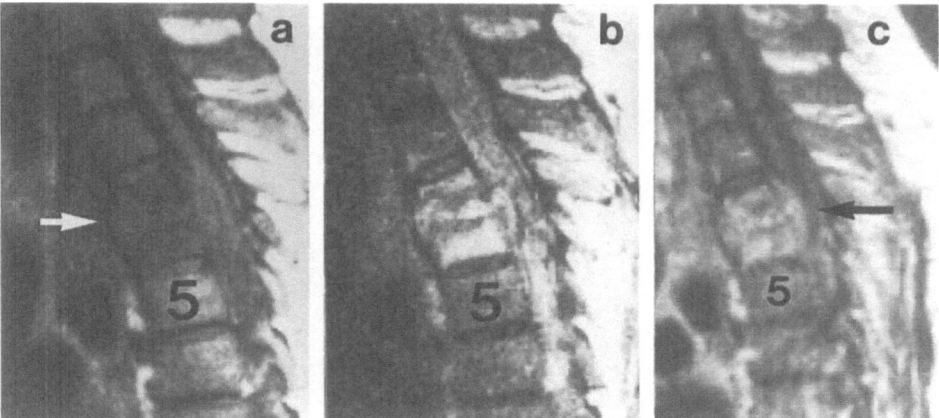

Fig. 1. Acute spondylitis of the thoracic spine
  a. TR 0.5/TE 30: Transdiscal signal decrease within the dilated segment
  b. TR 1.6/TE 90: High signal intensity confined by distal endplates
  c. Postcontrast scan: Better display of cord compression by epidural exudate

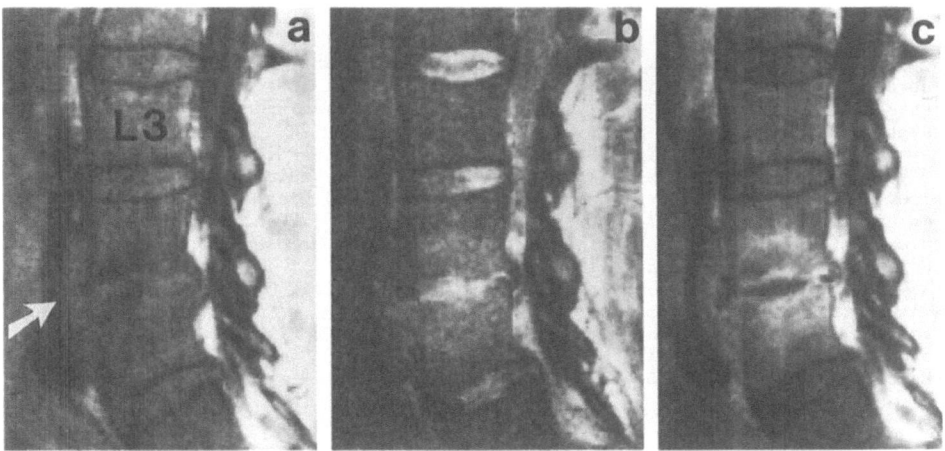

Fig. 2. Acute spondylitis of the lumbar spine
  a. TR 0.5/TE 30: Barrel-shaped segment without visualisation of vertebral contour
  b. TR 1.6/TE 90: High signal intensity of normal discs and inflamed segment
  c. Postcontrast scan: Superior exhibition of anatomical details compared with
     the other imaging modes

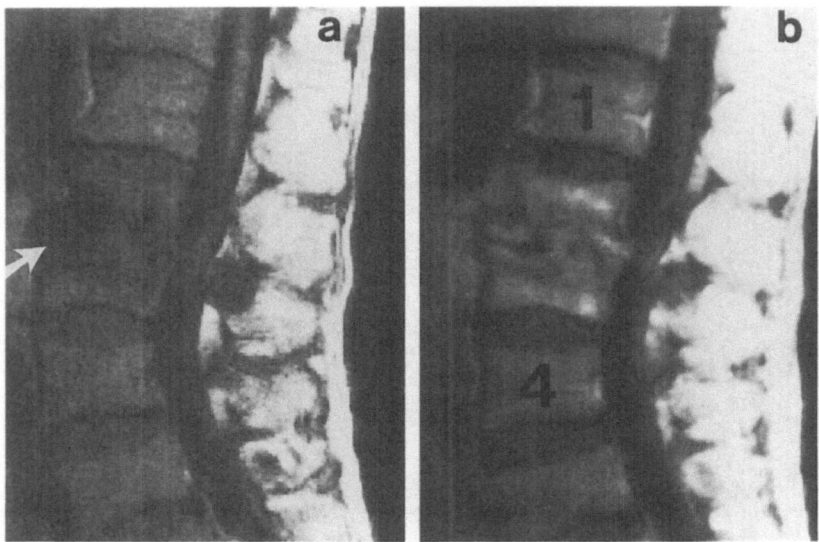

Fig. 3. Vertebral fusion following spondylitis
   a. TR 0.5/TE 30: Hypointense signal within the diseased lumbar segment
   b. Postcontrast scan: Superior discrimination of vertebral fusion and
      compression of the dural sac

REFERENCES

Angtuaco EJC, McConnell JR, Chadduck WM, Flanigan S (1987) MR imaging of spinal
   epidural sepsis. AJR 149:1249–1253
Brant-Zawadzki M, Norman D (1987) Magnetic resonance imaging of the central nervous
   system. Raven Press, New York, 315–319
Modic MT, Feiglin DH, Piraino DW, Boumphrey F, Weinstein PM, Duchesneau PM, Rehm S
   (1985) Vertebral osteomyelitis: assessment using MR. Radiology 157:157–166
Reiser M, Kahn Th, Weigert F, Lukas P, Büttner F (1986) Diagnostik der Spondylitis
   durch die MR-Tomographie. Fortschr. Röntgenstr. 145,3:320–325
Rodiek SO (1988) MR-Tomographie der unspezifischen infektiösen Spondylodiszitis.
   Fortschr. Röntgenstr. 148,4:419–425
Stark DD, Bradley WG,Jr (1988) Magnetic resonance imaging. C.V.Mosby, ST. Louis,
   Washington DC, Toronto, p 1364
Werner GT, Gadomski M, Goede G, Rodiek SO, Zwinck-Klas E (1988) Infektiöse
   Spondylitis – eine wichtige Differentialdiagnose beim Symptom "Rückenschmerz".
   Münch.med. Wschr. 130:456–458

MRI of Syringomyelia: Comparison of Pre-Postoperative Results with Clinical Symptoms

In pathology, *syringomyelia* (SM) is defined as a cavity of the spinal cord independent from the central canal, whereas *hydromyelia* has been reserved for dilatation of the central canal. Because, in most cases, it is impossible to differentiate these two entities syringohydromyelia or "syringomyelia in a generic sense" is used for both diseases, without implying a specific pathogenity.

MATERIAL AND METHODS

44 patients with intramedullary cavities of the spinal cord were examined with a 1,5 Tesla whole body imager (Siemens Magnetom). A quantitative evaluation was performed, using sagittal and axial T1-weighted spin echo images (SE/ 600ms/ 22ms) obtained in all patients and controls (N = 15). In addition, in 6 patients T2 values of the intramedullary fluid were calculated (CPMG-sequence, TR=2000ms, TE=30-480ms, linear regression of 16 echoes) and CSF motion was measured using ECG gated FLASH sequences (TR=75ms, TE=10ms, flip angle of 90 degree; analysis of magitude and phase). Intravenous GD-DTPA (Gadolinium-diethylenetriamine pentaacetic acid) was administered in a dosage of 0,1 mmol/kg to 16 patients.

RESULTS AND DISCUSSION

14 patients presented *accompanying intramedullary tumors* (5 astrocytomas, 2 ependymomas, 2 haemangioblastomas, 5 other tumors, not operatively proven). Preoperative administration of GD-DTPA displayed strong enhancement in all ependymomas and haemangiomas and was of great value in outlining solid tumoral masses of astrocytomas as well as in differentiating cyst and solid tumor. In low graded astrocytomas the enhancement was smaller or initially restricted to the margin of the tumor, followed by diffusion of the contrast agent into the cyst 30 to 60 min. later (Fig.3). In "idiopathic SM" neither enhancement of surrounding gliosis nor contrast diffusion into the cyst was detectable.

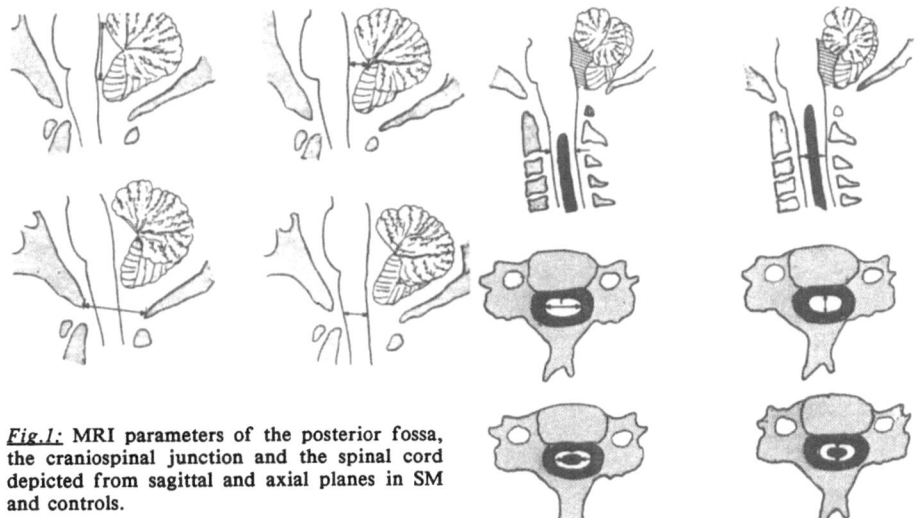

Fig.1: MRI parameters of the posterior fossa, the craniospinal junction and the spinal cord depicted from sagittal and axial planes in SM and controls.

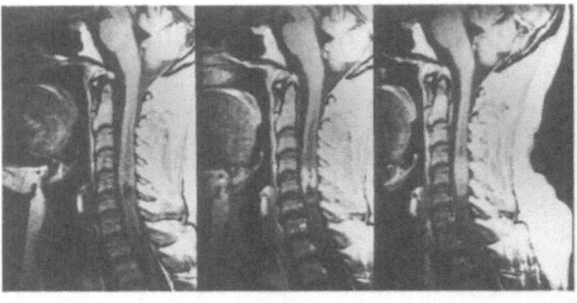

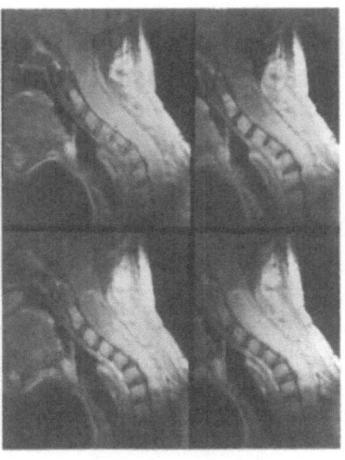

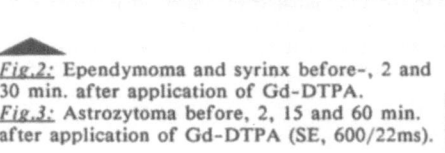

Fig.2: Ependymoma and syrinx before-, 2 and
30 min. after application of Gd-DTPA.
Fig.3: Astrozytoma before, 2, 15 and 60 min.
after application of Gd-DTPA (SE, 600/22ms).

4 patients had formerly suffered a *trauma with compression fractures* of vertebral bodies within the syrinx location. Arnold Chiari malformation (ACM) was not visible in this group as well as in the tumor associated group, but there was a striking similarity in the extension and MRI appearence of the cavities in all three groups.

27 patients did not have evidence of any preceding cause. In these patients quantitative evaluation was performed on the following parameters using a measuring circle and ruler (Rabone Chesterman Chrom Face No.27 R): position of the cerebellar tonsils compared to the level of the foramen magnum; sagittal diameter of the foramen magnum and medulla at the same level; size of the fourth ventricle, and maximal sagittal and transverse diameters of both syrinx and spinal cord in sagittal and axial cuts (Fig.1).

12/27 patients showed an Arnold Chiari malformation type 1. Thus, ACM may not be as frequent as reported by Gardner from operative evaluation (68 of his 74 cases).

Only one patient showed communicating SM with MRI visible (axial and sagittal planes) extension into the fourth ventricle (Fig.4). This patient, however, had no ACM, suffered from multiple intramedullary hemangioblastomas and showed no clinical signs suggestive of SM.

The diameters of the fourth ventricle, foramen magnum, and medulla were normal in all SM when compared to the control group.

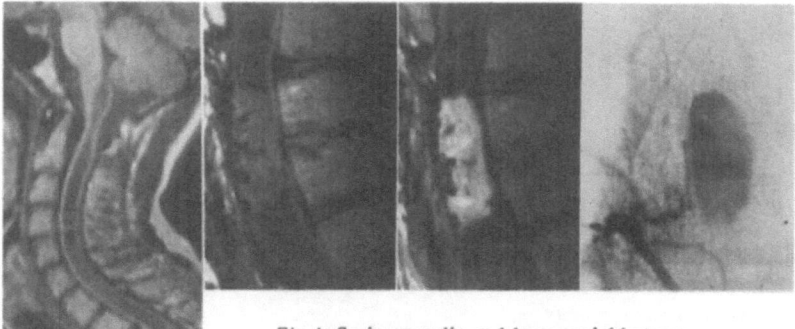

Fig.4: Syringomyelia and haemangioblastoma.
Left side: T1-weighted sagittal plane demonstrate the SM extension into the 4 ventricle. Right: One of two spinal haemangioblastomas before and after GD-DTPA (SE/400/30ms) and the corresponding angiography of the A.intercostalis TH 7.

Fig.5:

14/27 SM patients showed external cord diameters ranging within the normal limits even at the level of the maximal syrinx diameter, which was in almost all SM located between the cervical level C2 and C5. These would most probably present a normal myelogram, perhaps simulating a pronounced, physiological intumescentia cervicalis.

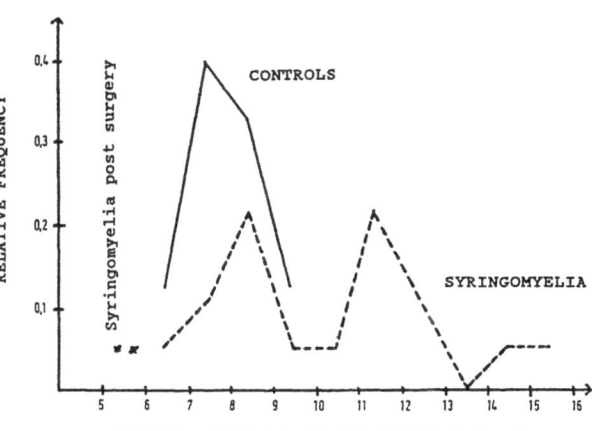

SAGITTAL DIAMETER OF THE SPINAL CORD (mm)

Only in about one third of the patients did the cranial SM extension correlate +- one segment with the most cranial neurological segment. As a rule, the cranial extension on MRI reaches two or three segments above the clinical level.

On axial MRI-planes all 8 syringes, examined postoperatively after insertion of a syringo-subarachnoid shunt, demonstrated a collapse in the anteroposterior direction, resulting in a transversely oriented, strongly oval shape, which remained unchanged on controls later on (follow up in MRI up to 4 years). This may be explained by the lateral fixation of the collapsing cord by the denticulate ligaments (Fig. 6). Despite small residual intramedullary cavities, in 3 patients the external spinal cord diameters ranged postoperatively below the 95th percentile of normal controls, indicating a gliomatous atrophy of the surrounding spinal cord.

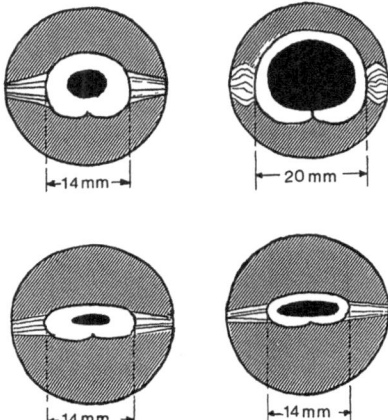

Fig.6: Shape of the spinal cord on axial MRI before (top) and after (bottom) shunt implantation. Whereas small cavities collaps in anteposterior direction only (left side), there is an additional reduction of the frontal diameter in large syringes, which may be explained by loosening of the denticulate ligaments.

There was no relationship between the maximal cyst diameter and clinical signs, independently determined using a patients disability and distress score. However it is noteworthy, that 5 patients, who were not operated on also showed strongly oval cavitations. All of them were most severely and chronically disabled by their disease, thus spontaneous collapse may be conceivable in these cases.

Postoperatively no improvement of clinical and neurophysiological signs (electromyography, evoked potentials from the tibial and median nerves) was detectable However, with respect to the impression of some patients, a slow down of the preoperative aggravation of the symptoms may be possible.

Compared with the spinal subarachnoidal spaces, intrasyringeal CSF flow (analysed by T2 changes and ECG gated FLASH images) is slight. Cardiac and respiration related CSF pulsations were detectable only in capillary columns connecting greater cysts.

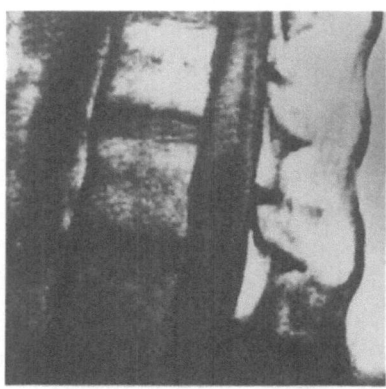 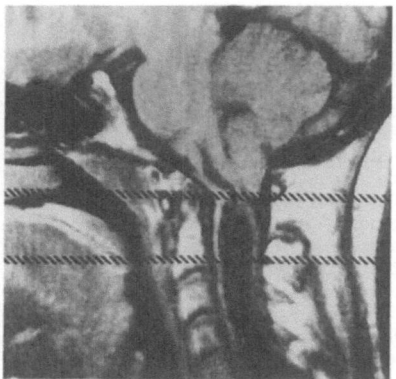

Fig.7 (left side): Capillary connection between large cavities in the thoracical and lumbar (conus medullaris) spinal cord. Cardiac related fluid motion was detectable inside the capillary cavity, therefore shunt implantation was performed into the cavity of the conus resulting in a collapse of the cervical and thoracical parts of the syrinx.

Fig.8 (right side): ACM associated Syringomyelia and -bulbia. Whereas cardiac related motion was detectable inside the capillary syringobulbia (despite an extension into the 4th ventricle could not be confirmed on axial planes) no motion was detectable in the syrinx cavity at level C2/3.

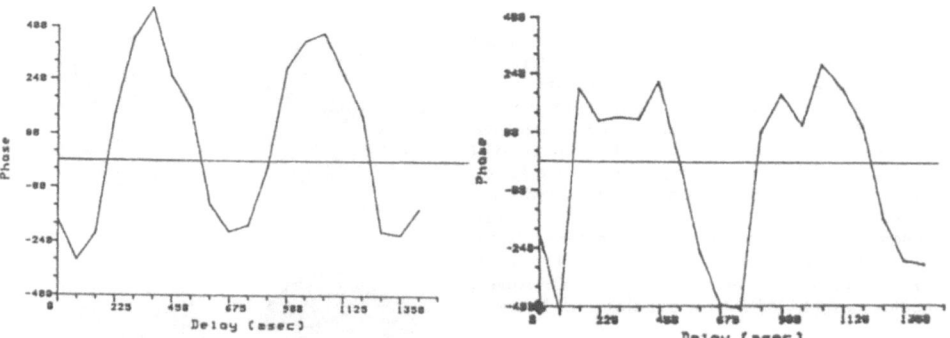

Fig.9: Plot of CSF motion as a function of R-wave delay of the ECG in the cerebral aqueduct (left) and the capillary extension of the Syrinx into the medulla oblongata (right) shown in Fig.8. Flow downwards is encoded as negative phase. The almost synchroneous oszillation of the syringeal fluid precedes the aquaeductal flow for about 50 msec, indicating that the syringeal pulsation can not be the result of pulsations of the ventricular system.

REFERENCES:

Du Boulay G.H. et al. (1974), Br.J. Radiol. 47: 579-587.
Gardner W.J. (1965), J. Neurol. Neurosurg. Psychiatry 28: 247-259.
Grant R. (1987), J. Neurol. Neurosurg. Psychiatry 50: 1008-1014.
Grant R. (1987), J. Neurol. Neurosurg. Psychiatry 50: 1685-1687.
Pojunas K. et al. (1984), Radiology 153: 679-683.
Schroth G. et al. (1988), Fortschr. Röntgenstr. 149: 23-29.
Scotti G. et al. (1984), J. Neuroradiol. 11: 239-248.
Sherman J.L. et al. (1986), AJNR 7: 985-995.
Steinmetz H. et al. (1988), Adv.Neurosurg.16: 206-210.
Tashiro K. et al. (1987), J.Neurol. 235: 26-30.
Tator et al. (1982), J. Neurosurg. 56: 517-523.
Yeates A. et al. (1983), AJNR 4: 234-237.

Low Flip Angle Gradient Echo MRI of the Cervical Spine at 0.3 Tesla

S. Holtås, F. Ståhlberg, E.-M. Larsson, and S. Cronqvist (Lund, Sweden)

Using the gradient echo technique in MR imaging of the cervical spine, the effect on contrast of changing flip angle and repetition time was evaluated in five volunteers. A 0.3 T Fonar β-3000 M scanner and solenoid surface coils were used in the study. Short TR/TE (300/12 msec) sequences with a flip angle of 10° provided the best contrast. CSF and discs had a high signal while cord, epidural space and vertebrae had a low signal. The image thus had the same myelographic appearance as on long TR/TE spin echo (SE) sequences, but could be obtained using a shorter acquisition time. Furthermore, it was possible to separate gray and white matter and no artifacts were caused by CSF pulsation. The limitation of the technique is the rather low signal/noise, which is, however, well compensated by the superior contrast. Ten patients with degenerative disease were studied with this technique and short TR/TE (300/16 msec) SE sequences. The low flip angle sequences were superior in visualizing narrowing of canal and compression of cord and it was in general easier to discriminate between bone and disc herniation. In five patients with lesions in the cord visualized on long TR/TE (2000/60 msec) SE sequences, the lesions were also visualized using the low flip angle gradient echo technique. In conclusion: 10° flip angle gradient echo (TR/TE 300/12 msec) sequences provides images with:

1. myelographic effect with separation of cord, CSF, epidural space, disc and bone,
2. separation of gray and white matter in the cord,
3. demonstration of lesions in the cord.

MRI Detection of Intramedullary Ischemia Due to Cervical Spondylosis

G. C. Dooms, P. Mathurin, G. Cornelis, and P. Hulcelle (Brussels, Belgium)

A retrospective study was performed to assess the value of MRI for detecting intramedullary ischemia due to cervical spondylosis and to assess its clinical significance. One hundred consecutive unselected patients (70 males and 30 females, mean age 62 years) were included in the study. All the patients were surgically treated, either by anterior discectomy and corporectomy or by posterior laminectomy. Clinical follow up for up to 2 years was available for every patient. MR was performed with a superconducting magnet Philips Gyroscan S15 operating at 1.5 Tesla. Sagittal T1 weighted (TR = 0.45 sec and TE = 30 msec) and cardiac gated T2 weighted (TR ≥ 1.2 sec and multiple TE of 50, 100, 150 and 200 msec) images were obtained in every patient. Cervical spondylosis was exquisitely demonstrated by MRI in every patient. By using the sagittal plane, its full extent and the degree of canalar stenosis was easily appreciated on T2 weighted images. A hyperintense intramedullary lesion was detected preoperatively in 24 of the patients and corresponded presumably to ischemic, edematous and/or necrotic damage to the cord. It was usually located at the level or just below the level where the most severe canalar stenosis was demonstrated; it was identified only on T2 weighted images. By comparing the clinical outcome of the patients after surgery, there was a striking difference between the groups of patients without and with intramedullary lesions. In the first group, the remission of symptoms surgery was partial or complete. In the other group, the clinical outcome was poor and remission of symptoms nearly absent. In conclusion, MRI is a sensitive modality for demonstrating necrotic intramedullary changes due to cervical spondylosis which may be a prognosis factor concerning the surgical results and clinical outcome of the patients.

Computer Aided Analytic Morphometry of Posterior Intervertebral Articulations

P. D'Aprile, G. Farchi, V. Pesce Delfino, and A. Carella

INTRODUCTION

The articular apophyses contribute to the posterior intervertebral articulation through the facet joints. The interapophysal articulations are flat arthrodies that allow a limited sliding movement. The spatial arrangement of the facet joints depends on the vertebral tract considered in light of its functional role. Many studies on the orientation of the facet joints are to be found in medical literature(N. Hermanus 1983, J.P.J. Van Schaik 1985).
However, a field of study as yet relatively unexplored is that relating to the possibility of evaluation of curvature and morphology of the facet joints.
To this end the S.A.M.(Shape Analytical Morphometry) work station was used since it affords real-time images from the C.A.T.(compterized axial tomography) either via TV camera or through direct link-up.

DESCRIPTION

The profiles of the facet joints (Fig. 1) were digitized by a semi-automatic procedure aided by a program for manual outline tracing where a light point is guided round the profile under examination on a screen. The result obtained is a file of points of known co-ordinates.
Before being digitized, every profile undergoes both standardization and normalization (Fig. 2).
Standardization in this research was effected by placing the extreme points of the profile vertically so that the first and last points present the same abscissa value. Dimensional normalization allows us to present the profiles each with the same number of luminous points modifying the image enlargement so that the profile is described in 190 points. This procedure guarantees the possibility of confrontation evidencing differences exclusive to shape. The analytic procedure which the files thus obtained then undergo includes a few stages.
 The first stage is the description of the so-called fundamental form through the use of high level polynomial equations. The coefficients of the equation are calculated according to the "lowest squares" method.

$$y = b_k x^k + b_{k-1} x^{k-1} + \ldots\ldots\ldots + b_3 x^3 + b_2 x^2 + b_1 x + b_0$$

Once all contours of the descriptive polynomial equation have been determined a new curve, a "fundamental" curve is obtained; it depicts the function curve of the original profile with respect to which the "smoothing" effect will be clearly evident(Fig. 3). The two curves - the original and the fundamental - are compared and from their file match many parameters are available the most sensitive and synthetic of which is represented by the square root of the mean quadratic error. In practice translation of one profile with respect to the other is carried out until the point which corresponds to the minimum distance between them is found (Fig. 4).

The second stage of the analytic procedure is represented by Fourier's harmonics analysis which in its classic form examines every profile as an irregular curve obtained by summing up sinusoids of different amplitudes, period and phase that represent the harmonics of the function data. The typical Fourier function may be described as:

$$y = a_0 + a_1 senx + b_1 cosx + a_2 sen2x + b_2 cos2x + \ldots a_k senkx + b_k coskx$$

Thus, what happens in practice is that each profile is analized in terms of sinusoidal components to the sum of which the curve under examination will correspond. The maximum number of evaluable harmonics for the normalization used is 94 (Fig. 5).

The third stage of the analytic procedure is based on the so-called "Janus" ("Giano") method named after the two-faced Roman god. The method is used especially in order to evaluate the degree of symmetry of the left and right facet joints (Fig. 6). The comparison is rendered visually by the parabola that forms between the two.

CONCLUSIONS

In the first phase of research – aimed at testing the applicability of such procedures to the study of computerized tomography – comparative evaluations were carried out between each articular facet and its counterlateral, a valuation for general classification purposes. The analytic instruments used turned out to be sensitive means describing the form of the articular facets examined.

The possibility offered by the various types of parameters suggests further applications towards individualizing pathogenetic mechanisms able to cause different anomalies in the behaviour of the said contours and of studying the incidence of such pathologies.

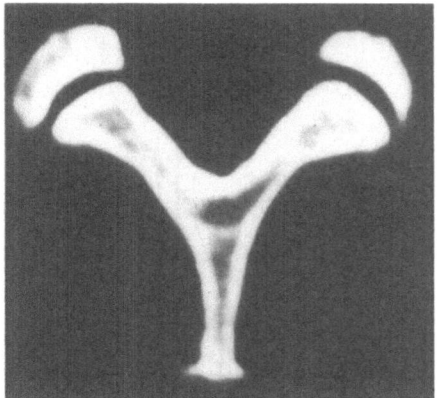

Fig.1 . Axial CT scan at L4-L5 level showing clearly articular profiles.

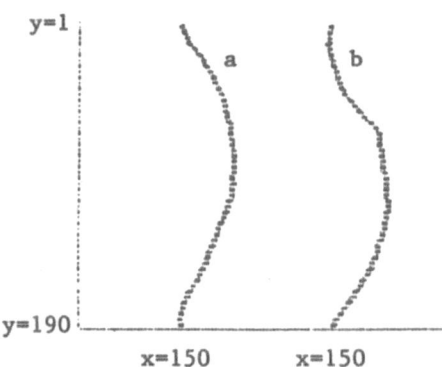

Fig.2 . Extreme points of the profiles are placed vertically and present the same abscissa value(standardization), each profile is described in 190 points (dimensional normalization)

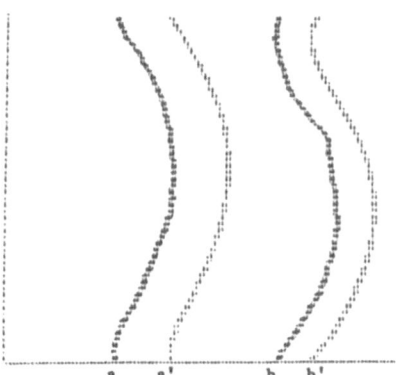

Fig.3 . Comparison between original curves(a and b) and the curves described by polynomial functions (a' and b'):smoothing effects are clear

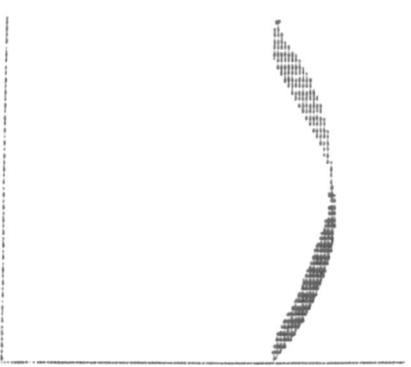

Fig.4 . Translation was carried out to reach the point which corresponds to the minimum distance between the two profiles

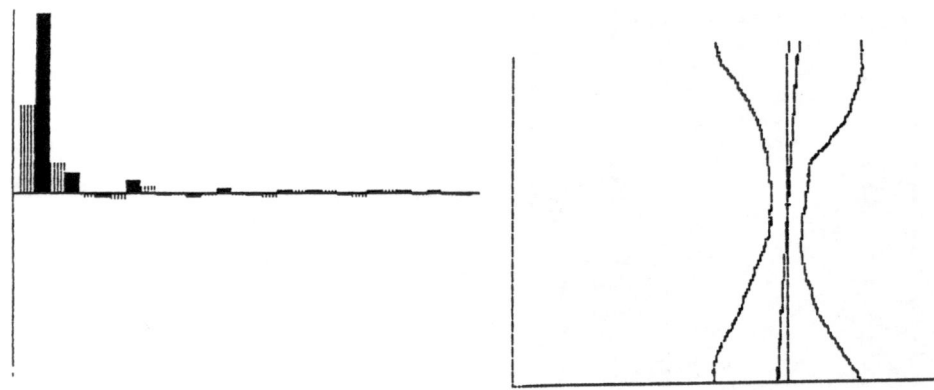

Fig.5 . Graphic representation of
Fourier spectrum

Fig.6 . "Janus"(Giano) comparison
is visualized by the parabola that
forms between the two curves

REFERENCES

Carrera GF (1980) Lumbar Facet Joint Injection in Low Back Pain and Sciatica.
   Radiology 137:661–667.
Carrera GF, Williams AL, Haughton BM (1980) Computed Tomography in Sciatica.
   Radiology 137:433–437.
Hermanus N, De Becker D, Baleriaux D, Hauzeur JP (1983) The Use of CT scanner for
   the study of Posterior Lumbar Intervertebral Articulations. Neuroradiology 24:
   159–161.
Pesce Delfino V, Ricco R (1985) Morfometria Analitica nello studio di forme biolo-
   giche: illustrazione della procedura e di soft-ware dedicato. Pathologica 77:
   77–86.
Van Schaik JPJ, Verbiest H, Van Schaik FDJ (1985) The Orientation of Laminae and
   Facet Joints in the Lower Lumbar Spine. Spine, vol 10, 1:59–63.
Van Schaik JPJ, Verbiest H, Van Schaik FDJ (1985) Morphometry of Lower Lumbar
   Vertebrae as seen on CT scans: newly recognized characteristics. AJR 145:327.

Spinal Cord Puncture: Diagnostic and Therapeutic Aspects

D. Tampieri, D. Melanson, and R. Ethier

ABSTRACT

Previous reports on spinal cord puncture (SCP) have stressed the usefulness of this procedure to differentiate cystic tumours from syringomyelia. Myelocystography with gas and/or positive contrast has been found a valuable technique of outlining the medullary cyst completely. The advent of MR imaging has decreased the need to use this technique, but we have found it still useful in certain circumstances for understanding cysts and their physiopathology. The aim of this paper is to report our personal experience with this technique on 77 punctures both for diagnostic and therapeutic purposes.

MATERIALS AND METHODS

46 patients harboring intramedullary cystic lesions of the spinal cord underwent spinal cord puncture in our Institute over the past 17 years. 28 patients were suffering from syringomyelia while 18 patients had an intramedullary tumour. A total number of 77 spinal cord punctures were carried out since 17 patients underwent more than one procedure. The punctures were performed under fluoroscopic control using a 2 needle set (25G and 20G) or a single needle (22G) when the cyst was expected larger. In several cases (16 patients), after removal of the fluid, an injection of dye was done for diagnostic purposes.

TECHNIQUE

The spinal cord puncture (SCP) is carried out under fluoroscopic control with the patient lying in prone position. Two different sets of needles may be used in accordance with the expected size of the cyst. When the cyst appears to be small, we use a 2 needle set, the leader needle being a 2 1/2 inches length and 20 Gauge diameter and the inner needle a 3 1/2 inches and 25 Gauge. The approach is posterior between the spinous processes; the leader needle is inserted on the midline as vertical as possible and is advanced to the CSF space.

Then the inner needle is introduced and advanced; eventually the
patient can experience some paresthesias in the trunk or the legs
when the needle passes in between the posterior columns of the
spinal cord. In order to stabilize the inner needle within the
leader a small rubber stopper may be used. Under fluoroscopic
control the tip of the inner needle is advanced in the center of
the spinal canal. Then the stylet is removed, a small plastic tube
is connected and gentle aspiration is performed in order to
facilitate the fluid collection. Sometimes, because of the
pressure, there is a spontaneous flow of the fluid and no
aspiration is required. If the intramedullary cyst is known to be
of a large size only a 3 1/2 inc. 22G. needle is used.

RESULTS

Syringomyelia

The 28 patients of our series with syringomyelia underwent 37 SCPs
since 9 of them were submitted to 2 procedures. The SCP allowed
aspiration of fluid in 25 of 28 cases. In all these cases but one,
the fluid aspirated was clear because of the low protein content.
In only one case the fluid aspirated was yellow. Since this group
of patient was investigated before the advent of MRI, the SCP had a
main diagnostic role. In fact, the aspiration of clear fluid, its
chemical and cytological analysis and the injection of dye allowed
the diagnosis of syringomyelia. Contrast medium was injected in 15
out of 25 cases. After the injection the patient is tilted in
Trendelbourg and anti-Trendelbourg positions and under fluoroscopic
control the movements of the contrast are evaluated. Usually the
dye moves freely within the cavity which extends to the two
extremities of the spinal cord. The syringomyelic cavity presents
a beaded appearance and sometimes double cavities were observed
(Fig. 1). In no case we were able to demonstrate the passage of
the dye from the spinal cord cavity to the 4th ventricle, through
the obex. The SCP failed to be therapeutic in this group of
patients. In fact in no case a subjective or objective relief of
symptoms was observed.

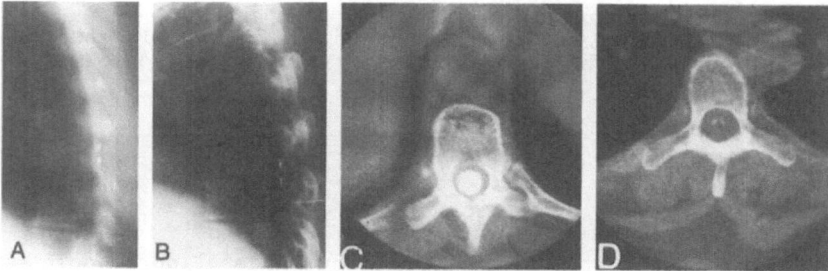

Fig. 1. Tomogram after myelogram (a), in a patient previously
treated with electrods implant at T8-T9 level shows enlargement of
the spinal cord below T9. The intramedullary cyst is punctured (b)
at T9 level. The CT after myelocystography demonstrates a large
cavity below the electrods level (c) and a double cavity above (d).
The latter one extends up to the cervical level. These findngs are
consistent with acquired syringomyelia.

Intradural intramedullary tumours

The group of intramedullary tumours is represented by 18 patients who underwent 40 SCPs. In this group of patients the SCP reached its two main goals: the diagnostic and the therapeutic. The aspect of the fluid and its cytological analysis associated with the appearance of the cyst allowed the diagnosis of intramedullary tumour. The fluid aspirated had a yellow-amber appearance because of the high protein content. In order to assess the walls of the cyst, contrast was injected in 2 patients. In both cases the cyst presented as an irregular cavity of limited extension (Fig. 2). Since the SCP permitted the aspiration of fluid in 8 patients, the procedure was repeated several times in order to obtain a relief of the symptomatology. Usually the improvement occured immediately after the SCP, and lasted for a mean of 6 weeks. A 62 year old male, with cystic cervical ependymoma, underwent 10 SCPs with improvement, starting usually within an hour after the procedure and persisting for 2-3 weeks. In all cases, improvement was noted within the next 24 hours.

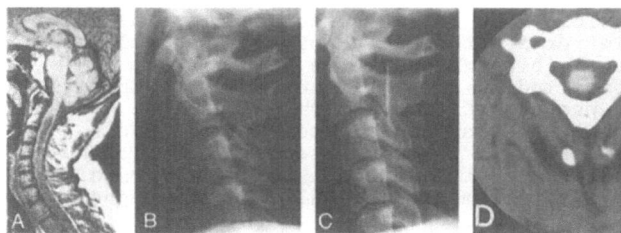

Fig. 2. T1-weighted image (TR 400, TE 30) of a 32 year old man harboring a cystic astrocytoma (a). The upper portion of the cyst is punctured at C3 level (b) and 1cc of Omnipaque 180 is used to outline the anterior surface of the cyst which appears to be irregular (c). Later the CT documents the cervical cyst (d).

COMPLICATIONS

In no case of our series transitory or permanent complications related to the SCP were observed. Before the advent of MRI, in 10 patients with intramedullary tumours, the SCP failed the fluid aspiration; we assumed that the needle was placed in a solid part of the tumour. In spite of that no worsening of symptoms occured in this group of patients. In order to prevent hemorrhagic accidents or intradural hematomas the needle must be on the midline to avoid the two postero-lateral spinal arteries. The tip of the needle has to reach the center of the spinal canal but any further advance must be gentle to stay away from the anterior spinal artery. The only complication we ever observed was related to an inadvertent intramedullary injection of 6cc of Metrizamide 180 in a lumbar syringomyelic cavity during a myelogram.
The patient presented acute paraplegia which progressively resolved within 48 hours. In our opinion the paraplegia was due to the toxic effect of a large amount of dye in the spinal cord and not to the puncture itself.

DISCUSSION

Several descriptions of SCP, using different approaches, have been done since the first procedure by Vitek in 1928 (Vitek 1928). In the past, mainly because of the lack of possibilities offered by the imaging, the literature (Westberg 1966) stressed the two main goals of the SCP: the diagnostic and therapeutic.
The chemical, microbiological and cytological analysis of the fluid and the myelocystography allowed the differential diagnosis between syringomyelia and intramedullary tumours (Ellertsson 1969; Quencer et al 1976). Since the advent of MRI, the role of the SCP has changed dramatically giving new perspectives to this procedure. In fact, while the diagnostic aspect has almost disappeared, the therapeutic one has increased its potentiality in patients with intramedullary cystic tumours. The site of puncture, which represented a laborious choice (Quencer 1980), is early detected by MRI because of the possibility to distinguish between the cystic and solid parts of the tumour. In fact, because of the long T1 and T2 relaxation times of the fluid, the cyst is nicely demonstrated and one or multiple sites of aspiration may be chosen. The removal of fluid improves the objective and subjective symptoms in the patient without complications. In patients who received multiple SCPs, we observed a relief of symptoms which progressively lasted less because of the irreversible damage of the spinal cord eventually occured. These findings lead to the fact that the cyst plays a main role in the production of the clinical picture distinct from that of the coexisting solid tumour (Booth and Kendall 1970). Moreover, MRI is a practical tool for the follow-up of these patients. Whenever the patient complains of a worsening associated with a larger cyst documented by MRI, the SCP represents a useful and recommended procedure. Finally, we think that the possibility to inject anti-neoplastic drugs within the cavity, after the fluid removal, opens new perspectives for the treatment of intramedullary tumours.

REFERENCES

Booth AE, Kendall BE (1970) Percutaneous aspiration of cystic lesions of the spinal cord. J Neurosurg, vol 33, No 2: 140-144.

Ellertsson AB (1969) Syringomyelia and other cystic spinal cord lesions. Acta Neurol Scand, vol 45, no 4: 403-417.

Quencer RM, Tenner MS, Rothman LM (1976) Percutaneous spinal cord puncture and myelocystography. Radiology 118: 637-644.

Quencer RM (1980) Needle aspiration of intramedullary and intradural extramedullary masses of the spinal canal. Radiology 134: 115-126.

Vitek J (1928) Dorsal puncture of syringomyelic cavities. Diagnostic injection of Lipiodol into cavities (Jirasek method) Casop Lek Cesk 67: 201-205.

Wesberg G (1966) Gas myelography and percutaneous puncture in the diagnosis of spinal cord cysts. Acta Radiol suppl 252: 1-67.

Clinical Relevance of Surface Coil Images Corrected by Homomorphic Filtering

F. E. Zanella, H. Lanfermann, W. Steinbrich, and J. Bunke

INTRODUCTION

Surface coils in MRI have the advantage of a high signal to noise ratio in the region of interest near to the surface coil (1,2). Their disadvantage is considerable variation in sensitivity over the measured object, resulting in intensity inhomogeneities in the acquired MR image. As a consequence tissues at moderate depth suffer from considerable sensitivity and contrast fall-off (Fig. 1a).

Clinically this is particularly disadvantagous, when the object of interest lies at moderate depth, as for instance the optic nerve or parts of the spinal canal.

It is desirable that contrast is chiefly determined only by T1 and T2 differences and not affected by such a sensitivity fall-off. This can be achieved by applying homomorphic filtering (Fig. 1b).

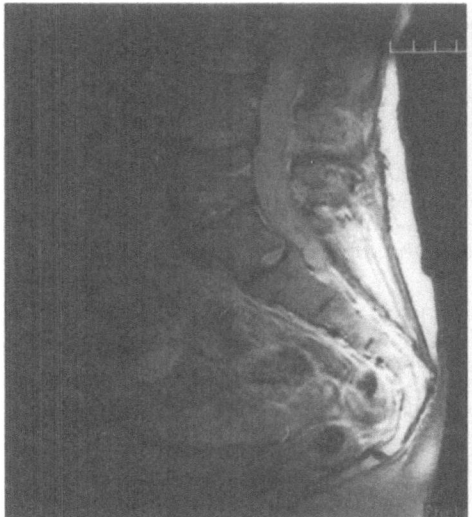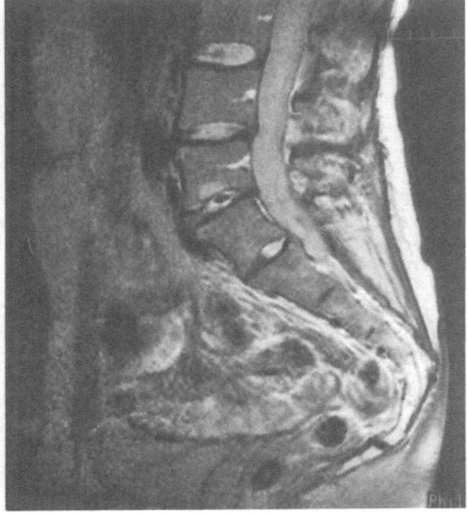

Fig. 1a, b; Normal lumbar spine: considerable contrast loss and sensitivity fall off in the anterior part of the spine on the original (Fig. 1a). Better demarcation of the low signal intesity of parts of the disks and better demonstration of a fatty area within the body of L4 on the corrected image (Fig. 1b).

METHODS

a) *theoretical*

The surface coil correction is based on the knowledge of the nature of the artifacts, namely a smooth multiplicative error over the object part of the image. This error can be eliminated by the use of a homomorphic filtering (4). The coil-induced intensity variations contain mainly low spatial frequencies, hence a very smooth function, and the useful tissue information contains mainly high spatial frequencies.

This method theoretically consists of three steps (3). First the logarithm of the image is taken. This step converts the multiplicative error into an additive error. In a second step this additive error is estimated by means of low-pass filtering. After correction by this estimated error an exponention is performed to undo the logarithm in the first step.

The whole algorithm can be summerized as:

$$C = W.exp\left(ln(I) - \frac{Smooth\ (W.ln(I)}{Smooth\ (W)}\right)$$

I, W and C are image arrays. I is the original image, C the corrected image and W the weights image. Smooth is a low-pass filtering operator. The filtering processing time is only about 2 seconds per image more than it is need for a normal reconstruction.

Independently of the correction factor the algorithm will also supress the background noise. This occasionally can lead to suppression of tissue regions with very low signal to noise ratio.

b) *practical*

All examinations were performed by a 1.5 Tesla system (GYROSCAN, Fa. Philips). All available surface coils were tested; ring-shaped surface coils with different diameters, rectangular-shaped surface coils with different length and wrap around surface coils.

After performing the usual examination raw data were saved. In case of a pathologic finding immediate reconstruction followed. There is a correction factor, to be set by the user: 0 means no correction, 1.0 means maximal correction. We use the correction factor 0.7. The additional time for this correction - which is unnecessary, if no comparison with the originals is required - depends on the number of slices and needs on an average 6 - 8 minutes.

The slices showing the pathologic findings best were selected; two radiologists trained in reading MR images compared independently the original with the image following surface coil intensity correction.

RESULTS

Up to August 1988 *automatic surface coil intensity correction* was used in 156 examinations of the spine performed with surface coils. Concerning the comparison between originals and images following surface coil correction in no case the corrected image missed or hid the pathologic finding. Looking at the general impression of the images, corrected images were superior in all cases by reason of better contrast (Fig. 2a,b), better demarkation of fat (no over-enhancement) and virtually comparable contrast of identical tissue located both close by the surface coil and in the depth (especially fat tissue).

No additional pathologic lesion was found by using the surface coil intensity correction. However, in most cases both radiologists felt that the corrected images demonstrated the lesions better (Abb. 3a,b); only in 18 cases the lesion was seen equally well on the originals.

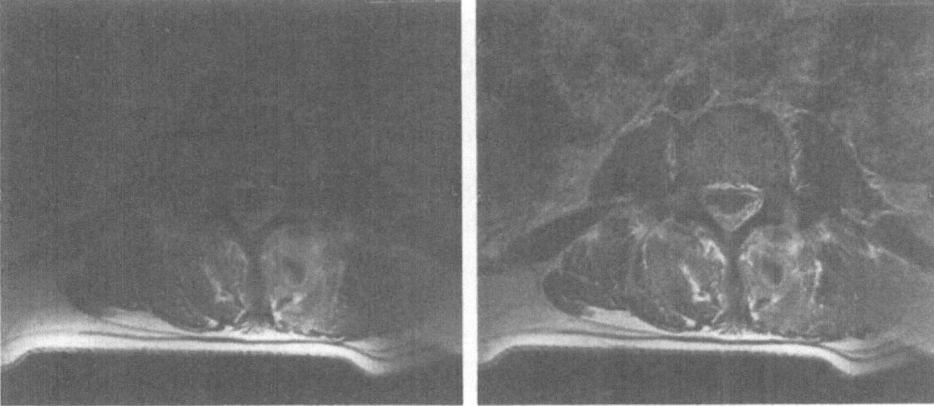

Fig. 2 a,b ; Purulent meningitis following peridural anesthesia: considerable enhancement of the meninges and the nerve roots after Gadolinium DTPA as an expression of the inflammation. Better delineation by using corrected images (Fig. 2b). Note also the inflammation and the abscess in the soft tissues.

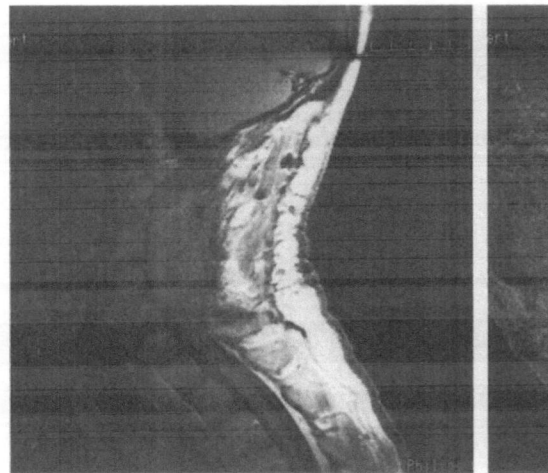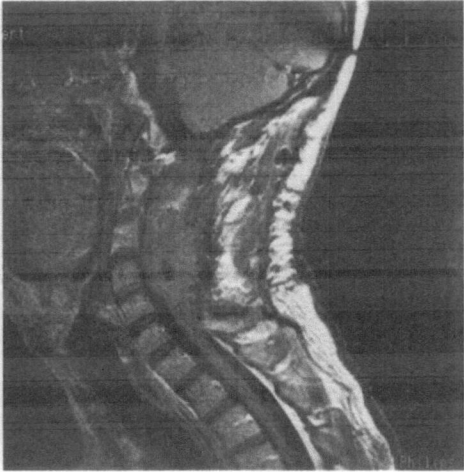

Fig. 3 a,b ; Recurrence of a cervical astrocytoma: well defined enhancement after administration of Gadolinium DTPA. The filtered image shows better definition of the enhancing tumor, the accompanying cyst and the calcifications (Fig. 3b). Superior visualisation of the cervical spine and of the structures of the soft tissues of the neck.

CONCLUSIONS

* Corrected images by homomorphic filtering show considerable contrast improvement at depth.
* Contrast is achieved virtually identical to that obtained with a head or body coil.
* The method gives good results for all surface coils.
* The number of patient examinations per day and the cost are not affected, because the filtering requires no operator interaction and processing time is only about 2 seconds per image more than it is need for a normal reconstruction.
* Clinical results with surface coil images show that homomorphic filtering facilitates diagnosis, because the typical intensity comes much closer to the equivalent body coil image than to the original surface coil image.

REFERENCES

1. Axel L (1984) Surface coil magnetic resonance imaging. J Comput Assist Tomogr 8:381-384
2. Edelstein WA, Schenck JF, Hart HR, Hardy CJ, Foster TH, Bootomley PA (1985) Surface coil magnetic resonance imaging. JAMA 253:828
3. Fuderer M, van Est A (1987) Abstracts of the SMRM 6
4 Gonzales RC, Wintz P (1977) Digital image processing. Addison Wesley, 1977

Effects of Gadolinium Complexes on Spinal Cord Cell Cultures

M. Allard (Bordeaux, France)

In various tissues, gadolinium (Gd^{3+}) has been shown to modify cal-
cium-influx-related metabolic functions and to block the binding of
calcium to the plasma membrane. The question arises as to whether
magnetic resonance (MR) contrast media are able to interact with
plasma-membrane calcium binding sites or calcium channels. The object
of this study was to investigate the possibility of a fixation of
gadolinium at the neuronal cell surface, and/or its penetration inside the cell. To distinguish the effect of ionic gadolinium from that
of complexed gadolinium and to improve sensitivity, we used radioactive compounds: MR contrast media were labelled with gadolinium 153
(γ) and carbon 14 (β). In all experiments cultured mouse spinal cord
cells were used. The techniques of preparing dissociated cell cultures have been previously described by Allard et al [J. Neurochem.
48, 1553-1559 (1987)]. Cells were plated in Falcon plastic tissue
culture dishes 3.5 mm diameter at a density of 2×10^6 cells/dish in
1.5 ml of nutrient medium at 37° C. After 8 days, cell cultures were
incubated for 3 days in 0.5 ml of nutrient medium containing 0.3 mCi
of DTPA [153] Gd or DOTA [153] Gd (at a final concentration of 50 nM)
or 0.4 mCi of [^{14}C]DTPA Gd or [^{14}C]DOTA Gd (at a final concentration
of 50 nM). Then, the supernatant was transferred into vials to
quantify radioactivity. Each well was rinsed twice with 200 µl of
medium, then the radioactivity of the pellet was measured. The structural integrity of the cells was assessed by morphological criteria
and the leakage of cytoplasmic lactate dehydrogenase. The pellet containing spinal cord cells contained 1 to 2% of the initial radioactivity. These results show that neuronal cells and MR contrast media interact.

Gadolinium Enhancement in MR of Suspected Spinal Multiple Sclerosis

E.-M. Larsson, S. Holtås, O. Nilsson, and S. Cronqvist (Lund, Sweden)

The potential of gadolinium DTPA (Gd) to determine the activity of spinal lesions compatible with multiple sclerosis plaques was evaluated. Five patients with elongated high signal intensity lesions in the cervical spinal cord, demonstrated on long TR/TE MR images, were examined after intravenous injection of Gd. Cervical MR was performed using a 0.3 T permanent/resistive magnet imaging system with a vertical magnetic field using a solenoidal surface coil. Short TR/TE (500/16 msec) and long TR/TE (2000/84 msec) spin echo images were obtained before and up to 50 minutes after Gd injection (0.1 mmol/kg body weight, Schering AG). No enhancement was seen in three patients who had clinically inactive disease. In two patients with symptoms of active disease enhancement was seen on short TR/TE images obtained 50 minutes after Gd injection but not on early post-injection scans. These patients were followed with MR with Gd injection until the enhancement had disappeared. The decrease of enhancement correlated well with the decrease of clinical symptoms. In conclusion, Gd-enhancement seems to reflect the activity of the spinal cord plaques.

The Role of MRI in the Assessment of Lesions of the Conus and Lower Cord

B. S. Worthington, A. R. M. Wilson, T. Jaspan, and I. M. Holland

EMBRYOLOGY AND ANATOMY

The lower lumbar and sacral segments of the spinal cord are formed
from the caudal cell mass in the second and third months in utero
by a process of secondary canalisation. The lumbar enlargement
of the cord is produced by expansion of the spinal grey matter
supplying the lower limbs. The lumbar enlargement normally
extends from T11 tapering to form the conus medullaris at the
L1 level. The conus medullaris contains the sacral segments of the
cord.

CLINICAL ASPECTS

The Conus Syndrome

Lesions involving the sacral region of the cord result in a
particular symptom complex including "saddle" anaesthesia (S3-5),
pain referred to the sacral dermatomes and flaccid paralysis of the
muscles of the pelvic outlet. Additional involvement of S2 may also
cause sensory deficit of the posterior aspect of the thigh. S1 is
not usually involved but loss of the ankle jerk and weakness of the
feet can be a feature of extensive lesions.

Lesions of the cauda equina will produce similar signs and symptoms.
However, lesions of the cauda tend to also involve varying numbers
of lumbar nerves producing more widespread neural deficit extending
to higher levels.

Pathology in 38 patients with pathology involving the conus and
lumbar enlargement of the cord.

Congenital spinal dysraphism - diastamatomyelia
(14 patients)   - conus cavitation
                           - conus lipoma and dermoid

Acquired neoplasia intramedullary   Glioma
                   (4 patients)   Ependyoma
                   extramedullary   Meningioma
                   (3 patients)   Neurofibroma
                        Extradural Metastases and primary tumours
                   (5 patients)

Degenerative   Disc prolapse
(3 patients)

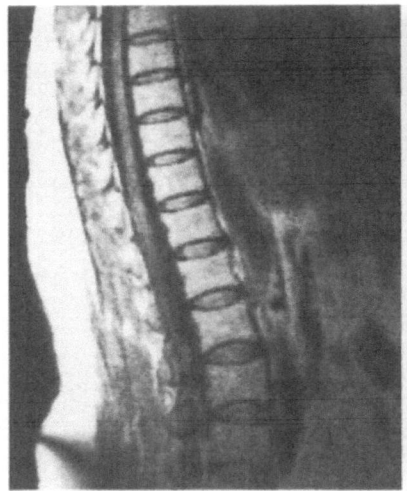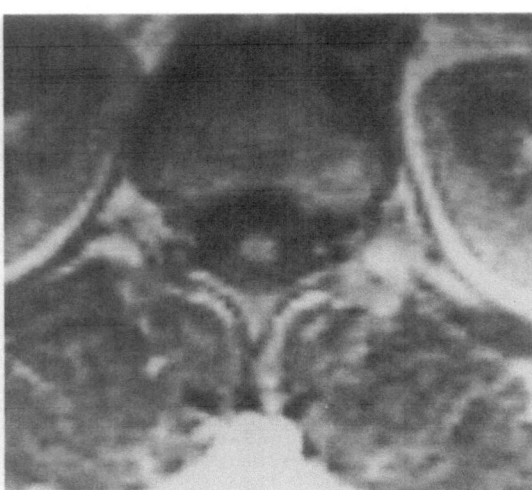

Fig. 1. Normal Conus. (SE 500/40)

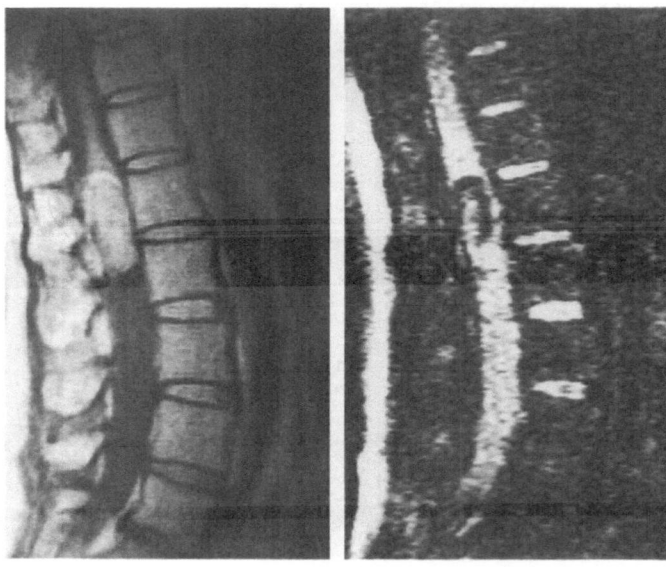

Fig. 2. Dermoid. (a) SE (500/40)   (b) STIR

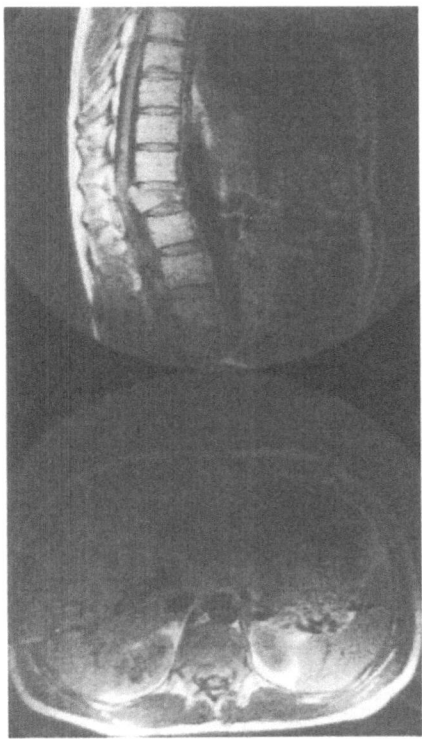

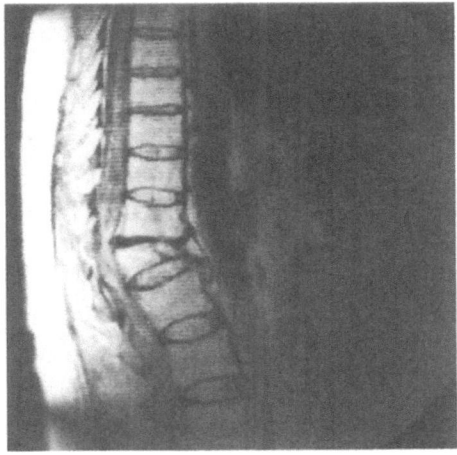

Fig. 4. Fracture of D12 with associated
traumatic syrinx (SE 500/40)

Fig. 3. Fracture of L1 with conus compression
(SE 500/40)

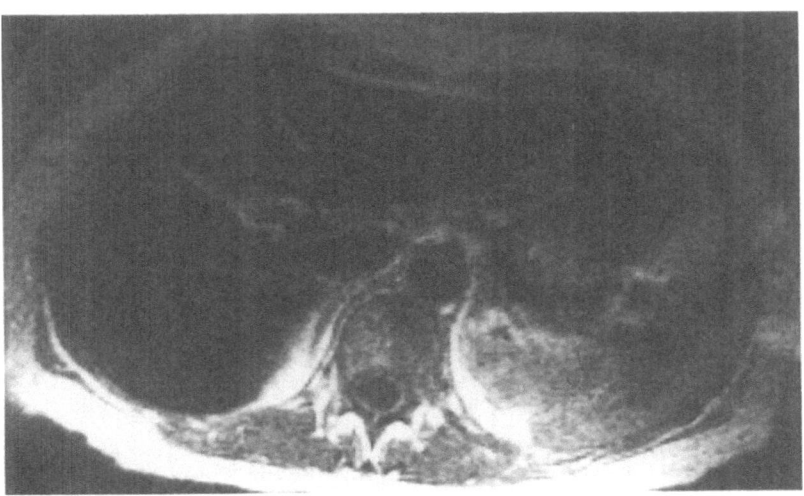

Fig. 5. Cystic conus glioma (SE 500/40)

Trauma
(7 patients)
Inflammatory   Infection
(2 patients)

IMAGING

Normal Appearances

On T_1 weighted spin echo sequences the spinal cord shows a uniform signal of medium intensity and its smooth contours are well defined by the low signal of the surrounding CSF. The conus normally lies posteriorly at the level of L1. The proximal cauda equina below this has a lower signal than the conus due to CSF between the roots.

On T_2 weighted spin echo and short tau inversion recovery sequences there is clear demonstration of the CSF-extradural interface and disc hydration.

PATHOLOGY

For the anatomical delineation of pathology a T_1 weighted spin echo sequence carried out in the sagittal plane is the most valuable initial examination. Having determined the level of the abnormality a multislice set of transverse axial sections is carried out with the same sequence; this is particularly valuable in determining the relationship of extrinsic lesions to the cord and for demonstrating focal abnormalities such as cavitation within the cord. Coronal sections are particularly helpful in assessing the shape and level of the conus in spinal dysraphism particularly in the presence of a scoliotic deformity. Other pulse sequences such as inversion recovery and STIR are used to achieve a measure of tissue characterization.

SUMMARY

MR imaging is the imaging technique of choice in the initial investigation of suspected lesions of the conus and lumbar enlargement of the spinal cord. The technique allows clear demonstration of the lower cord and adjacent structures in several imaging planes with inherent tissue contrast. MR imaging often provides more information than conventional invasive procedures allowing definitive management decisions to be made with minimal patient morbidity.

REFERENCES

Brodal A (1969) Neurological anatomy in relation to clinical medicine. Oxford University Press, New York and London, pp 629-633

Fitzgerald MJT (1985) Neuroanatomy basic and applied. Bailliere Tindall

Masaryk TJ and Modic MT (1988) The lumbar spine in magnetic resonance imaging. Eds, Stark DD and Bradley WGB, C V Mosby Company, St Louis, Washington and Toronto, pp 632-666

MR and Radionuclear Bone Scan in Evaluation of Spinal Metastases

G. Krol, S. Yeh, G. Sze and L. Ginsberg

INTRODUCTION

Radionuclear bone scan is presently a widely accepted method of screening for skeletal metastases. Infiltrative lesions of the bone marrow have abnormal metabolism and are depicted as areas of increased or decreased concentration of activity. Demonstration of marrow abnormalities by MR is based on a replacement of a fat tissue by an infiltrative process, giving rise to a decreased intensity of the involved areas, as opposed to a relatively high intensity of the normal vertebra. The aim of this investigation is a comparison of these two modalities in the detection of the spine pathology in patients with suspected metastases.

MATERIALS AND METHODS

Seventy-four patients with known malignant neoplasms and clinically suspected spinal metastases underwent MR and radionuclear bone scans. MR studies were limited to the area of clinical interest. Twenty-three examinations were performed on Technicare .5 Tesla unit using body coil and 51 patients were examined on 1.5 Tesla GE Signa scanner utilizing surface coils. Sagittal and axial and/or coronal sections of the area of interest were obtained. Only T1 weighted images (echo time TR/TE 500-800/20-32) were utilized for analysis. Radionuclear studies were obtained on Gamma camera, using radioactive agent Technicium 99 mTcMDP.

The studies were interpreted independently by two neuroradiologists and a nuclear medicine physician. Vertebral levels and number of the vertebral segments involved in the region encompassed by MR examinations were assessed on both MR and nuclear scans. The extent of the disease was expressed by a number of the segments involved.

RESULTS

There was agreement as to presence, absence of disease and the extent of metastatic process in 44 patients (59.4%) In five patients (6.8%) with negative radionuclear scan MR demonstrated a typical abnormal signal consistent with metastases (Fig. IA and B.) Additional lesions were diagnosed on MR in 15 patients (20.3%). The disease was considered to be more extensive as demonstrated on bone scan in eight patients (10.8%). In two patients, MR examinations were negative while bone scan was positive (Fig. 2). In 12 patients, a management of the patient was significantly altered on the basis of MR study. These changes usually involved the adjustment of treatment ports, decision whether surgery or radiation should be employed or decision whether treatment should be given because available studies were nonspecific.

DISCUSSION

Radionuclear bone scan constitutes a routine screening procedure for detection of metastatic disease to the bone. Within the spine, metastatic lesions appear predominantly as areas of increased activity and occasionally, as areas of decreased concentration of activity (1,2,3). On MR, normal bone marrow of vertebra is homogeneously hyperintense. Marrow replacement by infiltrative process results in loss of intensity as observed on short echo sequences (9,5,6). The appearance on T2 weighted images is variable. With prolongation of TR/TE intervals on spin echo sequences there is progressive increase of intensity of metastatic lesions of the vertebrae. With adjacent normal vertebrae as reference, metastases may remain hypointense (although to a lesser degree), become isointense (and therefore not visualized) and hyperintense. Our previous experiences suggest that T1 weighted images with time intervals in the range of 400-600/20-30 msec are optimal for visualization of bony metastases (7). Greater sensitivity of MR in detection of spine was noted previously (8,9). Our material, limited to patients with histologically proven neoplasms and clinical evidence of spinal metastases demonstrates that both modalities can give false negative results although these are less likely to occur with MR. MR demonstrates more extensive disease as compared to bone scan in approximately 20% of cases. Involvement of additional adjacent vertebral segments does not necessarily result in change of treatment. However, the management is usually altered when a distant focus of disease is found. Within our group, the addition of MR study accounted for adjustment of patients treatment in 16% of cases.

SUMMARY

The study indicates that in the assessment of spinal metastases, the results of MR and radionuclear bone scan agree in 60% of cases. Additional lesions are demonstrated on MR as compared to bone scan (and vice versa) in 20 and 11%, respectively. False negative studies occur on both modalities although less commonly on MR (7% versus less than 3%).

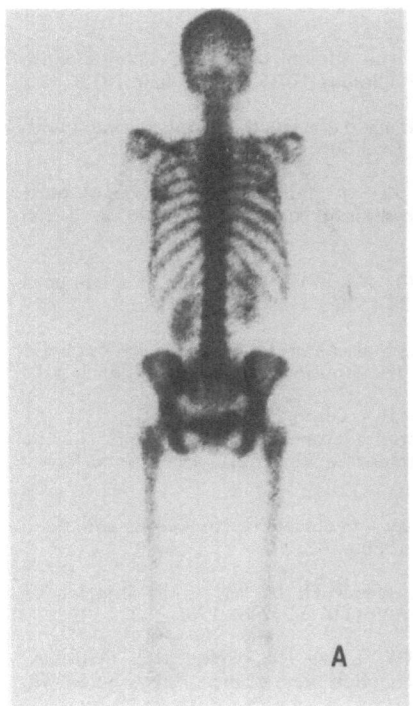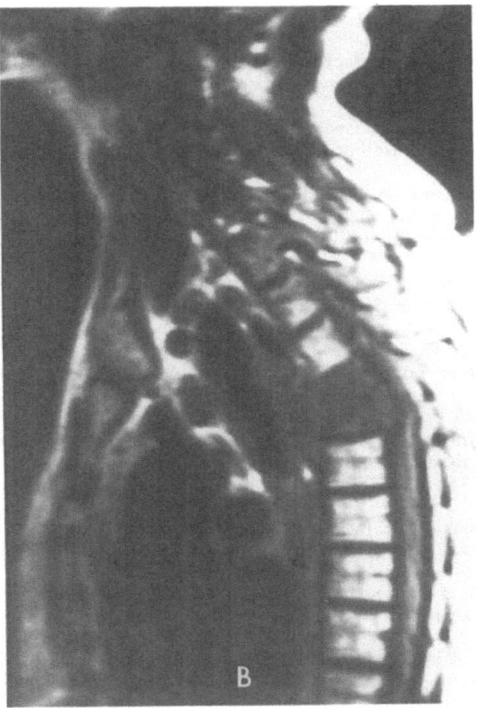

Fig. 1. Metastatic breast carcinoma.
A. Gamma camera view, PA. The scan was interpreted as normal.
B. Sagittal MR, TI weighted, 600/20. There is destruction of T4 and T5 vertebral with paraspinal soft tissue mass.

Fig. 2. Metastatic breast carcinoma. There was increased acivity of L4 vertebra (pedicle). Fine sections of the lumbosacral spine in axial and sagittal planes (A) showed no abnormality.

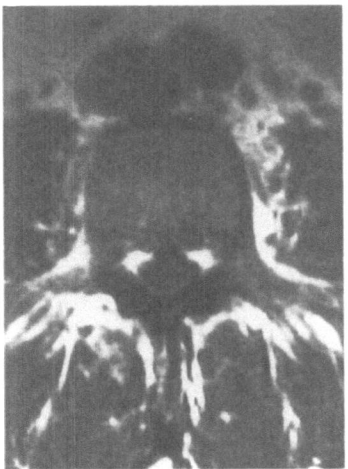

REFERENCES

1. Pendergrass HP, Potsaid MS, Castronovo FP: The clinical use of Tc-diphosphonate (HEDSPA). A new agent for skeletal imaging. Radiology 107:557-562, June 1973.

2. Citrin DL, Greig WR, Calder JF, et al: Preliminary experience of bone scanning with Tc-labelled polyphosphate in malignant disease. Br J Surg 61:73:75, Jan 1974.

3. Desaulniers M, Lacourciere Y, Lisbona R, et al. A detailed comparison of bone scanning with Tc-polyphosphate and radiographic skeletal surveys for neoplasm. J Can Assoc Radiol 24:340-343, Dec 1973.

4. Ramsey RG, Huckman MS, Russell EJ, Levine RS. MR in the evaluation of spinal cord compression (Meeting Abstract). Radiology. 1984 153(P) P 292.

5. Yu E, Sarpel SC, Ezdinli E. Early diagnosis of spinal epidural metastases by Magnetic Resonance Imaging (MRI) (Meeting Abstract). Proc-Am-Soc-Clin-Oncol. 1986 5. p10.

6. Colman L, Redmond J III, Dunning D, Porter B. Olson D. Stimac G. CT, CT metrizamide Myelography (CT-M) and Magnetic) Resonance Imaging (MR) in the diagnosis of metastases to the axial skeleton (Meeting Abstract). Proc-Annu-Meet-Am-Soc-Clin-Oncol. 1987 6. PA20.

7. Krol G, Ginsberg L, Sze G. Vertebral metastases - evaluation with routine spin echo sequences. Twenty-Sixth Annual Meeting. May 1988 p. 42.

8. Utz J, Durham NC, Herfkens RJ, Fram EK, Woodruff, III WW. MR imaging of vertebral metastases. RSNA Scientified Program Vol (161) P, Nov 1986.

9. Emory TH, Albuquerque NM, Orrison, Jr. WW, Lowe BA, Eckel CG, Dell LA. Comparison of Gd-DTPA MR imaging and radionuclide bone scans. RSNA Scientific Program Vol 165 (P), Nov 1987.

Improvement of Myelography by Application of Digital Radiography

B. Haubitz, W. Döhring, and H. Becker

Introduction

The recently developed technique of digital radiography enables
digital image processing with a greater dynamic range than with the
conventional film-screen combination. The system is based on the
principle of storing the radiation pattern obtained from the patient
using conventional X-ray equipment as image information on a luminescent screen.

In a study of 37 comparative conventional and digitally produced myelo-
graphs (1 cervical, 9 thoracic, 27 lumbar) we have investigated the advantages of the new method.

Method

Using conventional X-ray equipment instead of cassettes including normal film-screen combinations, the new system produces images with
cassettes containing a luminescent screen. This screen stores the radiation pattern as a latent image, with the radiation exposure at
each point represented by excited electrons in the crystal lattice
of the luminescent layer, which is scanned by a laser beam, causing
the electrons to return to the ground state and emitting light as
they do so (Sonoda et al. 1983). This emitted light is detected by
a photomultiplier, and the digitalized image information is passed
to the image processor according to various characteristics. The digital radiographs are produced photographically in a hard-copy unit
connected to the image processor. The cassettes in standard format
containing the luminescent screens are reusable, as the image information can be erased by intense exposure to light. Therefore,
prior to exposure, the luminescent screens were placed on a light
box to return all the excited electrons in the crystal lattice on the
ground state.

The digital imaging system enables postprocessing techniques to be
applied in order to obtain images with different characteristics,
while only one radiation exposure of the patient is needed for producing the primary image. The use of appropriate processor programs,
such as high-pass filtration and gray-scale adaptation, enables such
characteristics as density and contrast to be manipulated in the resulting images. Recently, image manipulations have become controllable
by a monitor.

The results of conventional and digital radiographs were evaluated and
compared. Both the conventional and the digital images were exposed
on the same conventional X-ray equipment.

The conventional radiographs were made with a film-screen combination
(Agfa RPI film with Siemens Tital 2U screens), while the digital myelographic images were obtained with a prototype of the FCT 101 digital
radiography system (Fuji, Tokyo, Japan).

Results

The luminescent screen has a much greater dynamic range than that of
the conventional film-screen combination (Haubitz et al. 1987). The
fibers of the cauda equina in standard radiographs are shown much more
clearly in the new technique than in conventional radiographs (Fig.1).
For example, a compression of the origin of a spinal nerve root by a
herniated intervertebral disc can be seen more clearly on the digital
radiograph. A further advantage of the new imaging system lies in the
imaging of the thoracolumbar and cervicothoracic transitions. This is
a decisive advance, caused by the greater dynamic range of digital radiography in this problem of conventional myelography. In the region
of the thoracolumbar transition the digital techniques gives a better
visualization of the conus medullaris. The spinal cord in the thoracic
and cervical regions is more clearly visualized in the new method than
in conventional radiographs, even when the contrast medium is injected
in the lumbar dural sac. The lack of soft tissue in the cervical region is a major problem with cervical myelography in the conventional
technique; the resulting overexposure with conventional radiographs
can be improved with the new technique. Digital radiography also provides sharper imaging of the slice plane when tomography is used for
myelographic examinations. The extent of surrounding structures is
shown more clearly in the digital radiography. A decisive advantage
of digital radiography over conventional radiography is the possibility of correcting for incorrect exposure by electronic postpro-

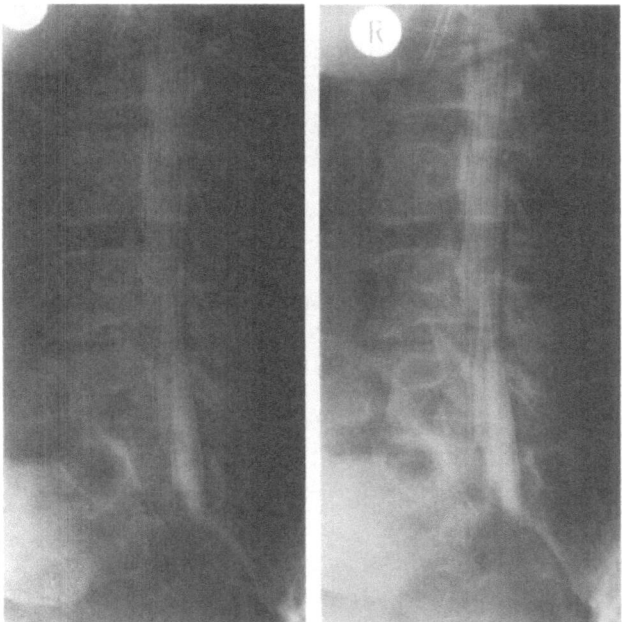

Fig.1a,b. Improved visualization of the fibers of the cauda equina in the lumbar dural sac by digital radiography in a case of spinal stenosis. a: Digital radiograph. b: Conventional radiograph

cessing; there is no need for repeating the examination. Even severe over- und underexposure can be manipulated to provide usable images. The resulting reduction in the radiation exposure of the patient and the work load of personnel are further advantages of the digital system. This possibility is a factor of increased efficiency with digital radiography. Finally, the digital technique offers the possibility of making radiographs with significantly less exposure than that required for conventional radiography using digital postprocessing. Particularly by high-pass filtration in regions of low optical density, a reduction to about one-third of that required for conventional images would be possible. Nevertheless, even the use of digital radiography could not adequately compensate for insufficient contrast in the dural sac due to the examination technique.

Conclusions

In contrast to other authors (Yang et al. 1988), we believe that digital radiography has many advantages over conventional radiography in myelography. In neuroradiology, digital radiography should be used in all cases in which myelography is still indicated.

References

[1] Haubitz B. Döhring W, Becker H (1987) The application of digital radiography in myelography. Medicamundi 32: 66-71
[2] Sonoda M et al. (1983) Computed radiography utilizing scanning laser stimulated luminescence. Radiology 148: 833-838
[3] Yang PJ, Seeley GW, Carmody RF, Seeger JF, Yoshino MT, Mockbee B (1988) Conventional vs computed radiography: evaluation of myelography. AJNR 9: 165-168

The Value of MRI in the Pre- and Postsurgical Evaluation of Cervical Spine Disease

F. E. Zanella, W. Gross-Fengels, and A. Koulousakis

INTRODUCTION

MRI has quickly been accepted as a diagnostic tool in neuroradiology and neurosurgery (2,6,7,9). After four years experience with magnetic resonance imaging there is no doubt that MRI is the method of choice in most cases of presurgical and postsurgical evaluation of cervical spine disease. We want to emphasize this by demonstration of some interesting or difficult findings and of unusual complications.

METHODS

MRI pulse sequence selection is critical in the examination of the spine, as certain processes may be demonstrated only by a particular technique. Measurements were carried out on an imaging system with a superconductive magnet, operating at 1.5 Tesla. We always start by obtaining a transversal rapid "scout" image to select the imaging planes for the sagittal images.

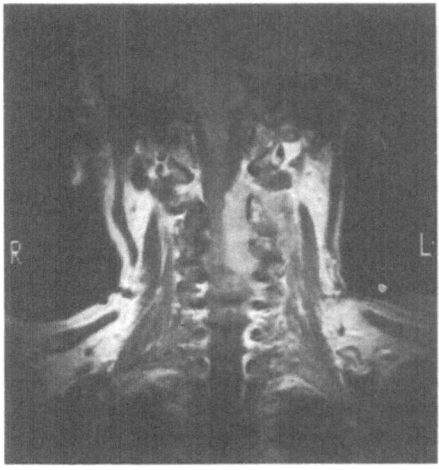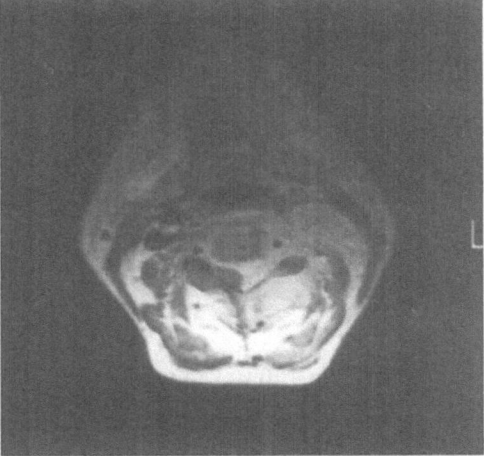

Fig. 1 a,b ; Malignant lymphoma in a 54 year old woman; progressive tetraplegia. The images following Gadolinium DTPA reveal a mass in the left paravertebral region. Note the exact delineation of the vertebral artery, surrounded by neoplastic tissue. The multiplanar slices show exactly the extension of the tumor through the foramina on the left side into the intraspinal space.

The spin-echo technique can provide T1 or T2 weighted images, depending primarily on the echo time (TE). The *T1 weighted images* are neccessary for sufficient soft-tissue contrast and anatomic details. The cerebrospinal fluid is of low signal intensity because of its long T1. *T2 weighted images* allow the separation of the two intervertebral disk components into the nucleus pulposus producing a higher signal intensity than the surrounding annulus fibrosus and show intramedullary lesions best.

RESULTS

MRI has become more and more important in the *presurgical evaluation* of cervical spine disease. Main advantages of MRI are:

* the excellent distinction between intra- and extramedullary lesions (Fig. 1 a,b),
* the exact delineation of the extent of a tumor (Fig. 1 a,b),
* the superior visualization of anatomic relationships and
* the demonstration of abnormalities in cervical spine alignment (Fig. 2 a,b).

Degenerative disease, disk herniation and canal stenosis are clearly seen with MRI. Posttraumatic changes to the cord are demonstrable in several planes with MRI.

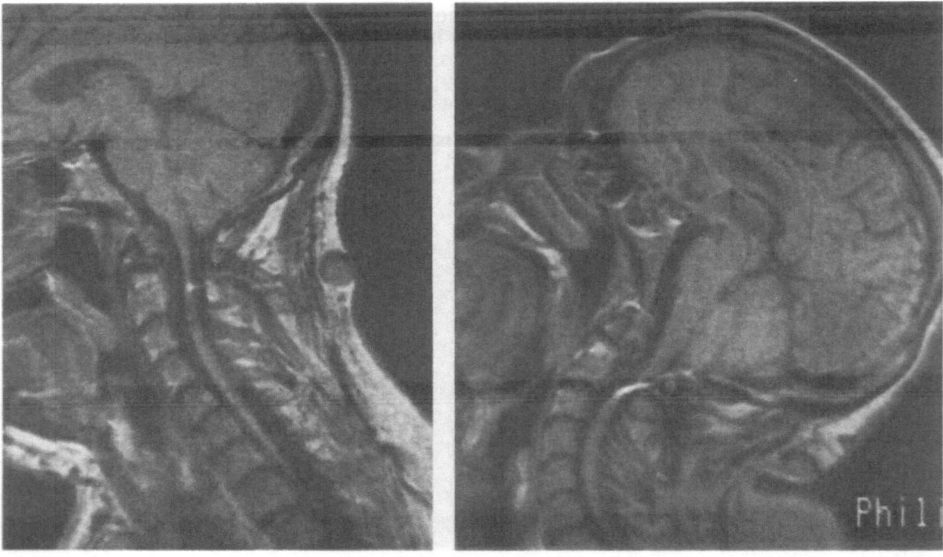

Fig. 2 a,b ; Pseudo-arthrosis of the dens. Flexion sagittal T1-weighted images demonstrate the anterior impingement on the craniocervical junction, which is reduced with extension, accompanied by marked atrophy of the upper cervical cord. Following this dynamic study, the neurosurgeons performed an operation to stabilize this region.

MRI also has become more important in the *postsurgical period*, especially concerning early detection of recurrent disease (Fig. 3 a,b), infection, postsurgical haemorrhage and dislocation of surgical material (Fig. 4 a,b). Postsurgical haemorrhage sometimes is difficult to recognize, especially if the examination is done within the first three days after surgery.

MRI examinations often display image artifacts in the area of surgery (Fig. 5). The artifacts are caused by minute metallic shavings; the presence of minute iron particles explain the loss of signal in patients after the CLOWARD procedure. These artifacts limit the value of MRI.

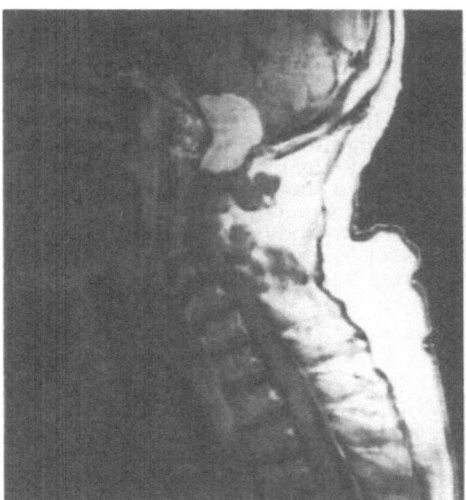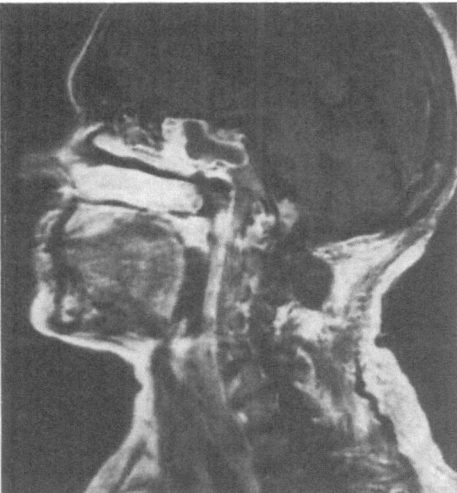

Fig. 3 a,b ; Examination some weeks after surgery of a large meningioma of the craniocervical junction (Fig. 3a). The MRI revealed residual meningioma well demarcated by enhancement following Gadolinium DTPA (Fig. 3b).

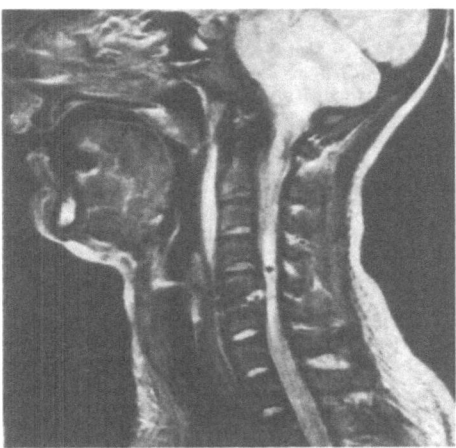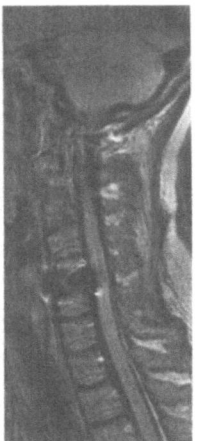

Fig. 4 ; Dislocation of surgical material into the spinal canal following fusion of C5 and C6 by Cloward procedure. It was easily located by MRI removed by the neurosurgeons.
Fig. 5 ; Artifacts after Cloward procedure: it is impossible to diagnose a recurrent disk herniation, but also impossible to rule it out.

222

DISCUSSION

The postoperative changes recognized by MRI will depend on the temporal relationship with the procedure and the nature and extent the primary lesion. Post-op studies can be performed to evaluate the operative effects in the neural canal, to determine the reestablishment of patency from stenosis, to show residual or recurrent tumor mass, to rule out a postsurgical cord hemorrhage, edema or compression, to demonstrate a disc herniation in a non-operated segment, to show an infection of the vertebral bodies , the intervertebral discs and the surrounding soft tissues or to deliniate a foreign body in the spinal canal (1,3,8).

Limitations may arise from image artifacts caused by metallic implants or by minute metallic shavings and from prolonged imaging time (4,5). Ferromagnetic life support devices may cause further problems. MRI may miss a small hemorrhage in the very early post-operative stage. Also smaller bone fragments are more difficult to be recognized as compared to CT, which also gives a better orientation of the traumatic destruction of the vertebral body, though MRI will demonstrate more clearly the secondary changes of the spinal cord. The problem with distinguishing a recurrent disc herniation from a postoperative scar though still remains unsolved by MRI.

CONCLUSIONS

MRI of the cervical spine is the image modality of choice in pre operative planing and post operative follow-up. There is no other imaging method in this setting, which will provide for itself as much complex and clinical relevant information as MRI does. If pre- or postsurgical neurologic symptoms cannot be explained by conventional X rays, magnetic resonance is now the diagnostic method of choice.

REFERENCES

1. Friedburg H, M Schumacher, J Hennig: Pathologie des kraniozervikalen Übergangs in der magnetischen Resonanztomographie. Fortschr Röntgenstr 145:315-320, 1986.
2. Friedmann G: Sinnvoller Einsatz und Wandel bildgebender Verfahren bei Erkrankungen des Zentralnervensystems. Röntgen Bl:39:303-307, 1986.
3. Hackney DB, R Asato, PM Joseph, MJ Carvlin, JT McGrath, RI Grossmann, EA Kassab, D DeSimeone: Hemorrhage and edema in acute spinal cord compression: demonstration by MR imaging. Radiology 161:387-390, 1986.
4. Heindel W, G Friedmann, J Bunke, B Thomas, R Firsching, RI Ernestus: Artifacts in MR imaging after surgical intervention. J Comput Assist Tomogr 10:596-599, 1986.
5. Larsson EM, Holtas S, Cronquist S (1988) Emergency magnetic resonance examination of patients with spinal cord symptoms. Acta Radiologica 29:69-75
6. Mc Ardle CB, Wright JW, Prevost WJ, Dornfest DJ, Amparo EG, Calhoun JS (1986) MR imaging of the acutely injured patient with cervical traction. Radiology 157:273-274
7. Modic MT, TJ Masaryk, GP Mulopulos, C Bundschuh, JS Han, H Bohlman: Cervical radiculopathy: prospective evaluation with surface coil MR imaging, CT with metrizamide, and metrizamide myelography. Radiology 161:753-759, 1986.
8. Quencer RM, JJ Sheldon, MJD Post, RD Diaz, BM Montalvo, BA Green, FJ Eismont: MRI of the chronically injured cervical spinal cord. AJR 147:125, 1986.
9. Zanella FE, W Steinbrich, G Friedmann, A Koulousakis: Magnetische Resonanztomographie (MR) bei spinalen Raumforderungen. Fortschr Röntgenstr 145:326-330, 1986.

Spinal Cord Lesions Due to Cervical Myelopathy.
Pre- and Postoperative MRI Findings

D. Kühne, H. C. Nahser, D. de Silva, A. Feldges, W. H. Heienbrok, and J. Lalik

Just as the pathophysiology and biomechanics of cervical myelopathies are not clear, the patho-anatomical changes in the spinal cord, caused by prolonged compression are varied (Bedford et al. 1952; Hashizume et al. 1983; Ono et al. 1977). The patho-anatomical findings are a diffuse shrinking or a reduction of tissue substance in the region of the ventral horns. On myelo-computertomograms tissue necroses were supposed, in some cases above and below the level of the compression (Iwasaki et al. 1985; Jinkins et al. 1986). It is correspondingly difficult to estimate and to correlate the prognosis from the clinical findings.

The value of NMR in the diagnosis of cervical canal lesions as well as in cervical myelopathies lies in demonstrating degenerative bone and disc lesions and more important the demonstrating and evaluating of parenchymal changes in the compressed cord (Al-Mefty et al. 1988; Masary et al. 1986; Norman et al. 1983; Steiner and Kunze 1986).

The aims of our work with our 3o cervical myelopathy patients, with degenerative spine and disc changes, was to correlate the NMR changes, pre- and post-op., the clinical findings and the duration of the problem. In each case we compared the grade of the stenosis with the duration of the complaint and the pre- and post-op. symptoms using 4 grades of severity. The intra-medullary parenchymal changes such as oedema, necrosis, cavitation and gliosis were likewise compared with the severity of the clinical symptoms pre- and post-op. and their duration.

The NMRs were performed on a Fonar scanner with a o,3 T permanent magnet using solenoid surface coils. The slices were 3.5 mm thick with 1.5 mm spacing, on a 256 x 256 matrix: T 1 and different T 2 weighted spinecho sequences were used.

The assessment of the degree of spinal canal stenosis was "eye balled" into 3 categories. The examination modalities permitted adequate demonstration of the extents of the dural sac as well as that of the spinal cord, from surrounding pathological structures such as the bony osteophytes and displaced disc material. The deformity of the dural sac and the loss of the subarachnoidal space were best demonstrated on the axial views. The high signal soft tissue changes on the T 2 views were only significant when seen in two planes (mostly sagittal and axial).

The age distribution showed a maximum involvement between the age 5o to 6o yr (Fig.1). The sex distribution (Fig.2) shows a 74 % male predominance as opposed to a 23 % female involvement.

The causes of the cervical myelopathies were in most cases diffuse bony encroachment on the spinal canal which often involved more than one level. The disc prolapses were found in all age groups except in those patients who were over 7o yrs. old (Fig.3).

Comparisons of the duration of the problems and the pre-operatively demonstrated spinal canal stenoses were not related (Fig 4). Likewise, there was no definite relationship between the degree of the stenosis and the pre-operative neurological findings (Fig.5).4 patients who appeared to have severe canal stenoses on NMR, had only slight neurological symptoms.

Comparison of the T 2 weighted parenchymal changes and duration of symptoms showed no correlation. Also, where there had been long standing symptoms, we find all grades of T 2 changes, ranging from normal to severe (Fig.6). A somewhat closer relationship was seen between the T 2 parenchymal lesions and the pre-op. neurological findings

(Fig.7). Cysts and atrophy were more frequently seen in patients with a longer duration of symptoms (Fig.8). Reasonable prognostic evidence was possible when comparing duration and the post-op. T 2 changes. The normal or slight changes were commoner in patients with shorter histories (Fig.9). When the T 2 changes had not regressed post-op. and actually become more prominent, it meant that the neurological improvement was unlikely (Fig. 1o).
When pre-op. the hyperintensive changes were severe and were seen over several segments the prognosis was worse, (Fig. 11), than in the other cases.

No worthwhile correlation was seen between the degree of pre-op. stenosis and between the post-op. neurological findings and their total duration (Fig.12).

Two clinical cases are presented. In the first patient (Fig.13) the pre-op. T 2 images (TE 6o, TR 15oo and TE 84, TR 3ooo) showed severe parenchymal high signal changes at and below the level of the maximum cord compression (a). Post laminectomy on the T 2 weighted images, sagittal and axial (TE 6o,TR 15oo), the high signal intensity lesions persisted (b). This corresponded with no significant clinical alteration in the neurological status.
In the 2nd case (Fig. 14), pre-op. T 2 images (TE 6o, TR 15oo and TE 6o,TR 4ooo) showed moderate high signal lesions just below the level of the severe stenosis (a). Post laminectomy the cord is markedly decompresses (sagittal T 1, axial T 2)(b), but demonstrated hemiatrophy with high signal changes in the atrophied part, in association with an unchanged clinical status.

Discussion and Summary
_____

The unsatisfactory treatment results of the operative management of cases of cervical myelopathies due to spinal stenosis and degenerative changes are well known. The causes of this are however not understood.
Patho-anatomical and modern imaging methods show, that in combination with narrowing of the subarachnoidal space and deformity of the spinal cord, there are additional intramedullary soft tissue lesions with or without cyst formation. These agreed with in vivo lesions, shown on the myelo-computertomograms (Iwasaki et al. 1985; Jinkins et al. 1986; Karnaze et al. 1987). There are also NMR spinal cord finding of different forms and extents: These medullary lesions are not always at the level of the maximum compression but in contrast also above and below this level (Al-Mefty et al. 1988).
The treatment and prognosis of these patients who have pre-op. irrepairable changes, largely means that it is likely that they will not have a worthwhile improvement post decompression. This evidence is interesting, as in the literature individual patients are reported, whose clinical condition has stabilised without operative management.
By comparing the clinical and NMR parameters in our 3o patients, we were suprised to find that there was no significant correlation between the degree of the stenosis and the post-op. clinical situation. In patients with a longer history after decompression we observed more cases of diffuse atrophy and localised cyst formation in the cord.
The clinical improvement post-op. was however definitely seen in those where the T 2 parenchymal changes were less marked. Where the high intensity signal changes persisted post-op.,the long term prognosis was uniformly worse.

A prognosis of the post-op. clinical situation cannot be made only from the degree of pre-op. cord compression.
A present NMR,as a non-invasive method, can ascertain if besides the cord compression, there are other associated lesions and can therefore be used for prognosis too. Similar information is obtained from the myelo-computertomogram though this examination is time consuming and is invasive for the patient. A disadvantage of NMR is that when the cord is severely narrowed,the resolution is not high enough to show and localise small cord lesions. New methods of investigation and new pulse sequences will however soon remove this NMR disadvantage.

References

Al-Mefty O.,Harkey. L.H.,Middleton T.H.,Smith R.R.,Fox J.L. (1988) Myelopathic
cervical spondylotic lesions demonstrated by magnetic resonance imaging
J.Neurosurg. 68: 217-222

Bedford P.D., Bosanquet F.D., Russel W.R. (1952) Degeneration of the spinal cord
associated with cervical spondylosis. Lancet 2: 55-59

Enzmann D.R., Rubin J.B., Wright A., (1987) Cervical Spine MR Imaging:Generating
High-Signal CSF in Sagittal and Axial Images. Radiology 163 : 233-238

Hashizume Y., Iljima S., Kishimoto H., et al. (1983) Pencil-shaped softening in
the spinal cord. Pathologic study in 12 autopsy cases. Acta Neuropathol. 61 :
219-224

Iwasaki Y., Abe H., Isu T., et al. (1985) CT myelography with intramedullary
enhancement in cervical spondylosis. J.Neurosurg. 63 : 363-366

Jinkins J.R., Bashir R., Al-Mefty O., Al-Kawi M.Z., Fox J.L. (1986) Cystic
Necrosis of the Spinal Cord in Compressive Cervical Myelopathy . AJNR 7 :693-7o1

Karnaze M.G., Gado M.H., Sartor K.J., Hodges III F.J. (1987) Comparison of MR
and CT Myelography in Imaging the Cervical and Thoracic Spine. AJNR 8 : 983-989

Masary T.J.,Modic M.T., Geisinger M.A., Standefer J., Hardy R.W., Boumphrey F.,
Duchesneau P.M. (1986) Cervical Myelopathy: A Comparison of Magnetic Resonance
and Myelography. Journal of Computer Assisted Tomography 1o (2) : 184-194

Norman D., Mills C.M., Brant-Zawadzki M. et al. (1983) Magnetic resonance imaging
of the spinal cord and canal: AJR 141 : 1147-1152

Ono K., Ota H., Tada K. et al. (1977) Cervical myelopathy secondary to multiple
spondylotic protrusions. A clinicopathologic study. Spine 2 : 1o9-125

Ross J.S., Masaryk T.J., Modic M.T. (1987) Postoperative Cervical Spine: MR
Assessment. Journal of Computer Assisted Tomography 11 (6) : 955-962

Steiner H.H., Kunze St. (1986) Kernspinresonanztomographische Befunde beim
zervikalen Bandscheibenvorfall. Neurochirurgica 29 : 186-188

Teresi L.M. Lufkin R.B., Reicher M.A., Moffit B.J., Vinuela F.V., Wilson G.M.,
Bentson J.R., Hanafee W.N., (1987) Asymptomatic Degenerative Disk Disease and
Spondylosis of the Cervical Spine : MR Imaging . Radiology 164 : 83-88

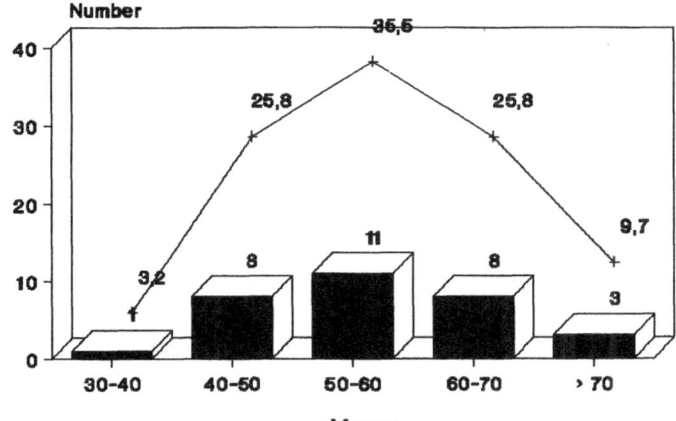

Age Distribution
Cervical Myelopathy

Sex Distribution
Cervical Myelopathy

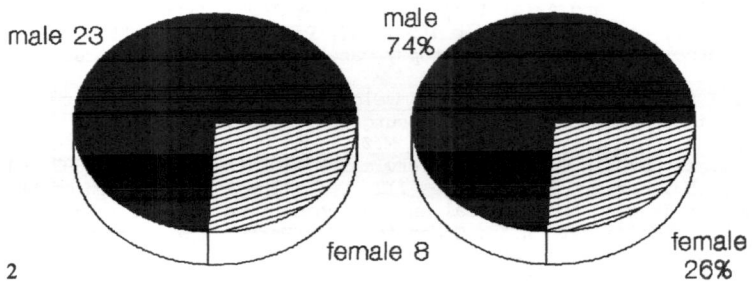

Age and Morphology
Cervical Myelopathy

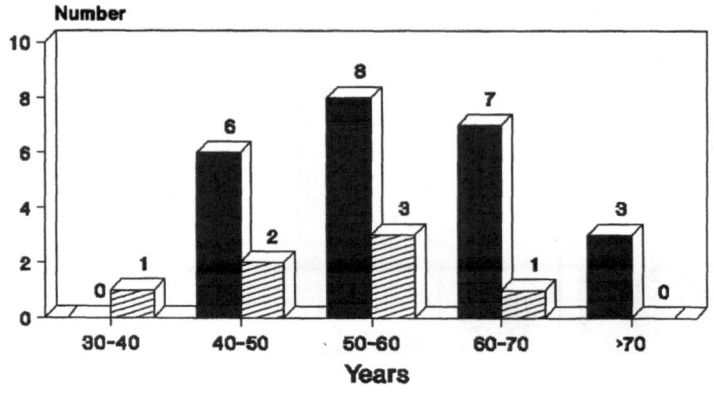

Anamnesis and preop T1
Cervical Myelopathy

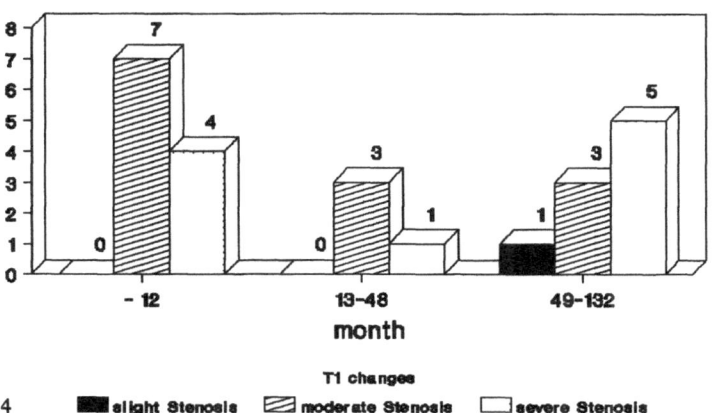

month

T1 changes

4 ■ slight Stenosis ▨ moderate Stenosis ☐ severe Stenosis

Preop T1 and preop Neurology
Cervical Myeolopathy

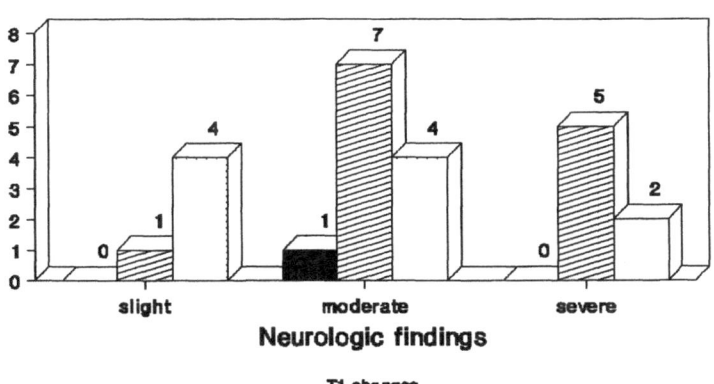

Neurologic findings

T1 changes

5 ■ slight Stenosis ▨ moderate Stenosis ☐ severe Stenosis

Anamnesis and preop T2
Cervical Myelopathy

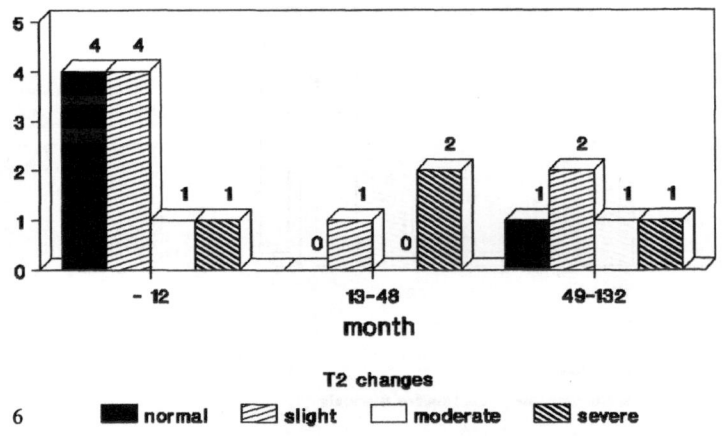

6

Preop T2 and preop Neurology
Cervical Myelopathy

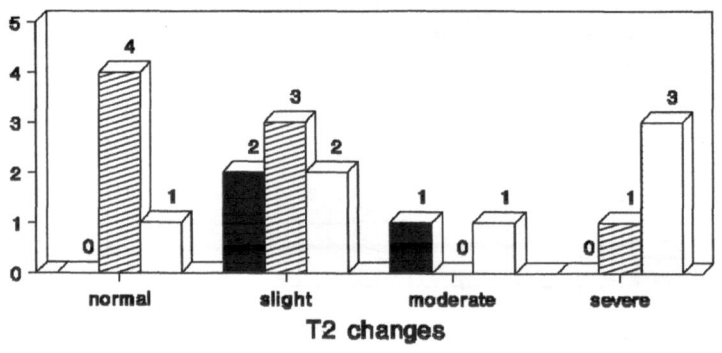

7

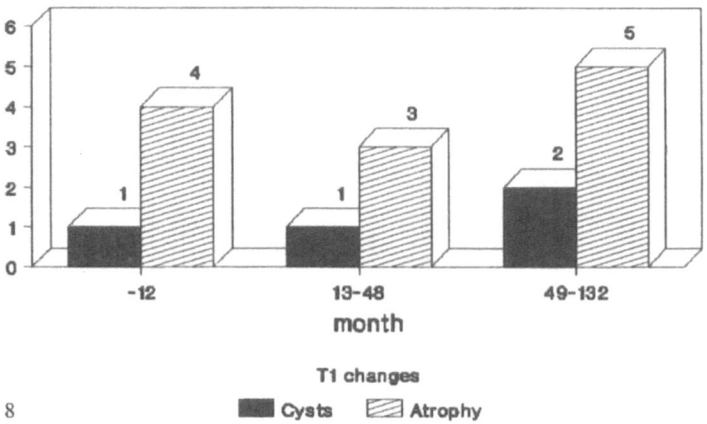

Anamnesis and postop T1
Cervical Myelopathy

month

T1 changes
Cysts   Atrophy

8

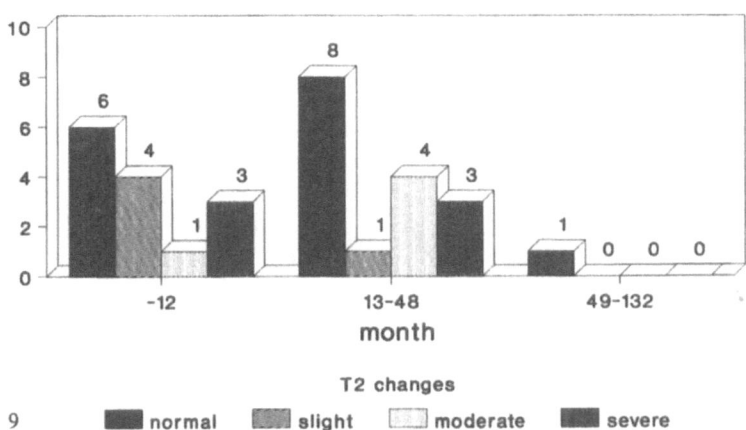

Anamnesis and postop T2
Cervical Myelopathy

month

T2 changes
normal   slight   moderate   severe

9

Postop Neurology and postop T2
Cervical Myelopathy

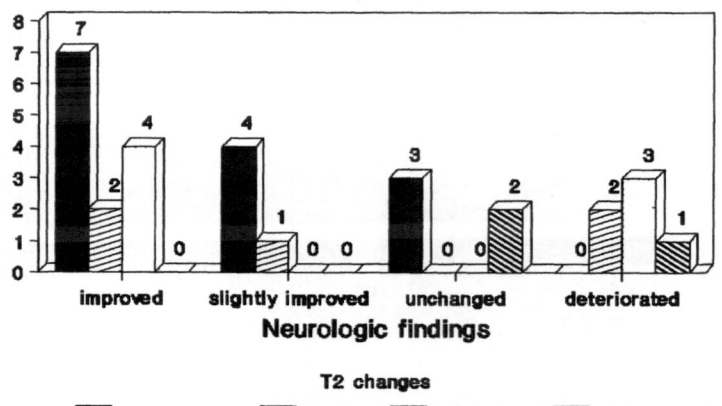

Neurologic findings

T2 changes

10   ■ no changes   ▨ slight   ☐ moderate   ▧ severe

Preop T2 and postop Neurology
Cervical Myelopathy

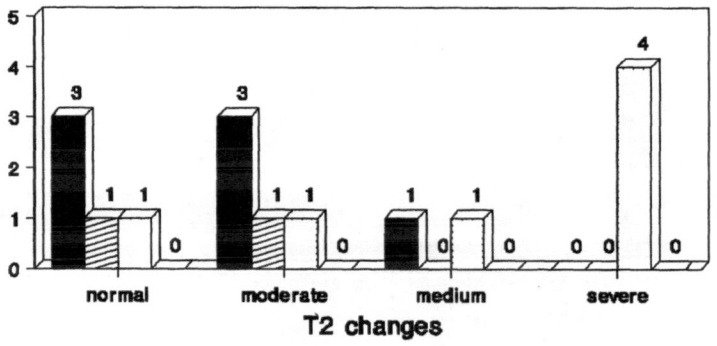

T2 changes

Neurologic findings

11   ■ improved   ▨ moderately improved   ☐ unchanged   ▧ deteriorated

Postop Neurology and preop T1
Cervical Myelopathy

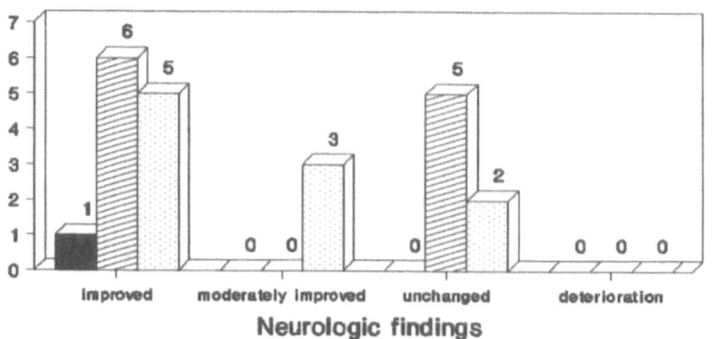

Neurologic findings

T1 changes

12   ■ slight Stenosis   ▨ moderate Stenosis   ▢ severe Stenosis

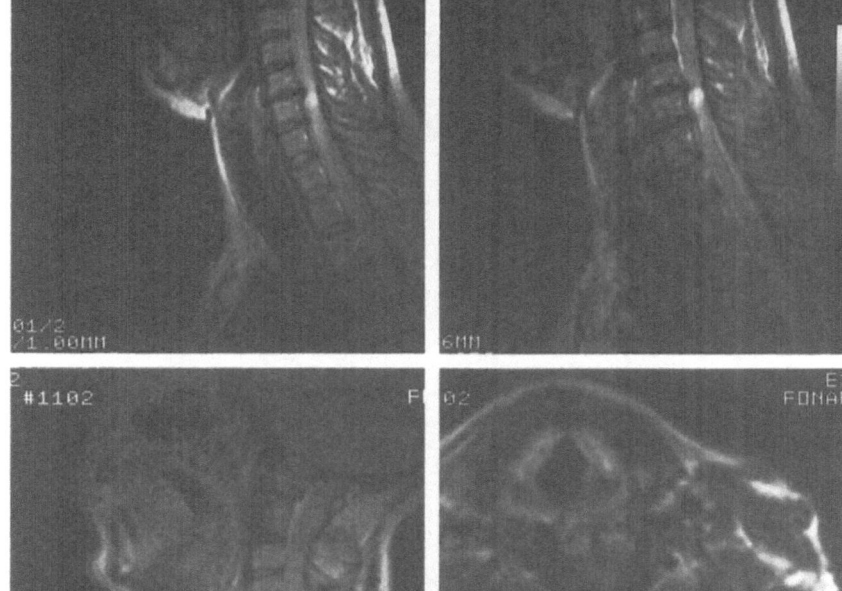

13

14

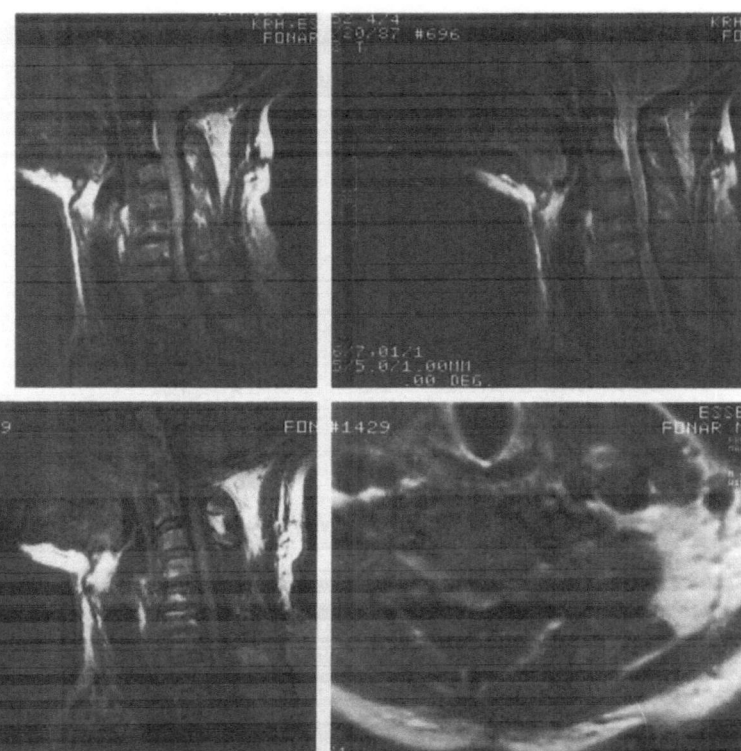

Delay of Tibial F-Wave Response after Lumbar Myeloradiculography

N. Prey, G. Kubina, Th. Staudacher, and P. Stoeter

INTRODUCTION AND METHOD OF EXAMINATION

In order to examine the effect of contrast medium (CM) on nervous structures the F-wave latencies of the tibial nerve of both legs were measured
before, 2 hours and 2 days after lumbar myeloradiculography in 24 patients.
The results were compared with the latencies of the somatosensory evoked
potentials (SEP) of the tibial nerve and theF-wave of the median nerve
The patients were unselected and suffered from disc disease with different
neurological deficits. All patients received iotrolan (Isovist[R], Schering)
in a dose of 10ml (25o - 3oo mgJ/ml), a dimeric non-ionic water soluble
contrast medium. After examination all patients were kept in bed in
horizontal position for 24 hours. Identical measurements were carried out
in a control group of 1o patients after lumbar puncture alone.

Results:

2 hours after CM application we saw a significant lengthening of the
tibial nerve F-wave latency and a normalisation to the original level after
2 days in every case (Fig. 1). The latencies of the SEPs of the tibial
nerve and the F-wave of the median nerve were also prolonged but to a
smaller degree (Fig. 2,3), whereas no significant change (Table 1)
of latency was found in measurements following lumbar puncture alone.
There were no neurological deficits after myelography.

Table 1. Increase of latencies
Before/ 2 hours after myelography

	n	$\bar{x}$(msec)	σ_{n-1}	t*	t^*_α = 1%
F-wave N. tib.	24	2,45	1,17	12,34	2,o7
F-wave N. med.	24	o,33	o,49	3,o4	2,81
SEP N. tib.	17	o,58	o,93	4,49	2,72

Before/ 2 hours after LP alone (control group)

	n	$\bar{x}$(msec)	σ_{n-1}	t*	t^*_α = 1%
F.wave N. tib.	1o	o,o2	o,88	1,53	2,88

* Standard Student T-test

234

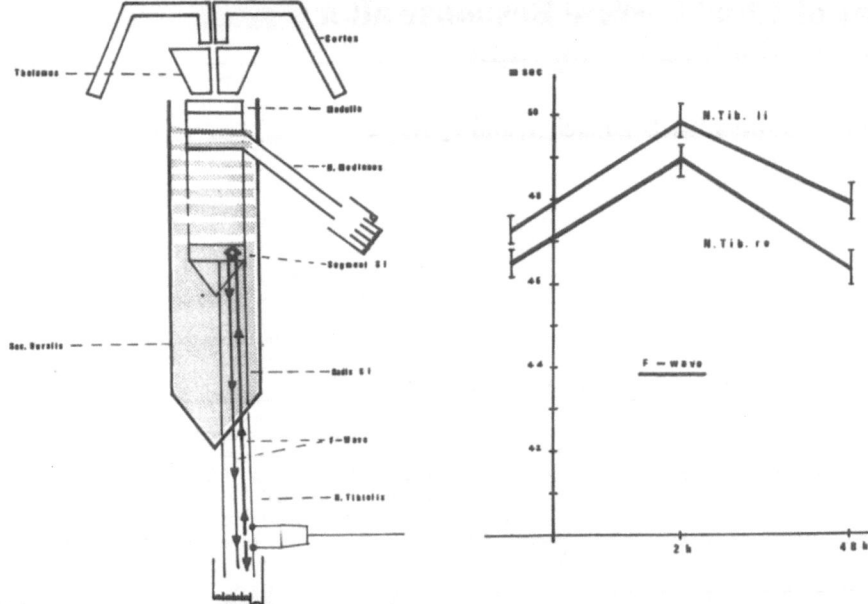

Fig. 1. Anatomical schematogram of the tibial nerve F-wave. Tibial
F-wave latency before, 2 hours and 48 hours after CM application.

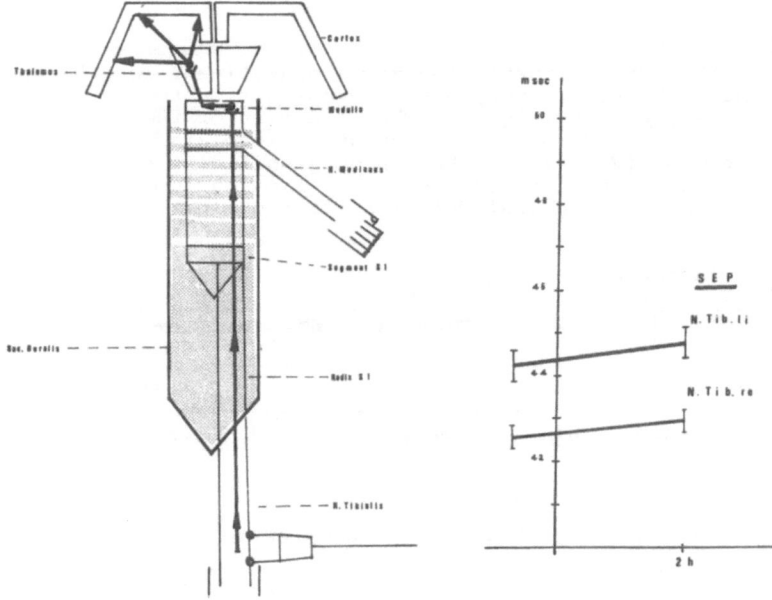

Fig. 2. Anatomical schematogram of the SEP's of tibial nerve.
Latencies before and 2 hours after CM application.

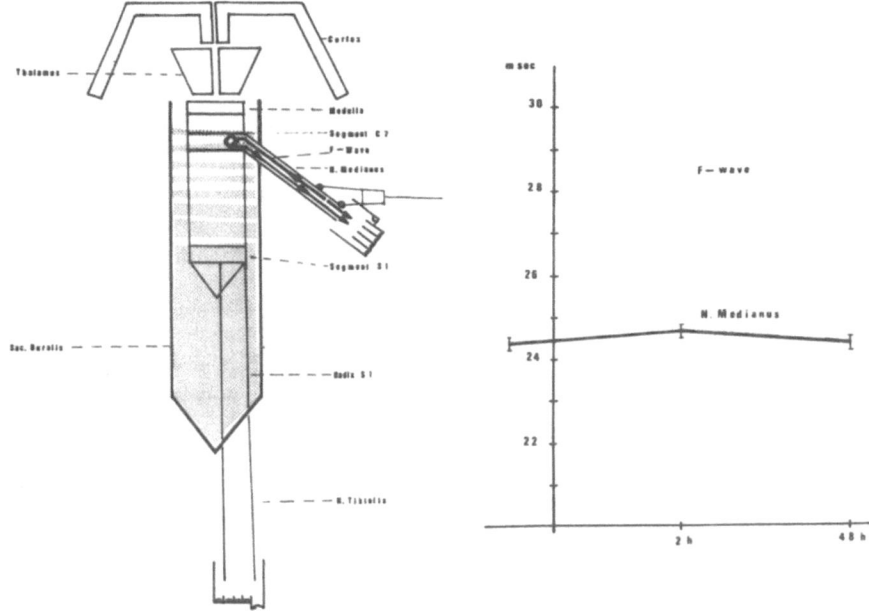

Fig. 3. Anatomical schematogram of the median nerve F-wave.
Latencies before, 2 hours and 48 hours after CM application.

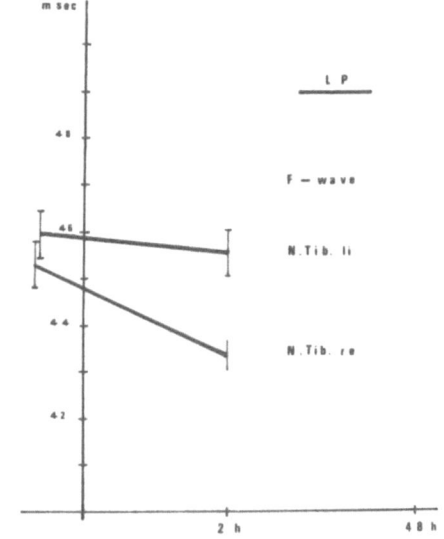

Fig. 4. Latencies of the tibial nerve F-wave before and 2 hours
after LP (no significance).

Discussion and conclusion

The introduction of non-ionic CM for intrathecal use has been regarded as an advance although adverse reactions such as abnormal EEG, seizures and acute psychosis have been reported (Schmidt 198o). As shown by other authors water soluble CM may affect the latency of the visual and other evoked responses dose related, tending to be more marked when CM is allowed to enter the cranium (Broadbridge et al 1984).

A delay of the H-reflex response after subarachnoid CM application was shown in cats (Allen et al 1976) but up to date not in man. As for the F-wave the impulse of the H-reflex passes twice the CM pool within the lumbar dural sac.

The delay of the tibial nerve F-wave response is more pronounced and of higher significance as compared to those of the median nerve and the SEPs. We suggest three possible reasons for this finding:
1. The maximum CM concentration is found in the lower lumbar dural sac.
2. The whole length of the cauda equina fibers is sourrounded by this pool of CM.
3. The fibers of the cauda equina have to be passed twice by the action potential of the F-wave.
Especially for these reasons measurement of tibial nerve F-wave latency may be used as a clinical indicator for the neurotoxicity of CM in clinical practice.

REFERENCES

Allen WE, Van Gilder JC, Collins WF (1976) Evaluation of the Neurotoxicity of Water-Soluble Myelographic Contrast Agents by Electrophysiological Monitors. Radiology 118: 89 - 95
Broadbridge AT, Bayliss SG, Firth R, Farrel G (1984) Visual evoked response changes following intrathecal injection of water soluble contrast media: a possible method of assessing neurotoxicity and a comparison of metrizamide and jopamidol. Clin. Radiol. 35: 371 - 373
Schmidt RC (198o) Mental disorders after myelography with metrizamide and other water soluble contrast media. Neuroradiology 19: 153 - 157

MR Imaging and Gadolinium Enhancement of Spinal Epidural Sepsis

M. Boukobza, L. Feldman, B. Chenesseau, and J. Metzger (Paris, France)

Eight patients with spinal epidural sepsis were examined with MR imaging. The lesions were best visualized with spin echo technique and gadolinium enhancement. Sagittal and axial planes were imaged and sagittal views are sufficient to delineate the extent of the lesions. Comparison with contrast-enhanced CT showed that MR is more sensitive in demonstrating the abscesses, and in showing their longitudinal extent and the spinal cord compression.

Intramedullary Lipoma

B. Appel, R. Crols, E. Moens, and A. Lowenthal (Antwerp, Belgium)

A 17-year-old man with a swan neck, familial pes cavus and recent gait disturbances was referred for MRI of his cervical cord for possible heredodegenerative disease. An intradural, partially intramedullary, lipoma C0-C4 with distal hydromyelia was discovered. Standard XR disclosed a congenital spina bifida occulta C1. CT confirmed the intramedullary components (level C3) of the dorsal located lipoma. No myelography was needed.

Surgery on the large extramedullary part of the tumor was successfully followed by relief of the neurological symptoms. Around this case report, completed with a review of the literature, the pathophysiological behavior of intraspinal lipomas will be discussed.

- Is this case a true spinal tumor or a part of spinal dysrafism (C1)?

- Why did neurological deficits appear at the age of 16?
  - Hormonal changes of puberty and influences on lipogenesis and lipolysis.
  - Influence of obesity on the growth of intraspinal lipoma can not be taken in consideration in this thin patient.
  - Cervical growth is finished, no more enlargement of the spinal canal can be expected, so that further tumor expansion will induce medullary compression.

Embryonal and Fetal Vascularisation of the Spinal Cord: Microangiographic Examinations

A. Thron, P. Stoeter, C. Hauss, R. Dietz, U. Drews, and W. Sonntag

In contrast to the well-known anatomy of the spinal cord´s blood
supply in adult man (Thron 1988) and the prenatal vascularisation
of the brain (Voigt and Stoeter, 1980), only few studies are
concerned with the embryonal and fetal development of spinal cord
vessels. Intramedullary capillarisation starts in the 4th week in
mammal embryos (Hoskins 1914, Craigie 1955) and the extramedullary
arteries are formed from a preceeding network by the end of the
second month (Di Chiro et al. 1973, Torr 1957). Reports on the
development of medullary veins do not exist to our knowledge.

Technique of examination

13 bovine embryos of a vertex-breech-length (VBL) of 20-130 mm were
removed from the slaughtered maternal animals and their umbilical
arteries were injected with an aqueous solution of barium sulphate
and gelatin. After fixation and decalcification or removal of the
spinal cord from the vertebral column, the specimens were dehydrated
in paraffine and cut into longitudinal and transverse slices for
microradiography and histology. For details, see Thron (1988) and
Stoeter et al. (1980).

RESULTS

5 th week (1 embryo, VBL 20 mm):

The anlage of the vertebral arch surrounds the neural tube, and a
dense vascular network of a circular and longitudinal orientation
is injected within the subarachnoid space (Fig. 1 a). In the cervical
cord, some intramedullary capillaries are opacified in the dorsal
part of the broad mantle layer. This layer contains the neuroblasts
which originate from the avascular ependymal layer surrounding the
oval-shaped central canal (Fig. 1 b). Although no afferent arteries
are visible they undoubtedly have pentrated through the small marginal
layer of nervous fibres. No intramedullary vessels are opacified
within the dorsal and lumbar region at this stage.

7 th week (2 embryos, VBL 45-50 mm):

Due to the enlargement of the mantle layer, the dorsal part of the
central canal is compressed and on the anterior aspect of the cord,
a shallow groove, the later anterior median fissure, is folded in.
Numerous immature vessels of an irregular caliber and broad branching
segments invade the cord mainly from its dorso-lateral side and form

a dense periependymal network in the inner part of the mantle layer
(Fig. 2 a). The vascular density is higher in the lower parts of the
spinal cord, but the pattern of a predominant invasion of the
arteries from the dorsal aspect of the cord is similar (Fig. 2 b).

8 th - 9 th week (4 embryos, VBL 65-80 mm):

Parallel to the enlargement of the anterior horns, the vascular
density increases mainly in the anterior part of the mantle layer.
In the cervical cord, the anterior and posterior roots are used as
main entrance areas of the afferent arteries (Fig. 3 a). In the
dorsal and lumbar region, an increasing number of arteries originates
from the anterior fissure (Fig. 3 b).

10 th - 11 th week (5 embryos, VBL 100-130 mm):

Now also the cervical part of the cord receives its main blood supply
from anterior sulcal arteries. These vessels originate from a single
longitudinal artery in front of the sulcus, the anterior spinal artery
and show prominent centrifugal branches   in the horizontal and
vertical plane (Fig. 4 a). The vascular network of the lateral and
dorsal parts of the mantle layer is less prominent than that of the
anterior horns and is supplied mainly by separate strong and branching
perforators. In addition, a number of small and radially orientated
vessels enters the marginal layer of nervous fibres (Fig. 4 b). As
in the previous stage, the pattern of a higher vascular density within the anterior horns is more pronounced in the dorsal and lumbar than
in the cervical parts of the cord. A dense vascular network is
opacified in the spinal ganglia.

SUMMARY AND CONCLUSION

As in the brain the vascularisation of the spinal cord depends on the
cytoarchitectonic maturation and the metabolic demands (Craigie, 1955).
After first capillary opacification in the 5th week, the initially
dense vascular network in the periependymal zone of the mantle layer
may be initiated by the high metabolic rate of the cell-producing
matrix. The subsequent enlargement of the anterior horns shifts the
main source of blood supply to the anterior aspect of the cord. In
contrast to the dense network of vessels within the mantle layer, the
marginal layer of nervous fibres remains in a stage of poor
vascularisation. Thus, a pattern of spinal blood supply which is
comparable to that of adult man is reached at the end of the 3rd
embryonal month.

ACKNOWLEDGEMENT

We thank Dr. Tutzer from the Veterinäramt in Ravensburg for the
animal embryos.

REFERENCES

Craigie EH (1955) Vascular patterns of the developing nervous system. In: Waeksch H (ed) Biochemistry of the developing nervous system, Academic Press, New York, p. 28-51

Di Chiro G., Harrington T., Fried LC (1973) Microangiography of human fetal spinal cord. Am J Roentgenol 118:193-199

Hoskius ER (1914) On the vascularisation of the spinal cord of the pig. Anat REc 8:371-391

Stoeter P, Schmidt-Lademann S., Voigt K (1980) Embryonal and fetal development of capillaries: microangiographic investigatoins. I. The brain stem. Diagnostic Imaging 49:131-140

Thron AK (1988) Vascular anatomy of the spinal cord. Neuroradiological investigations and clinical syndromes. Springer, Wien - New York

Torr JBD (1957) The arterial supply of the fetal spinal cord. J Anat London, 91:576

Voigt K, Stoeter P (1980) Neuroradiologie der embryonalen Hirnent-wicklung. Enke, Stuttgart

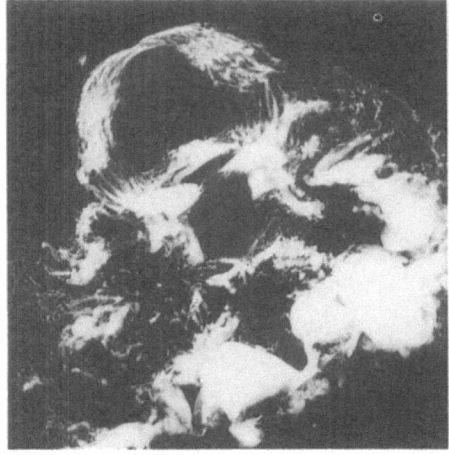
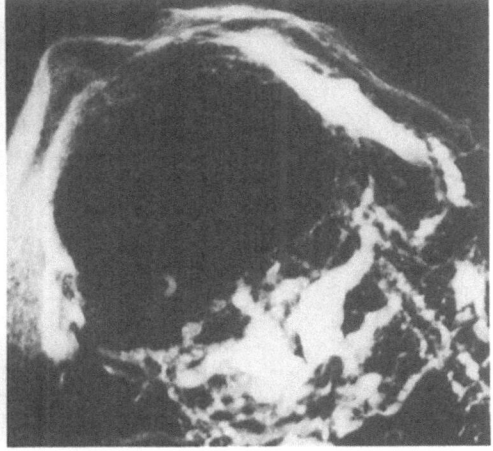

a)   b)

Fig. 1. Gestational age (GA) 5 weeks. Vertex-breech-length (VBL) 20 mm. Within the dense vascular network surrounding the neural tube (a) some intramedullary capillaries are opacified (b).

242

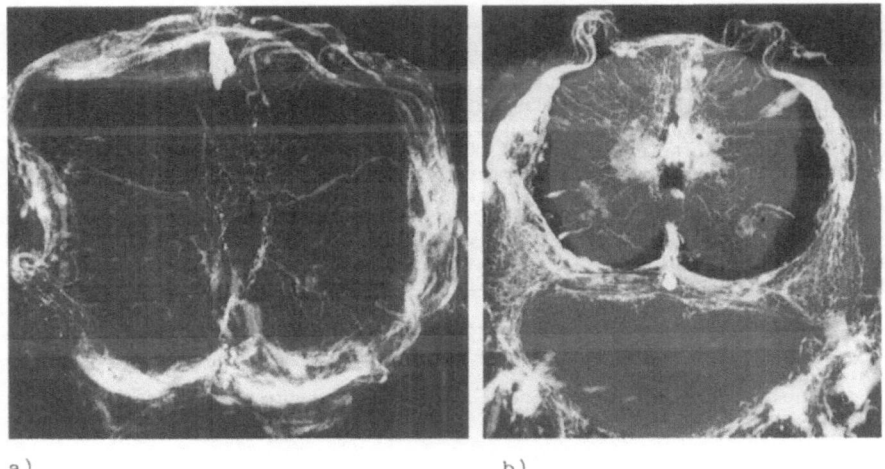

a) b)

Fig. 2. GA 7 weeks. VBL 45-50 mm. For explanations see text.

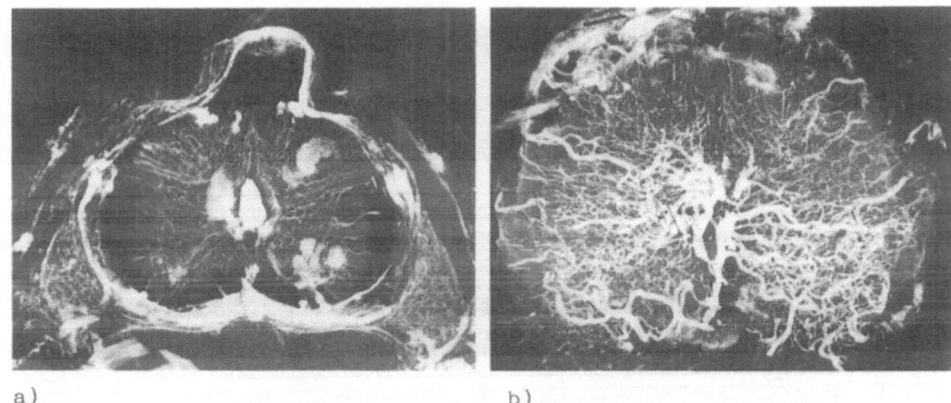

a) b)

Fig. 3. GA 8-9 weeks. VBL 65-80 mm. For explanation see text.

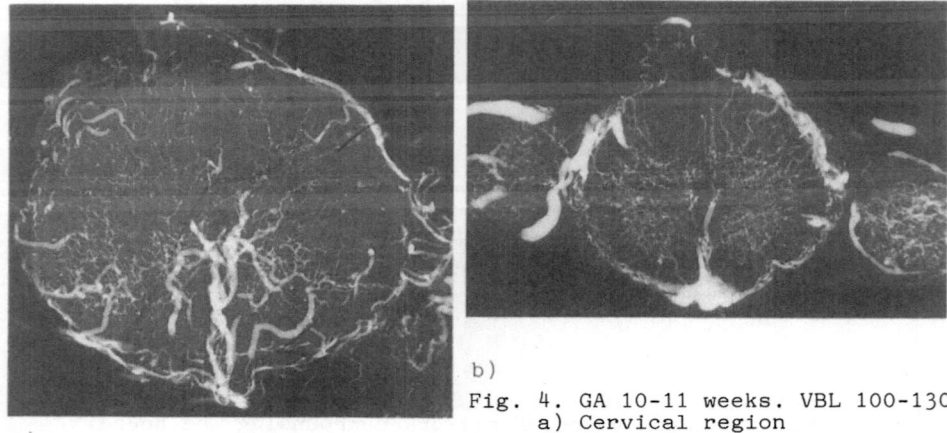

b)

Fig. 4. GA 10-11 weeks. VBL 100-130 mm
        a) Cervical region
        b) Thoracic region

a)

Spinal Cord Sonography in Post-Laminectomy Tumour Patients

U. Mende, A. Aschoff, P. Fritz, and H. Betz

SUMMARY

30 laminectomized tumour patients underwent 68 transcutaneous sonographic examinations of the spinal contents in the laminectomy region.
Good to excellent visualization of the spinal cord was found in 67% of
the patients. Insufficient or lacking demarcation of the spinal cord
in 23% of the patients was due to tumorous processes. Only in 10% incomplete visualization was based on other reasons (bone fragments,
keloid formation, short postoperative interval).
Noninvasive, inexpensive, efficient and dynamic, often superior to other
imaging methods postoperative sonography should become a standard procedure in diagnosis of residual tumours or recurrences, therapy-monitoring, follow-up and posttherapeutic care.

INTRODUCTION

The diagnosis of intraspinal space-occupying processes is based on
clinical examinations and the imaging methods with conventional X-ray,
tomography, myelography, CT and increasingly MRI. The advantages of
percutaneous realtime sonography, widely used in other fields, are
usually rather limited due to the high acoustic reflection and attenuation of ultrasound by the mature intact bone. The situation is completely different when extensive osteolytic destructions or surgical laminectomy provide the acoustic window through which the vertebral canal
and its contents can easily be evaluated.
Based on the experience with 30 post-laminectomy tumour patients who
had been examined by transcutaneous postoperative sonography this contribution discusses the advantages and limitations of this imaging
method for follow-up, therapy-monitoring, and diagnosis of tumour recurrence.

MATERIALS AND METHODS

Between December 1984 and June 1988, 30 patients (24 male, 6 female)
after laminectomy because of tumorous intraspinal processes underwent
examinations by high resolution real-time sonography (N=68; frequency
1 to 12 times) either routinely for postoperative follow-up and therapy-
monitoring under chemo- or radiotherapy or because they were showing
clinical signs of a recurrent tumour.

The mean age was 49.9 ± 18.4 years, ranging from one to 81 years.
Histologically the space-occupying lesions were astrocytoma, ependymoma (4), lymphoma (4), metastases of hypernephroma (4), unknown primary (4), breast cancer (3), bronchus carcinoma (3), other malignancies (7), and exostosis (1). The examinations were performed with the patients in prone, sitting or lateral decubitus positions on a Picker LSC 7000 device with 5 (or 7.5) MHz linear array transducers using water soluble gel as coupling agent. Representative sagittal and transverse sections of the pathological findings, measured in size and analyzed in structure (grey-scale histogram) were documented on video imaging film.

RESULTS

20 patients (66.7%) with 54 examinations (79.4%) presented good or excellent visualization of the spinal contents (Fig. 1A). Sonographic demarcation of the spinal cord from the neighbouring structures was incomplete in 4 patients (13.3%) with 8 examinations (11.8%) due to tumorous involvement. Artefacts and attenuation based on bone fragments,too short postoperative interval and expressed keloid formation were technical reasons for incomplete visualization in another 3 cases (10 and 4.4% resp.). Nonvisualization of the spinal cord was found in 3 examinations (4.4%) of 3 patients (10%) with tumour recurrence only(Fig. 1B).

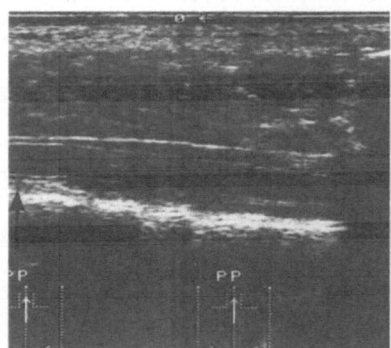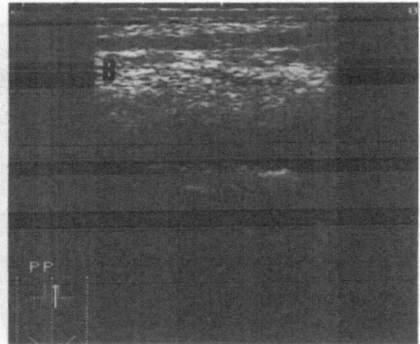

Fig. 1. Visualization of the spinal cord. Sagittal sonograms.
A) 26-year-old male, Hodgkin's disease IV. Intraspinal manifestation in the thoraco-lumbar spine. Small residual tumour (arrow), excellent visualization after laminectomy. B) 69-year-old female, carcinoma of the breast. Intraspinal metastases in the thoracic spine. 7 months after laminectomy, hypoechoic recurrent tumour. No visualization of the spinal cord.

DISCUSSION

Whereas intraoperative spinal sonography is gaining growing importance as standard procedure in many neurosurgical centers, postoperative spinal sonography hs not become a routine method yet (Braun et al. 1983, Horii and Raghavendra 1986, Montalvo and Quencer 1986, Pasto et al. 1984).
As in expensive and available method, noninvasive, without the risks of contrast medium nor the need for radiation protection it is repeatable in optimal planes giving excellent evidence due to its high structural resolution. Bearing in mind its limitations with diagnostic

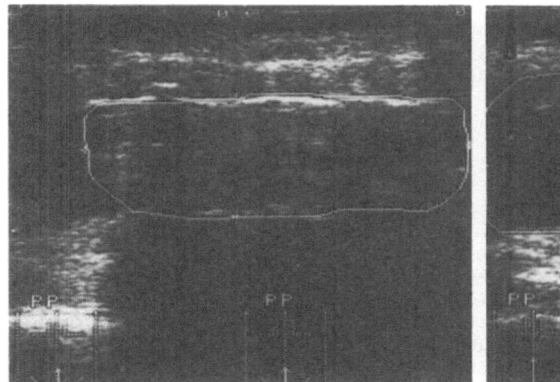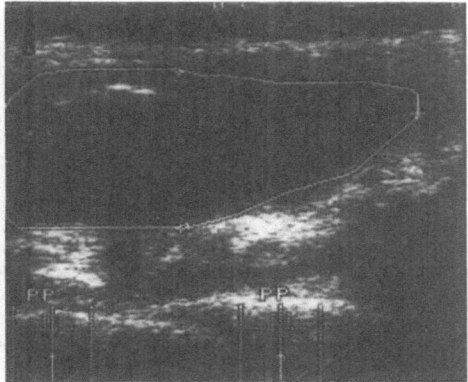

Fig. 2. Recurrent pseudomeningocele. Sagittal sonograms.
46-year-old patient with recurrent ependymoma of the lumbar spine.
Pseudomeningocele.
A) after puncture
B) recurrence 11 days later

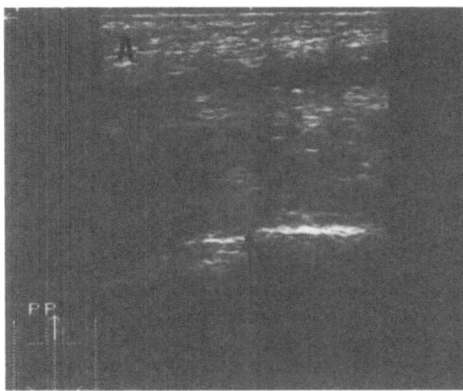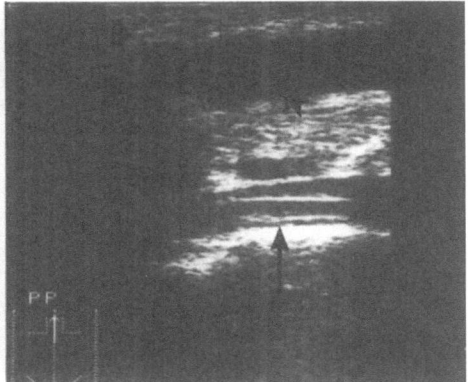

Fig. 3. Sonographic control under radiotherapy. Sagittal sonograms.
20-year-old male with Hodgkin's disease. Intraspinal manifestation
in the thoracic spine.
A) 2 weeks after laminectomy. Badly defined spinal cord; residual
tumour (arrow).
B) Excellent visualization of the spinal cord, no rest tumour (arrow)
after radiotherapy. Secundary findings: Seroma in the soft tissues of
the back (*).

problems in case of short laminectomy, obscuring foreign material, extreme keloid formation, short postoperative interval and unsatisfactory visualization of deep-lying structures with high-frequency transducers as well as nonvisualization of changes beyond the laminectomy gap this method offers many advantages.
It will not only show metrics and structure of the spinal cord and its relation to its environs including bone lesions. Moreover as **the dynamic "real-time" method** (superior to static CT and MRI) it offers the fourth dimension that is the motility of the cord by visualizing its movements induced by variations of the intraspinal pressure and arterial pulsations or its absence in presence of infiltrating or large spaceoccupying processes of the soft tissue or the bones. Postoperative changes as hematoma, seroma, abscess or pseudomeningocele can easily be visualized(Fig. 2A,B). Especially in case of questionable radicality position, size and structure of residual tumours as well as its relation to the spinal cord can be well documented. The analysis of changes in size and structure of these processes will objectify the response to chemo- and radiotherapy (Fig. 3A,B). Even in cases where other imaging methods give equivocal evidence these criteria will help to differentiate between tumour recurrence (mostly hypoechoic if extramedullary) and non-tumorous processes like keloid formation and fibrosis (mostly hyperechoic), cyst-formation (mostly anechoic) and atrophy in the follow-up and posttherapeutic care.

CONCLUSION

Based on these results transcutaneous sonography appears as the imaging method of choice for the postoperative spine in tumour patients. Noninvasive, efficient and with a good cost-benefit-relation, occasionally superior to other imaging methods it often makes more costly diagnostic procedures unnecessary in postoperative follow-up, therapy-monitoring and diagnosis of a recurrent tumour.

REFERENCES

Braun IF, Raghavendra BN, Kricheff II (1983)
  Spinal cord imaging using real-time high-resolution ultrasound.
  Radiology 147: 459-465
Horii SC, Raghavendra BN (1986) Transcutaneous sonography of the
  postoperative spine. Neuroradiology 28: 599-607
Montalvo BM, Quencer RM (1986) Intraoperative sonography in spinal
  surgery: current state of the art. Neuroradiology 28: 551-590
Pasto ME, Rifkin MD, Rubenstein JB, Northrup BE, Cotler JM, Goldberg BB
  (1984) Real-time ultrasonography of the spinal cord: Intraoperative
  and postoperative imaging. Neuroradiology 26: 183-187

MR Evaluation with Gadolinium of the Spine in Spinal Cord Compression Secondary to Metastatic Disease and Posttreatment Control

J. Metzger, M. Boukobza, N. Bouayed, A. Arzimanoglou, M. Poirier and R. Roy-Camille (Paris, France)

50 patients with symptoms of spinal cord compression secondary to metastatic disease of the spine were studied by MR with gadolinium enhancement to evaluate the number of metastatic lesions and the degree of impingement on the cord. 27 patients had epidural lesions. In 18 cases CT was also performed. Generally, epidural tumor extension was visible without contrast and MR is demonstrated to be superior to CT. In some cases, lesions not well defined or not visible without contrast were easily seen after administration of gadolinium.

Postoperative and post-radiation therapy MRI was performed in 15 cases and is very useful to appreciate the results, even with artifacts due to plate.

Compression of the Cervical Spinal Cord in Mucopolysacharidosis

D. Wagner and P. Stoeter (Ravensburg, FRG)

A 39-year-old man suffering from mucopolysacharidosis type II (Runter disease) developed cervical myelopathy mainly with disturbance of gait. CT and myelography showed an important hyperdense enlargement of the dura with severe compression of the spinal cord and the surrounding subarachnoid space from the foramen magnum to the level of C5. For decompression, laminectomy C1-C3 and dural splitting with plastic reconstruction was performed. The patient improved for 1 month following operation and has now been stable for 2 years.

The findings and course of this case are compared with the few reports in the literature.

Lumbar Facet Joint Syndrome. A Randomized Prospective Trial

E. M. Laasonen, G. Lilius, A. Harilainen, P. Myllynen, and G. Grönlund

Chronic low back pain (LBP) is a major cause of disability and sick-leaves in many Western countries (Frymoyer and Cats-Baril 1987). Pathogenesis of LBP can be clarified in only 15-20% of cases (Nachemson 1985). Great interest has been focused on the intervertebral disc, obviously because a specific diagnostic entity and therapy mode are at hand. Another topic attracting growing interest is facet joint syndrome (FJS), although its definition is most vague as yet (Fairbank et al. 1981; Lippitt 1984; Eisenstein and Parry 1987; Mooney 1987). Facet joint injections (FJI) of steroids and/or local anaesthetics have been recommended for therapy in FJS (Destouet et al. 1982; Theron et al. 1983; Carrera and Williams 1984; Lynch and Taylor 1986). The number of patients in these publications has varied from 20 to 100 and the favourable results up till six months from 20 to 58%. No previous randomized, placebo-controlled study has come to our attention and we now report the results of such a study.

PATIENTS AND METHODS

An orthopaedic surgeon and a physiatrist together selected 109 patients for this study, according to the following criteria:
- unilateral low back pain ≥ 3 months,
- - in 57% combined with radiating pain (above the knee),
- local paralumbar tenderness and muscle spasm,
- no actual neurological symptoms or signs,
- failed previous therapy with analgesics and/or physiotherapy,
- - in 25% (27 pat.) previous disc surgery.

These 109 patients were randomized into three injection groups:
- 6 ml bupivacaine hydrochloride (Marcain[R]) mixed with 2 ml (80 mg) methylprednisolone acetate (Depo-Medrol[R]), altogether 8 ml into each of the two facet joints (28 pat.),
- the same mixture pericapsularly around two facet joints (39 pat.),
- 8 ml physiological hydrochloride (saline) into two ipsilateral facet joints (42 pat.).

The ipsilateral facet joints L3 - 5 were injected in 14, and L4 - S1 in 94 patients.

Altogether 53 subjective and objective criteria (or combination scores of them) were recorded before the injection, one hour, two weeks, and six weeks after the injection, and the subjective criteria were recorded three months later by letter. Neither the

patient nor the recorders of the objective criteria knew which
medium was used and where the patient had been injected. The
following criteria revealed significant improvements or were of
interest for other reasons (the ones with best consistency
underlined): work status, subjective pain scale (0 mm = no pain,
100 mm = intractable pain), pain drawing (= an areal sketch of
subjective pain), diminution of pain during flexion, extension, or
rotation of the back, subjective verbal evaluation of the effects of
the injection, length of pain relief assessed by letter at 3 months,
objective disability score combined during physical examination of
standing, walking, sitting, dressing, climbing onto the examination
table, and sitting with legs extended (a score from 6 to 18 points),
spinal flexion, extension, lateral bending to the painful and
painfree sides (Moll and Wright 1971), rotations alike, short and
long Schober tests measured using a measure band, inappropriate
signs (IAS) and symptoms, side effects of injection, and
degenerative changes in lumbar spine films. The IAS consisted of
nonanatomic tenderness, over-reactions, simulation, inappropriate
distraction pain, and inappropriate regions of pain (Waddell et al.
1984). If the patient revealed $\leq$ 2 signs during the physical
examination, she was included in the low IAS group (65 pat.); $\geq$ 3
signs meant inclusion in the high IAS group (44 pat.).

RESULTS

Table 1. Most consistent improvements in the assessed criteria in
109 patients with facet joint syndrome and subjected to fact
joint injection

Criterion	Improvement	Difference in improvement	
	In the whole material	Between IAS groups	Between injection groups
Work status	p < 0.001	n.s.	n.s.
Subjective pain scale	p < 0.0001	p = 0.0186	n.s.
Pain relief 3 months or longer	36%	n.s.	n.s.
Objective disability score	p < 0.0001	p = 0.0202	n.s.

Altogether 25 patients from the whole material group returned to
work during the follow-up of 3 months, five patients went on sick-
leave and three retired. A shortening of the subjective pain scale
(= improvement) was also marked at follow-ups one hour, two and six
weeks after FJI (all, p < 0.001). In addition, a statistically
significant diminution in subjective pain during flexion, extension
and rotation was observed in the whole material. However, the
objective measurements of spans of these movements did not change
significantly.

Paradoxically, the patients <u>without</u> degenerative changes in their lumbar films were more often on sick-leave (p < 0.05). Other differences between these two groups were insignificant.

Eleven low IAS patients returned to work during follow-up, as well as nine high IAS patients (N.s.). However, the work status of the latter group was worse both at the beginning (p < 0.05) and at the end of the study. The high IAS group had a more pathological pain drawing both before the injection (p = 0.0186). The situation was almost the same in the objective disability score (p = 0.0607 and 0.0202, respectively). The diminutions of subjective pain during flexion, extension and rotation did not differ in the two IAS groups. On the other hand, the high IAS patients bent their backs less both on the painful and pain-free sides, and also extended their backs (p = 0.00111, = 0.0002, and = 0.0458, respectively).

When comparing the abnormalities on the subjective pain scale, pain drawing, inappropriate symptoms and IAS, significant correlations were found between all of them (from p < 0.001 to p = 0.039), suggesting that they all reflected the same personal (psychic ?) aspects of a patient.

The three injection groups did not differ with regard to age, sex, marital status, duration of symptoms, work status, operations, or distribution of pain before the study. There were no differences with respect to clinical findings, subjective pain scale, or IAS. After injection, the three injection groups did not differ from each other in any of the 53 criteria recorded. There were two exceptions: the patients with intra-articular cortisone-anaesthetic mixture extended (p = 0.0433) and rotated (p = 0.0380) their backs more easily than those to whom the same mixture was administered pericapsularly.

DISCUSSION

The choice of FJS patients was as vague as in earlier publications and our material is not identical with any of them. We avoided patients with symptoms and signs indicating disc herniation or spinal stenosis. We preferred patients in a subchronic phase and at risk of chronic, debilitating disease.

The search for relevant criteria for improvement was a complicated process. We correlated enormous amounts of data and arrived at a great number of statistical significancies, of which many were controversial. We cannot therefore be 100 % certain that all of our criteria are correct. However, our main purpose was to help the patient to return to work.

We are able, however, to emphasize some general trends. A significant proportion of the patients returned to work during our study and also improved according to other criteria. This was the case both in the low and the high IAS groups, irrespective of which drug was injected and regardless of the site of injection. This occurred in spite of the fact that the high IAS group was both subjectively and objectively poorer both before and after FJI. We even dare to claim that the relative improvement in the high IAS group was of the same magnitude between the end-points, as in the low IAS group. What could be the reasons for such success? Could the psychological influence of the doctor's presence have played a part, or could an impression have been created by the semi-dark examination room with its flickering TV monitor? Could the deep pain and discomfort inflicted by the injection have had a psychological effect also? Were the psychological factors dominating the whole FJI play?

The subjective and objective improvement results measured by various movements of the lumbar spine did not lead to consistent results. Our material may have been too limited for them to have yielded convincing results.

We conclude:

- it is difficult to choose a patient material that unequivocally represents FJS,
- it is difficult to choose objective criteria to reveal and quantitate the benefit found or affected among FJS patients,
- if FJI is the correct therapy, the choice of drugs is still controversial,
- the beneficial effect after FJI is temporary and a long-standing effect is dependent on the patient's somatic and psycho-social resources for self-induced cure,
- the high IAS patients are poorer both before and after FJI, but the relative improvement between the two extremes is the same.

REFERENCES

Carrera GF, Williams AL (1984) Current concepts in evaluating of the lumbar facet joints. CRC Crit Rev Diagn Imaging 21:85-104
Destouet JM Gilula LA Murphy WA Monsees B (1982) Lumbar facet joint injection: indication, technique, clinical correlation and preliminary results. Radiology 145:321-325
Eisenstein SM Parry CR (1987) The lumbar facet arthrosis syndrome. Clinical presentation and articular surface changes. J Bone Joint Surg (Br) 69B:3-7
Fairbank JCT Park WM McCall IW O'Brien JP (1981) Apophyseal injection of local anaesthetic as a diagnostic aid in primary low back syndromes. Spine 6:598-605
Frymoyer JW Cats-Baril W (1987) Predictors of low back pain disability. Clin Orthop 221. Clin Orthop 221:89-98
Lippitt AB (1984) The facet joint and its role in spine pain. Management with facet joint injections. Spine 9:746-750
Lynch MC Taylor JF (1986) Facet joint injection for low back pain J Bone Joint Surg (Br) 68B:138-141
Moll MJH Wright V (1971) Normal range of spinal mobility. Ann Rheum Dis 30:381-386
Mooney V (1987) Facet joint syndrome. In: Jayson MIV (Ed.): The lumbar spine and back pain, 3rd Ed. pp 370-382. Churchhill Livingstone, London
Nachemson AL (1985) Advances in low-back pain. Clin Orthop 200: 266-278
Theron J Blais M Casaco A Courteoux P et al. (1983) Lumbar spine: therapeutic radiology. J Neuroradiol 10:223-230
Waddell G Bircher M Finlayson D Main CJ (1984) Symptoms and signs: Physical disease or illness behaviour? Brit Med J 289:739-741

Width of the Cervical Spinal Canal in Multiple Sclerosis and Its Significance for Therapy

M. Muessig, W. Trabert, K. Schimrigk, and G. Huber

The width of the Cervical Spinal Canal (CSC) had already been measured in healthy persons and different groups of patients because it is an important pathogenetic factor for Cervical Myelopathy. If patients with Multiple Sclerosis (MS) get symptoms of a damage of the cervical spinal cord and show a narrow CSC in the lateral spine X-ray, it is not clear if the symptoms are due to Cervical Myelopathy or to plaques of MS in the cervical spinal cord.

Before presenting our results according to this problem it is necessary to agree upon some definitions to avoid misunderstandings:
    1.) Only the sagittal width of the CSC is measured, because it is narrower than the transverse width.
    2.) The width measured from the midpoint of the dorsal surface of a vertebral body to the next point of the spine of the same vertebral body will be called "dispositional width" of the CSC at that vertebral level. Spondylophytes are neglected in this measure.
    3.) The width from the tip of a dorsal spondylophyte to the next dorsal point of the CSC will be called "minimal width" of the CSC at that vertebral level.

Up to now most authors preferred to measure the "dispositional width" of the CSC and thus neglected the influence of dorsal spondylophytes. The two main reasons for this approach were:
1.) Spondylophytes are a result of degenerative processes and thus their occurence depends on age and environmental factors. The "dispositional width" therefore seems to reflect the genetically determined width of the CSC.
2.) Theoretically it is possible to confound spondylophytes, which are sited in the lateral part of the CSC with medial sited spondylophytes. In this case the CSC would be assessed to be too narrow, because the real sagittal width of the CSC was not measured.

Our impression was, however, that this approach lead to the reverse error: by using the "dispositional width" the width of the CSC was estimated to be too wide.

To prove that we compared the lateral spine X-rays and the lateral spine-tomographies of 35 patients with MS. In the X-rays we measured "dispositional" and "minimal" width, and in the exact median layer of the tomographies we measured the "minimal width", which in this case we called "true minimal width".
Fig. 1 shows the deviation of the "dispositional width" and the "minimal width" from the "true minimal width" in the 35 patients.

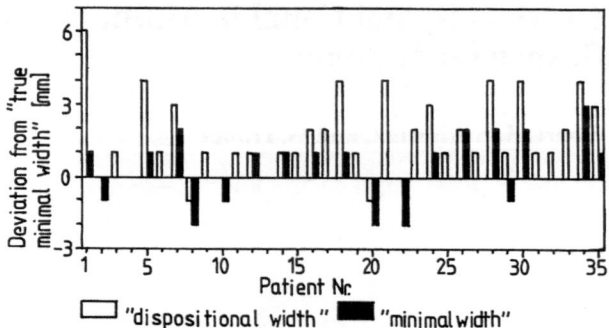

Fig. 1 shows "dispositional width" and "minimal width" compared to
"true minimal width" in 35 patients with Multiple Sclerosis. Positive
values indicate that the CSC was measured too wide, negative values
indicate that it was measured too narrow.

The results confirm our theory that using the "dispositional width"
leads to a greater error than using the "minimal width". The mean
error using the "dispositional width" was 1.8 mm, but using the
"minimal width" it was only 0.66 mm.
If it is especially intended to discover patients with pathologically
narrow CSC, the "dispositional width" leads in most cases to
overestimation of the width of the CSC.

For these reasons we measured in our study of 98 patients with MS who
had been admitted to our hospital between 1982 and 1985 the "minimal
width" to detect the pathogenetic important factor of narrowing of the
CSC and also the "dispositional width" to get values, which could be
compared with the values of other authors.

To our surprise we found that patients with MS had a significantly
wider CSC at all vertebral levels than healthy people (values for
healthy people were taken from Losch (1968)). The significance was
0.0001 at all vertebral levels (C1-C7), except C2, where it was 0.001
(see Fig. 2).
We also took into account that values for the width of the CSC in
patients with MS already had been published by Lurati and Mertens in
1971. These authors found values for the width of the CSC in MS which
were nearly identical with our values, but they did not mention the
difference to the width in healthy people.

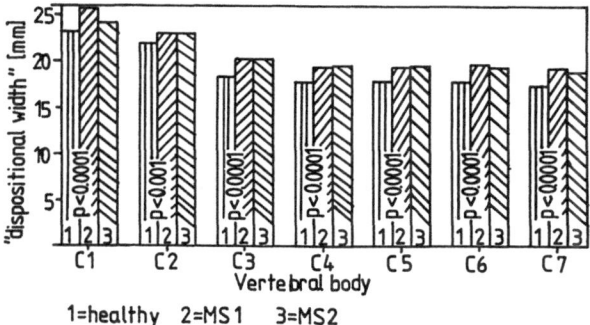

Fig. 2 shows the width of the CSC in healthy people (Losch 1968) and in two groups of patients with Multiple Sclerosis (MS1 = own group, MS2 = Lurati and Mertens 1971).

Thus in two independent studies it could be shown that the CSC is wider in patients with MS than in healthy persons. The width of the CSC was measured in the two MS groups with exactly the same method as in the healthy people.

Why patients with MS have a wider CSC than healthy persons is an open question. A genetic reason could be possible, but further studies are necessary to give an answer.

The real interest of our study, however, focused on patients with MS and a very narrow CSC.
If these patients get symptoms of a damage of the cervical spinal cord, it is not clear if the symptoms are due to Cervical Myelopathy or to plaques of MS in the cervical spinal cord.
It is also possible that patients with demyelinisation of the cervical cord due to MS are especially susceptible to mechanical damage of the cervical cord due to a narrow CSC.
This leads to the important question whether patients with MS and narrow CSC should have Clowards operation or a laminectomy.
To answer this question we selected the patients with the narrowest and with the widest CSCs out of the 98 MS-patients of our study. The case histories of these patients were analysed to see if there were symptoms of the damage of the cervical spinal cord.
The result was that there was in both groups the same frequency of patients with symptoms of damage of the cervical spinal cord.
To get further information we investigated all MS patients in our hospital who had either a Clowards operation or a laminectomy in the years between 1962 to 1986. There were 12 patients and their histories and postoperative courses were analysed in detail.

In 8 of these 12 patients the operation was not successful. In two patients there was a temporary improvement of the preoperative complaints and in only two patients the improvement was permanent. In one of the two patients with long lasting improvement, however, this improvement did not start until one month postoperatively and during intensive physiotherapy. In the other patient there was complete improvement of the preoperative complaints for three years but then symptoms of a damage of the cervical spinal cord accured again. Nine years after the first operation a second operation was necessary, which was unsuccessful.

Altogether Clowards operation and laminectomy seem not to be very promising to patients with MS and narrow CSC.

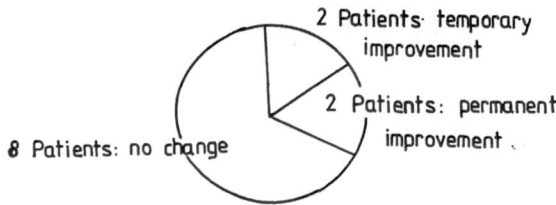

Fig. 3 shows the postoperative outcome in 12 patients with Multiple Sclerosis in whom Clowards operation or a laminectomy was carried out.

CONCLUSIONS

1.) If it is intended to estimate the width of the CSC in a lateral X-ray, it is necessary to take into account the influence of dorsal spondylophytes.
2.) Patients with MS have a wider CSC than healthy persons.
3.) Patients with MS and narrow CSC do not have more frequently symptoms of damage of the cervical spinal cord than patients with MS and wide CSC.
4.) Clowards operation or laminectomy are rarely successful in patients with MS.

REFERENCES

Losch A (1968) Röntgenuntersuchungen über den sagittalen Durchmesser des Zervikalkanales bei gesunden Erwachsenen. Dissertation an der medizinischen Fakultät Hamburg.
Lurati M, Mertens HG (1971) Die Bedeutung der anlagebedingten Enge des Cervicalcanales für die cervicale Myelopathie. Z Neurol 199:46-66.

Tethered Spinal Cord: Reliability of Conventional Myelography and Postoperative Follow-up in 30 Patients

H. O. M. Thijssen, J. L. Merx, and S. H. Bakker-Niezen

The aim of this investigation is to evaluate the reliability of the diagnostic parameters of the radiological features, especially in conventional lumbar myelography, since these will be used in the future as golden standard for new developing diagnostic methods (1) like ultrasonography (US) and magnetic resonance imaging (MRI) and to evaluate the results of surgical intervention in the same group of patients. In earlier communications we described the execution of conventional myelography in these patients. Myelograms have to be of high quality because errors are easely introduced (2-3).

MORPHOLOGY

Three types of spinal cord tethering can be distinguished although often combinations are found:

1. Pathological filum terminale the most simple form; a short filum terminale, attached to the periost of the sacral arches, holds the conus in an abnormal low position.
2. Intradural lumbosacral lipomas, which can be divided into three forms:
a) the lipoma of the filum terminale can be considered as a very broad filum. The conus tapers into a filum terminale that shows a progressive thickening into a lipoma.
b) the conus lipoma is an intradural lipoma in the neighbourhood of the normally closed conus medullaris and is adherent to it. In most cases the filum terminale is present as a distinct structure, caudally from the lipoma.
c) the lipomyeloschisis is a pathological entity in which the incompletely closed end of the cord, the myeloschisis, is embedded in a lipoma. Inside the lipoma are many fibrous septa and an interface between cord and lipoma is absent.The lumbosacral roots originating from the edge of the open neural plate are running through the lipomatous mass and are often hypoplastic and asymmetrical in length. In most cases there is no distinguishable filum terminale.
In these three forms of intradural lumbosacral lipomas tnere is an extension of the intradural part of the lipoma through a defect in the dura mater into the extradural tissue, which tethers the conus in an abnormal low position (4).
3. Diastematomyelia, total schisis and fixation of the cord due to an osseous, fibrous or fibrocartilagineous septum connected with the ventral and/or dorsal osseous border of the spinal canal. Both legs of the totally split cord reunite to one conus that often tapers in a pathologically short filum terminale.

MATERIAL AND METHOD

In 31 patients conventional myelography was carried out, 30 of them were positive for a tethered spinal cord and surgically treated. The prevalence of the disease in our hospital is high: 0.96. The findings in the myelography and the surgical inspection were correlated.

RESULTS

Findings in radiological examination and surgical inspection are listed in table 1.

Table 1. Radiological and surgical findings.

	plain X-ray films 30 patients	conventional myelography 30 patients	CT myelography 20 patients	surgical findings 30 patients
open lumbar arches	18			19
open sacral arches	28			28
fused arches	7			5
block vertebra	3			
butterfly vertebra	1			
bony spur	5		4	5
sacral hypoplasia	11			
scalloping of vertebrae	9			
scoliosis	8			
wide dural sac		28		
meningocele		11		14
pathologic filum terminale		14	5	20
lipoma of filum terminale		6	5	6
lipoma in or near conus		9	10	14
diastematomyelia		6	4	6
abnormal course of nerve roots		18	7	16
asymmetric location of cord		9	9	15
dorsal location of cord		16		

Comparing these findings the following conclusions can be drawn. All patients had a form of spina bifida or dysplasia on plain X-ray films of the lumbar spine, what means that the sensitivity is high although the specificity is low.

In general conventional lumbar myelography is a reliable method of investigation for determination of the normal and abnormal position of the conus. In case of a lipoma however it can be difficult or impossible to locate the tip of the conus, but in these cases the exact location of the conus does not influence the indication for surgery.
The meningocele was always found on myelography, unless an earlier meningocele repair had resulted in a disconnection between the cele and the dural sac. Myelography showed a reasonable reliability in the detection of an abnormal conus position due to a pathological filum terminale. The false negative findings were due to a very thin filum, that could not be distinguished from a nerve root, while a false positive finding appeared to consist of adherent sacral roots. In these cases however the low position of the conus already formed an indication for surgery.
Because we could not differentiate in most cases between a conus lipoma or a lipomyeloschisis, we combined these as a group called conus lipoma. The diagnosis of a conus lipoma was not always possible in case of an earlier operation or if the border between nerve tissue and lipoma was located outside the dural sac. Also a lipoma of the filum terminale in close relation with the dural sac, due to adhesions, can be missed. The cases of diastematomyelia were always found during myelography. The diagnostic quality parameters for the conventional lumbar myelography are listed in table 2. The mainly high predictive values indicate that conventional myelography is a reliable method of investigating the TSC syndrome in our hospital.

Table 2: Diagnostic quality parameters. Prevalence 0.96.

	sens	spec	PWpos	PWneg
Position of the conus	0.83	0.94	0.91	0.89
Meningocele	1.00	1.00	1.00	1.00
Path. filum terminale	0.60	0.89	0.92	0.50
Filum terminale lipoma	0.83	0.96	0.83	0.96
Conus lipoma	0.64	1.00	1.00	0.76
Diastematomyelia	1.00	1.00	1.00	1.00
Total	0.82	0.96	0.94	0.85

CT myelography was not carried out in all patient and most of these investigations were done on a second generation CT scanner. However, the information of the anatomic derangements in the transverse plane was of great value for the surgeon, especially in case of a diastematomyelia. We also got the impression that CT myelography with a 3rd or 4th generation CT scanner facilitates the diagnosis in cases of lipomyeloschisis.

SURGICAL FOLLOW-UP

The aim of the surgical intervention of the tethered spinal cord is to prevent or stop progression of functional disturbances of legs and bladder and to treat the coexisting pain. If this succeeds, the treatment has fulfilled its purpose; it is even better if improvement of funcional disturbances occurs after the operation. Gait disturbances improved in 74% of the patients with this symptom while in 21% of these patients the progressive deterioration came to an end. Bladder disturbances improved in 67% of the patients with this symptom, while the pain disappeared in 75% of the 25% patients with pain. In only 1 patient the operation resulted in bladder disturbances, due to a complication. Of the other 29 patients operated upon in 8 patients a normal clinical situation was retained, in 14 patients an improvement was established, while in 7 patients a pre-existent progression came to an end. As a result the overall succes rate in our 30 patients comes to 97% (5-6). The follow-up time was 1 to 5 years.

CONCLUSION

In patients with a tethered spinal cord an early operation can prevent or stop progressive neurologic, orthopedic and urologic symptoms; therefore, diagnostic radiology should be done as early as possible. We do advocate an early lumbar conventional and CT myelography in patients with external signs of occult spinal dysraphia and osseous anomalies in the lumbar region, even if clinical symptoms are lacking. The diagnostic quality parameters as mentioned indicate to our opinion that conventional myelography can be used as "golden standard" in the preoperative evaluation of the TCS. Future studies have to prove the same accuracy for new developing diagnostic procedures like US and MRI.

REFERENCES

1. Naidich TP, Fernbach SK, McLone DG, Shkolnik A (1984) Sonography of caudal spine and back: congenital anomalies in children. AJNR 5: 221-234

2. Bakker-Niezen SH, Walder HAD, Merx JL (1984) The tethered spinal cord syndrome. Z Kinderchir (Suppl 11) 39:100-103

3. Merx JL, Thijssen HOM, Bakker-Niezen SH (1983) Tethered conus medullaris in metrizamide myelography. Diagnostic Imaging 52: 179-188

4. Naidich TP, McLone DG, Mutluer S (1983) A new understanding of dorsal dysraphism with lipoma (lipomyeloschisis): Radiologic evaluation and surgical correction. AJNR 4: 103-116

5. Bakker-Niezen SH (1986) Tethered spinal cord. Academic thesis, Nijmegen

6. Merx JL, Bakker-Niezen SH, Thijssen HOM, Walder HAD. The tethered spinal cord syndrome; a correlation of radiological features and peroperative findings in 30 patients. Presented for publication in Neuroradiology

Myelographic Presentation of Meningeal Carcinomatosis

G. Krol, M. Malkin, N. Imam, and J. Posner

INTRODUCTION

Metastatic involvement of the spine occurs frequently in neoplasms (1). A bone marrow of the vertebrae constitutes a favorite target. Involvement of leptomeningeal membranes represents an unusual form of spread of metastatic disease. It occurs in malignancies arising within the central nervous system and, less commonly, as a complication of systemic neoplasms. Specific diagnosis is provided by cytological examination of cerebrospinal fluid. Myelography, although less sensitive, outlines the distribution of the lesions and extent of the involvement.

MATERIALS AND METHODS

Myelographic studies of patients with proven neoplasms and positive CSF cytology were reviewed. There were twenty-nine positive examinations. All were complete myelograms, performed via lumbar (25) or lumbar and cervical (4) approach. Pantopaque was used in nine patients and water soluble contrast was employed in the remainder. The following myelographic findings were defined:

1. Thickening of the roots of cauda equina.

2. Nodular filling defects within the subarachnoid space.

3. Irregularity of the surface of the spinal cord.

4. Scalloping of the periphery of the subarachnoid space.

5. Enlargement of the spinal cord.

RESULTS

The lumbar subarachnoid space was involved in all patients. Additional areas of involvement (thoracic, cervical) were present in seven patients. The most common mode of presentation consisted of abnormal thickening of nerve roots of cauda equina which was identified in 18 patients. This occurred as a single finding in seven patients, four with diagnosis of lymphoma. It was commonly associated with other radiographic abnormalities of subarachnoid space. The second most common radiographic finding consisted of a single or multiple filling defects within the subarachnoid space of various size which occurred in 14 patients. Large nodular lesions with substantial compromise of the spinal canal were found in three patients. Diffuse involvement with disease found in all three regions was identified in five patients, four with primary diagnosis of medulloblastoma.

DISCUSSION

Metastatic involvement of leptomeninges may occur in a course of primary CNS neoplasm as well as a complication of tumors arising at the distant site. Clinical presentation is that of multifocal neurological deficits, headache and change of mental status (3). The diagnosis of meningeal metastases is usually made by cytological examination of CSF. Radiographic assessment of the extent of the disease includes myelography, computed tomography of the head and, more recently, contrast enhanced MR examination of the spine and head. Myelographic abnormalities of meningeal carcinomatosis include thickening of the roots of cauda equina, single or multiple nodular filling defects within the subarachnoid space, localized enlargement of the spinal cord, irregularity of the surface of the spinal cord and the periphery of the subarachnoid space (4). Pathologically, these are due to infiltration of the neural structures by the tumor or growth of the tumor within or on the surface of roots, spinal cord or meningeal membranes (5). There appears to be some correlation between the type of primary diagnosis and the above described patterns. Patients with lymphoma are more likely to present with thickening of the roots while this is less likely in other types of tumor. Large nodules may occur in systemic as well as primary CNS cancers. However, together with diffuse involvement of spinal subarachnoid space, they are more likely to occur as a complication of medulloblastomas.

SUMMARY

Meningeal infiltration by metastases may pose a difficult diagnostic problem and may even mimic benign disease. Myelography is diagnostic a procedure of choice and reveals variable presentation of root thickening, multiple nodular filling defects, scalloping of the spinal cord and subarachnoid space. It should be obtained even if noninvasive tests (including MR) are negative.

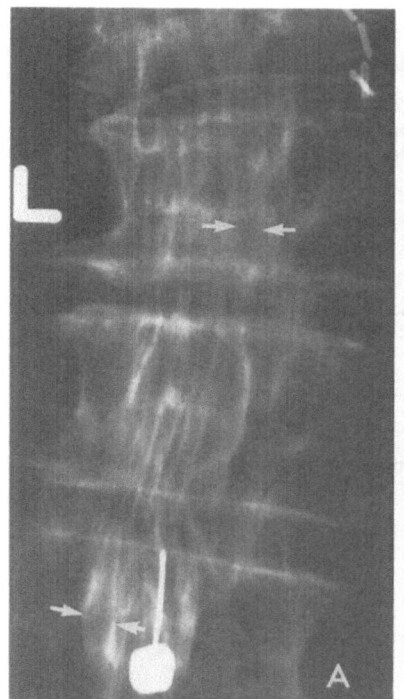

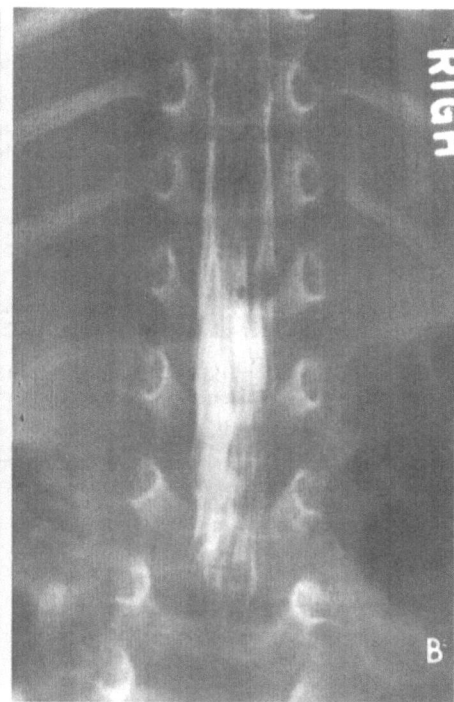

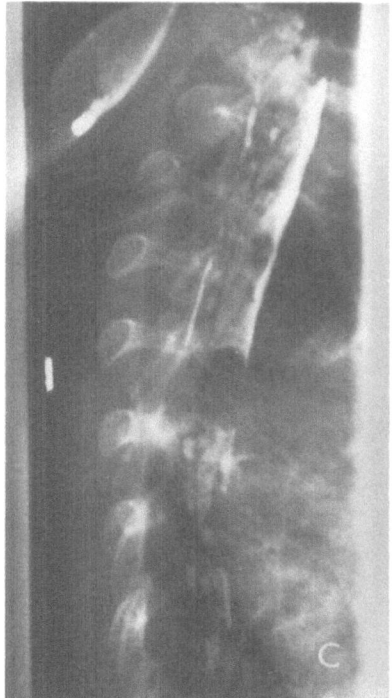

A. Metastatic lung carcinoma. There is diffuse crowding and thickening of the roots of cauda equina. Discrete "beaded" appearance of the individual roots is noted (arrows).

B. Medulloblastoma. Small individual nodules are identified within lumbar subarachnoid space. In addition there is enlargement of the conus medullaris.

C. Medulloblastoma. Single, large nodule is identified in mid thoracic region.

REFERENCES

1. Spinal metastases: Current status and recommended guidelines for management. P Black. Neurosurgery 5 #6 1979 pages 726-746

2. Spinal metastases with neurological manisfestation. Review of 600 cases. JP Constanse, D Divitiis, R Donzelli, R Spaziante, JF Meder C Haye. Journal of Neurosurgery 59:111-118 (1983)

3. Diagnosis and treatment of leptomeningeal metastases from solid tumors: Experience with 19 patients. WR Wasserstrom, JP Glass, JB Posner. Cancer 49:4 pages 759-772, 1982

4. Spinal leptomeningeal infiltration by systemic cancer: Myelographic features. KS Kim, Su Ho, PE Weinberg, C Lee, AJNR May-June, 1982 139:361-365

5. Myelographic diagnosis of radiculomeningeal metastases of carcinomas. P Cauquil, D Doyon, J Metzger, M Thibierge, G Crouzet, M Hurth. Journal of Radiology, 64:11 pages 607-613.

6. MR of cranial and spinal meningeal carcinomatosis: Comparison with CT and myelography. Krol G, Sze G, Malkin M, Walker R. AJNR, 1988;9:709-714.

Interventional Neuroradiology

Interstitial Nanoradiology

Endosaccular Treatment via the Endovascular Approach of the So-called Surgical Subarachnoid Aneurysms: A New Technique

J. Moret, L. Picard, P. Derome, J. Lepoire, L. Castaings, and A. Boulin

Introduction

The introduction of the detachable balloon technique by Serbinenko in 1974 [6] and by Debrun in 1975 [1] opened the way toward the endosaccular treatment of aneurysms [2,3,7]. To date the most extensive experience regarding this therapeutic approach has been published by Romodanov in 1982 [5]. However, multiple obstacles have slowed down applications of the technique:

The detachment system in association with the valve mechanism [4] at the balloon neck had to be mode "softer" and more reliable.

The flexibility and the navigation control of the catheter had to be improved in order to allow access to aneurysms at the circle of Willis or beyond.

The balloon material had to develop toward a polymerizing substance, as suggested by Taki in 1980 [8], in order to prevent balloon deflation, which occurs in time and can lead to aneurysm recanalization.

After 14 years of progressive improvements we are now able to propose a simple, efficient and reliable technique for definitive treatment of subarachnoid aneurysms.

Materials and Methods

The first of the recent advances in endovascular treatment of aneurysms was the use of polymerizing substances which can be mixed with con-

---

* This paper received the Schering Award of the European Society of Neuroradiology 1988

trast medium, such as HEMA (2-hydroxyethyl-methacrylate)[1]. This substance, described by Hieshima and Goto (to be published), combines almost all the properties required: (1) Its viscosity before the beginning of polymerization is almost the same as that of water. (2) It is a hydrophilic material which mixes perfectly with water-soluble contrast medium. (3) Its polymerization characteristics can be reliably controlled at body temperature, especially the time between mixture preparation and the beginning of polymerization. This enables us to work for 20-40 min, depending on the mixture concentration, with a very fluid material, i.e. with very small catheters (size below 2F).

The second recent advance is the introduction of microcatheters with progressive suppleness, variable flexibility and steering capacity[2], which has transformed and tremendously extended the potential for brain navigation without a guidwire, a _sine qua non_ when working with a blind-ending catheter.

Despite these technical advances, the endosaccular treatment of aneurysms by endovascular approach still faced a barrier:

Although HEMA seems to be the most suitable material for balloon inflation, its preparation must follow very strict rules to obtain reliable and reproducible results: (1) The concentration of catalyzed HEMA in the final mixture must be superior to 42% to ensure that polymerization will occur. (2) The mixture of catalyzed HEMA and contrast medium must be perfectly homogeneous to avoid partial polymerization inside the balloon, which induces partial balloon deflation because of osmotic exchanges between the nonpolymerized part and the surrounding tissues, or because of insidious leaking through the valve mechanism.

Although microcatheters with progressive suppleness and variable flexibility allow cerebral navigation with good manual control of progression and direction, even through small vessels, their dead space is too big regarding the volume of small aneurysms. This makes it impossible to replace contrast material by a polymerizing substance

---

[1] I.T.C., 389 Oyster Point Bvld, Suite 5. So., San Francisco, CA 94080, USA

[2] "Magic catheters" from Balt (10 rue Croix-Vigneron, 95160 Montmorency, France)

inside the balloon. The problem of dead space in any kind of micro-catheter has been a tremendous barrier to the spread of the balloon occlusion technique. A simple 2F microcatheter of 1.50 m length, used via the femoral approach, has a dead space of around 0.25 ml, which is quite a large volume when dealing with berry aneurysms. Hieshima has proposed a technique of "exchange" between contrast medium and HEMA through the microcatheter. He uses several inflations and deflations of the balloon as an exchanging and mixing mechanism. Doing this, one must take into account the volume of the catheter dead space and the necessary volume of the balloon for aneurysm occlusion, in order to calculate the best mixture of HEMA and contrast medium according to the above-mentioned parameters of HEMA preparation.

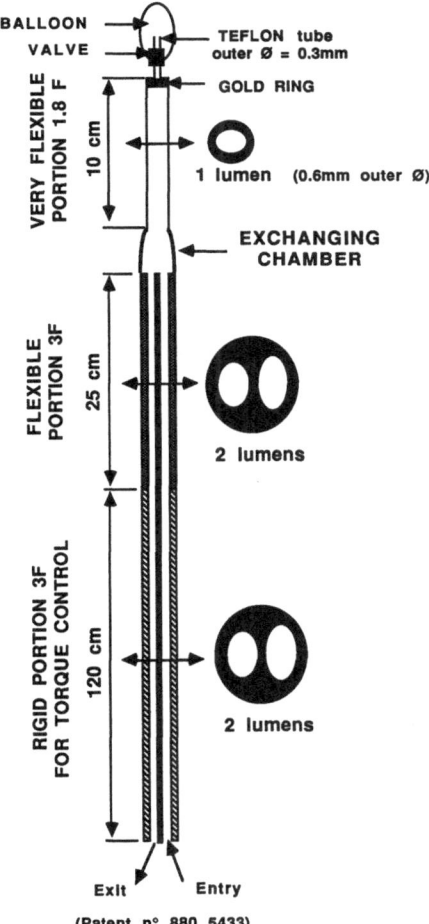

Fig.1. Schematic representation of the catheter described herein

Until now this technique has been the only one available to "ex-change" contrast material and HEMA, but still has not enabled treatment of berry aneurysms whose volume is lower then that of the micro-catheter dead space. One again this technique did not represent a true exchange but rather an "intra-balloon blending." This led to a partially intra-balloon preparation of the HEMA mixture with consequent difficulties in ensuring corrent and reliable mixing. Also, inflations and deflations of the balloon represent a potential risk of weakening the aneurysmal sac, therefore increasing the risk of rupture.

Taking advantage of recent advances in microcatheter technology, we have now developed a catheter which combines progressive suppleness, variable flexibility, steering capacity, a double lumen and an exchanging chamber between the two lumens (Fig.1), and is specially devoted to endosaccular treatment of aneurysms by the endovascular approach.

Discussion

This catheter, produced by Balt (Magic BD 2L). has kept all the intrinsic qualities of the "magic" catheters (torque control during catherization, thermoplastic properties allowing shaping of the catheter tip according to individual anatomical pattern, easy and safe valve mechanism for detachment), and for the first time overcomes the difficult problem of dead space, permitting true and total exchange between contrast material and any kind of polymerizing substance. The exchanging chamber has been positioned close to the catheter tip, and not actually at the tip, for two reasons: (1) The exchanging maneuver uses only the double lumen portion of the catheter and, by the way, can be performed completely outside the balloon, avoiding potentially risky manipulations inside the aneurysmal sac. (2) The single outlet of the exchanging chamber on which the balloon is fixed is very narrow (1.8 F) and has a negligible dead space of 0.01 ml. This very flexible distal portion of the catheter preserves the possibility of hyperselective catherization of vessels at the circle of Willis and beyond.

Because of this new technology, the HEMA mixture can be totally prepared in vitro and simply exchanged with contrast medium. This clears up the above-mentioned problems concerning the HEMA preparation. As a matter of fact it is easy to get a very reliable mixture regarding ho-

mogeneity and percentage of catalyzed HEMA when preparing it in vitro.
Personally we use the following mixture (Polymeran, Balt); solution A:
2.45 ml HEMA mixed with 0.05 ml ethylenglycldimethacrylate[1] and 0.05 ml
of H_2O_2 at 30%; solution B: 50 mg ammonium ferric sulphate with 1 ml
bidistilled water. Eight drops of solution B are put into solution A
and 1.5 ml of 200 mg/ml nonionic contrast medium is added. After
blending, the mixture is ready for exchange.

At body temperature this solution allows 25 min to perform the exchange
and a control angiogram before being unable to deflate the balloon
because of polymerization. This is plenty of time, as the exchanging
maneuver itself needs just 2 min. If a longer exchanging time is needed,
for a more precise control angiogram, one can use only four drops of
solution B without changing any other parameters. This gives an exchanging time of around 40 min. The Polymeran mixture has the key advantage of keeping its volume exactly when drying after polymerization.

Because the mechanism of detachment induces slight traction on the
balloon, we prefer in most cases to detach the balloon before waiting
for complete polymerization of the mixture. In this way, if the
balloon is moved during detachment, we can deflate it and reposition
it.

Results

Seventeen "surgical berry aneurysms" whose size ranged from 4 to 10 mm
were treated by endosaccular occlusion via the endovascular approach
using the new technology and according to the technique we have described. Eight of these aneurysms arose from the intracranial carotid
artery, at the carotid bifucation (Fig.2) or in the carotido-ophtalmic
position (Fig.3) or close to it; three from the tip of the basilar artery; two from the posterior communicating artery (Fig.4); two from the
middle cerebral artery (Fig.5); and two from the anterior cerebral and
anterior communicating arteries.

Three patients were treated in the acute phase between the 3rd and the
10th day after the onset of the hemorrhage. One of them presenting with
a basilar tip aneurysm died 3 days later from ischemic complications,
but had an extensive and marked spasm. The two others did well and are
cured.

---

[1] Merck, Darmstadt, West Germany

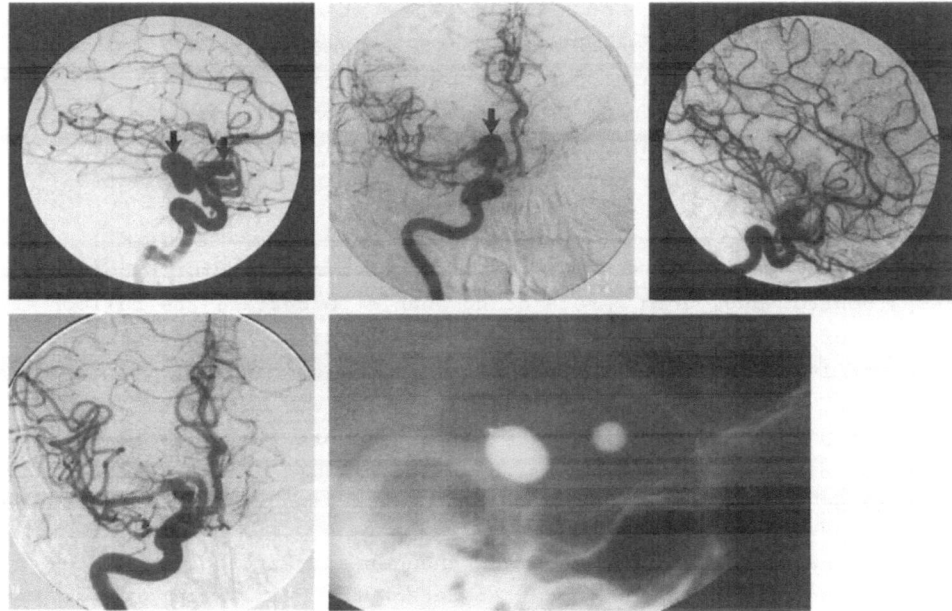

Fig.2. a,b: Internal carotid injection lateral (a) and AP (b) projections in a patient presenting with two aneurysms (arrows) at the
carotid bifurcation. c,d: Control angiogram after treatment showing
cure of the aneurysms. Internal carotid injection lateral (c) and
AP (d) projections. e: Plain film in lateral projection showing
balloons in the aneurysmal sacs

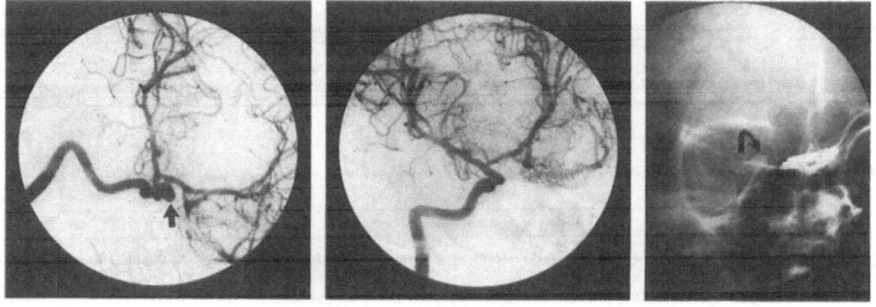

Fig.3. a: Carotido-ophthalmic aneurysm (arrow) seen on an oblique
internal carotid injection. The patient had been operated on previously for a similar aneurysm on the opposite side. b: Control
angiogram after balloon occlusion showing cure of the aneurysm.
c: Plain film of the skull in oblique projection showing the balloon
(curved arrow) and metallic clips

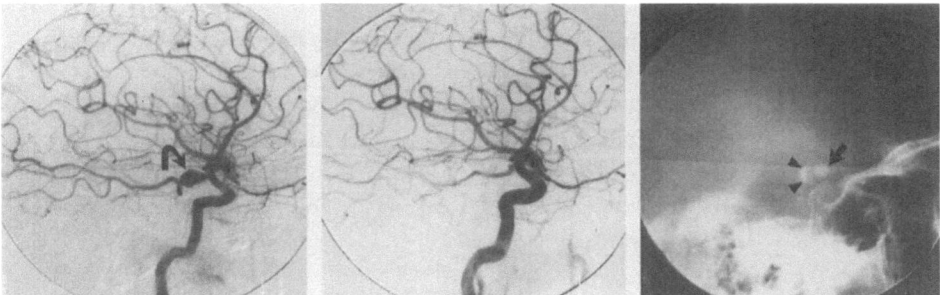

Fig.4. a: Aneurysm of the posterior communicating artery (curved arrow) seen on a lateral internal carotid injection. b: Control angiogram after balloon occlusion showing cure of the aneurysm. c: Plain film of the skull in lateral projection. Note the positioning of the balloon (arrow) just at the aneurysmal neck, far away from the bottom (arrowheads)

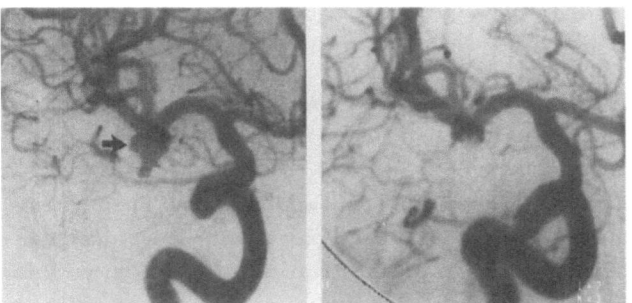

Fig.5. a: Aneurysm of the middle cerebral artery bifurcation (arrow) seen on an oblique internal carotid injection. b: Control angiogram in the same projection showing cure of the aneurysm after balloon occlusion

Four patients had never bled - the aneurysm was discovered by chance. One of them, with an anterior cerebral artery aneurysm, could not be treated by the endovascular approach because of technical problems and was operated upon. The three others did well and are cured.

Ten patients were treated in the late subacute phase between the 4th and the 8th week after hemorrhage. Two of them got neurological complications: (1) Hemianopia caused by clotting in the supraclinoid internal carotid artery and embolism through the posterior communicating artery, although the patient was fully heparinized and despite the immediate injection of urokinase. Because of a very small aneurysmal neck, a

double-balloon technique was used in order to force balloon penetration
into the sac. The length of the procedure and the two catheters in
the same internal carotid artery were the cause of the complication.
(2) Hemiplegia by occlusion of the anterior cerebral artery after treatment of an aneurysm of the anterior communicating artery which was
giving rise to both anterior cerebral arteries (this patient had been
operated upon twice prior to embolization). The eight other patients
of this group did well and are cured.

At this point, eleven of our patients have had a control angiogram
around 4 months after endovascular treatment, confirming definitive
occlusion in all cases.

Beside the above-mentioned anatomical results, which are tremendously
encouraging, one must emphasize two points which clearly reflect the
technical advances: in all cases whatever the location of the aneurysm,
balloon detachment could be performed without any problem and total
replacement of contrast medium by a polymerizing substance could be
achieved.

Endovascular treatment of berry aneurysms in emergency during the acute
phase of hemorrhage does not seem to pose more problems if the patient
has no spasm. Although we need more experience, we can already say
that the trauma involved in endovascular treatment of the aneurysmal
sac is probably less than that with surgical treatment, as endovascular therapy does not change the external environment of the aneurysm.
In fact the counterpressure applied by the brain on the aneurysmal sac,
which is one of the major factors in warping the breach after bleeding,
is kept intact during endovascular treatment. The "inner trauma" to
the aneurysmal sac which can be charged to endovascular treatment may
exist, but its importance is mainly theoretical. In practice, two
things make this risk much lower than expected: (1) The use of digital
substraction angiography associated with the road mapping technique
allows almost perfect control of balloon fitting in the sac. (2) Experience shows that it is often possible to occlude an aneurysm by
placing a small balloon just at the neck, without filling the sac
completely (Fig.4). Doing so, one can avoid inducing pressure on the
bottom sac which is well known to be the weakest point.

We have never experienced aneurysmal rupture. This does not mean
that the risk does not exist, simply that careful management of the
technique, use of the appropriate tools and adequate training are the
best guarantee of safety. To be able to act if a rupture happens we

always have glue (Histoacryl), prepared in advance, which can be immediately injected (either through the balloon catheter after detachment, or through another catheter) to try to stop the bleeding. We have performed such a "life-saving" maneuver in a rupture of an anterior communicating artery aneurysm which occurred during selective catheterization for treatment of a corpus callosum angioma.

Conclusion

In 1 year we have moved from the hope of being able to treat berry aneurysms definitely by endosaccular occlusion to the reality. The results, technically speaking, exceed all expectations. The clinical results reported here are tremendously promising. It appears that endosaccular treatment of berry aneurysms via the endovascular approach can already compete with neurosurgical treatment. We believe that aneurysms in difficult surgical locations, such as basilar tip or carotido-ophthalmic aneurysms, must be treated first via the endovascular approach. There is no doubt that in the very near future more and more aneurysms, even in emergency, will benefit from treatment using this new technique.

Summary

Endosaccular treatment of berry aneurysms via the endovascular approach has hitherto still faced technical problems which limited the safeby and reliability of clinical application. This paper describes a new concept of catheterization which gives the possibility of: (1) reaching small aneurysms of the circle of Willis; (2) totally exchanging the contrast medium in the balloon with a polymerizing substance in order to prevent balloon deflation; (3) detaching the balloon using a simple, smooth and reliable valve mechanism. Highly promising clinical results are reported based on the treatment of 17 small berry aneurysms via the endovascular approach with preservation of the parent vessel. Three of the patients were treated during the acute phase of the hemorrhage. This new technological advance has already dramatically changed the indications for endovascular treatment.

References

[1] Debrun G, Lacour P, Caron JP, Hurth M, Comoy J, Keravel Y (1975) Inflatable and released balloon technique experimentation in dogs: application in man. Neuroradiology 9: 267-271
[2] Hieshima G, Higashida RT (1986) Intracranial embolotherapy; plugging aneurysms with balloons. Diagn Imaging 8: 90-94
[3] Hieshima G, Higashida RT, Wapenski J, Halbach V, Bentson J (1987) Intravascular balloon emboliyation of a large midbasilar artery aneurysm. J Neurosurg 66: 124-127
[4] Laitinen L, Servo A (1978) Embolization of cerebral vessels with inflatable and detachable balloons: technical note. J Neurosurg 48: 307-308
[5] Romodanov AP, Shcheglov VI (1982) Intravascular occusion of saccular aneurysms of cerebral arteries by means of a detachable balloon catheter. In: Krayenbühl (ed) Advances and technical standards in neurosurgery, Vol 9. Springer, Vienna New York, pp. 25-48
[6] Serbinenko FA (1974) Balloon catherization and occlusion of major cerebral vessels. J Neurosurg 41: 125-145
[7] Taki W, Handa H, Yamagata S, Matsuda I, Yonekawa Y, Ikada Y, Iwata H (1979) Balloon embolization of a giant aneurysm using a newly developed catheter. Surg Neurol 12: 363-365
[8] Taki W, Handa H, Yamagata S et al (1980) Radiopaque solidifying liquids for releasable balloon technique: a technical note. Surg Neurol 13: 140-142

Endovascular Treatment of Intracranial AVMs by Means of Wing Microcatheter: Technique, Clinical and Pathological Results

A. Benati, A. Beltramello, R. Colombari, A. Maschio, S. Perini, E. Piovan, R. Da Pian, A. Pasqualin, R. Scienza, L. Rosta, A. Scarpa, and G. Zamboni

INTRODUCTION

In the embolization of brain AVMs dissatisfaction both for balloon-catheter systems and for bucrylate, led us to the search for new safer alternative materials of catheterization and embolization.
This paper deals with our new microcatheter system and with the pathological aspects of cerebral arteriovenous malformations surgically resected after embolization with Polylene threads.

MATERIALS AND METHODS

Embolization technique: Our personal technique is a modification of the Debrun balloon catheter system (Debrun et al. 1982), but the distal end of the silastic microcatheter is completely open and exposed. Small latex wings surround the tip of the catheter; these "floating" wings increase the area exposed to the blood stream and consequently traction of the microcatheter along the blood flow direction is strengthened (Ingenor, Paris, France) (Benati et al. 1987). Intravascular navigation is flow dependent and is obtained by a propulsion chamber. Once the microcatheter has reached the desired position, superselective angiograms of the vascular feeders are obtained without blocking the blood flow, with high precision and no damage to the vascular walls. As embolic agents, both fluids and particles can be used with our multi-purpose microcatheter: therefore, it is suitable both for AVM embolization and for drug injections. Our experience is mainly based on the use of threads, which can be injected in our own catheter as in other ones commercially available: Pursil and Tracker. Polyfilament polylene 3-0 threads (2 metric: 0,2 mm. in diameter) cut 1,5-2 mm. are discharged into the artery by 1,5-2 ml. of saline. As this technique carries out a progressive form of embolization, the higher-flow shunts are the first to close, followed by the slower flow ones; only when shunt flow is markedly reduced, a few threads may be deposited on the walls of the arterial pedicles, very close to the AVM. In any case the procedure can be suspended, if necessary, at any moment. At the end of each procedure, a superselective angiography of the embolized feeder is carried out by the means of the same microcatheter. Once one feeder is embolized, the same microcatheter can be moved to other feeders: in this way, more pedicles can be embolized in the same session. Control angiograms with the outer coaxial polyethylene catheter are carried out during the various phases and at the end of the procedure without removing the microcatheter.

Patient Population : 51 patients with symptomatic "critical" brain AVMs underwent 77 embolization procedures, carried out with our wing-microcatheter. Clinical status was tested before and after embolization. For each embolization the estimated amount of nidus obliteration was recorded. According to the results obtained by embolization treatment, patients were then submitted to surgery, radiosurgery or scheduled for further embolization sessions.

Pathology : The tissues were fixed in formalin 10% and embedded in paraffin. From each block we obtained sections, 5 microns thick, for routine hematoxylin-eosin examination and for immunohistochemistry.

To characterize the nature of inflammatory cells eventually present around Polylene threads, we analyzed immunohistochemically the paraffin sections just following those obtained for routine hematoxylin-eosin examination. Every case has been treated with a panel of antibodies reactive in routinely fixed paraffin-embedded tissue, including LN1, MB2,UCHL1 and anti-Vimentin antibody, that discriminate between B and T lymphocytes and recognize fibroblasts.

RESULTS

Clinical results : Among the 51 patients embolized in 77 procedures with Polylene threads by means of our silastic microcatheter, 31 patients had completed their treatment. Partial obliteration of the lesion permitted surgery in 22 patients while 9 critical angiomas were reduced to less than 2 cm in diameter: a size suitable for radiosurgery. Operated patients were particulary important in order to study the pathological aspects of resected AVMs previously embolized with Polylene threads. Mean age of the 22 patients operated on was 34 years (range 10-49). AVMs were always located in eloquent areas of the brain (12 left; 10 right). 5 patients experienced previous hemorrhages. Seizures were present in 11 patients, headache in 7. Only one patient presented with a neurological deficit, a left homonymus hemianopia resulting from previous bleeding. Embolization was performed only once in 12 patients, twice in 7, more than twice in 3 cases. The interval between embolization(s) and surgery ranked from 4 to 30 weeks. Intracranial navigation failed twice. Regarding complications only four, totally reversible, minor deficits were noticed with our microcatheter and embolization with threads. In all cases in which a significant decrease (50% or more) in the AVMs size was obtained (18 out of 22), the surgeon felt that pre-operative embolization had consistently helped the surgical removal of the angioma. Surgery caused 3 persisting neurological deficits; in one patient seizures significantly worsened, in another one his previous deficit persisted immodified. For the 17 remaining patients post-operative follow-up was completely normal.

Pathological results : Routine sections of arteriovenous malformations showed Polylene threads in a varying, but frequently small, number of vascular channels. The threads appeared as a colourless material, birifrangent in polarized light, put together in multiple fascicules, mimiking a beehive in transversal sections. In tissues examined from 6 weeks after embolizing therapy, every Polylene fiber was surrounded by varying amount of granulation tissue, with a rich component of mononuclear and foreign body giant cells, that was gone through by many small capillary vessels. The mononuclear inflammatory infiltrate consistently diminished in tissues resected from 12 weeks after embolization; from this time, in fact, the Polylene threads were surrounded by a thin cushion of connecttive tissue with scant mononuclear inflammatory cells and foreign-body giant cells, that filled and completely occluded the vascular lumen. Necrosis of vascular channel walls was never found, nor threads were discovered in the neuroglial parenchyma that commonly lies in the interstices of the vascular channels. In three cases aggregates of polymorphonucleates (PMN) were present in the wall of some AVM channels, far from the threads emboli.

Immunohistochemical methods permitted us to characterize the mononuclear infiltrate, previously described. Around Polylene fibers we always found a great number of T-lymphocytes, UCHL-1 positive and a variable number of spindle-shaped Vimentin positive fibroblasts; instead we never found any LN-1 and MB-2 positive cells, markers of B-lymphocytes.

DISCUSSION

Various proposed techniques for embolization of brain AVMs cannot be considered fully satisfactory and as a result a "gold standard" of proven efficacy and safety does not exist. Recently, various Authors have tried to avoid the risks of vascular damage linked to the inflation of the balloon attached to the tip of the microcatheter (Rufenacht and Merland 1987). But, above all, many doubts still exist about the best embolizing agent. Bucrylate, being fluid, would be the ideal substance but many problems arise both as its practical use (abrupt solidification, complicated calculation of the right polymerization time) and its long term effects are concerned. Besides the suspicions of cancerogenecity, long-term pathological follow-up of brain AVMs treated by embolization with bucrylate have shown patchy transmural necrosis of portions of vessels treated days or weeks before with IBC embolotherapy (Vinters et al. 1985). On the contrary the hallmarks of the inflammatory response to Polylene threads are the presence of both mononuclear cells and foreign body giant cells and the absence of PMN infiltrates. The presence of PMN infiltrates is very important as it is the only reproducible parameter to evaluate the presence of wall necrosis being the structure of vascular channels within AVMs highly abnormal. Differing from what has been reported for IBC (Klara et al. 1985; Vinters et al. 1983, 1985), we found PMN infiltrates only in three cases where they were present in the wall of AVM channels far from the threads emboli. This inflammatory reaction may have occured in response to necrosis, induced by occlusion of the major blood supply to the AVM, as what reported for AVMs resected after balloon embolizations, in which no embolic substance was injected (Lamman et al. 1988).

At immunohistochemistry the absence of LN-1 and MB-2 positive cells around Polylene threads permitted us to state that B lymphocytes were not involved in this inflammatory process: in other words, the immunological process taking place in response to this type of foreign substance is not an humoral one. On the contrary, both many UCHL-1 positive T lymphocytes and Vimentin positive fibroblasts are present: as in other better known granulomatous inflammatory responses, we can postulate that T lymphocytes would give origin to a chain reaction leading to a self-maintaining process, acting until the fibrosis sets in.

CONCLUSIONS

Embolization by means of our microcatheter system associated to Polylene threads proved to be a useful and reliable tool to achieve, in conjunction with surgery, the complete cure in a significant number of critical AVMs. Morbidity and technical failures are both so low as to justify the embolization as the first step in the treatment plan of the majority of critical AVMs. Pathological studies of brain AVMs resected after embolization have demonstrated the absolute absence of angionecrosis; a moderate inflammatory response can be seen, with a tendency towards spontaneous end by the fourth week. The immunological response to threads emboli is cell-mediated, not humoral in type: it gives origin to a self-maintaining granulomatous fibrotic process, taking place from the first month and peaking at the third month. Threads can therefore be usefully employed as embolizing agents for brain AVMs, thanks to their effectiveness and absence of toxicity.

REFERENCES

Benati A, Beltramello A, Maschio A, Perini S, Rosta L, Piovan E (1987) Endovascular treatment of intracranial AVMs. Combined embolization with a multipurpose mobile-wing microcatheter system. J Neuroradiol 14: 99-113

Debrun G, Vinuela F, Fox AJ, Drake CG (1982) Embolization of cerebral arteriovenous malformations with bucrylate. Experience of 46 cases. J Neurosurg 56: 615-627

Klara PM, George ED, McDonnell DE, Pevsner PH (1985) Morphological studies of human arteriovenous malformations. Effects of isobutyl 2-cyanoacrylate embolization. J Neurosurg 63: 421-425

Lamman TH, Martin NA, Vinters HV (1988) The pathology of encephalic arteriovenous malformations treated by prior embolotherapy. Neuroradiology 30: 1-10

Rufenacht D, Merland JJ (1987) Superselective catheterization using very flexible, formed catheters. Acta Radiol; Suppl 369: 600-602

Vinters HV, Galil KA, Lundie MJ, Kaufmann JCE (1983) Long-term pathological follow-up of cerebral arteriovenous malformations treated by embolization with bucrylate. N Engl J Med 314: 477-483

Vinters HV, Galil KA, Lundie MJ, Kaufmann JCE (1985) The histotoxicity of cyanoacrylates. Review article. Neuroradiology 27: 279-291

Embolization of Brain AVMs with Flow-Independent Microcatheters

A. Valavanis (Zurich, Switzerland)

The introduction of flow-independent microcatheter systems (e.g. Tracker-microcatheter) represents a significant progress in the endovascular approach to and obliteration of brain AVMs. This is mainly based on three factors: (1) the possibility to catheterize and embolize the terminal prenidal segments of the feeding arteries, with preservation of small branches of the feeding arteries not participating in the supply of the nidus but supplying normal surrounding brain; (2) the possibility to safely catheterize feeders thought to be mostly inaccessible with the flow-guided calibrated-leak microballoon catheters; (3) the simplicity in the use of these systems, which makes possible obliteration of multipedicular AVMs in one session.

This paper reviews the experience obtained from the application of flow-independant microcatheter systems for the angioarchitectural evaluation and embolization of 42 cases of brain AVMs.

Balloon Occlusion of Internal Carotid for the Treatment of Giant Inoperable Aneurysms

W. S. Tan, J. J. Jafar, R. Abejo, R. M. Crowell, and D. Spigos (Chicago, IL, USA)

Fifteen patients with inoperable giant aneurysms of the internal carotid system were treated by proximal balloon occlusion of the internal carotid. Each patient was assessed with I.V. xenon 133 cerebral
blood flow (rCBF) before and during test balloon occlusion. One patient had a low CBF less than 40 ml/100 gm/min and received an EC-IC
bypass before balloon occlusion. He developed a transient weakness of
upper extremity following balloon occlusion. The weakness recovered
completely within one hour and was considered probably related to embolism. Three patients had low CBF and had their CBF augmented with
manitol (to 40 ml/100 gm/min), followed by balloon occlusion of
internal carotid. Every patient was clinically assessed for tolerance
during balloon test occlusion of the internal carotid before the balloon was detached. One patient had a mild stroke during catheterization and the procedure was terminated. One posterior communication
artery aneurysm and one supraclinoid aneurysm with a persistent trigeminal artery did not thrombose completely. Otherwise the patients
are doing well on a six month to four year follow up.

Endovascular Treatment of a Giant Fusiform Aneurysm of the Basilar Artery. Case Report.

A. Aymard, D. Rufenacht, D. Reizine, F. Woimant,
and J. J. Merland (Paris, France)

A giant partially thrombosed fusiform aneurysm involving the entire
basilar artery presented clinically as a severe, rapidly progressive
tumoral syndrome of the posterior fossa. Treatment by detachable
balloon was performed with an excellent result at a five year follow
up. Treatment methods and the result will be discussed.

Cerebral Arterio-Venous Fistulas Treated by Endovascular Procedure

A. Biondi, D. Rufenacht, and J. J. Merland (Paris, France)

Embolization of cerebral arterio-venous fistulas (AVFs) were performed in 7 patients.

These lesions can be isolated or associated with an arterio-venous malformation (AVM). The associated AVM can be easily recognized in diagnostic angiography, but in some cases it is identified only after occlusion of the fistula because of the dilated venous pouch hiding the AVM.

Clinical findings were progressive neurological deficit or hemorrhage.

Due to advances and progress in technical aspects and microcatheters used, these lesions can be safely treated using an endovascular approach. In our series AVFs were occluded by detachable or undetachable balloons. During embolization, because of high flow in the AVF, the risk of involuntary detachment of the balloon exists. This can be avoided by a second balloon, temporarily inflated behind the first one. This allows a diminished blood flow and so a safe embolization. The use of the undetachable balloon represents an alternative and easier procedure.

Indications, technical aspects and results will be discussed.

The "Creeping Balloon": An Alternative Technique for the Treatment of the Difficult Carotid-Cavernous Fistulas

W. J. Huk

INTRODUCTION

The carotid-cavernous fistula has been the crux for neurosurgeons for a long time. Today it can also be the crux for the neuroradiologist who uses endovascular techniques.

Fistulas, which turn out to be crucial cases, are often high flow fistulas with a wide communication between the artery and the cavernous sinus.

In such a case of a large and difficult fistula, the occlusion of the fistula could finally be achieved with the help of a "creeping" balloon.

CASE REPORT

An 18-year-old woman was admitted to the hospital after a head injury with a pulsating proptosis of her left eye and a loud pulsating murmur.

Angiography of the left carotid artery revealed a large, high-flow carotid-cavernous fistula with steal effect from the circle of Willis into the fistula as was shown by angiography of the right carotid and the vertebral arteries.

The initial plan was to place a detachable balloon through the fistula into the cavernous sinus in order to preserve patency of the internal carotid artery.
Via a direct approach to the left carotid artery in general anaesthesia, a large balloon was brought up to the intracavernous portion of the carotid artery, where it was sucked into the fistula immediately. When inflated, no significant reduction of flow could be observed. A second and, finally, a third balloon were brought into the cavernous sinus across the fistula, which did not succeed in the occlusion of the fistula when inflated simultaneously to their maximum volume and when different positions of the balloons were tried.

However, since I was afraid of inducing oculomotor palsy and because the risk of cerebral embolism from a pseudoaneurysm could not be excluded, no additional balloons were put into the cavernous sinus.

Occlusion of the carotid artery at both ends of the fistula as alternative solution was not possible, as the balloons could not be brought across the large fistula against the retrograde flow from the distal portion of the carotid artery; they were always washed into the fistula.

Finally all three balloons, which were not yet detached, were removed, and a special non-detachable balloon was built intraoperatively, which was designed to achieve distal and proximal occlusion of the carotid artery and the fistula. This balloon was about two cm long when uninflated; upon inflation, the balloon started to enlarge at its proximal end, and with further inflation it was gaining length to the shape of a sausage (Fig. 1).

This balloon was brought up into the syphon and inflation was started about 1,0 - 1,5 cm proximal to the fistula. With further inflation the balloon crept across the fistula - stabilized and guided by the walls of the carotid artery - until it reached the distal intact portion of the syphon (Fig. 2); inflation was stopped before the ophthalmic artery branched off. Now the fistula was occluded, and all symptoms disappeared during the following days.

Since the arterial supply of the left hemisphere through the collateral flow was sufficient while the fistula with its steal effect from the circle of Willis was patent, it was more so after this steal effect was no longer effective.

As this "creeping" balloon was successful in a second, similar case of a problematic carotid cavernous fistula, it may offer a possible alternative technique for the treatment of these crucial cases.

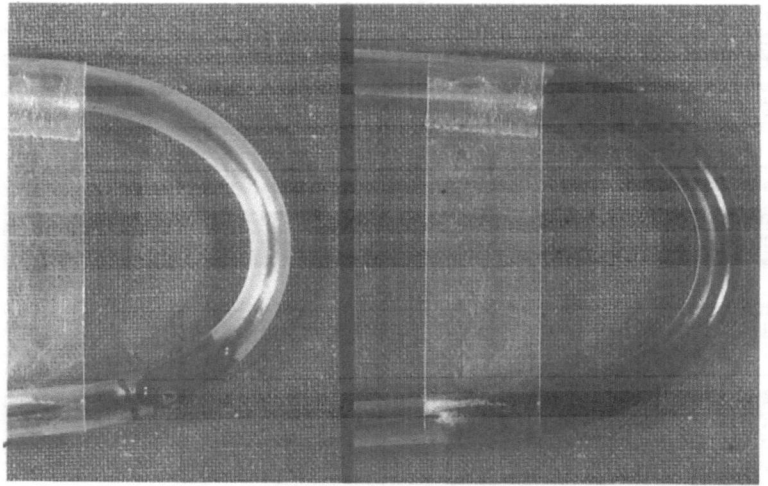

Fig.1: Experimental model of the balloon in a plastic tube. With continuing inflation the ballon "creeps" around the curve.

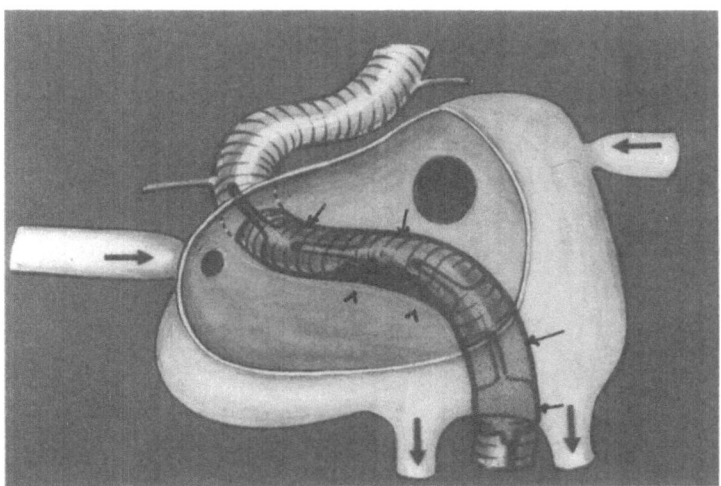

Fig. 2: Drawing of the carotid artery in the cavernous sinus. The balloon (arrows) crossing the fistula (arrowheads) is shown in different stages of inflation.

Embolization of Cerebral AVMs: Experience with Nine Cases

G. Guglielmi, M. Feliciani, G. Guidetti, and P. Silipo

Introduction

The management of cerebral AVMs has been improved and extended by the advent of endovascular embolization techniques which represent preoperative or preradiosurgical procedures. This makes it possible to achieve a reduction in the size of the AVM; sometimes an improvement in progressive neurological deficits, if present, can be expected. In this paper we report our experience with nine cases of cerebral AVMs, in which embolization was attempted as a primary preoperative therapeutic method in order to reduce intraoperative bleeding.

Material and Method

Nine patients (4 men, 5 women) who showed the presence of cerebral AVMs were treated: three AVMs were parietal, two frontal, two deep temporal, one occipital, and one prerolandic. Six patients were referred to our department following bleeding from the AVM, two sufferend from seizures, and one patient complained of intractable headache (Table 1).

All patients underwent a three-vessel (bilateral carotid and one vertebral) angiographic investigation, with a 2 films/s arterial phase evaluation and, when needed, geometrical magnification and photographic image subtraction.

In all cases, after the superselective cannulation of the feeding pedicle(s) and immediately prior to the embolization, an Amytal test was performed under EEG recording and clinical observation. In six cases (nos. 1-6), the superselective cannulation of the feeding pedicle(s) was performed with a Tracker or Pursil catheter, and the embolization was done by injecting an Ivalon-33% ethanol-avitene embolic mixture ("Los Angeles cocktail"), as indicated by Dion et al. (1988). In case no. 9 a Silastic microcatheter was used to inject silk threads into the largest feeding pedicle of the AVM. Case

Table 1. Description of cases

Case no.	Age	Sex	Clinical picture	AVM localization, trunks involved	Embolized pedicles	Embolizing substance	Clinical complications
1	23	F	Severe headache	Right parietal, MCA/ACA	2	L.A.cocktail	None
2	40	M	SAH	Left prerolandic, MCA/ACA	3	L.A.cocktail	None
3	26	F	SAH	Left occipital, PCA	1	L.A.cocktail	None
4	15	M	Seizures	Right parietal, MCA	1	L.A.cocktail	None
5	12	F	SAH	Left parietal, MCA/ACA/PCA	4	L.A.cocktail	None
6	35	F	SAH	Right frontal, MCA/ACA	1	L.A.cocktail	None
7	32	M	Seizures	Left frontal, ACA	1	IBCA	None
8	16	F	SAH	Left deep temporal, MCA/PCA	1	IBCA	None
9	35	M	SAH	Left deep temporal, MCA/PCA	1	Silk threads	None

SAH, subarachnoid hemorrhage; MCA, middle cerebral artery; ACA, anterior cerebral artery; PCA, posterior cerebral artery.

nos. 7 and 8 were treated in a less recent period, using a Silastic calibrated-leak balloon microcatheter (Kerber catheter) and injecting isobutyl-2-cyanoacrylate (IBCA).

Results

A total of 15 feeding pedicles were embolized in the nine treated cases. In seven out of the nine cases (the six treated with the Ivalon-33% ethanol-avitene embolic mixture and the one treated with silk threads) we were able to obtain a marked reduction in the blood flow through the nidus of the AVM (Figs.1-3). In the two cases treated with IBCA there was only a poor reduction in the size of the AVM. The maximum number of embolized pedicles in a single case in the same session was four; in case no. 1, in which the AVM was fed by two pedicles, one pedicle was embolized twice in two different sessions while the other was embolized once. In two cases the optimal positioning of the microcatheter was reached only after more than one session.

No clinical complications occurred during or after the embolization. Four cases underwent surgical removal of the AVM shortly after embolization (nos. 3,4,6,7). In two cases a radiosurgical procedure

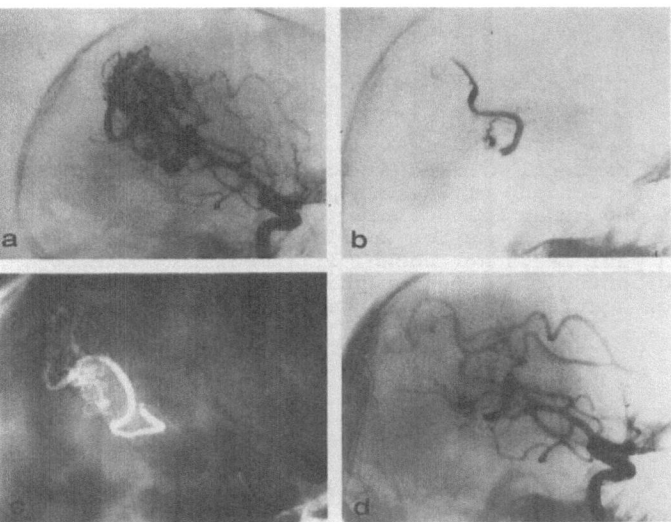

Fig.1. a: Right parietal AVM fed by two main pedicles from MCA and one minor from the anterior choroidal artery. b,c: Superselective angiography and embolization of the two main pedicles with the Los Angeles cocktail. d: Postembolization angiogram showing a persistent feeding from the anterior choroidal artery

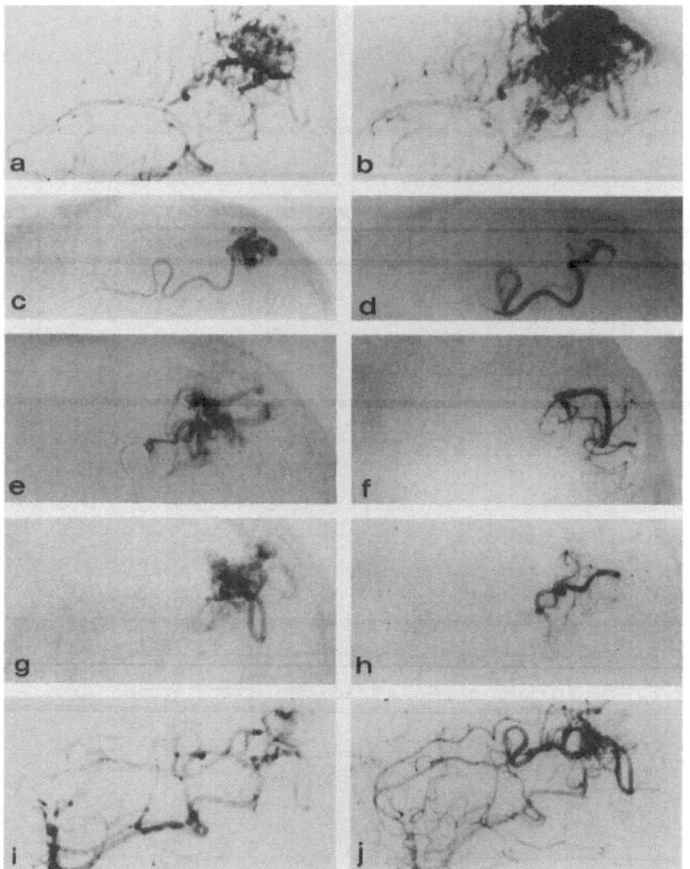

Fig.2. a,b: Large left parietal AVM fed by four pedicles (ACA, MCA, PCA). Superselective angiography of one ACA pedicle (c,d), of one MCA pedicle (e,f), of the other MCA pedicle (g,h) before (<u>left</u>) and after (<u>right</u>) embolization with the Los Angeles cocktail. Embolization of the other ACA pedicle is not shown. i: Immediate postembolization angiographic control. j: Angiographic control 2.5 months after the embolization (patient refused surgery)

was performed (nos. 8,9). Two patients refused the neurosurgical intervention after embolization (nos. 1,5); these underwent a control angiograph 2.5 months after the embolization which confirmed the reduction of the AVM nidus (Figs.1,3). Case no. 2 was considered inoperable due to the volume and depth of the AVM; in this patient further embolizing sessions are planned.

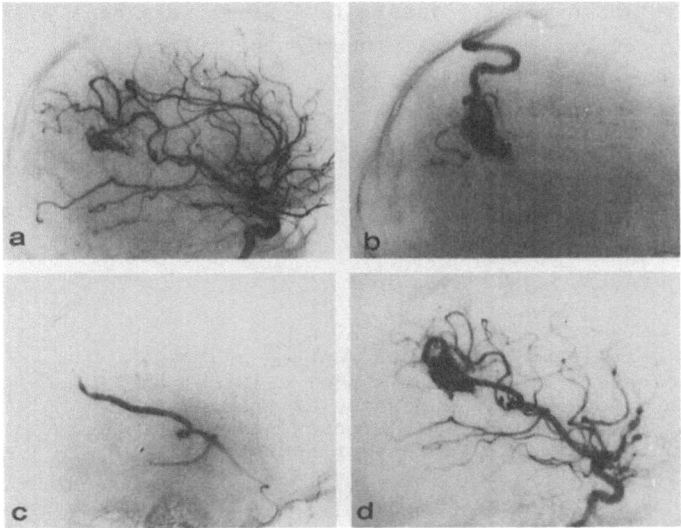

Fig.3. a: Right parietal AVM fed by one main trunk from MCA. Superselective angiography before (b) and after (c) embolization with
the Los Angeles cocktail. d: Postembolization angiogram showing
the persistence of small portion of the nidus fed by tiny branches
of MCA

Discussion

In the majority of cases presented in this paper the Ivalon-33% ethanol-avitene mixture (L.A. cocktail) was used as an embolizing substance; the rationale for its use is based on the hypothesized action
of its components: ethanol acts as a sclerosing agent, avitene pro-
motes platelet aggregation in the distal arterial nidus, while
Ivalon occludes the proximal arterial nidus. By using this mixture,
the extremely distal cannulation of the feeding pedicle(s) is not
as imperative as with IBCA. Furthermore, more than one pedicle can
be cannulated and embolized with the same microcatheter in the same
session. Compared with IBCA, another advantage of the L.A. cocktail
is that there is no risk of glueing of the catheter tip into the
arterial lumen. The partial failure in the two cases treated with
IBCA might be ascribed to the unavailability of effective and ma-
nageable catheters at the time of the intervention and to the fact
that the risks related to the use of acrylic glues did not allow
the injection of an adequate amount of IBCA.

While the Ivalon-33% ethanol-avitene embolic mixture seems to be
effective in treating cerebral AVMs due to its efficacy, manage-

ability, and low risks (Dion et al., 1988), IBCA still retains a
role in embolizing procedures, especially when an arteriovenous
shunt is present inside an AVM.

Acknowledgement. This work was supported by a grant of Ministero
della Pubblica Istruzione (1983-2-12-1).

Reference

[1] Dion JE, Vinuela F, Lylyk P, Lufkin P, Bentson J (1988)
    Ivalon-33% ethanol-avitene embolic mixture: clinical ex-
    perience with neuroradiological endovascular therapy in
    44 arterioveneous malformations. In: Proceedings of the 26th
    Annual Meeting of the American Society of Neuroradiology,
    Chicago, May 15-20, p 220

Therapeutic Embolization of Vascular Malformations of the Head and Neck: Indications, Technique, Results

J. Stojanović, A. Kamler, M. Turić, J. Unušić, and B. Malenica

Introduction

In the 1970s French authors, led by Djindjian, developed superselective angiography and the vascular malformation (VM) embolizing
technique (Djindjian et al., 1972; Merland, 1973; Djindjian, 1974;
Merland and Djindjian, 1975; Natali and Merland, 1976; Natali et
al., 1976; Djindjian and Merland, 1978). Nowadays the angiographic
technique, using mainly the microcatheter system, provides a significant contribution in clinical and hemodynamic VM studies. Better
understanding of VMs led to advances in their classification and to
improvement in treatment efficiency by choosing an adequate thera-
peutical procedure for each case and in accordance with embolization, surgical treatment, and reconstructive surgical procedures.
Angiography, supported by CT and US (pulsed Doppler), shows the
feeding arteries and allows an estimation of VM flow capacity. It
also shows the location and extension in various surrounding anatomic structures irrigated by branches of the external carotid artery (ACE). This artery and other arteries, manifestly or latently,
irrigate through collaterals the head and neck regions of VMs.

Materials and Methods

This study included 15 patients (9 women, 6 men) treated and
followed-up in the RTG Department of CHC Rebro and CIT, University
of Zagreb, since 1983. Ages ranged from 11 to 61 years. Treatment
was performed mostly in younger patients aged 20-40. Routine laboratory tests were followed by CT and US examination, which provided
data necessary for analysis of the location, width, and depth of
VMs, as well as involvement of neighboring and distant structures.

Embolization

Embolization was performed according to the standard therapeutic procedure, most often via the femoral artery. It was carried out in the same session as angiography if the malformation was not irrigated by many feeding arteries. In cases where many feeding arteries were present the embolization was performed in the second or third session, but only when the efficiency of previous embolization was revealed.

As a rule, nonresorbing embolizing materials were used, taking into consideration the hemodynamic characteristics of each VM. In all cases Ivalon particles were used (ca. 250-1000 μm) in combination with other materials (Marbagelan, dura, silk).

In two cases of venous malformation, angiographic and embolizing procedure were performed percutaneously. Final embolization was performed with Ivalon particles mixed with hypertonic glucose solution.

Results

The topographic distribution breakdown of VMs treated in the period 1983-1988 is as follows: four in forehead, scalp, pavillon; three in cheeks, chin, lips, eyelids; two in tongue, cheek, soft palate; two in scalp, calvaria, meninges; and four in neck, nuchal region, scalp.

Angiographic aspects of VMs included the following types of malformation: eight with angiomatous mass with active AV fistulas; three with angiomatous capillary venous mass, without active AV fistulas; two with large venous malformations (cavernoma); and two with mixed malformations. In terms of hemodynamic characteristics, the "active" form of AV shunt was dominant in most cases.

Discussion

The VM embolization technique, at any site, is used increasingly as a sole therapeutic method or as a method of treatment in combination with surgical procedures.

The first step in treatment is devascularization. Many publications present the advantages of this mode of treatment. Each case of VM requires its own embolization technique. Consequently, every angioradiologist must be informed about the best materials and embolization techniques to be able to perform a specific therapeutic embolization. In 11 out of 15 cases of VMs in the region of the head and neck subjected to therapeutic embolization from 1983 and followed up until 1988, the feeding arteries originated in the ACE.

In four cases selective and superselective angiography revealed a complex vascular malformation, irrigated predominantly from ACE branches but also from branches of the internal carotid, vertebral, and deep and ascending cervical arteries.

In all cases the aim of therapeutic embolization was reduction of lesion volume and/or total ablation of the lesion.

In all patients the therapeutic results obtained can be considered positive. Up to now no evident revascularization or recanalization of VMs has been recorded in 12 cases. In three cases the therapeutic embolization was incomplete. It was performed only via ACE branches.

Complications

In numerous papers both the reasons for and various complications in connection with therapeutic embolization are discussed. In our study, although in a small number of cases, no severe complications were recorded, in spite of the fact that the therapeutic material used was not always of the best quality. Also we were presumably not able to prevent distal embolus migration in all cases using our embolization technique.

Conclusion

Each case of VM must have multidisciplinary diagnostic and therapeutic evaluation. None of the embolizing materials that we have used for embolization of complex lesions has produced totally satisfactory results.

Probably the explanation is the "aggressiveness" of the malformation and also the impossibility of filling it with therapeutic material. Results of embolization with less extended lesions could be considered as very good.

References

[1] Djindjian R (1975) Indications, contraindications and complications in embolization of the external carotid artery. J Neuroradiologie 2: 173-200

[2] Djindjian R, Merland JJ (1978) Superselective arteriography of the external carotid artery. Springer, Berlin Heidelberg New York

[3] Djindjian R, Cophignon J, Theron J, Merland JJ, Houdart R (1972) L'embolisation en neuroradiologie vasculaire. Technique et indications. A propos de 30 cas. Nouv Presse Med 1: 2153

[4] Merland JJ (1973) Superselective arteriography of the external carotid branches. Thesis, Paris

[5] Merland JJ, Djindjian R (1975) Embolization of angiomas in the external carotid territory - techniques and results. J Neuroradiol 2: 201-232

[6] Natali J, Merland JJ (1976) Superselective arteriography and therapeutic embolization of vascular malformations (angiodysplasia). J Cardiovasc Surg 17: 465-472

[7] Natali J, Merland JJ, Bories J (1976) Arteriographie superselective et embolisation therapeutique dans les angiomes. J Mal Vasc (Paris) 1: 19-27

Thrombus Formation: Structure and Evolution in Intracranial Aneurysms Treated by Balloon Occlusion

V. Graves, C. Strother, C. Partington, Y. Kikuchi, and P. Eldevik

Nine Patients with intracavernous (N=S) or supraclinoid (n=4) carotid aneurysms were treated by occlusion of the ipsilateral carotid artery with detachable ballons placed as near the origin of each aneurysm as possible. All patients had serial evaluation with CT scans, angiography, and magnetic resonance (MR). Since not all of the nine patients were examined with MR exactly at the same follow up interval, patients were divided into those studied pretreatment (n = 6), within 48 hours of treatment (n = 6), 5-10 days after treatment (n = 4), 4-6 weeks after treatment (n = 4), and at greater than 11 months after treatment (n = 4).

MR was performed using a 1.5-Tesla General Electric Signa Unit. Images were obtained in at least two orthogonal planes. T-1 weighted images (T1WI) were obtained using a spin echo sequence (TR = 600 ms, TE = 20 or 25 ms). Proton density weighted images (PDWI) and T-2 weighted images (T2WI) were obtained using a spin echo sequence TR = 2000 ms, TE = 20 and 90 or 120 ms). the matrix size was 256x256 and slice thickness ranged between 3 and 10 mm.

Two distinct types of thrombi were identified within the aneurysms studied. Spontaneous thrombus which was present on the pretreatment MR scans and induced thrombus which appeared within the aneurysm lumen following balloon occlusion. Each had very different MR characteristics and evolution. While it is impossible to predict how a particular thrombus will evolve, the recent report by Kwan et al 1988,(3) and the sequential MR studies done in this group of patients provides some insight into their evolution. Thrombus evolution is governed by its degree of contact with flowing blood and the state of the vessel wall in which it has formed.

PRETREATMENT MR FINDINGS: Five of the six aneurysms studied with MR before treatment showed evidence of partial thrombosis, on T1WI and PDWI. All of these thrombi were laminated in appearance with thin (< 2mm) layers of irregularly alternating zones of hypointensity, isointensity and hyperintensity (Fig. 1A) On T2WI the bulk of the thrombus became markedly hypointense.

The aneurysm lumen was generally identified by an area of signal void on all pulse sequences (Fig. 1A). In some aneurysms the MR signal within the lumen was heterogeneous with varied signal intensities. These corresponded to intraluminal areas of slow or turbulent blood flow or inflow jet phenomenon as demonstrated by angiography.

POST TREATMENT MR FINDINGS: Following treatment by parent artery balloon occlusion, evidence of new induced thombus within the lumen of the aneurysm was demonstrated in all nine aneurysms.

MR CHANGES WITHIN 48 HOURS: Six of the nine aneurysms were studied within 48 hours after treatment. All showed marked changes in the MR signal characteristics of the aneurysm lumen from the pretreatment MR. In all instances the induced thrombus in the lumen was similar in appearance being isointense or minimally hypointense to grey matter on T1WI (Fig. 1B) and markedly hyperintense on PDWI and T2WI (Fig. 1C).

In all six cases studied within 48 hours, the spontaneous pretreatment thrombus showed a few new areas of hyperintensity on T1WI (Fig. 1B). These were most prominent around the periphery of the thrombus. T2WI demonstrated continued hypointensity (Fig. 1C). There was a small but consistent increase in the mass associated with the aneurysm in all cases. Two cases showed changes in the brain adjacent to the aneurysm consistent with edema.

MR CHANGES WITHIN 5-10 DAYS: Four of the nine aneurysms were studied within 5-10 days of treatment. The bulk of the induced thrombus within the aneurysm lumen became hyperintense on T1WI. Previously homogenous and hyperintense on both PDWI and T2WI the induced thrombus became heterogeneous and hyperintense on PDWI and homogeneous and markedly hypointense on T2WI.

The pretreatment spontaneous thrombus showed some increase in volume on T1WI. This was primarily due to an increase in a band of hyperintensity around the outer margin of the spontaneous thrombus. Varying signal is evident within the spontaneous thrombus on T2WI, but generally remains hypointense.

MR CHANGES WITHIN 4-6 WEEKS: Four patients were examined at an interval between 4-6 weeks post treatment. In all cases the induced thrombus has become homogenous and hyperintense on all pulse sequences (Fig.2 A&B).

The spontaneous thrombus continued to remain inhomogenous but contained large areas of hyperintensity on T1WI and PDWI. The bulk of these areas become hypointense on T2WI. Two cases showed a definite decrease in the mass effect of the aneurysm.

MR CHANGES WITHIN 11-24 MONTHS: Four patients were examined at intervals greater than 11 months. Three of the four aneurysms showed dramatic decrease in their size and mass effect. In two cases it was almost impossible to demonstrate any residual mass. One case showed only a minimal area of heterogeneous signal in the area of the aneurysm. The one aneurysm in this group that did not show a decrease in size was the only one which had MR changes consistent with incomplete thrombosis. This patient continued to have an area of persistent signal void on all pulse sequences which enlarged on follow up MR exams done at 18 and 24 months. This corresponded to a persistent and enlarging aneurysm lumen demonstrated on angiography.

DISCUSSION: A thrombus differs significantly from a hematoma. Depending on its etiology, site of formation and the blood flow, the composition of a thrombus is a spectrum ranging between those composed of primarily platelets and fibrin, and those with a much larger component of red blood cells.(5)(6) A direct relationship exists between the rate of blood flow and the proportion of a thrombus which is composed of platelets. Those thrombi forming in areas of rapid blood flow have the greatest amount of their bulk composed of platelets and fibrin.(2) A hematoma is a collection of blood outside the vasculature and unlike a thrombus is made up of all elements of the blood in proportion to their abundance in the circulation. Thrombus formation and evolution is a dynamic process.

The induced thrombus formed in the lumen of the aneurysm following balloon occlusion is probably initiated because of blood stasis. The hypo or isointensity on T1WI and the hyperintensity on PDWI and T2WI within the first 48 hours after treatment are consistent with those of non flowing blood, the erythrocytes of which still contain oxyhemoglobin.(7) No sedimentation levels were observed in any patients suggesting that within the first 24-48 hours of being isolated from the circulation, blood within the aneurysm is organized. The physical state of the thrombus, along with the stage of erythocyte lysis and hemoglobin degradation combine to determine its MR signal characteristics.(8)(9) Over the interval of 5-10 days post treatment the induced thrombus assumes some of the characteristics of parenchymal hematomas. By 4-6 weeks the induced thrombus was hyperintense on all pulse sequences, a finding consistent with a

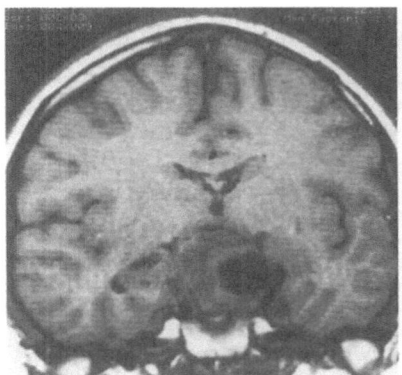
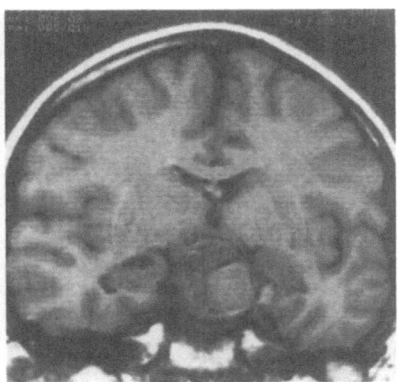

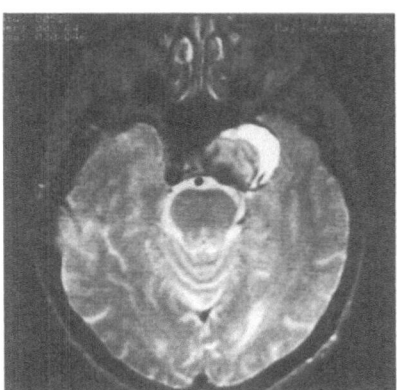

Fig. 1: A. Pretreatment (T1WI) spontaneous thrombus inhomogeneous with thin laminations. Aneurysm lumen and patent carotid are identified by discrete areas of signal void. B. Post treatment T1WI (24-48 hours) induced thrombus in aneurysm lumen isointense to grey matter. Spontaneous thrombus shows scattered areas of hyperintensity. C. Post treatment T2WI (24-48 hours) induced thrombus hyperintense. Spontaneous thrombus hypointense. Fig. 2: Post treatment (4-6 weeks). A. T1WI. B. T2WI peripheral induced thrombus homogenous and hyperintense on T1WI and T2WI. Spontaneous thrombus isointense on T1WI and T2WI. Note in (B) persistent aneurysm lumen posteriorly (signal void) and second smaller aneurysm on right.

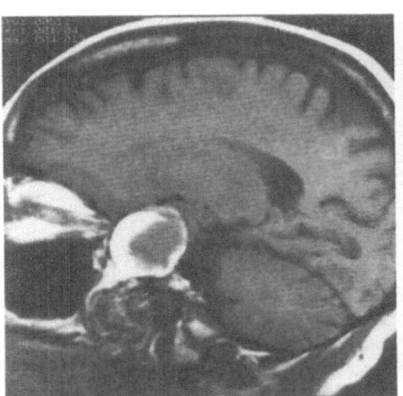
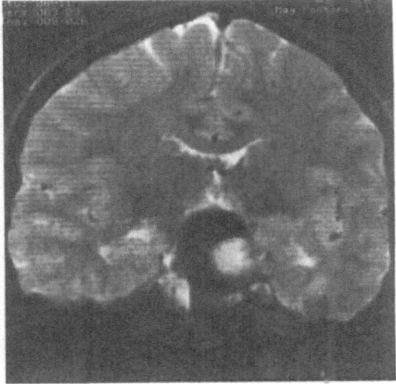

predominance of extracellular methemoglobin. Follow up at intervals greater than eleven months showed these thrombi to continue to evolve in a manner similar to that of parenchymal hematomas.

The spontaneous thrombi in these aneurysms was very different from the induced thrombus both in its initial appearance and in its evolution. A thrombus may undergo lysis, growth or organization. In fact all these processes maybe occurring simultaneously in different areas of a given thrombus.(4) They may organize and be converted into collagen and fibrin.(6) This organization process probably accounts for the laminated and heterogeneous MR appearance of the spontaneous thrombus on T1WI. This is supported by correlation of autopsy material and MR exams.(1) After isolation from the circulation the spontaneous thrombus underwent changes which acted to shorten its T1 and lengthen its T2. These changes became apparent on the initial post treatment MR of 24-48 hours. There were similar but more extensive changes on scans done 5-10 days post treatment. By 4-6 weeks after treatment the bulk of the spontaneous thrombus was comprised of tissue having hyperintense signal on T1WI and PDWI and hypointense signal on T2WI. These changes maybe due in part to the degradation of red blood cells mixed with platelet debris, fibrin and collagen. This explanation is at best speculative and lacks histopathologic correlation.

Reduction in aneurysm mass effect was easily detectable with MR. In those aneurysms which underwent complete thrombosis following balloon occlusion there was marked reduction in mass effect.

REFERENCES

1. Atlas SW, Grossman RI, Goldberg HI et al. Partially thrombosed giant intracranial aneurysms: correlation of MR and pathologic findings. RAD 1987;162:111-114
2. Baumgartner HR. The role of blood flow in platelt adhesion, fibrin deposition, and formation of mural thrombi. Microvascular Res. 1973; 5:167-179
3. Kwan ESK, Wolpert SM, Scott RM, Runge V. MR evaluation of Neurovascular lesions after indovascular occlusion with detachable balloons. AJNR 9: 523-531, 1988
4. Artmann H, Vonofakos D, Muller H, Grau H. Neuroradiological and neuropathologic findings with growing giant intracranial aneurysm. Review of the literature . Surg Neurol 21: 391-401, 1984
5. Welch WH. Thrombosis. In Albutt TC: A System of Medicine. Vol 6: 155-228. New York, Macmillan, 1889
6. Freiman DG. The Structure of Thrombi; Colman RW, Hirsh J, Marder VJ, Salzman EW. Editors, Hemostasis and Thrombosis, Basic Principles and Clinical Practice. JB Lippincott, Philadelphia, 1982
7. Olsen KL, Kucharczyk W, Keyes WD, Newton TH. Magnetic resonance characterization of non-flowing intravascular blood. Acta Radiol [Diagn] (Stockh) 1986; 369: 63-66
8. Gomori JM, Grossman RI, Hackney DB, et al. Variable appearances of subacute intracranial hematomas on high-field spin-echo MR. AJNR 8: 1019-1026, 1987
9. Sostman D, Pope CF, Smith GJW, Carbo P, Gore JC. Proton relaxation in experimental clots varies with method of preparation. Invest Rad 22; 509-512, 1987

Silk Suture Embolization of High Flow Vascular Malformations

S. T. Hecht and J. A. Horton (Pittsburgh, USA)

The extremely high flow rates observed in some vascular malformations reduce the probability of embolic agents within the nidus and increase the probability of deposition of embolic agents on the venous side. Reduction of flow helps to assure successful embolization of the nidus. For safety during embolization, a superselective catheter position within the feeding pedicles must be achieved, requiring a very distal placement of a microcatheter. Only liquids and solids with a tiny cross section can pass through a microcatheter. We have found silk suture material both easy to inject through a microcatheter and effective in reducing the flow rates of high flow lesions. Following substantial reduction of flow with silk, small particulate emboli are often used to further embolize. We have successfully used the Tracker micro-catheter system to deliver silk suture emboli to high flow vascular malformations in more than 20 patients. Angiographic and pathologic follow-up will be presented.

Local Intraarterial Fibrinolysis in the Carotid Territory. Risk Factors

J. Théron, P. Courtheoux, A. Casasco, and F. Alachkar (Caen, France)

A series of 14 cases of intraarterial local fibrinolysis in the carotid territory is presented. A schematic classification into three groups of the different types of occlusions, based on their location on the angiogram, is proposed. The most risky group for using fibrinolysis is the one with involvement of the lenticulostriate arteries in the occlusion. The time factor is particularly critical in this group to minimize the risk of hemorrhagic complications. A marked dilatation of the freshly revascularized lenticulo-striate arteries seems partly responsible for the higher hemorrhagic risk in this group. Rapid transportation of the stroke patients is recommended to rapidly perform CT and complete angiography before making the decision about using fibrinolysis.

Advances in the Endovascular Treatment of Cerebral AVMs

B. Richling, E. Knosp, E. Öztürk, and G. Bavinzski

Introduction

During the past year advances in the treatment of cerebral AVMs
have been achieved in two ways. Technical evaluation has brought
us flow-independent microcatheter systems, making the use of flow
chambers unnecessary. Products with an increasing degree of softness, either with guidewire (Tracker System, Target Therapeutics,
California, USA) or without (Magic, Balt, Paris: Minitorquer,
Ingenor, Paris), allow the examination of vascular areas without the
help of a pathologically increased blood flow. For use in cerebral
blood vessels, specially designed microguidewires have been further
improved by softer tips and a Teflon surface. Technical advances
have also been seen in the evaluation of embolizing materials. Because of reports that cyanoacrylates are toxic and because of un-
certainty regarding the setting mechanism, attempts were made to
develop new materials or combinations for endovascular embolization.

In addition to technical improvements, changes in the strategy of
the treatment of AVMs have been seen. Especially in neurosurgical
units with a high quality of microvascular surgery, comprehension
of the endovascular treatment of cerebral AVMs has risen and this
has led to improved strategic planning in such patients.

Technical Improvements

An example is presented here which demonstrates the advance in the
flow-independent catheter technique and the evaluation of new types
of microguidewires. While some operators declare the use of cerebral
guidewires as unnecessary, others demonstrate approaches to very
peripheral, narrow, and slow-flow areas.

In using the microguidewire at a intracerebrally deep location, not
only the softness of the tip but also the length of the soft catheter segment is important. Figure 1 shows the endovascular approach to a

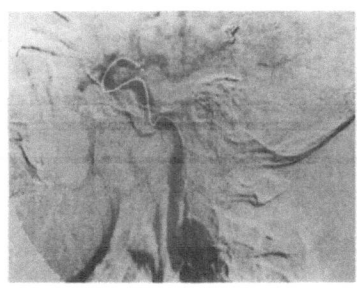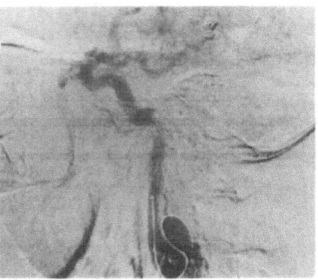

Fig.1. Taper guidewire in the kinked part of the carotid and the
siphon

left parieto-occipital AVM and one of its feeders. The distance
between the internal carotid and the left occipital target territory would - by use of a normal Taper guidewire (Target Therapeutics) - bring the stiff segment of the wire to the level of the
carotid siphon. The bending of this segment both in the extensive
carotid kinking of this patient and higher up in the siphon would
hinder movement of the catheter tip and therefore diminish the
guiding effect of the wire. High friction between the bent stiff
segment of the wire and the catheter also leads to a reduction of
sensitivity in handling the tip of the wire in the cerebral vessels.
Specially designed new guidewires with a long soft segment (18 cm)
reduce the friction in the curved catheter and allow smooth movements and torque. In the case referred to, they allowed a close
approach of the catheter to the high-flow fistula (Fig.2).

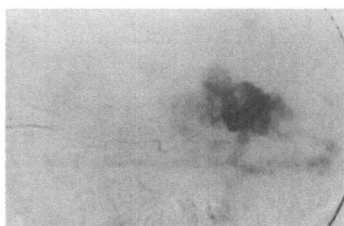

Fig.2. Tracker catheter located in a high-flow fistula (guided by
a special long-tip guidewire) over the kinking and via the communicating posterior artery

A further step in the evaluation of cerebral guidewires was achieved
with the evaluation of the Seeker wire (Target Therapeutics). This
guidewire has a Teflon-based variable surface finish (VSF), reducing

the friction between wire and catheter. This new guidewire allows
precise torque-controlled movements of the tip, even through a catheter bent several times. Unfortunately, since the radiopaque part
is only 2 cm long, it does not show all the movements of the wire
on the videoscreen. Figure 3 shows the radiopaque tip of a Seeker
approaching the AVM mentioned above via the right carotid and anterior cerebral artery. The tip remains capable of torque even above
the kinking of the right carotid artery and the long and bent distance to the pericallosal territory. Figure 4 demonstrates the result of endovascular treatment after having occluded territories
from the right anterior; Figure 5 does the same from the left posterior cerebral artery.

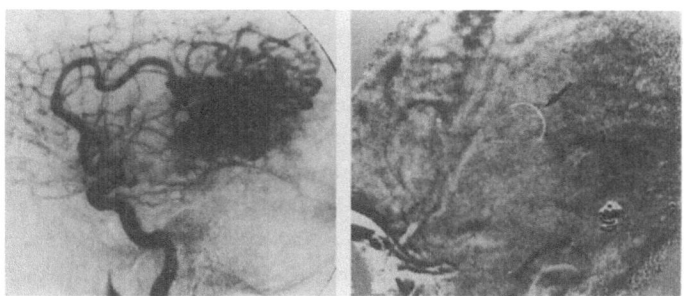

Fig.3. AVM feeder via the right internal carotid. The tip of a
Seeker wire can be advanced close to the AVM and remains capable
of torque even after multiple bendings

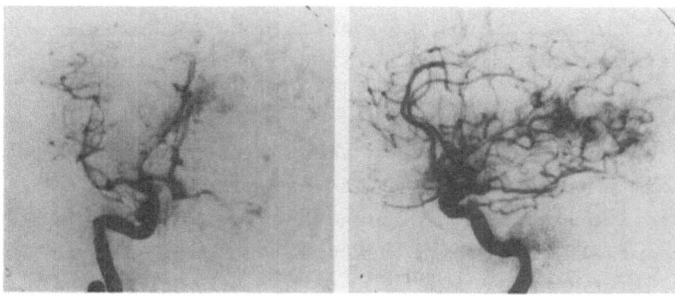

Fig.4. Result after embolization via the right approach (pericallosal artery). Remaining flow into the left middle cerebral
artery and its feeders to the AVM

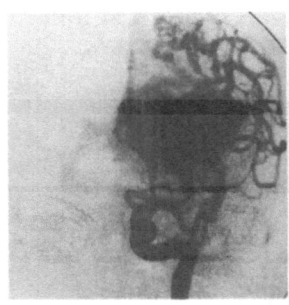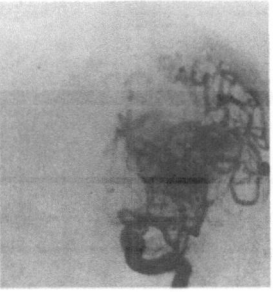

Fig.5. Angiogram via the left internal carotid artery before and after embolization via the communicating posterior artery

While clinical and industrial researchers have made substantial efforts to improve catheter technique, only little advance has been achieved in the evaluation of embolizing materials. Despite reported toxic side effects, cyanoacrylates mixed with contrast material are still commonly used as embolizing substances for cerebral AVMs. Especially under nonblocked flow conditions (which is the rule with the use of balloonless catheters), calculation of the setting point of the cyanoacrylate is sometimes difficult. Blocking of the draining veins may occur as well as early occlusion of a feeding artery.

Following the suggestion of Vinuela we now use a mixture of alcohol 96% (2 ml), Iopamidol 300 (4 ml), Ivalon (90-250 ml) and the collagen Avitene (50 mg). Using this mixture, we embolized a series of 17 cases of AVMs in the period from May to September 1988. The mixture, designed to be a preoperative material, allows stepwise occlusion of the territory, building up the embolus from the fistula to a total filling of the nidus. Control angiograms done on four patients up to 10 weeks after the first embolization showed the material to be stable.

The stepwise filling of an AVM nidus (with the patient awake and cooperative) to perform a total occlusion of the malformation represents a safe procedure and avoids the "gunshot" effect of bucrylate. Despite the expected instability of the mixture, our angiographic controls after 10 weeks showed the material to be persisting. The high level of safety during embolization motivates us to perform a series of "Los Angeles cocktail" embolizations of AVMs and to analyze angiographic results. In the case of insufficient stability we should try to increase the stability of the mixture by changing its components rather than to go back to the bucrylate method.

Conclusion

The philosophy of therapy of cerebral AVMs has changed more during the past year than have the technical details of endovascular treatment. The old idea of performing complicated, sometimes heroic surgical interventions or rejecting the patient from therapy at all has changed. Increasingly, endovascular procedures are being included in the therapeutic concept, and the priority of the endovascular approach to the cerebral AVM in most patients is now becoming accepted.

Therapeutic Embolization in Vertebrospinal Vascular Malformations – Ten-Year Experience

J. Stojanović, A. Kamler, S. Šimunić, B. Malenica, M. Vidović, and J. J. Merland

Introduction

Criteria for treatment and follow-up in vertebrospinal arteriovenous malformations (AVMs) are well known (Houdart et al. 1975; Djindjian et al. 1977, 1978, 1981; Kendall and Logue 1977; Merland et al. 1980, 1987a, 1987b; Riche et al. 1983, 1984; Laredo et al. 1986; Gueguen et al. 1987; Stojanović et al. 1987; Thorn 1988). There are three methods used in the treatment of vertebrospinal AVMs: surgery, irradiation, and embolization. No matter what type of treatment is chosen, it is essential to ensure the continuity of blood supply through the anterior spinal artery as well as the vascularization of the normal medullary areas around the malformation. Technical innovations in diagnosis and treatment of AVMs, mainly using coaxial microcatheter systems, have enabled embolization of even distal areas. In this paper we describe therapeutic procedures performed in the period from 1978-1988 in 102 patients with vertebral angiomas, 52 with spinal AVMs, 13 with complex vertebroparavertebral and spinal AVMs, and 4 with spinal hemangioblastomas.

Material and Methods

In a 10-year period, 167 patients with vertebrospinal AVMs and four with spinal hemangioblastomas were treated. The ages of patients with vertebral angioma (65% female, 35% male) ranged between 18 and 72 years (mean 44.7 years) and of those with spinal AVMs, between 6 and 58 years (mean 31.8 years) (63.4% male, 36.6% female). Pretherapeutic diagnostic studies included standard anteroposterior and lateral radiographs in all patients, myelography (using Metrizamid, lately Iohexol, Nycomed) complemented by CT (CT myelography) or CT with intravenously administered contrast media, spinal angiography, and MRI.

The embolization technique used depended upon the angiographic status of the afferent vessels and the status of the anterior spinal artery. Various materials were used for therapeutic embolization of vertebrospinal AVMs. As a rule, nonresorbing material was given, taking into consideration the hemodynamic characteristic of the individual AVMs. Polyvinyl alcohol (Ivalon) was used in more than 90% of cases (particles 149-590 μm), alone or in combination with other materials (fibrospum, dura, silk). Bucrylate alone was used in two cases.

Results

Vertebral Angiomas
Out of 102 patients with vertebral angiomas, 46 were irradiated, 40 were embolized, and 16 underwent no treatment.

Therapeutic Procedure
Out of 46 irradiated patients, 36 were treated without diagnostic spinal angiography. In nine patients no clinical improvement was observed. Following completed radiation therapy, spinal angiography performed 18-24 months later showed a characteristic, pathologic vascular supply of angioma in six cases. Three showed stenotic occlusive disturbances of segmental arteries and a. Adamkiewicz originated at the level of the irradiated angioma (postirradiation arteritis? ischemic myelopathy?). As expected, their clinical status was worsening. No evident clinical improvement was observed in two of six irradiated patients in whom spinal angiography had been performed before treatment. Spinal angiography revealed persistent pathologic vascularization. Patients were treated with a mean therapeutic dose of 4200 cGy. Clinical and neurological results in 46 irradiated patients were good in 76.1%, and insufficient or poor in 23.9%.

Therapeutic Procedure - Embolization
Therapeutic embolization of vertebral angiomas in the dorsal and lumbar regions was performed in 40 patients, with marked clinical improvement in 34 and only slight improvement in six. Six patients underwent spinal angiography, which revealed angioma "activity" via a collateral nonembolized artery. In the same session re-embolization was successfully carried out.

In 16 patients with vertebral angiomas, no treatment was given. In eight patients spinal angiography showed spinal angioma type C. In five cases the origin of a. Adamkiewicz was at the level of the angioma and in three cases at the neighbouring level. Consequently, in those 16 patients neither embolization nor irradiation was recommended.

Spinal AVMs

Out of 52 patients with spinal AVM; 31 were embolized, eight were both embolized and operated on, and 11 underwent surgical treatment only.

Therapeutic Procedure - Embolization

Out of 31 embolized patients, very good or good therapeutic results were obtained in 23 (78%), insufficient in five (16%), and poor in three (6%).

In four patients with medulary and/or perimedulary AVMs and involvement of the anterior spinal artery, embolizations were performed through a. Adamkiewicz with the help of free blood flow ("flux liber"). Marked improvement was observed in two patients, satisfactory results in one, and poor in one. All were paraplegic before treatment. Control spinal angiography revealed arteriovenous fistulae and/or malformations, nidus occlusion and sufficient blood flow through a. Adamkiewicz.

In the group of embolized and surgically treated patients (N = 8), therapeutic results were good in five and poor in three.

In one particular case with an intramedullary AVM irrigated by the anterior spinal artery via a. Adamkiewicz, surgery was performed in the first session in another hospital. In the postoperative period, no clinical improvement was recorded (paraplegia remained). Embolization through a. Adamkiewicz was carried out later. One month after embolization, the first signs of clinical and neurological improvement were observed. In patients treated only surgically (11), good therapeutic results were obtained in six, and poor or unsatisfactory in five.

Out of 13 patients with complex vertebroparavertebral and spinal AVMs, eight were embolized and five both embolized and operated on.

Ten patients from this group had several embolizing sessions, with very good final therapeutic results. Out of four patients with hemangioblastoma, two were successfully embolized (later they were surgically treated) and two were only operated on.

Discussion

All patients included in this study (from 1978-1988) had long-lasting pain in the spinal region and in the upper and/or lower extremeties.

Obvious neurological deficits were present in 48% of patients with a
vertebral angioma, and in 92% of those with spinal AVMs. Vertebrospinal AVM topography distribution is similar to that described by
various authors (Schmol and Junghanns 1971; Merland et al. 1980,
1987; Riche et al. 1984; Stojanović et al. 1985, 1985a; Laredo et al.
1986; Thorn 1988). As regards spinal AVMs, most often diagnosis was
established and embolization performed in type B vertebral angioma
(40.8%), meningeal AV fistula (42.3%), and perimedullary intradural
AV fistula (28.8%). Cases in which embolization was not performed
were combined AVM and aneurism (7.7%) and isolated aneurisms (1.9%).
In embolized cases, the technique of superselective catheterization
of segmental and/or pedicular arteries was used, aiming at occlusion
of AV fistula, angioma nidus and pedicular artery; embolizing material was given by free flow (flux liber) and/or directly into the
pedicular artery via a coaxial microcatheter. The size of the nonresorbing particles was chosen according to the width of the AV
fistula, pedicular artery and the hemodynamic capacity of the angioma nidus. Therapeutic results of embolization were better than
those of irradiation by 10%. Also, the criteria used for selection
for embolization were more strict than those for selection for irradiation (86% of irradiated cases had no previous spinal angiography). In most patients with spinal AVMs the effect of therapeutic
embolization was good (78%) and usually appeared quickly. In a
small number of cases the improvement was slow, and in four patients
with long-lasting paraplegia, there was hardly any improvement.

Complications

In some cases a localized pain was recorded in the area of embolized
segments during embolization, but it was usually of short duration.

In four cases of spinal AVM in which several pedicular arteries were
embolized during the procedure, a transient worsening was recorded,
lasting for several hours after treatment. However, the final results were good. No other severe complications were recorded.

Conclusion

Therapeutic embolization, technically not too difficult to perform,
has some advantages over irradiation and surgical treatment. In any
case, in each case treated one should take into consideration the
characteristics of the AVM, contraindications, and possible compli-

cations of each of the procedures. Good practice and experience have led to a low rate of complications. Although the advances in microneurosurgery are evident, therapeutic embolization is by no means the method of choice in treatment of vertebrospinal AVMs.

References

[1] Djindjian R, Houdart R, Hurth M, Cophignon J, Rey A, Thurel C (1975) Embolisation dans les angiomes de la moelle. J Neuroradiol 2: 73-172
[2] Djindjian R, Meland JJ (1978) Place de l'embolisation dans le traitement des malformations arterioveineuses medullaires a propos de 30 cas. Neuroradiology 16: 428
[3] Djindjian R, Merland JJ, Djindjian M, Stoeter R (1981) Angiography of spinal column and spinal cord tumors. Thieme, Stuttgart
[4] Gueguen B, Merland JJ, Ricje MC, Rey A (1987) Vascular malformations of the spinal cord: Intrathecal perimedullary arteriovenous fistulas fed by medullary arteries. Neurology 37: 969-979
[5] Houdart R, Djindjian R, Hurth M (1966) Vascular malformations of the spinal cord: The anatomic and therapeutic significance of arteriography. J Neurosurg 24: 583-594
[6] Kendall BE, Logue V (1977) Spinal epidural angiomatous malformations draining into intrathecal veins. Neuroradiology 13: 181-189
[7] Laredo JD, Reizine D, Bard M, Merland JJ (1986) Vertebral hemangiomas: radiologic evaluation. Radiology 161: 183-189
[8] Merland JJ, Riche MC, Chiras J (1980) Les fistules arterioveineuses intracanalaires, extra-medullaires a drainage veineux medullaire. J Neuroradiol 7: 271-320
[9] Merland JJ, Reizine D, Assouline E et al. (1987) Le malformazioni vascolari vertebro-midollari. In: Pistolesi GF, Bergamo Andreis IA (eds) L'imagining dianostico del rachide. Edizioni libreria, Cortina, pp 522-562
[10] Riche MC, Melki JP, Merland JJ (1983) Embolization of spinal cord vascular malformations via the anterior spinal artery. AJNR 4: 378-381
[11] Riche MC, Reizine D, Melki JP, George B, Rey A, Merland JJ (1984) Treatment of vascular malformations of the spinal cord. Surg Rounds 60-75
[12] Schmorl G, Junghanns H (1971) The human spina in health and disease. Grune and Stratton, New York
[13] Stojanović J, Papa J, Buljat G, Tetičković E, Bradač GB (1985) Ein Beitrag der spinalen Angiographie zu Diagnostik eines Wirbelangioms. Fortschr Röntgenstr 141: 348-350
[14] Stojanović J, Šamija M, Papa J et al. (1987) Therapeutic embolization of spinal (N = 22) and vertebral (N = 31) angiomas. VI European congress of radiology, Portugal, Lisbon, 31 May-6 June 1987, p 271
[15] Thron AK (1988) Vascular anatomy of the spinal cord. Neuroradiological investigations and clinical syndromes. Springer, Vienna New York

Spinal Aneurysms Associated with Spinal Cord AVMs

A. Biondi, M. C. Riche, J. P. Bruvo, and J. J. Merland (Paris, France)

Spinal aneurysms (SAs) are rare lesions usually associated with AVMs. This association in spinal cord AVMs has been reported with an incidence varying between 6% and 7.7%, and only few cases of isolated SAs have been documented. In our series we have found 11 SAs associated with AVMs (usually intramedullary AVMs). The lesions were located in the cervical (6 cases), dorsal (4 cases) and dorso-lumbar (1 case) regions. The relationships between the site of the SA and the feeding arteries to the AVM were studied. The patients were 4 males and 7 females. In all cases the clinical onset was subarachnoid hemorrhage and in 6 cases repeated bleeding occurred before treatment. The incidence of subarachnoid hemorrhage seems to increase when the AVM is associated with SA. It remains unsettled, however, whether the bleeding is from the AVM or from the SA. Sometimes angiographic diagnostic problems with tortuosities of the dilated vessels, mimicking saccular formations, can exist; both frontal and lateral projections are always needed to confirm the diagnosis and angiotomography may clearly define the aneurysm and its location.

Three main hypotheses on the genesis of this association can be suggested: 1) both lesions are expressions of a developmental vascular anomaly, 2) a hemodynamic factor, 3) a mere coincidence. A definitive understanding of the interrelationships of the 2 lesions is still elusive.

MR study was available in 7 cases.

Endovascular treatment was performed in 10 cases. Indications, technical considerations, complications and results are reported.

Endovascular Treatment of Intramedullary Dorsal Angiomas. Report of 35 Cases

S. Bien, A. Biondi, F. Gelbert, E. Assouline, and J. J. Merland (Paris, France)

The endovascular treatment of 35 dorsal intramedullary AV malformations is described. The most common clinical presentation in our series was a subarachnoid hemorrhage, although in the literature this is reported as rare and usually associated with spinal aneurysms. Endovascular treatment was performed in all cases: One or more embolizations have been performed in each case, varying in number from 1 to 14.

Clinical and angiographic follow-up were obtained. Clinical improvement was usually observed after the treatment. Although partial revascularization of the lesions was often detected, the risk of rebleeding seems to be very unusual. Materials used were dura mater, ivalon, gelfoam and only in very few cases IBCA.

Endovascular Treatment of Hemangioblastomas

A. Biondi, S. Bien, E. Cervigon, and J. J. Merland (Paris, France)

In our series of 22 patients, presenting solitary or multiple hemangioblastomas located in posterior fossa and/or in the spinal cord, 8 underwent endovascular treatment. The location of the lesions was posterior fossa (2 cases), cervical spinal cord (3 cases) and dorsal spinal cord (3 cases).

The patients were 3 males and 5 females ranging in age from 25 to 63 years.

Embolization was performed before surgery in 6 cases. In all patients endovascular treatment allowed reduction of tumoral vascularization and clinical improvement, immediately after the embolization, in 7 cases.

No complications related to the endovascular prodedure was observed, also in the patients with lesions fed by medullary or cerebellar arteries. After embolization the surgical approach is facilitated and blood losses are reduced, particularly in large, hypervascularized tumors. Indications, technical aspects and results are discussed.

The Cobb – Syndrome or Metameric Angiomatosis

E. Garcia-Cervigon, S. Bien, A. Biondi, and J. J. Merland (Paris, France)

Since S. Cobb first described the combination of a spinal with a cutaneus angiomatosis in 1915, only a few other cases have been published. We will review the clinical and radiological signs and symptoms, and our experience with the endovascular treatment of 32 cases of Cobb syndrome.

The duration of the symptoms varied from 2 months to 16 years before treatment.

In ten cases there was a subarachnoid hemorrhage, the other 22 patients suffered from a spinal cord deficit syndrome. All our patients underwent endovascular treatment with particles (dura mater, ivalon, gelfoam). Most of the patients improved with treatment.

Pre-operative Embolization of Naso-pharyngeal Angiofibromas. Report of 58 Cases

E. Garcia-Cervigon, S. Bien, B. Tran Ba Huy, and J. J. Merland (Paris, France)

58 patients with a juvenile nasopharyngeal angiofibroma have been treated by a combined neuroradiological-surgical method. In the cases with smaller tumor extension, fed only by the external carotid arteries or with only slight participation of the internal carotid arteries, the external carotid arteries alone have been embolized using particles. In the cases with marked participation of the internal carotid arteries embolization of these feeding pedicles was also performed. In the first group there were no complications and no recurrences. In the latter, (31 cases), there have been three temporary minor complications and 11 recurrences.

Embolization: A Definitive Treatment for Meningiomas? (Three Cases)

A. Laurent, P.Y. Gobin, A. Rogopoulos, S. Bien, and J. J. Merland (Paris, France)

The first case, a cavernous sinus meningioma diagnosed by CT scan and angiography was embolized with particles. Followup CT scan and angiography 5 years later showed complete disappearance of the mass.

The second case, a convexity meningioma diagnosed by CT scan and isotope scan, also had particulate embolization. Isotope scan, four days later, revealed a clear decrease in image size. At surgery, 10 days later, an almost completely necrosed meningioma was found. The third case, diagnosed as a middle fossa meningioma by CT scan and angiography, was completely embolized in one session and showed CT evidence of necrosis in the following weeks. Indications and modalities for embolization of meningiomas are discussed.

Endovascular Treatment of Mandibular Arteriovenous Angiomas

A. Aymard, M. C. Riche, E. Garcia-Cervigon, and J. J. Merland (Paris, France)

The mandibular angiomas are of particular interest due to the dramatic hemorrhagic episodes. Ligation of the external carotid artery has proved to be ineffective. Surgery requires a resection of the hemimandible, an operation which is a dangerous as it is mutilating. The progress in developing superselective catheter materials allows an mebolization which obviates the need for an operation. We report three cases of complete healing with percutaneous treatment.

Percutaneous Angioplasty of Supraaortic Arteries – Experiences with 120 Patients

K. Mathias (Dortmund, FRG)

Percutaneous angioplasty of supraaortic arteries has developed to a valuable treatment modality characterized by a high technical success and low complication rate. Vessels suited for angioplasty are: subclavian, innominate, vertebral as well as common, internal, and external carotid arteries.

In a series of 81 patients with subclavian obstruction 76 could be improved by catheter dilatation. All 8 innominate artery stenoses could be removed. In 8 of 9 patients a vertebral artery stenoses was treated successfully. A comparable result was obtained in 21 of 22 patients with carotid artery stenoses. 9 patients suffering from multiple vessel disease were treated in different vascular territories at one session. Angioplasty was combined with vascular surgery in 8 cases.

The obstructed neck arteries could be opened in 113 of 120 (94%) patients with a 3-year patency rate of 78%. Neurological complications were rare with only 2 transient ischemic attacks. One patient developed a false aneurysm after dilatation of a subclavian artery stenoses.

Embolization in Untractable Epistaxis

M. Schumacher, J. Strutz, and K. Kutluk

INTRODUCTION

Episodes of epistaxis are a common event in about 60 % of the normal population requiring treatment in only 6 % (Small et al. 1982). Most of the cases can be controlled by cautery or a anterior nasal packing being localized in the accessable septal area. In the group requiring medical care in less than 1/5 th (Schaithin et al. 1982) there is a demand for further treatment, e.g. Bellocq tamponade, cryotherapy and arterial ligation. Though Sokoloff et al. already in 1974 mentioned the advantages of selective embolization in severe epistaxis the method has not been widely adopted in ENT concepts for treatment (Feldmann 1981).

In 39 patients of severe epistaxis we established a therapeutic protocol escalating step by step from arterior packing to artery ligation depending on the circumstances and according to the specific case.

MATERIALS AND METHODS

39 patients were admitted to our hospital from 1985 to 1988 suffering from severe epistaxis requiring hospitalization. The age ranged from 23 to 76 with a mean of 48 years. 23 patients were treated by packing or cautery, two of them additionally with arterial ligature at the very first time, when embolization was not systematically used. In 16 cases embolization was performed. The etiology of the latter group is listed on table 1.

Table 1. Etiology of epistaxis in embolization group

Postoperative	6
Hypertension	3
Unknown (hypert. episode?)	3
Traumatic	1
Angioma	1
Angiofibroma	1
Rendu Osler disease	1

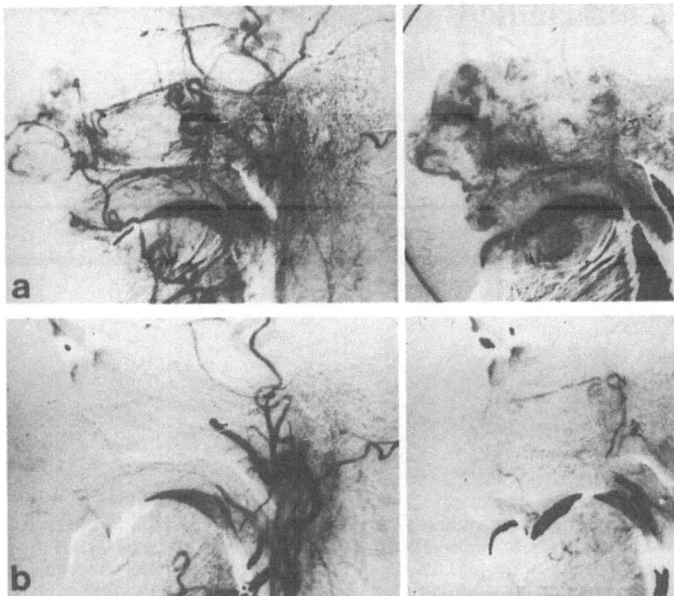

Fig. 1. Rendu Osler disease. Multiple teleangiectatic nodules fed by internal maxillary, facial, lingual and superficial temporal artery before (a) and after (b) embolization.

All patients were treated initially by anterior packing. If necessary, because of permanent bleeding an endoscopic cauterization was performed, followed by a posterior package (Bellocq tamponade) if cautery was insufficient. In all cases involving rebleeding after removal of the posterior package, angiography and embolization was done. Before embolization again a Bellocq tamponade was placed to tide over the critical time up to the definite occlusion of the bleeding source. One day after embolization the package was removed.

In most cases embolization was carried out with a 4F vertebral catheter, in the last 4 patients a tracker catheter was used. Only nonremovable material was applicated (PVA 150 - 590 micron, size adjusted to the bleeding cause and angiographic finding).

RESULTS

In all cases where patients were embolized unilaterally (all cases except one) we successfully stopped the bleeding. This patient was cured by embolization on both sides. Another patient required a second embolization due to rebleeding. Except the patient with bilateral embolization the clinically predicted side of the bleeding correlated well with the angiographic verification of the bleeding and the therapeutic effect. Arterial ligature after embolization was done in an early case of the series without trial of a second embolization as we would do today. Two patients had undergone arterial clipping during the initial operation (sup.thyreoid, lingual, facial and pharyngeal artery in a case of carcinoma of the tongue and palate; ethmoidal arteries in a case of Rendu Osler disease).

In 5/16 the internal maxillary artery was embolized, in one patient only the lingual artery was treated. In the remaining 10 cases several branches had to be embolized including the facial, ascending pharyngeal, descendend palatine, transverse facial, superficial temporal and profund cervical artery. The point of bleeding could be defined by angiography in 7/16 (4 postoperative, 1 Rendu Osler disease, 1 traumatic, 1 angioma).

Besides minor side effects like muscle pain, trismus and slight fever there were no complications. In one patient with a generalized arteriosclerotic process, repeated TIA's in the post, highgrade respiration insufficiency and severe blood loss a hemiparesis developed immediately before angiography and embolization started.

DISCUSSION

Severe epistaxis may be a life threatening event, whether idiopathic or caused by surgical complications, hypertension, trauma, vascular malformations, tumors or hemostasis disorders. Though in conservative therapy the failure rate varies from 26 to 52 % with a complication incidence from 2 to 50 % (review in Schaithin et al. 1987) the primary treatment should be anterior and/or posterior nasal packing (Davis 1986, Merland et al. 1980). This correlates well with a successful medical therapy in 59 % of our patients.

The bleeding point may be exactly defined in some patients. Those needing a ligation of the ethmoidal arteries, which are inaccessible by embolization, should be separated. In our series there was a demand for arterial ligature in about 8 %. Compared with the literature (2 % in Federspil 1971) the higher incidence may be explained by the higher quota of cases, which were admitted from other hospitals after surgical problems.

4 French transfemoral catheters normally will be adequate to reach selectively enough the vessels to be embolized. Only in single cases a flow independent 2 to 3 F inner catheter may be used in order to achieve a more selective position or to prevent arterial spasm. Differing from Davis (1986) bilateral angiography seems to us not generally necessary. It depends on the accuracy of the clinician in presuming the side of bleeding. Only in 1/16 of our series the prediction was wrong. Beyond it recurrence from revascularization developes ipsilaterally (Lasjaunias et al. 1979).

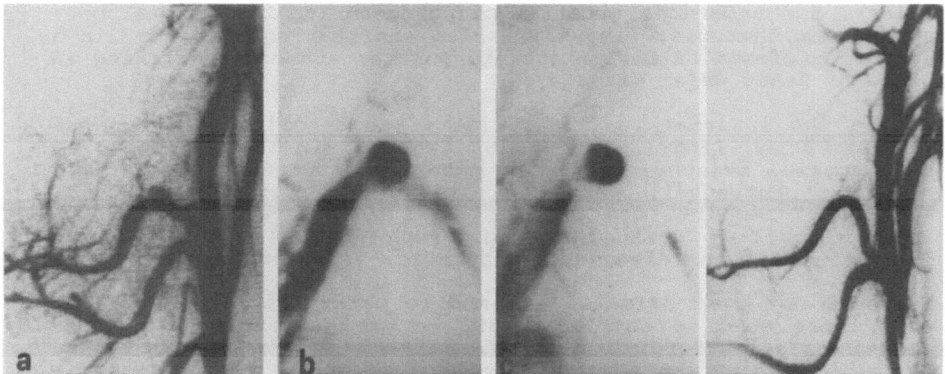

Fig. 2. Postoperative (tonsil-removal) bleeding due to false aneurysm of the lingual artery (a). Late phase showing persistent
intrasaccular contrast medium (b, c). Angiographic control after
embolization with 250 - 590 micron PVA.

To achieve a permanent occlusion we used a various sized PVA
according to the size of the involved vessels and the presence of
dangerous anastomoses. Though other embolic material is available
we chose nonresorbable agent also in hypertensive and unknown
bleedings, since in the history of these patients recurrent epistaxis had often occured. Even in two aneurysms embolization with
particles stopped bleeding and occluded the aneurysm although the
vessel remained patent (fig. 2). Treatment with a detachable balloon therefore seems to be redundant in false aneurysms of that
vascular territory.

REFERENCES

Davis RK (1986) Embolization of epistaxis and juvenile nasopharyngeal angiofibromas. AJNR 7:953-962
Feldman H (1981) Notfälle im HNO-Gebiet. Springer, Berlin Heidelberg New York, p 2-13
Federspil P (1971) Die Gefäßunterbindung bei unstillbarem Nasen-
bluten. HNO 199:171-175
Lasjaunias P, Marsot-Dupuch K, Doyon D (1979) The radio-anatomical basis of arterial embolization for epistaxis. J.Neurora-
diol. 6:45-53
Merland JJ, Melki JP, Chiras J, Riche MC, Hadjean E (1980) Place
of embolization in the treatment of severe epistaxis. Laryngoscope 10:1694-1704
Schaithin B, Strauss M, Houck JR, Hershey PA (1987) Epistaxis:
medical versus surgical therapy. A comparison of efficacy, complications and economic considerations. Laryngoscope 97: 1392-
1396
Small M, Murray J, Maran A (1982) A study of patients with epistaxis requiring admission to hospital. Health Bull.40:24-29
Sokoloff J, Wickbom J, Mc Donald D, Brahme F, Goergen TG, Gold-
berger LE (1974) Therapeutic percutaneous embolization in intractable epistaxis. Radiology 3:285-287

PTA of Carotid Artery Stenosis – Clinical Neuroradio-logical and EEG-Findings Before and After Treatment

R. D. Koch, G. Freitag, J. Freitag, D. Müller, and P. Heinrich

Abbreviated as PTA, percutaneous transluminal angioplasty is well established in the treatment of arterial stenoses and even short-length occlusions of the lower extremity, the kidneys, coronary arteries, and recently the subclavian artery alike. To date, however, fear of cerebral embolisms has been an obstacle to an equally wide use of ballooning the carotid arteries.

After the PTA of carotid arteries was upscaled from the animal experiment to clinical application by Mathias in 1981, we have since 1982 given PTA treatment to eighteen patients aged 34 to 76 years with carotid stenoses of which five were stenoses of the external carotid artery and one of the vertebral artery.

Instrumented preliminary examinations and follow-up applied were Doppler sonography, electroencephalography, measurement of regional cerebral blood flow, and computed tomography, while electro-encephalography was used for cerebral function monitoring during the treatment.

This range of methods is recommended as one has to be sufficiently certain in deciding whether the stenosis has given rise to the clinical symptoms, or if it is asymptomatic. It is just computed tomography that helps us in differentiating between the ischaemic insults due to micro- or macroangiopathy, or a combination of both.

Of the twelve patients with stenoses of the internal carotid artery, seven were subjected to a clinical and instrumented follow-up after one to three years. Neurologic follow-up revealed a marked improvement in four out of seven patients which was in accord with the anamnestic data. Two of them were symptom-free, and one patient remained unchanged.

For seven patients followed up electroencephalographically, the focal findings after PTA clearly decreased, and even normal EEG findings were obtained for two of them. It was merely in two of the patients followed up that moderately severe functional disorders persistedt.

Regional cerebral blood flow measurement demonstrated stenosis-related pathological blood flow conditions in all cases. Following angioplasty, perfusion normalized in five cases. In one patient, the pathologically changed readings remained unaltered.

It is evident that computed tomography was not expected to demonstrate regression of the previously noted morphological changes. On the other hand, no progression was seen the atrophies detected prior to therapy. Neither were insult regions or even sequelae of embolisms revealed.

To summarize and draw a few conclusions:

PTA can be successfully applied to treat carotid artery stenosis. In selecting the patients, classing into micro- or macroangiopathic lesion patterns should be given due consideration in addition to the four-stage classification. Complications abserved during PTA were only those which are known to result from a conventional cerebral angiography.

The small number of carotid artery dilatations performed so far does not lend itself to reliably assessing the risks involved. It is important to note that, for the already greater number of dilatations of subclavian arteries, no embolisms have been reported. Also, in angioplasty of pelvifemoral arteries, 1.1 percent embolisms occurred exclusively after recanalisation of occlusions, but not in dilatation, whereas the mortality after surgery has been reported to be several percent.

We believe that, compared to vascular surgery, the PTA is advantageous in that
- there is less discomfort for the patient;
- the treatment is performed under local anaesthesia;
- blood flow is interrupted intermittently and for a shorter interval, and
- we permanently cooperate with the patient while monitoring the EEG.

Restraint should be exercised in indicating PTA for patients with ischaemic insults in microangiopathy. For these, even the cerebral angiography necessary involves a greater risk.

REFERENCES

Freitag G, Freitag J, Koch RD Perkutane transluminale Angioplastik von Karotisstenosen. Fortschr Röntgenstr 150:209-212

Freitag G, Freitag J, Koch RD, Wagemann W Percutaneous angioplasty of carotid artery stenoses. Neuroradiology 28:126-127

Mathias K, Mittermayer Ch, Ensinger E, Neff, W Perkutane Katheter-dilatation von Karotisstenosen. Tierexperimentelle Untersuchungen. Fortschr Röntgenstr. 133:258-261

Mathias K Perkutane transluminale Katheterbehandlung supra-aortaler Arterienobstruktionen. Angio 3:47-50

Mathias K, Bockenheimer St, v.Reutern G, Heiss HW, Ostheim-Dzerowaycz W Katheterdilatation hirnversorgender Arterien. Radiologe 23:208-214

Percutaneous Transluminal Angioscopy of Supraaortic Branches and Angioscopical Control of PTA

A. Beck and D. Ott

INTRODUCTION

Percutaneous transluminal angioscopy has been realized in the last 2 years by developing ultrathin endoscopes with less than 2 mm of diameter. In our clinic this procedure has been introduced using various prototypes of scopes raging from 1.2 - 2.4 mm outer diameter. The main problem of obtaining angioscopic view is to diminish blood flow. Many animal trials have been necessary to obtain the first evaluable pictures. To obtain pictures we use perfusion of the vessel with NaCl solution. The results are documented by using quick - shot cameras or recently by using a video unit.
In 14 patients an angioscopical control of angiographical findings in supraaortal vessel pathology could be performed.

MATERIAL AND METHODS

Various prototypes of endoscopes with an outer diameter ranging from 1,2 - 2.4 mm have been used.The access is transfemorally only. First a sheath - set (F 9) is placed. Then a selective catheter is positioned into the origin of the supraaortic vessel.
Through this F 8 selective catheter the F 4 - 6 endoscope can be inserted until the region of interest (fig.1). The endoscope itself disposes of 3 channels : 2 light channels and 1 working channel. Through the working channel either a guide wire or saline can be advanced. The NaCl - solution is promoted by a mechanical pump.For one spot of several seconds an amount of 5 - 10 cc saline is needed. Saline - infusion in one patient should not exceed 200 cc. Documentation can be obtained by quick shot cameras with minimally 2 exposures/ sec. Recently we use a video unit with permanent registration. The major part of the pictures is not useful for diagnostic purposes due to artefacts caused by blood-flow.

RESULTS

First of all it must be mentioned that the quality of angioscopically achieved pictures cannot be compared to that of the gastroenterologic standard. The quality of pictures is influenced by the disturbing blood flow and by the small diameter of the scopes which dispose of less light - fibers than big ones. Furthermore all pictures are taken through NaCl - solution - they are all " water - pictures ".
Arteriosclerotic lesions of all stages can be diagnosed easily. Even when angiography is still without pathological findings, angioscopy can reveal vessel pathology. Arteriosclerotic lesions

could be found in almost all patients. Angiographically invisible
lesions angioscopically showed as alteration of intimal colour:
The intima is normally pink. Early arteriosclerotic lesions
appear as white spots or plaques in the intima. In progressive
arteriosclerosis the initially flat plaques become prominent
(fig.5,6). In late stages of disease the prominent plaques occlude the vessel more or less. The kind and degree of the disease
can be diagnosed more exactly by angioscopy than by plain film or
even by digital - subtraction angiography. Arteriosclerotic lesions often move in the NaCl - stream which can be observed by
video-documentation: This proves the instability of some plaques.
Even by using a hard tip of a guide wire or a catheter tip these
particles can be loosened and embolize in the periphery. This
fact has to be borne in mind when performing any kind   of
intervention in all vessel regions.After perforation of the
stenosis by the guide wire the dilatation balloon - catheter is
placed under fluoroscopic control. The vessel wall after dilatation shows the following aspects: The arteriosclerotic plaques
are mainly longitudinally cracked on the whole length of the
balloon catheter. The longitudinal cracks can be found in the
whole circumference of the vessel wall. The architecture of the
arteriosclerotic vessel wall becomes instable and destroyed (fig.
2-4). If sufficient blood flow can not be obtained after PTA,
this instable structure can collapse: Thereby the technically
successful dilatation of an arteriosclerotic lesion with subsequent early re - occlusion can be explained easily.
Furthermore thrombotic lesions can be found in the niches of
arteriosclerotic alterations before intervention. Immediately
after dilatation such thrombotic lesions can be detected in the
cracked arteries. NaCl - solution cannot wash away these thrombi
in or near the cracked vessel - walls. An important mechanism of
early re - occlusion after successful dilatation is thereby ex-
plained:the local thrombotic occlusion is caused by the cracked
walls, which induce formation of thrombi.
The complication rate of angiography combined with angioscopy is
not higher than using angiography alone.

DISCUSSION

The first publications on angioscopy report vessel alteration
under surgical conditions (Fleisher 1986; Grundfest 1985; Litvack 1985; Mehigan 1986; Cortis 1984). Only recently percutaneous transluminal proceeding has become possible, using ultrathin endoscopes and NaCl- perfusion (Beck 1987; Ferris 1985).
Angioscopy is useful diagnosing different degrees of arteriosclerosis and is therefore superior to angiography. Nevertheless
angioscopy can only be performed under fluoroscopic control and
therefore it is an additional method only until now. Angioscopy
can also distinguish between local thrombotic and embolic lesions. The degree of vessel alterations caused by balloon dilatation can be detected by angioscopy only. The so far unknown
cause of early re - occlusion after successful dilatation can be
clarified by angioscopy.The destroyed vessel architecture as well
as the thrombogenicity of the cracked arteriosclerotic plaques
can only be diagnosed by angioscopy.
Percutaneous transluminal angioscopy is still in the beginnings
of its possibilities. A lot of problems are still to be solved:
size of endoscopes, fragility of glass - fibers, optical problems, documentation modalities, insufficient blood flow dimi-
nution.The fascination of direct in vivo observation of vessel
pathology and future angioscopically monitored interventions will
help further development of this method.

fig.1
Procedure of angioscopy:
Through a guiding catheter
the scope is placed into
the subclavian artery.
The guide wire passes the
working channel of the
endoscope

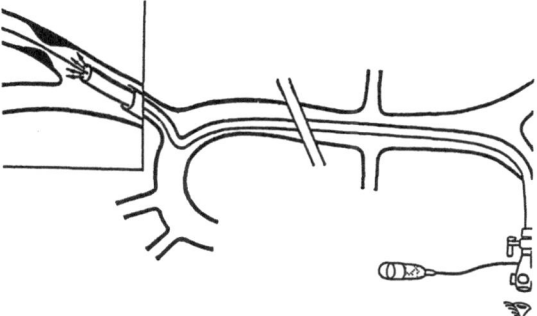

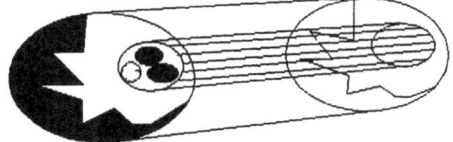

fig.2

ANGIOSCOPY OF ARTERIOSCLEROTIC LESIONS

BALLOON — DILATATION OF
ARTERIOSCLEROSIS

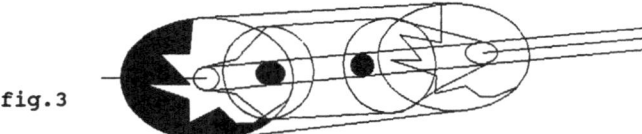

fig.3

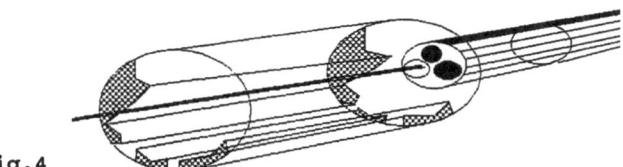

fig.4

Angioscopy after dilatation of arteriosclerotic lesions

332

fig.5
Severe arteriosclerotic
lesion of the subclavian
artery of a 65 year old
patient. Situation be-
fore PTA.

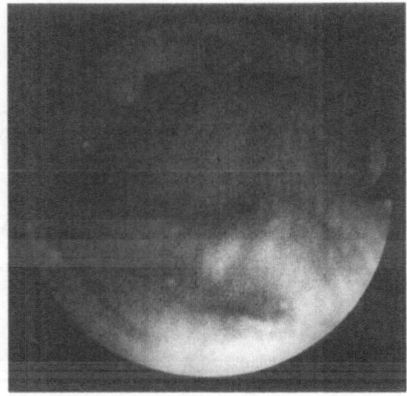

fig.6
Same patient as above:
Situation after PTA. The
lumen is widened but
still with severe arteriosclerotic lesions

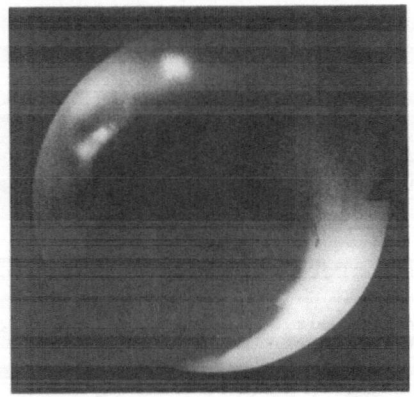

REFERENCES

Beck A (1987) Perkutane transluminale Angioskopie: Erste
    Ergebnisse einer neuen Methode. Der Radiologe 48: 123 –
    127
Cortis BS, Hussein H, Khandekar CS, Principe J, Tkaczuk
    RN(1984)
    Angioscopy in vivo. Cath. Cardiovasc.Diagn.10:493 – 500
Fleisher HL, Thompson BW, Mc Cowan TC, Ferris EJ (1986)
    Angioscopically monitored saphenous vein valvulotomy. J.Vasc.
    Surg. 4: 360 – 364
Ferris EJ, Ledor K, Ben Avi DD, Baker LL, Robbins KV (1985)
    Percutaneous angioscopy. Work in progress. Radiology 157:
    319   – 322
Grundfest WS, Litvack L, Sherman T (1985) Delineation of
    peripheral and coronary detail by intraoperative angioscopy.
    Ann. Surg. 202:394 – 400
Litvack L, Grundfest WS, Lee ME, Carroll RM, Foran R, Chaux A
    (1985) Angioscopic visualization of blood vessel interior
    in animals and in humans. Clin. Cardiol. 8: 65 – 70
Mehigan JT, Olcott C (1986) Video – angioscopy as an
    alternative   to intraoperative arteriography. Am. J. Surg.
    12: 139 – 145
Wenz W, Beck A, Richter GM, Nöldge G (1988) Neue Entwicklungen
    in der Angiographie. Jahrbuch der Radiologie,p 3 – 12

Long-Term Follow-up After Percutaneous Transluminal Angioplasty (PTA) of the Subclavian Artery

H. Brückmann, E. B. Ringelstein, and H. Zeumer

INTRODUCTION

A recent publication demonstrates that nowadays about 240 subclavian PTA have been performed (Mathias, 1988). The complication rate during angioplasty is very low (Zeumer, 1985); (Brückmann, 1987). Only 7 transitory complications have been reported (Mathias, 1988). This is partly due to the delayed reversal of vertebral artery blood-flow following PTA for subclavian steal syndrome (Ringelstein and Zeumer, 1984). In the following we report the results of the longterm follow-up of our patient group.

METHODS

Since December 1982 until December 1987 sixty-four PTA procedures have been performed in 52 patients suffering from subclavian steal syndrome due to proximal subclavian stenosis. All patients had complaints, which were considered to result from vertebrobasilar insufficiency. As 10 patients died during the follow-up period and 6 patients were not available, 36 patients remained for follow-up examinations. 8 of 10 patients died by cardiac infarction, one by bronchiogenic carcinoma, one by sinus thrombosis.

In the time period from 6 to 63 months (range 35 months) the patients were examined clinically and by Doppler Ultrasound. Relying on ultrasound findings, all patients presenting with subclavian steal syndrome were ranged according to the degree of the subclavian lesion and to the severity of steal effect.

At least 4 stages should be differentiated with respect to the hemo-dynamic effect of subclavian lesion on vertebral bloodflow (Ringelstein and Zeumer, 1984).

RESULTS

All of the 36 remaining patients were subsequently examined by ultrasound according to stage II or III. Fourteen belonged to stage II and twenty-two to stage III. Eleven of these fourteen patients had angiologically a very stable course and remained up to 56 months (in maximum) in stage I.

Twenty-two patients were preinterventionally ranged to stage III. In comparison to the other group it is evident that in this group not as many patients belonged to stage I after PTA. But an improvement was possible in 18 patients, in 4 patients no success was obtained.

Half of the patients (18/36) who had been treated by PTA never developed symptoms according to vertebrobasilar insufficiency in the follow-up period. Almost all members of this group improved angiologically. No patient deteriorated to stage III (Fig. 1).

In the group of all patients without clinical improvement only one half improved to stage I (Fig.2). A brainstem stroke occurred in two patients, one young male and one female. Both were stage III and had bilateral subclavian vertebral artery.

DISCUSSION

Theseresults indicate:
1. that the angiological course after PTA depends on the severity of preinterventional findings and
2. that the clinical course corresponds withthe angiological course.

This is confirmed by the fact that 8 of 10 patients in whom re-PTA was necessary belonged to stage III preceding PTA, as demonstrated by figure 2. Nevertheless, this data should not be overestimated.

So in a series of 91 patients examined with transcranial doppler monitoring with various degrees of subclavian steal only 13 showed severe disturbances of basilar artery blood flow namely either alternating blood flow during brachial hyperemia or even flow reversal during the whole cardiac circle. It should be noted that such severe flow disturbances occurred only in patients with bilateral subclavian vertebral artery lesions and not in those with merely unilateral subclavian artery stenosis (Ringelstein, 1987). Furthermore a recent contribution supports our oppinion that "subclavian steal phenomenon in a merely unilateral subclavian artery stenosis seems to be a common vascular disorder with rare neurological deficits" (Hennerici, 1987).

CONCLUSION

1. From the angiological point of view the indications for PTA of subclavian steal syndrome should be restricted to cases according to stage II or III with bilateral subclavian vertebral artery lesions with severe disturbances of basilar artery blood flow.
2. From the clinical point of view those cases are to be treated in which vertebrobasilar transient ischemic attacks occur frequently and in which arm claudication debilitate the patient.

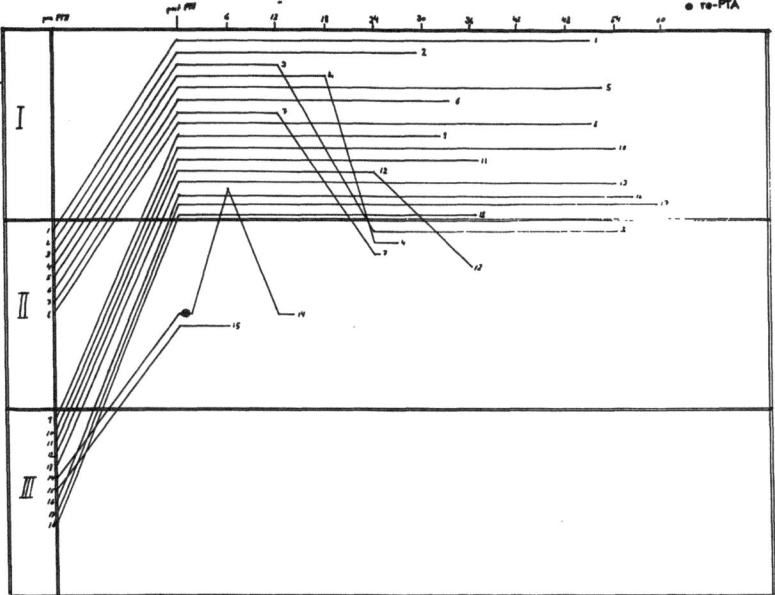

Fig. 1. Angiological course of the patients without complaints. The angiological stage is related to the time course (up to 60 months), no patient deteriorated to stage III.

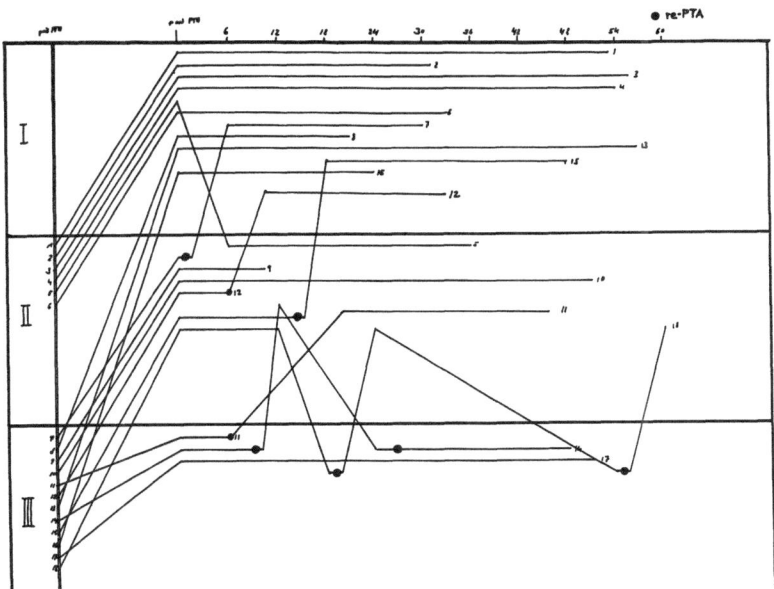

Fig. 2. Angiological course of all patients without clinical improvement. Only one half of the patients improved to stage III.

REFERENCES

Brückmann H, Ringelstein EB, Buchner H, Zeumer H (1987) Vascu
   recanalising techniques in the hind brain circulation. Neur
   Review 10:197-199
Hennerici M, Klemm C, Rautenberg W (1988) The subclavian stea
   phenomenon: A common vascular disorder with rare neurologic
   deficits. Neurology 38:669-673
Mathias K (1988) Perkutane Rekanalisation der supraaortalen G
   In: Günter R, Thelen M (eds) Interventionelle Radiolgoie. T
   Verlag, Suttgart, pp.73-87
Ringelstein EB, Zeumer H (1984) Delayed reversal of vertebral
   blood flow following percutaneous transluminal angioplasty
   subclavian steal syndrom. Neuroradiology 26:189-196
Ringelstein EB (1987) Transcranial Doppler Sonography. In: Po
   Ringelstein EB, Hacke W: New trends in diagnosis and manage
   stroke. Springer Verlag, pp. 3-28
Zeumer H (1985) Vascular racanalising techniques in intervent
   neuroradiology. J. Neurol 231:287-294

PTA of Subclavian Artery: A Special Technique, Short and Long Term Results 2–6 Years After Treatment

A. Beck and M. Schumacher

INTRODUCTION

4750 percutaneous transluminal angioplasties have been performed in the Department of Diagnostic Radiology and Neuroradiology since 1978. The total number of PTAs in the subclavian arteries amounts to 89. 54 have been performed in the left subclavian artery, 24 in the right subclavian artery, 7 in the axillary arteries and 4 in the brachial arteries. All patients have been controlled clinically, by Doppler sonography and partially by re - angiography. In all cases we used a special technique: A special guide wire with a gold - tip can be introduced through common catheters and be brought into the stenosed area. Rotating the wire manually the gold - tip passes the stenosis easily.

Material and Method

A special guide wire with a very smooth golden tip of 1 - 1.5 cm of length (12 - 22') and a rigid far - end can be placed in the subclavian artery (fig. 1-3).
By slowly rotating the rigid far - end of the guide wire manually, almost all stenoses and many occlusions can be passed easily. The manual manipulation of the guide wire is similar to the movement of a corkscrew. By this method perforation or penetration into the intima of the vessel can be avoided in most cases. The rigidity of the far - end of the guide wire guaranties a 1 : 1 movement of bottom to tip. The rigidity and the 1:1 movement result from the fact that the wire consits of one piece only. The golden tip is soldered to the rigid part of the wire in several points as not to loose the tip.
The access to dilatation of the subclavian, axillary and brachial arteries is usually transfemorally . Only in three cases the access was via the brachial artery.
The tip of the guide wire is positioned into the cubital area of the brachial artery and fixed externally by inflating a blood pressure cuff at the upper arm. The pressure needed is about 200 mm Hg for 4 minutes maximally. Thereby dilatation can be performed without dislocation of the guide wire and even hard and severe stenoses can be passed with the balloon catheter subsequently. The whole procedure should be finished within 15 minutes. The dilatation time itself is twice 20 seconds in the stenosis. All patients are controlled angiographically, clinically and by blood pressure - measurement immediately after the intervention. The following week another clinical control is performed (early PTA - results) . The long - term control is performed 2 - 8 years after the intervention by Doppler - sonography and clinical examination.

RESULTS

48 out of 54 patients with left subclavian artery stenosiss
showed good short-term results; 45 showed still good results at
long-term control (fig.4). 20 out of 24 patients with right
subclavian artery stenosis showed good results immediately after
dilatation; 18 showed good long-term results. In the axillary
artery 6 patients performed well short-term, 5 performed well
long-term. In the brachial artery 3 out of 4 patients showed good
long-term and short-term results. Alltogether 77 patients out of
89 showed good short-term results, 71 showed good long-term
results (fig. 5).
6 patients could not be dilated technically.
The complications of PTA of subclavian,axillary and brachial
arteries were as follows:

Inguinal hematoma (2 - 8 cm diameter)
- without surgical consequences   3

Inguinal hematoma (retroperitoneal hematoma)
- subsequent surgery   1

Embolization into peripheral arteries
of the hand   1

Vessel - dissection
- without surgical consequences   1

deterioration of angiographic situation:
- thrombotic occlusion   2

                                                            8

DISCUSSION

Since the first publications on dilatation (Dotter 1964; Grüntzig 1974) of the supraaortic branches (Mathias 1977,1980) this
interventional method became a wide - spread therapy. The complication rate is very low world - wide, so that the indications
could be taken wider than in the beginning. The mechanism of
dilatation could be clarified by the new method of angioscopy(
Beck 1987). The first publications on long term results of
dilatation and recanalization of peripheral and even central
arteries (Zeitler 1978; Beck 1988) showed a positive direction.
Dilatation of our own patients was very successful. One main
reason may be the atraumatic procedure with the smooth gold tip
of the guide wire, which cannot perforate and avoids subintimal
proceeding. The diameter of the inflated balloon never exceeds
the diameter of the angiographical lumen of the vessel. In our
experience the PTA must be performed as quick as possible. The
inflation time of the balloon only amounts to twice 20 seconds.
This contrasts to other publications.
In our opinion dilatation and recanalization of subclavian, axillary and brachial arteries should be the first adequate therapy
of stenotic arterial lesions in this area.

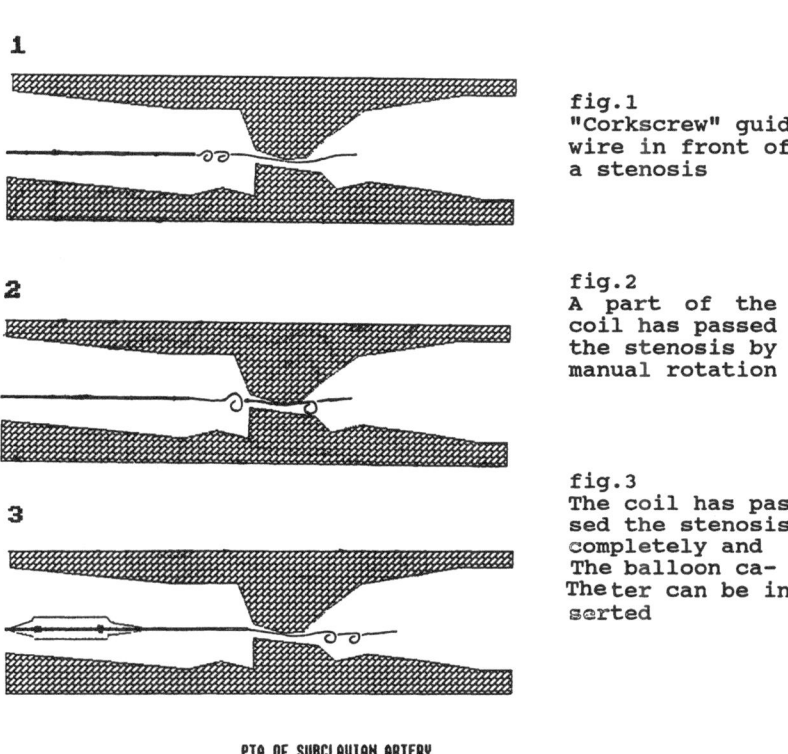

fig.1
"Corkscrew" guide
wire in front of
a stenosis

fig.2
A part of the
coil has passed
the stenosis by
manual rotation

fig.3
The coil has pas-
sed the stenosis
completely and
The balloon ca-
Theter can be in-
serted

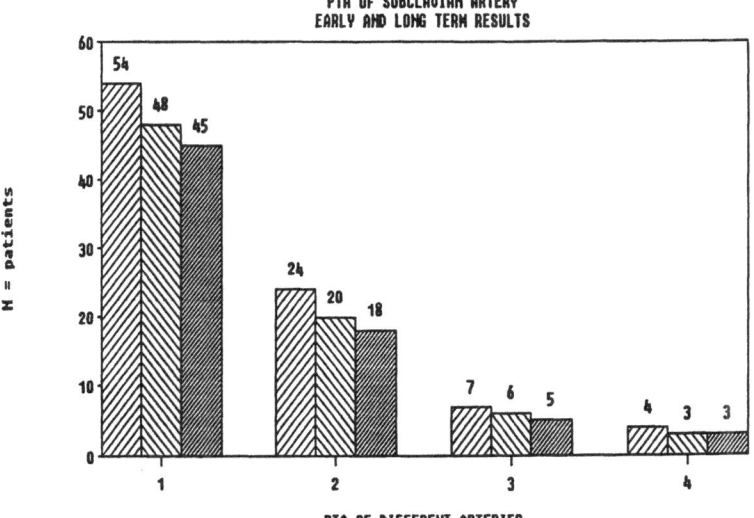

fig.4 Correlation between total number of patients, early
and long - term results of PTA.
1 = left subclavian artery
2 = right subclavian artery
3 = axillary arteries
4 = brachial arteries

340

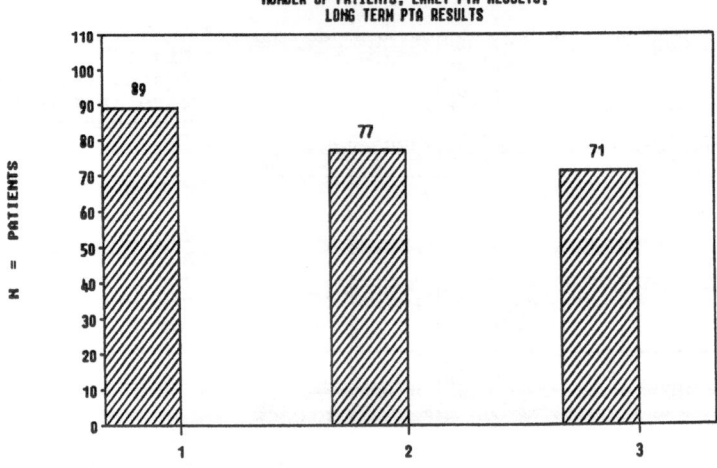

fig. 5 Short term and long term success of total number of
       patients dilated in all three vessel areas

REFERENCES
Beck A, Ostheim - Dzerowycz W, Grosser G, Heiss HW (1988)
   Clinical and angiographic long - term results of percutaneous
   transluminal angioplasty and local catheter lysis of the
   supraaortic, pelvic and lower limb arteries
   CORVAS 2: 77 - 86
Beck A, Ostheim - Dzerowycz W, Heiss G, Mühe A, Hasler K (1988)
   Long term results of 4750 dilatations and local lyses
   European Journal of Vascular Surgery (in press)
Beck A (1987) Perkutane transluminale Angioskopie:
   Erste Ergebnisse einer neuen Methode.Der Radiologe 48:123 -
   127
Dotter CT, Rösch MP (1964) Transluminal treatment of
   arteriosclerotic obstruction: Description of a new technique
   and a preliminary report of its application. Circulation 30:
   654-670
Grüntzig A, Hopff H (1974) Perkutane Rekanalisation chronischer
   arterieller Verschlüsse mit einem neuen Dilatationskatheter.
   Dtsch Med Wochenschr. 99: 2502
Mathias K (1977) Ein neuartiges Kathetersystem zur perkutanen
   transluminalen Angioplastie von Carotisstenosen. Fortschr Med
   95 (15): 1007- 1011)
Mathias K, Staiger J, Thron A, Spillner G, Heiss HW, Konrad-Graf
   (1980) Perkutane Katheterangioplastik der Arteria Subclavia.
   Dtsch Med Wochenschr 105: 16-18
Mathias K, Schlosser V, Reinke M (1980) Katheterrekanalisation
   eines Subclaviaverschlusses RÖFO 132: 346-347
Zeitler E, Grüntzig A, Schoop W (1978) Percutaneous vascular
   recanalization. Springer, Berlin, Heidelberg, New York

Percutaneous Nucleotomy of the Lumbar Disk: Method and Preliminary Results

U. Salvolini, U. Pasquini, F. Menichelli, and R. Rossi

Introduction

Percutaneous nucleotomy is a new method for decompressing herniated
lumbar disks and can be considered a new device in interventional
radiology. It is an alternative to traditional laminectomy in selected cases and is less invasive [3,4,5]. It is based on concepts of
percutaneous diskectomy, presented as an alternative to traditional
laminectomy [2] and to chemonucleolysis [1].

Material and Method

Percutaneous nucleotopy is performed with a specific device called
the nucleotome, furnished in a disposable kit. The method was first
described by Onik [4,5]. The nucleotome disk aspiration probe is
introduced transcutaneously in the center of the disk under local
anesthesia by means of a posterolateral approach, with fluoroscopic
control. Then the nucleus is automatically removed in little fragments. The patient does not need general anesthesia or analgesic
treatment and after the procedure does not need hospitalization.

Our present experience is based on 50 patients treated during the
period from October 1987 to September 1988. We operated on each of
them at one level: 47 patients at the L4-L5 and 3 patients at the
L5-S1 level. Our series included four patients with recurrence of
herniated disk, previously treated by laminectomy, and two patients
affected by narrow spinal canal, one of whom was affected also by
degenerative vacuum phenomena in a bulging disk.

Clinical evaluation was the main parameter for assessing the efficacy of treatment. All patients were evaluated by CT before and immediately after the percutaneous nucleotomy, and 3 months later.
Twelve were also evaluated by MRI before and after treatment.

Discussion and Results

The therapeutic effect of percutaneous nucleotomy is based on reduction in the volume of the nucleus by removing fragments using

the nucleotome probe. This reduces the compression of the anulus over the nerve roots, especially at the foraminal level.

We obtained good or satisfactory results in 39 of 50 patients and unsatisfactory results in 11. Three of the 11 were then treated by traditional laminectomy. CT controls showed no significant modification in the morphology or structure of the herniated disks in most cases (80%), independently of clinical results [6,7]. RMI controls also did not show any significant modification in the morphology of the diskal hernia after percutaneous nucleotomy, in either acute of chronic phases, in accordance with CT results [6,7]. However, herniated disks treated with chemopapain did show a change in the nucleus on RMI control in the chronic phase: the nucleus had a degenerative aspect with a low signal, in accord with our previous observations [6,7] and these at others [8]. In one case, a 22-year-old patient, a late RMI control after percutaneous nucleotomy showed a significant increase in the nucleus signal, especially in T2-weighted images. This finding is not unequivocally interpretable (rehydration?).

A critical point is represented by the indications for percutaneous nucleotomy. This method seems to have the best efficacy in the bulging disk and the uncomplicated herniated disk. However, it fails in the presence of a free fragment beyond the anulus. In our series the three patients operated by laminectomy after percutaneous nucleotomy for persistent symptomatology were all affected by transligamental herniated disk with free fragment. The role of diskography can be discussed for the diagnosis of the extraligamentous herniated disks.

The clinical results of percutaneous nucleotomy also do not seem to be satisfactory in chronic herniated disks, in severe degenerative facit disease with lumbar stenosis, and in previous lumbar surgery, as observed by Onik [5]. In these cases the nerve root compression is caused by fibrocalcified tissue, adherent scars, and nonelastic diskal anulus; thus, the removal of the nucleus has no effect on the nerve roots.

Conclusions

The relatively limited number of treated patients and the brief follow-up period in this study does not allow conclusive assessments. Nevertheless on the basis of our initial results we can state: (a) the procedure is well tolerated by the patient; (b) it is a safe and low-risk method in experienced hands; and (c) the clinical results are satisfactory in most patients in our follow-up period, if well selected. A long follow-up period and a greater number of patients are required for a definitive assessment about the efficacy of the treatment. A good patient selection requires strict clinical criteria for inclusion and exclusion.

References

[1] Friedman WA (1983) Percutaneous diskectomy: an alternative to chemonucleolysis? Neurosurgery 13: 542-547
[2] Kambin P, Gellman H (1983) Percutaneous lateral diskectomy of the lumbar spine. Clin Orthop 174: 127-132
[3] Onik G, Helms C, Ginsburg L et al. (1985) Percutaneous lumbar diskectomy using a new aspiration probe: porcine and cadaver model. AJNR 6: 290-293
[4] Onik G, Helms C, Ginsburg L, Hoaglund P, Morris J (1985) Percutaneous lumbar diskectomy using a new aspiration probe. AJNR 6: 290-293
[5] Onik G, Maroon J, Helms C et al. (1987) Automated percutaneous diskectomy: initial patient experience. Radiology 162: 129-132
[6] Salvolini U Pasquini U, Menichelli F (1988) Valutazione pre- e post-operatoria con TC e MR nella nucleoaspirazione discale lombare percutanea. Personal communication: 9th Carvat, Digital imaging modalities in clinical radiology, Rome February 1-5, 1988
[7] Salvolini U, Pasquini U, Menichelli F (1988) La nucleoaspirazione discale (NAD) percutanea lombare: tecnica e risultati preliminari. In: Smaltino F, Elefante R, Cirillo S (eds) Neuroradiologia Oggi. Atti VII Congresso Nazionale A.I.N. Idelson, Napoli
[8] Szypryt EP, Gibson MJ, Mulholland RC, Worthington BS (1987) The long-term effect of chemonucleolysis on the intervertebral disc as assessed by magnetic resonance imaging. Spine 12: 707-711

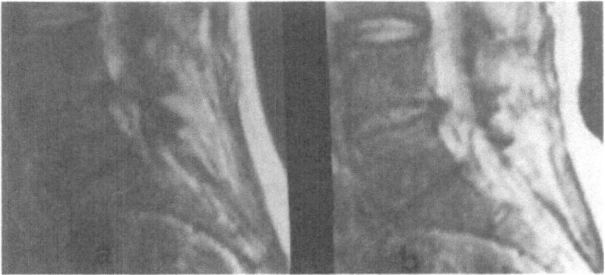

Fig.1. MRI controls before (a) and after (b) percutaneous nucleotomy at the L4-L5 level. The signal of the nucleus does not change in T2-weighted images

344

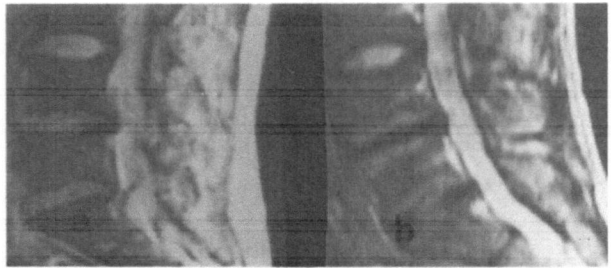

Fig.2. MRI controls before (a) and after (b) chemopapain at L4-L5
or L5-S1 levels. The signal of the nucleus became low in T2-weigh-
ted images, with a degenerative aspect, after chemopapain

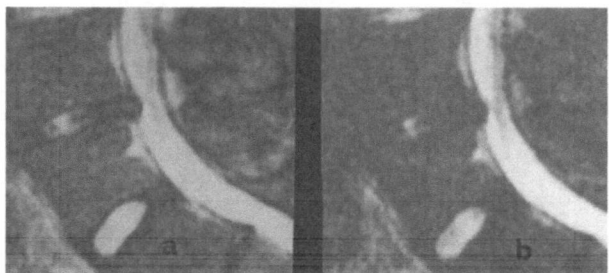

Fig.3. MRI control after percutaneous nucleotomy at the L4-L5 level.
The signal of the nucleus is bright in T2-weighted iamges. This
finding is not unequivocally interpretable (rehydration?)

Prognosis and Treatment Possibilities in Occipital Dural Arteriovenous Malformations

D. Kühne, D. de Silva, and H. C. Nahser

Of all intracranial AVMs, occipitomastoid dural AVMs of the posterior fossa are the most common, with 7% (Newton and Chronqvist 1969). The large number of treatment methods available, such as embolization with different embolic materials, operations, radiotherapy, and manual compression of the supply vessels, mirror the magnitude of the therapeutic problem (Halbach et al. 1987; Sundt and Piepgras 1983; Vinuela et al. 1983; Lasjaunias et al. 1983).

We present our experiences in treating 23 patients with dural AVMs situated in the occipitomastoid region and the efficacy of Ethibloc as an embolic material. They were treated over a period of time with repeated Ethibloc embolizations.

It is not the purpose of this paper to discuss their clinical presentation, although a few brief comments will be made. The main well-known clinical symptom is a persistent, mostly pulse-synchronous bruit, which in some patients leads to severe depression. Less common clinical features are enumerated in Table 1. We did not find involvement of cranial nerves as is seen with dural AVMs in the middle and anterior cranial fossae, especially in the region of the sinus cavernosus.

Table 1. Clinical manifestations in 23 patients

Bruit		17
Headache		13
Vertigo		7
Hemorrhage		6
Intracerebral	4	
Subarachnoid	3	
Subdural	0	
Epidural	0	
Tinnitus		5
Nausea and vomiting		4
Raised intracranial pressure		2

The typical angiographic finding was the involvement of multiple meningeal branches forming a network of fine pathological vessels which mostly drained directly into the transverse or sigmoid sinuses (Fig.1). The occipital artery was the dominant feeder in most cases. The involvement of branches of the internal carotid and other meningeal arteries, including those of the vertebral artery, make the situation more complex but do not cause any significant alteration of the clinical symptomatology. Among the 23 patients, six developed intracranial hemorrhages; four had intracerebral hematomas (one with an associated subarachnoidal bleed); and two had purely subarachnoidal bleeds. We saw no cases of subdural or epidural bleeds, in keeping with the findings of other authors (Table 1; Lasjaunias et al. 1986).

In all the patients who presented with intracranial bleeds, whether intracerebral or subarachnoid, the venous drainage was more complex (Fig.2). There were additional or exclusively venous pathways over cortical veins, or there were locally dilated venous sacs (Table 2). The danger of intracranial hemorrhages in this type of dural AVM is much higher, and their management requires rapid and special care (Lasjaunias et al. 1986; Vinuela et al. 1986). In the patients who had direct antegrade venous drainage along the sinuses and jugular

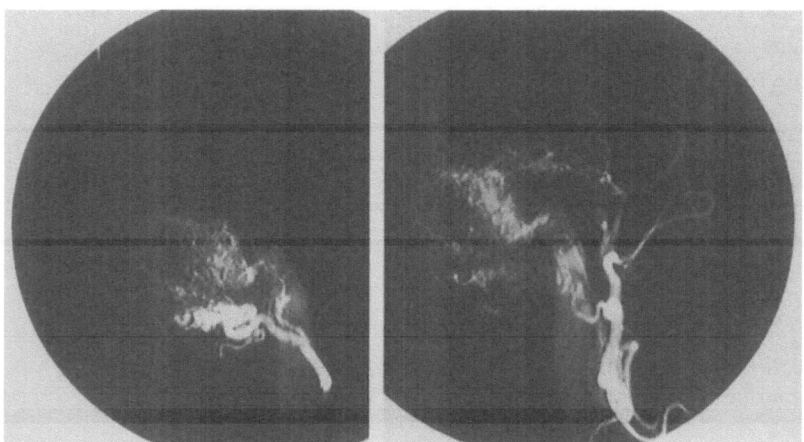

Fig.1. Selective lateral angiograms of the occipital (a) and the external carotid (b). Multiple meningeal arteries of the occipital, posterior auricular, and posterior branch of the middle meningeal arteries supply the dural AVM at the junction of the transverse and sigmoid sinuses

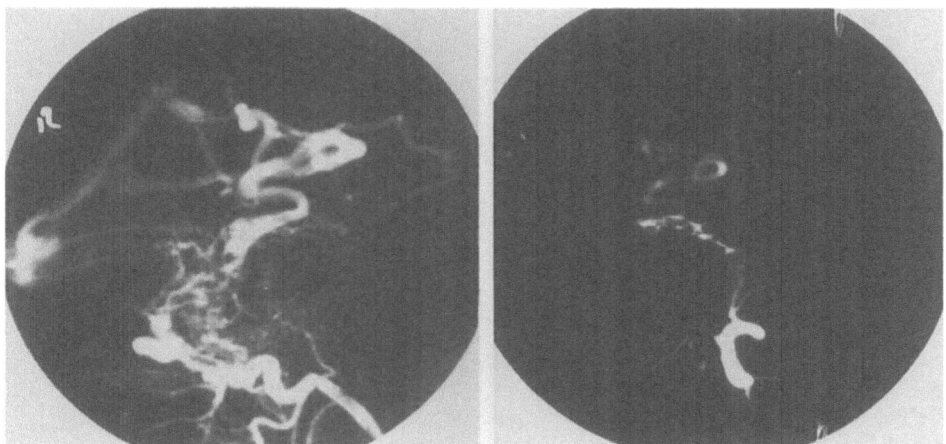

Fig.2. Lateral angiograms of the right occipital (a) and right
maxillary (b) arteries. The dural AVM drains primarily into the
superficial cortical and the deep cerebral vein

veins, we encountered no cases of intracranial bleeding. This was
also observed by other authors (Lasjaunias et al. 1986; Vinuela et
al. 1986).

Table 2. Routes of venous drainage

Directly into transverse or sigmoid sinus	15
Additionally into cerebral veins	8
Superficial 5	
Deep 3	
Intracerebral, associated with transverse sinus abnormalities	3

We have found no indications as to the etiology of these AVMs either
in the history or in the angiographic appearances. We have observed
sinus anomalies in three patients. In one patient with an intracerebral hemorrhage there were severely dilated cortical veins; the
transverse sinus was outlined only over a short segment, in the region of the AVM. This was maintained also during digital compression
of the opposite jugular veins and therefore suggested that there had
been thromboses in the nonopacified parts (Fig.3).

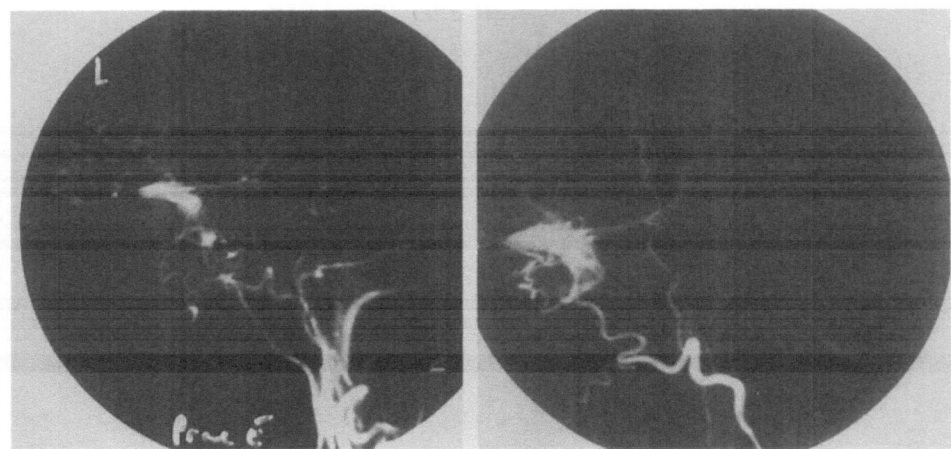

Fig.3. Lateral external carotid (a) and selective occipital (b)
arteriograms. The dural AVM draining into the junction of the
transverse and sigmoid sinuses, which are only partially filled,
most likely due to old thromboses. Cortical venous filling is also
seen

In a 24-year-old female patient who complained of severe headaches
we found that the large venous sinuses in the posterior cranial
fossa, bilaterally, were not opacified. Here, the venous blood filled
the superior sagittal sinus, draining anteriorily and also draining
anteriorily along the orbital veins (Fig.4).

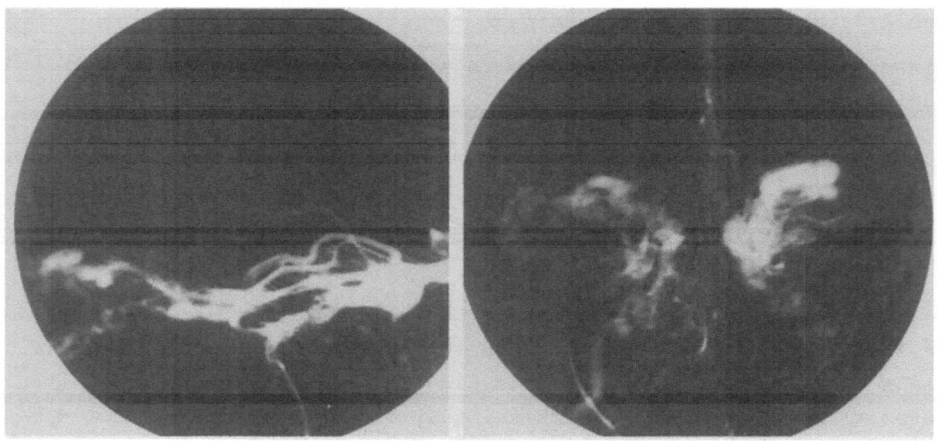

Fig.4. AP and lateral internal maxillary angiograms. The dural AVM
is supplied by the hypertrophied middle meningeal artery draining
into the transverse sinus, without filling of the sigmoid sinus
and jugular vein. Venous drainage occurs anteriorly (see text)

Table 3. Analysis of cases

Age (years)	Sex	Period of observation (years)	No. of vessels involved and Hemorrhages	No. of embolizations and other facts	Clinical results
4	M	1	1	1	Cured
24	M	2.5	2 + SAB	2	Improved
36	F	3	3	3	Cured
43	M	1.75	1 + ICB	2	Cured
43	M	3	2 + SAB + ICB	4	Cured
45	F	2	3	2 + RT	Cured
46	F	4	2	2	Cured
47	M	2	3 + ICB	2	Cured
50	M	3	3 + SAB	4	Cured
52	F	0.25	3	2	Cured
52	F	2.5	4	3	Cured
54	M	3	4 + ICB	4	Improved
60	F	1	2	1	Improved
61	F	3	3	4	Improved
61	F	5	3	5	Improved
62	M	3	4	3 + op	Improved
64	M	1.5	2	1	Cured
64	F	1.25	3	3	Improved
67	F	1	3	1	Cured
67	F	1.5	4	3	Improved
68	F	1	4	3	Cured
70	F	3	3	2	Cured
56	F	1	3	1	Improved

SAB, subarachnoidal hemorrhage; ICB, intracranial hemorrhage

The embolization took place over several sittings (up to five; Table 3) and the embolic material mostly used was Ethibloc, mixed with various volumes of Lipiodol. This was injected selectively through a coaxial catheter. In some cases polyvinylalcohol particles were used. Here we found that the effect was very shortlasting, with recanalization of the vessels and return of the clinical and angiographic features. After Ethibloc embolization recanalization of the occluded vessel was never seen. When recurrence occurred, this took place from the nonembolized proximal part. The findings of our series are included in Table 3.

In the 14 patients who were clinically cured, confirmatory angiograms were not always performed. Some patients however, were reexamined and showed an angiographic cure. The patient shown in Fig.5 had cortical venous drainage of the dural AVM associated with intracerebral hemorrhages. The occipital and ascending pharyngeal were embolized twice. Another patient (Fig.6) with multiple feeders was embolized five times and was clinically symptom free. The angiogram 1 year after the last embolization showed a slight fistulous connection over fine middle meningeal branches. The maxillary artery had been totally occluded after embolization.

In some cases following total embolization of the occipital and/or other dura-supplying vessels on one side, we found additional secondary supply from the opposite side which maintained a fraction of the

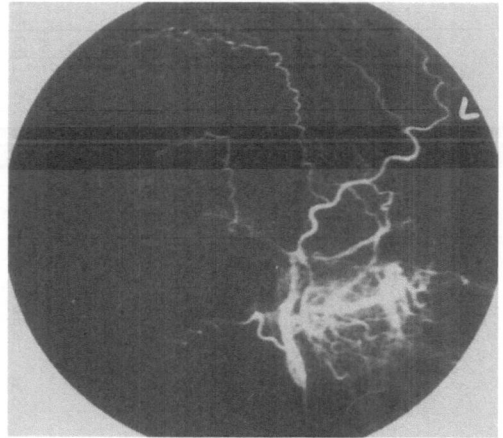

Fig.5. Lateral external carotid angiogram 1 year after embolization of a dural AVM with cortical drainage (preoperative, see Fig.3)

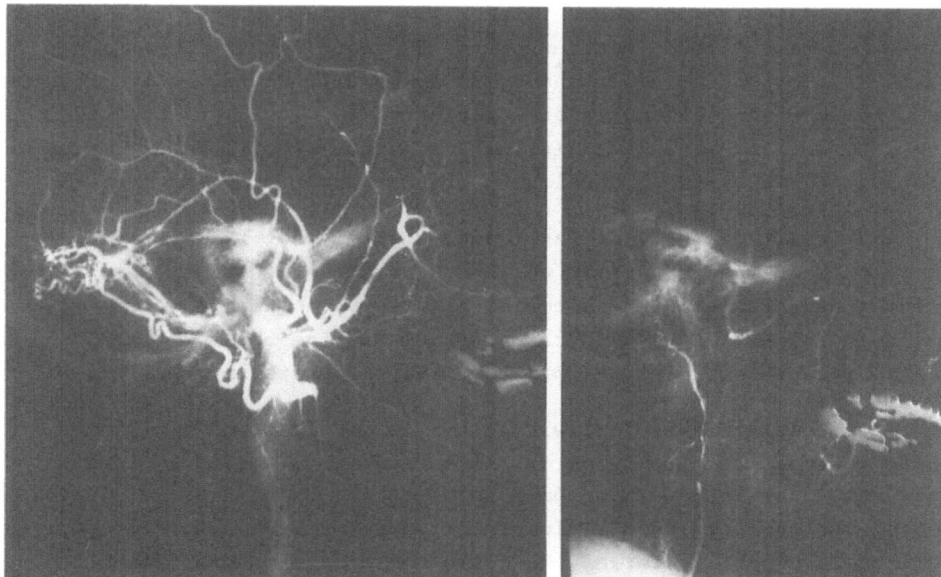

Fig.6. Selective right external carotid artery angiogram. Dural AVM supplied by the retroauricular and middle meningeal arteries drainage into the right transverse sinus. One year after several embolizations, the distal maxillary artery and middle meningeal arteries are filled over several collaterals with slight filling of the fistula. The patient was clinically asymptomatic

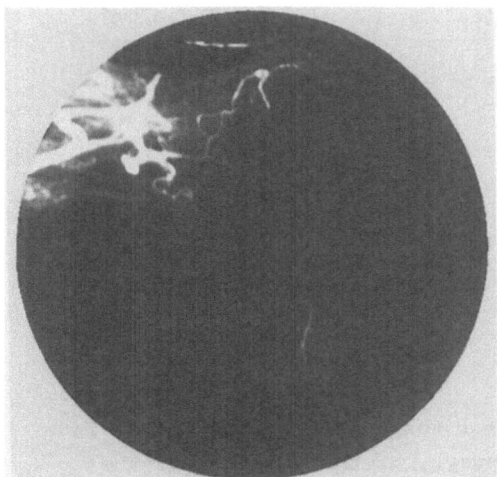

Fig.7. Right external carotid angiogram (AP) after embolization of the left external carotid dural AVM branches. Filling of a small residual nidus occurs via collaterals from the right occipital artery

AVM nidus (Fig.7). Despite this supply, this patient remained symptom free. Several of these patients (9 of 23) were clinically improved, with a reduction in the intensity of the bruit. We have not encounted hemorrhage in any of our treated patients up to this point in time. In one embolized patient additional radiotherapy of a small residual nidus supplied by a meningeal vertebral artery branch was performed.

A control angiogram 1 year later demonstrated that the AVM was totally closed. In one patient who had a partial resection of the AVM with ligature of the distal occipital artery, a massive recurrence was seen 1 year later, with reappeareance of the bruit. At this stage several embolizations produced only moderate improvement.

The complications seen following Ethibloc embolization are listed in Table 4. These complications in all our patients were only transitory. One patient developed paresis of the lower cranial nerves following the one sitting Ethibloc embolization of the ascending pharyngeal and occipital arteries. We would now change this approach, however, and wait a minimum of one week between the embolizations of vessels which supply cranial nerves. Ethibloc embolization causes a marked inflammatory reaction, producing pain and swelling in the region of embolization. The symptoms and signs usually improve in 3-4 days. We have never encountered a thrombosis of the venous sinuses.

Table 4. Complications after embolization (Ethibloc and Ivalon)

Pain	22
Swelling	20
Fever	7
Transient TM joint stiffness	5
Transient lower cranial nerve palsies	1
Tissue necrosis	0
Falling out of hair	0

Discussion and Conclusions

The purely dual AVMs of the posterior fossa are located mostly in the region of the large venous pathways, at the junction of the transverse and sigmoid sinuses (Houser et al. 1972; Newton and Chronqvist 1969; Newton et al. 1968). Several methods of treatment and sets of results have been discussed. Good long-term results are reported following total surgical resection of the abnormality.

but in one series of 27 patients, two deaths were reported (Sundt and Piepgras 1983). The proximal ligature of involved external carotid branches is fruitless, but sadly this method is still practiced. Some good results have also been reported by other authors following manual compression in the region of the occipital artery (Halbach et al. 1987). The most efficient and satisfying treatment of symptomatic dural AVMs seems to be their arterial embolization. This is confirmed by our study and collaborates the findings of other authors (Halbach et al. 1987; Lasjaunias et al. 1983; Vinuela et al. 1983). In our series 14 of 23 patients (61%) were markedly improved, especially with regard to the bruit, headache, and giddiness. The catheter technique today is so well developed that selective embolizations in the distributions of the vertebral and internal carotid arteries with microcatheters can be safely undertaken (Vinuela et al. 1983).

To achieve the best results, patience and a good liaison with the patients is important. This is due mainly to the complex nature of the malformations and to the need for repeated interventions, possibly over a considerable period of time.

Among the patients who have had intracranial bleeds abnormalities on the venous sides of the AVMs are common (Lasjaunias et al. 1986; Vinuela et al. 1986). Here additionally dilated cortical veins exist, from which the bleeding is most likely to have occurred. These patients should have their intervention with the minimum of delay and as radically as possible. If the embolization is not complete, other methods of supplementary management such as radiosurgery or resection should be instituted.

Summary

The therapeutic management of 23 cases of occipital AVMs is discussed. Treatment resulted in 61% cured and 39% improved after several embolizations with Ethibloc. Patients with intracranial bleeds developed no further hemorrhages. No permanent complications were encountered.

References

[1] Halbach V, Higashida RT, Hieshima GB, Goto K, Norman D, Newton TH (1987) Dural fistulas involving the transverse and sigmoid sinuses; results of treatment in 28 patients. Radiology 163: 443-447
[2] Houser OW, Baker HL, Rhoton AL, Okazaki H (1972) Intracranial dural arteriovenous malformations. Radiology 105: 55-64

[3] Lasjaunias P, Halimi P, Lopez-Ibor L, Sichez JP, Hurth M, Tribolet N (1983) Traitement endovasculaire des malformations vasculaires durales (MVD) pures "spontanées". Neurochirurgie 30: 207-223

[4] Lasjaunias P, Chiu M, ter Brugge K, Tolia A, Hurth M, Bernstein M (1986) Neurological manifestations of intracranial dural arteriovenous malformations. J Neurosurg 64: 724-730

[5] Newton TH, Chronqvist S (1969) Involvement of dural arteries in intracranial arteriovenous malformations. Radiology 93: 1071-1078

[6] Newton TH, Weidner W, Greitz T (1968) Dural arteriovenous malformation in the posterior fossa. Radiology 90: 27-35

[7] Sundt ThM, Piepgras DG (1983) The surgical approach to arteriovenous malformations of the lateral and sigmoid dural sinuses. J. Neurosurg 59: 32-39

[8] Vinuela F, Debrun GM, Fox AJ, Kan S (1983) Detachable calibrated-leak balloon for superselective angiography and embolization of dural arteriovenous malformations. J Neurosurg 58: 817-823

[9] Vinuela F, Fox AJ, Pelz DM, Drake CG (1986) Unusual clinical manifestations of dural arteriovenous malformations. J Neurosurg 64: 554-558

Stereotaxy Within the CT Scanner: A Safe and Fast Technique For Puncture and Biopsy

W. J. Huk

INTRODUCTION

Modern imaging techniques - CT and MRI - enable a direct diagnosis of intracranial disease at the time of initial neurological symptoms in many cases. In this early stage, when many lesions are still small, open surgery often is not indicated because of unjustified risks. Nevertheless, an operative intervention may be necessary or a histological diagnosis may be required to decide the further management of the patient.

For these purposes stereotaxic techniques have become the method of choice and they are employed more frequently today.

With the high spatial resolution of modern CT units it is only reasonable to use CT for the localization of intracranial targets for stereotaxic procedures. Today I will present our experience with a relatively simple targeting device in 250 cases, which makes possible stereotaxic procedures within the CT scanner under tomographic control.

METHOD

The apparatus consists of the actual targeting device and a phantom.

The targeting device consists of a head holder which is firmly attached to the CT table and which carries the targeting ring at its rear opening. Since we perform the procedure in general anaesthesia, the patient's head is immobilized sufficiently with firm plastic cushions.

The phantom consists of three coaxial rings which can be moved in relation to each other in order to simulate the spatial relationship between the lesion, the burr hole, and the needle (Fig. 1). When the coordinates are calculated with the help of a computer program, the phantom is no longer necessary.
The CT image of the needle in the center of the head holder is used as reference structure for all localization procedures. The burr hole and the target point within the lesion are related to this reference point by an angle and the distance (Fig. 2); these can be calculated with the standard soft ware of the scanner. The distance between the needle, the burr hole and the target are measured directly on the millimeter scale of the head holder by means of a calibrated light marker or laser.These data are transferred to the phantom to obtain the final coordinations for the needle, which in return are transferred to the identical sterile targeting ring at the patients head. Now the needle can be

advanced to the target point. After CT control of its exact
position, diagnostic or therapeutic procedures can be performed.

The duration of the operation varies between one und 1 1/2 hours
depending on the kind of procedure.
The accuracy of the system is +/- 1mm, the pixel size of the CT
image with a 256 x 256 matrix being 0.9 x 0.9 mm2.

Indications for this stereotaxic technique are:
- biopsy for histological diagnosis
- puncture and drainage of abscesses and cysts of various
  etiologies
- interstitial radiotherapy

RESULTS and CONCLUSIONS

The stereotaxic procedures performed in our series (n=250)
include:

- tumor biopsies	149
- drainage of cystic craniopharyngioms (-/+ Y-90)	34
- drainage of abscesses	8
- interstitial radiotherapy	47
- others (e.g. drainage of tumor cysts, hematomas)	12

Possible side effects, which are independent of the system, are:

1- intracranial/intracerebral hemorrhage
2- transient/permanent neurological deficits
3- infection

ad 1: There were no space occupying hemorrhages requiring
operative evacuation of the clot. Occasionally a little oozing can
be seen in the puncture canal and the area of the biopsy specimen.

ad 2: A slight transient deterioration was seen in two cases,
probably due to edema, but no permanent deficits. The procedure
should be performed with great caution in cases with a marked
increase of intracranial pressure. In these cases a single
puncture may raise the intracranial pressure to a critical level.

ad 3: There were no infections in the biopsy cases. In three out
of 47 cases where catheters loaded with iodine-125 seeds were
implanted for permanent or temporary interstitial radiotherapy,
and who had received long term treatment with dexamethasone,
cerebritis - in one case also ventriculitis - was seen. In one
girl with two catheters on either side for the drainage of
separate cysts of a craniopharyngioma, infection occurred five
months after the implantation of the last catheter.

Disadvantages of this system are:

- only supratentorial lesions (including brainstem) can be reached
  with the present version
- the need for approximately one hour of CT-time, which is an economical disadvantage

The advantages include:

- easy and fast calculation of coordinates with high accuracy
- quick and easy positioning of the patient without screws, when
  general anaesthesia is used. General anaesthesia ist preferred
  to local anaesthesia by the majority of our patients. When the
  procedure has to be done in local anaesthesia, the patients head
  can be immobilized with screws after a minor technical modification of the head holder
- intraoperative ("on line"):
  -- control of the position of the probe
  -- documentation of the origin of the biopsy specimen. Different
     areas of an inhomogeneous tumor can be located easily during
     the procedure to obtain the diagnosis most likely to be re-
     presentative for the tumor

  -- control of the position of the catheter in cystic lesions.
     The implantation of catheters may be difficult when the
     walls of cysts are very firm or very flaccid

  -- immediate intraoperative control of complications (e.g. he-
     morrhage)

CT guided stereotaxic procedures have become an important part of
the diagnosis of space occupying intracranial lesions and they are
a valuable alternative method for their treatment. When the rules
of the method are obeyed, its risks may be considered very low.

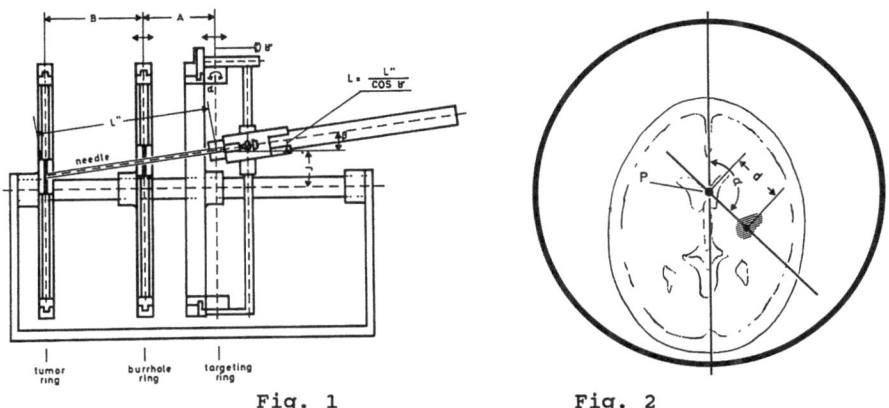

Fig. 1   Fig. 2

Fig. 1: The phantom with coaxial rings to simulate the spatial
relationship between the tumor, the burr hole, and the targeting
ring. The distance A and B can be measured on the millimeter scale
of the head holder.

Fig. 2: The CT-image of the needle (P) is the reference point for
the calculation of the coodinates (distance D and angle a) of the
target and the burr hole.

Specificity of CT Diagnosis Assessed by Stereotaxic Brain Biopsy. A Retrospective Analysis of 180 Cases

B. Dietrich and F. Alesch

Since CT has been employed as a clinical tool the aim has been not only to localize an intracranial lesion but also to come to a specific diagnosis by careful analysis of the entire criteria (Kazner et al. 1978; Nadjmi et al. 1981). The original expectations that a reliable CT diagnosis could be arrived at by subjective and objective analysis of densities before and after intravenous contrast and all other criteria were not fullfilled.
The aim of the study is a critical retrospective assessment of CT specificity confirmed by stereotaxic biopsy on a sample of intracranial lesions.

MATERIAL AND METHODS

In a 4 year period (1984 to 1988) 181 patients were selected to undergo stereotaxic biopsy after CT. These patients were subdivided into 6 groups according to the final histological diagnosis. Table 1 summerizes these groups. CT examinations were performed in the usual manner before and after intravenous contrast and sometimes with multiplanar reconstructions. The CTs were reviewed by the radiologists of the Institute of Neuroradiology.

The CT-based serial stereotaxic biopsies were performed by the Department of Stereotaxic Neurosurgery to confirm the diagnosis and/or to plan therapy. 6 to 10 specimens were taken at each biopsy and were examined by a neuropathologist. Stereotaxic biopsy was done on an average 20 days after the initial CT.
Comparison of the results of stereotaxic biopsy and CT diagnosis was related to conditions listed in Table 2.

RESULTS

Stereotaxic biopsy provided a definite histological diagnosis in 176 out of 181 patients.
Histological diagnosis was not possible in 5 patients although CT showed definite pathological lesions (2 abscesses, 1 metastasis, 1 glioblastoma, 1 ventricular tumor).

There was an overall agreement between stereotaxic biopsy diagnosis and initial CT diagnosis (point 1 Table 2) in 54 percent (n=94). Conditional agreement (point 2 Table 2) was seen in 24 percent (n=43). CT diagnosis failed (point 3 Table 2) in 22 percent (n=39).

Table 3 figures out the detailed results based on the 6 groups listed in Table 1. Best concordance was shown by the groups of anaplastic gliomas, the metastases and low grade gliomas. The group of lymphomas and "glioses" revealed a high rate of discrepancy. Group 6, "other intracranial lesions" included abscesses, bleedings chordomas, colloid cysts, craniopharyngeomas, epidermoids, and tumors of the pineal body.

DISCUSSION

This retrospective study demonstrates best agreement between stereotaxic biopsy diagnosis and initial CT diagnosis in the group of the most frequent lesions namely the anaplastic gliomas, metastases and low grade gliomas. CT specificity problems in the group of gliomas were due to over- and underestimating the grade of malignancy. The errors in the metastases'group were related to their solitary occurance. Additional causes of error were due to atypical location and pattern of the lesions.

Typical lymphomas are rarely evaluated by stereotaxic biopsy because their definite diagnosis is often proven by clinical follow-up under therapy. The distinct discrepancy in our 10 cases resulted from their having an atypical pattern.

Another misleading group were the lesions which were histologically confirmed as "gliosis". The CT diagnosis had suggested mostly a malignant lesion because of the frequent presence of contrast enhancement associated with (in some cases) perifocal decreased density.

CONCLUSIONS

This study confirms that CT's ability is limited in determining the specificity of histological diagnosis of cerebral lesions. Accuracy of CT depends greatly on the type of cerebral lesion.

Table 1. Patient's grouping according to biopsy diagnosis (181 patients)

1	Anaplastic gliomas	52
2	Low grade gliomas	43
3	Metastases	25
4	Lymphomas	10
5	Glioses	13
6	Other intracranial lesions	33
	Histological diagnosis not arrived at	5
		181

Table 2. Scheme for correlation between biopsy results and
        CT diagnosis

1	Unconditional agreement between histological and CT diagnosis
2	Conditional agreement i.e. the correct diagnosis was amongst the differential diagnosis offered by CT
3	No agreement

Table 3. Percentage of correlation between stereotaxic biopsy
        diagnosis and CT diagnosis (after scheme in Table 2)

	1 (Unconditional agreement)	2 (Conditional agreement)	3 (No agreement)
Anaplastic gliomas	60% (n=31)	31% (n=16)	9% (n= 5)
Low grade gliomas	53% (n=23)	26% (n=11)	21% (n= 7)
Metastases	60% (n=15)	32% (n= 8)	8% (n= 2)
Lymphomas	30% (n= 3)	10% (n= 1)	60% (n= 6)
Glioses	8% (n= 1)	8% (n= 1)	84% (n=11)
Other intracranial lesions	39% (n=13)	19% (n= 6)	42% (n=14)

REFERENCES

Kazner E, Wende S, Grumme TH, Stochdorph O, Felix R, Claussen C
  (eds) (1988) Computer- und Kernspin-Tomographie intrakranieller
  Tumoren aus klinischer Sicht. Springer, Berlin Heidelberg
  New York London Paris Tokyo
Nadjmi N, Piepgras U, Vogelsang H (eds) (1981) Neuroradiologische
  Atlanten. Kranielle Computertomographie. Ein synoptischer Atlas.
  Thieme, Stuttgart New York

Ultrasound Guided Biospy for Diagnosis and Treatment of Brain Lesions

M. Kopytek, B. Goraj, and Z. Jagodziński

Introduction

Recent advances in real-time ultrasonography enable neurosurgical
therapy in that they provide a safer and faster way of localizing
brain lesions and guiding their biopsy; there is still no way of
making an accurate diagnosis in many cases of intracerebral neoplasms without histological examination of the biopsy specimen. The
usefulness of US scanning in the localizing and biopsying of brain
lesions has been described by Collier et al. (1980), Tsutsumi et al.
(1982), and Sjölander et al. (1983).

Direct visualization of the potential needle pathways relative to
the ventricles and other major brain structures and vessels makes
placement of the needle safe and more accurate and thus increases
the diagnostic value of US-guided brain biopsy. This may also serve
as a therapeutic technique to puncture and aspirate brain abscesses
and other liquid intracranial collections.

The results of brain biopsy and further histological examinations
allow many patients with inoperable brain neoplasms to be treated
with chemo- and radiotherapy.

Clinical Material and Methods

Percutaneous US-guided needle biopsy of brain lesions was performed
in 22 patients (14 men and 8 women) aged 26-67 years through the
skull defect (acoustic window). Patients were divided into three
groups on the basis of initial investigations, including CT and
cerebral angiography in several cases (Table 1). Among the patients
with inoperable neoplasms there were persons with deep-seated tumors
(Fig.1) or multilobar tumors (Fig.2). The second group contained
patients with neoplasm recurrence (Fig.3), and the third, patients
with inflammatory tumors (Fig.4). The skull defect persisted in patients from the second group, and was especially made for the purpose
of needle biopsy in patients from groups 1 and 3. In patients in the

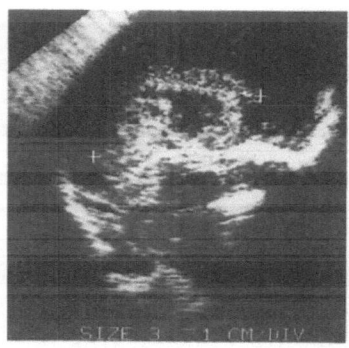
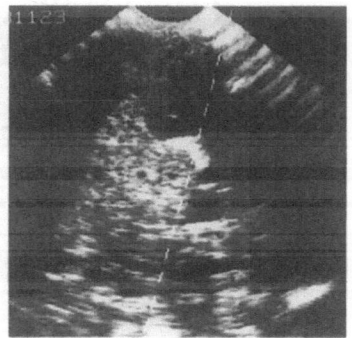

Fig.1. Deep-seated brain neoplasm. Nonresectable malignant glioma

Fig.2. Multilobar brain neoplasm. Nonoperative glioblastoma multiforme

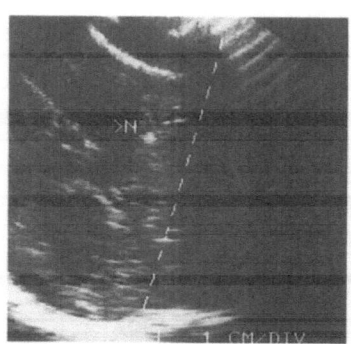
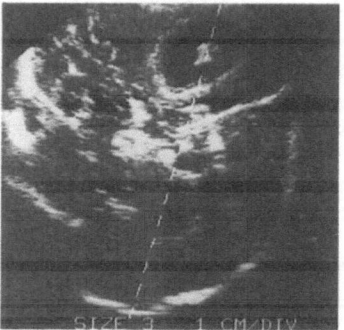

Fig.3. Recurrence of brain neoplasm

Fig.4. Brain abscess with well-developed capsule. In the center of
the abscess needle echo can be seen

first group with multilobar tumors decompressive craniotomy was also
performed. The minimum diameter of the skull defect was 3.0 cm.

For US examination a Brul-Kjaer 1846 sector scannor with 3.5 and
5.0 MHz transducers with 115° field of view was used. The transducers were fitted with a guide-tunnel for the biopsy needle. The biopsy was made with a Sure-Cut biopsy needle, 20 cm in length and 1.0 mm
in diameter. Prior to the puncture the transducer head with adapter
was immersed in an antiseptic solution for 20 min. After the skin was
surgically cleansed, the transducer was positioned over the skull
defect.

Table 1. Types of brain lesions and results of US-guided biopsy

Group of patients	Type of brain lesion	n	Procedure Procedure	Histological examination of biopsy specimen	n
Nonoperative neoplasms	multilobar neoplasm	10	External decompression	Glioblastoma multiforme + biopsy	7
				Glioma malignum	5
	Deep-seated neoplasms	6	Enlarged burr hole + biopsy	Astropcytoma anaplasticum	3
				Astrocytoma fibrillare	1
Operative neoplasms	Recurrent neoplasms	4	Biopsy + reoperation + aspiration of pseudocyst	Glioma malignum	3
				Astrocytoma anaplasticum	1
Inflammatory tumors	Brain abscess	1	Aspiration of pus + biopsy	Pus	1
	Granuloma	1		Granuloma	1

Ultrasound scanning was displayed on the monitor and the location of the tumor was ascertained. The transducer was then fixed at the position where the potential needle pathway, marked by a dotted line on the monitor, passed through the chosen part of the tumor echo. The needle was then inserted into the brain through the tunnel in the adapter after a small incision was made in the skin. The passage of the needle could be followed on the monitor, and special attention was paid to avoid crossing of the needle pathway with vessel echoes, which showed pulsative scintillation on the echogram. After positioning of the needle in the tumor, the stylet was withdrawn, and aspiration biopsy was performed. Three or two biopsy specimens were taken from the most strongly echoic parts of the tumor. All specimens were sent to laboratory for histological examination. In order to puncture and aspirate brain abscesses we used a needle with an outer diameter of 2.0 mm to enable better aspiration of the pus. In two cases with neoplasm recurrence in the posterior fossa, a liquid was aspirated from a subcutaneous pseudocyst. In two patients we observed bleeding complications of no significance after withdrawal of the needle; it appeared as a little area of high echogenicity on the needle path.

The results of histological examination are presented in Table 1. In 20 cases a specimen taken from a tumor allowed the establishing of accurate diagnosis of gliomas. There was the opportunity in ten cases to compare histological examinations of needle biopsy specimens with the tissue specimens obtained during decompressive operations in patients from group 1 and at extirpation of recurrence neoplasms in group 2. The results revealed complete concordance between these two groups. In one case in which deep-seated glioma was suspected on the basis of clinical examination and CT scan the needle biopsy specimen was histologically diagnosed as granuloma, which was treated medically. In the case of brain abscess the pus was completely removed, and the patient underwent antibiotic therapy.

Discussion

Kaufmann et al. (1985) suggest the following indications for brain biopsy: (a) no alternative procedures can provide the information desired, and (b) the information serves a useful purpose. In our patients with nonresectable neoplasms brain biopsy was the only way to give them a chance to be treated with chemo- and radiotherapy. As a result of needle biopsy and further histological examination of tissue specimens, seven patients from group 1 were admitted to the Oncology Center in Łódź to be treated with irradiation and chemotherapy. In patients from group 2 extirpation of recurrent brain neoplasms was performed. The diagnostic value of US-guided biopsy is high; in our investigations the results revealed total concordance between biopsy and the tissue specimens obtained in the other way.

Ultrasonography is a very attractive method for guiding transcutaneous needle biopsy in patients with skull defect. Several biopsy specimens can be taken from different parts of the tumor with great simplicity. Many cross-sections of the tumor can be rapidly obtained during real-time scanning. Since the technique is flexible and dynamic, it allows the neurosurgeon to study the brain in much greater detail than can be accomplished by most diagnostic procedures (Rubin et al. 1983). The real-time US biopsy is superior to the blind punctures used until now, for it shows the movement of the needle during its passage through the brain tissue and gives the possibility of immediate investigation of any bleeding complication during the brain biopsy. This technique allows introduction of the tip of the biopsy needle accurately into the tumor. Enzmann et al. (1984) showed that the specimen should be taken from the most echogenic region of the lesion.

Conclusions

The following advantages of transcutaneous ultrasound-guided needle biopsy in patients with skull defect have been identified: (a) US-guided biopsy is a simple, reliable, accurate and non-time-consuming diagnostic procedure, completely safe for patients; (b) the tissue samples taken by needle biopsy are sufficient to make proper diagnosis, which gives many patients the chance to be treated by chemo- and radiotherapy; and (c) this technique can serve additionally for puncture and aspiration of brain abscesses and other intracranial fluid collections.

References

[1] Collier BD, Seltzer, SE, Kido DK, Utsunomiya R (1980) Ultrasound directed placement of needles into brains of rhesus monkeys. Neuroradiology 19: 201-205
[2] Enzmann DR, Irwin KM, Fine M, Silvberger GM, Hanberry JW (1984) Intraoperative and outpatient echoencephalography through a burr hole. Neuroradiology 26: 57-59
[3] Kaufmann HH (1985) Diagnostic brain biopsy. In: Wilkins, RH, Rengachary SS (eds) Neurosurgery, vol. 1, part 3, sect D. McGraw-Hill, New York, p 289
[4] Rubin JM, Dohrmann GJ (1983) Intraoperative neurosurgical ultrasound in the localization and characterization of intracranial masses. Radiology 148: 519-524
[5] Tsutsumi Y, Andoh Y, Inoue N (1982) Ultrasound guided biopsy for deep seated brain tumors. J Neurosurg 57: 164-167
[6] Sjolander U, Lindgren PG, Hugosson R (1983) Ultrasound sector scanning for the biopsy of intracerebral lesions. J Neurosurg 58: 7-10

A Simple CT Targeting Device for Percutaneous Biopsy and Chemonucleolysis

G. Vogl

Introduction

Needle biopsy of the brain utilizing CT is an accepted diagnostic
technique that has been performed both with and without the aid
of stereotaxic fragmes (Goldstein et al. 1987). CT-guided biopsies
in the thorax, abdomen, retroperitoneum, pelvis, and spine have
been performed free-hand.

In order to save time and to increase safety, accuracy, and the
patient's comfort, a targeting device has been developed which
enables us to remove biopsy material or to carry out therapeutic
drainage and chemonucleolysis under stereotaxic conditions within
the CT under tomographic control. Previously reported body-stereotaxic systems (Wunschik et al. 1984) use a large metal ring placed
around the patient's body and attached to the CT table or use a
free-standing instrument beside the CT scanner and a localization
triangle (Onik et al. 1985).

Instrumentation

The aim was to develop a body-stereotaxic system which is simple
and fast to handle and needs no attachment. The system should be
inexpensive. To be independent in slice selection every available
gantry tilt should be possible, which means that the plane of the
needle holder must be combined with the gantry for simplicity.

For these reasons we attached a support base onto the CT gantry,
formed from a rollable cradle which can be moved horizontally on
rails at distinct distances. These rails are fixed on the top of
the gantry and are adjusted horizontally and parallel to the
scanning plane (Fig.1). A vertical rod is fixed onto this cradle
which allows vertical movements of the needle support. This support
renders independent angle movement for the attached needle holder
in and out of the scanning plane (Fig.2).

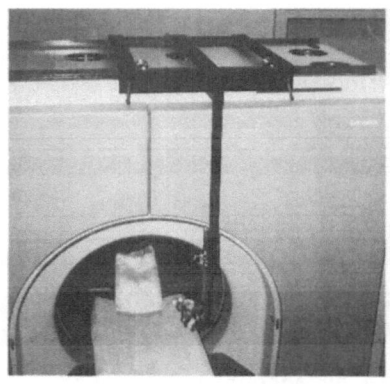 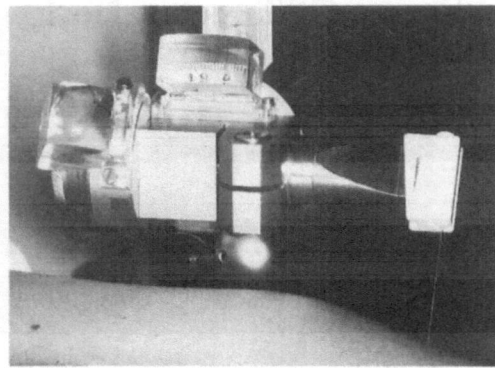

<u>Fig.1.</u> Support base on the CT gantry formed by a rolling cradle movable on rails

<u>Fig.2.</u> Needle support which enables compound angle movements of the sterilized disposable needle holder

A sterilized needle holder must allow for sudden motions of the patient. For this we use a quick-release disposable needle holder which is commercially obtainable for ultrasound transducers (Amedic). The plastic needle holder is put onto the needle support after accurate positioning.

Method

The patient's previous diagnostic scans are reviewed to determine the optimal placement of the entry point for the needle. If the center of the scan is maintained relative to the scales of the stereotaxic device, the horizontal and vertical adjustment as well as the needle angle can be determined quickly by the digitizing scale. In case of gantry tilt the position of the needle holder is additionally determined by the Pythagorean theorem (Fig.3). However, when the highest possible gantry tilt is insufficient for the needle procedure, which may be the case in discography or nucleolysis of the level L5/S1, compound angulation becomes important. At first, the angle in the scanning plane is determined, and reconstructions can be performed to confirm the chosen path. From this the second angle can be estimated. The position of the needle holder is determined by the coordinates of the aiming point and these two angles with the help of a simple computer program.

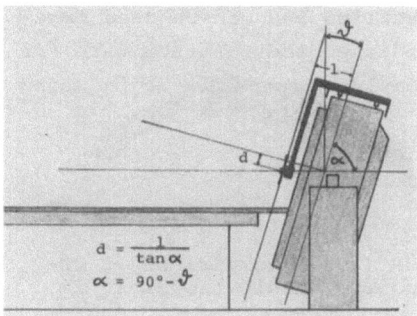

Fig.3. The needle holder position in case of gantry tilt. The distance must be added (or subtracted in case of negative tilt) to the targeted vertical position

To test the method of stereotaxis a phantom consisting of a melon with injected deposits of Duroliopaque was used. After localizing a spot on a scout view, a trajectory was calculated and the stereotaxis device positioned according to the desired coordinates and angle. After the 22-gauge 22-cm-long Chiba needle was placed, a 4-mm-thick confirmation scan was obtained at the same level as the localization scan (Fig.4).

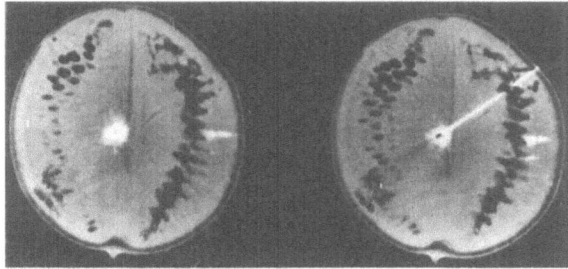

Fig.4. Watermelon with injected deposit of Duroliopaque (<u>left</u>) and after needle placement (<u>right</u>), with gas bubble at the point

Discussion

The stereotaxic system proved to be highly accurate in the phantom. It is capable of aiming at targets in all planes. It is inexpensive and adaptable to other CT scanners. Especially, it is fast to handle and needs no attachment as do other systems. No alignment in the plane of the scan by the positioning lights of the CT scanner is necessary. Our system is permanently installed and can be used immediately. At present we are developing modified and fast software for the routine; as soon as this has been completed, we will begin using the stereotaxic procedure in patients.

References

[1] Goldstein S, Gumerlock MK, Neuwelt EA (1987) Comparison of CT-guided and stereotaxic cranial diagnostic needle biopsies. J Neurosurg 67, 341-348
[2] Onik G, Cosman ER, Wells T, Moss A, Goldberg H, Costello P (1985) CT body stereotaxic instrument for percutaneous biopsy and other interventive procedures. Invest Radiol 5: 525-530
[3] Wunschik F, Georgi M, Pastyr O (1984) Stereotactic biopsy using computed tomography. J Comput Assist Tomogr 8: 32-37

Artificial Cerebrovascular Infarction in Baboons – A New Technique Using an Endovascular Approach

F. Brassel, C. Dettmers, A. Nierhaus, A. Hartmann, and L. Solymosi

INTRODUCTION

Transorbital occlusion of the middle cerebral artery (MCA) has been used to provoke focal cerebral ischemia in monkeys (Hartmann et al. 1981; Del Zoppo et al. 1986; Symon et al. 1979), cats (Shigeno et al. 1985, Rosner et al. 1986) and other animals (Fein and Molinari 1976). This approach was first described by Hudgins and Garcia 1970 for rhesus monkeys and by O'Brien and Waltz 1973 for cats and superceded the retroorbital approach as described by Sundt and Waltz 1966. The transorbital approach with either clipping or ligation of the MCA has been used in our laboratory for several years and has been proven to produce cerebral ischemia and cerebral infarction (Hartmann et al. 1982, Barbosa-Coutinho et al. 1985).
However, our own studies with measurement of focal cerebral blood flow using the microsphere technique have revealed, that in some baboons blood flow might drop after surgical widening of the optic foramen and opening of the dura before the clip had been installed. Therefore a new technique has been developed which permits occlusion of the MCA by an intravascular approach.

PROCEDURE

24 consecutive baboons of either sex with a weight between 9 and 30 kg were used for the experiments.
The procedure for catheterization was performed using a Tracker 18-Infusion Catheter System***. A 7 French Catheter Sheath Introducing System**** was positioned in the right femoral artery in percutaneous Seldinger technique. A 6 French Hink Headhunter Torque Control Femoral Cerebral Catheter***** (6F-Catheter) with its tip distally tapered over a length of 8 cm to 5 French and equipped with a 0.035 inch guide wire was introduced through the catheter sheath introducer system. The catheter was placed in one internal carotid artery under fluoroscopic control and the catheter's tip placed at the cervial level of the internal carotid artery. The catheter was permanently flushed by a pressure infusion with normal saline to avoid reflux of arterial blood.

The patency of the distal vascular bed was controlled by a cerebral angiogram.
The Tracker 18 Infusion Catheter* is a catheter with an increasing stiffness from a highly flexible tip to a semirigid proximal section over 3 segments. The proximal shaft has 3 French diameter, the distal shaft 18 cm length and 2.2 French diameter and the tip 1 mm length and 2.7 French diameter. This system was used in conjunction with a 0.018 inch torquable guide wire to facilitate access to distant tortuous vessels. The microcatheter tip is radio-opaque for fluoroscopic imaging.
The torquable guide wire with a small j-shaped tip together with the microcatheter was advanced step by step towards the proximal part of the MCA. Once the catheter was positioned with its tip in the M1-segment of the MCA, the 6F-catheter was redrawn into the aortic arch and a selective angiogram was performed through the microcatheter. Thereafter the liquid embolization was achieved (Fig. 1). The mixture with its short polimerization time consisted of n-Butyl-2-cyanaoacrylate (NBC) ** and tantal powder was added if necessary. Before injection into the microcatheter the system was flushed with 5% glucose to avoid early polymerization of the NBC within the catheter.
The distribution of NBC may be visualized by fluoroscopic control, if tantal powder has been added to NBC. After injection the catheter system has to be withdrawn immediately and rapidly to avoid fixation of the microcatheter by rapid polymerization inside the vascular bed. A control angiogram may be performed (Fig. 1).
Alternatively embolization can be performed with Polyvinylalcohol (PVA)-particles with a size between 150 and 250 micron. They are injected pulsesynchronously using a 1 ml-Luer-lock-syringe. The result of embolization can be verified by another selective angiogram over the microcatheter which is still in place during this alternative procedure.

RESULTS

In 21 baboons the procedure using NBC was completed without any severe complication. In all animals autopsy or a computer tomogram of the brain revealed infarcts in the territory of the MCA of different size (Fig. 2).Size and location of the infarcts depend on the location of the occlusion. With proximal isolated occlusion of the MCA stem small deeper infarcts could be provoked with preservation of the cortical surface, whereas occlusion of proximal and more distally located main branches of the MCA produced larger infarcts reaching the cortical surfaces. In some animals transient bradycardia was provoked during passing of the 6F catheter at the carotid bifurcation. In 3 animals embolization was not possible using this technique due to athero-sclerotic narrowing at the orifice of the internal carotid artery or due to kinking and coiling of the internal carotid artery. In one of these 3 baboons the technique could be performed by direct puncture of the ICA after a small cervical cut.
Since this technique was used in conjunction with another protocol to test drug effects, longtime studies have not been performed. However, during the 24 hour-protocol none of the 21 animals died due to effects of the technique. 5 animals died 14 - 17 hours after embolization due to massive brain edema in the territory of the MCA with consecutive herniation at the tentorium

---

*   Target Therapeutics, Los Angeles, USA
**   Braun-Dexon GmbH, Spangenberg, FRG

DISCUSSION

Experimental infarcts have provided new insights into pathophysiology of cerebral ischemia (Hayakawa and Waltz 1975: Spetzler et al. 1980; Symon et al. 1974; Diaz and Ausman 1980). However, direct trauma to the brain must be minimal to guarantee changes of cerebral blood flow and pathology which are caused only by intended focal ischemia.

With the transcranial approach (Waltz et al. 1965; Crowell et al. 1970; Molinar and Laurent 1976) mechanical forces may alter the "natural" course of ischemia. Opening of the cranium (even by the transorbital approach) may alter cerebrospinal fluid dynamics during preparation and thus influence the pressure gradients which develop during cerebral ischemia (Hayakawa and Waltz 1975; O'Brien and Waltz 1972).

Symon et al. 1974 used both the transcranial and the transorbital approach and found no differences between both techniques with respect to size of the ischemic area.

The transorbital approach which we have used for many years is a reliable method to produce cerebral ischemia and infarcts. Transient clipping of the MCA is possible with this (Hartmann et al. 1983; Hayakawa and Waltz 1975) and other techniques (Spetzler et al. 1980). However, the technique involves removal of one eye, opening of the dura, possible damage to the arachnoidea and in most cases widening of the optic foramen. Own studies have revealed that in some animals after the transorbital removal and opening of the dura (even without opening of the subarachnoideal space) cerebral blood flow as measured with the microsphere technique may decrease. Further the autonomic fibers which accompany the MCA may be interrupted thus altering physiological autoregulation or its changes by focal ischemia.

Intravascular occlusion with silastic material has been used by other groups (Molinari et al. 1974; Levinthal et al. 1979; Dujovny et al. 1976; Osgood et al. 1976). However, the technique requires direct surgical opening of the common or internal carotid artery in the neck of monkeys (Molinar et al. 1974) or dogs (Levinthal et al. 1979; Dujovny et al. 1976), and the site of the occlusion may not be voluntarily selected.

In the technique described here the distal end of the microcatheter marks the site of the occlusion. With alteration of the polymerization time of the NBC-material, which may be altered by additional Durolyopaque*, the length of the occlusion in the MCA may be altered. Prolongation of the polymerization time is in most cases not of advantage, since the material may pass the capillaries before polymerization.
If PVA particles instead of NBC are used for embolization the particles must be injected synchronously with the pulse to avoid reflux and involuntary filling of territories other than the MCA.

---

* Ingenor, Paris, France

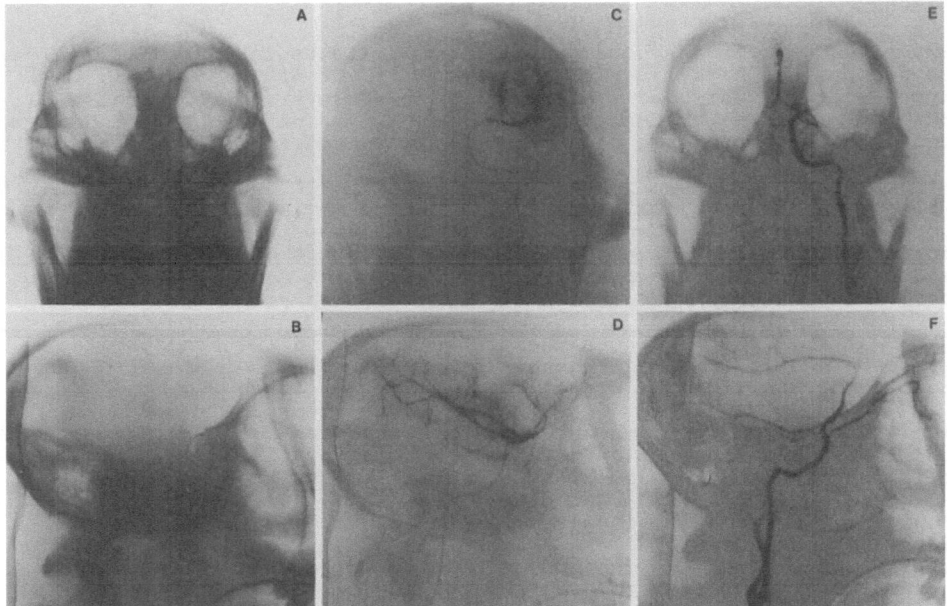

Fig. 1: Selective embolization of the middle cerebral artery (MCA) in
the baboon. Upper row: anterior-posterior view, lower row:
lateral view. A, B: microcatheter with its radiopaque end
placed in the patend MCA. C, D: selective angiogram of the
patent MCA with the microcatheter. E, F: post-embolization
angiogram of the internal carotid artery.

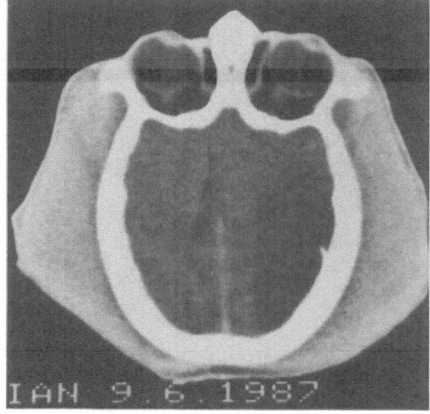

Fig. 2: Cranial CT of a baboon after proximal embolization with NBC
in the left MCA 18 hours after embolization. Fresh infarct
in the MCA-territory.

REFERENCES

Barbosa-Coutinho LM, Hartmann A, Hossmann KA, Rommel T (1985) Effect of dexamethasone on serum protein extravasation in experimental brain infarcts to monkeys. An immunohistochemical study. Acta Neuropathol, Berlin 65:255-260

Crowell RM, Olsson Y, Klatzo I, Ommaya A (1970) Temporary occlusion of the middle cerebral artery in monkeys. Clinical and pathological observations. Stroke I:439-448

Del Zoppo GJ, Copeland BR, Waltz TA, Zyroff J, Plow EF, Harker LA (1986) The beneficial effect of intracarotid urokinase on acute stroke in a baboon model. Stroke 17:638-643

Diaz FG, Ausman JI (1980) Experimental cerebral ischemia. Neurosurg. 6:36-445

Dujovny M, Barrioneuva PJ, Laha RK, Osgood CP, De Castro S, Maroon J, Hellstrom R (1976) Experimental middle cerebral artery microsurgical embolectomy. Microsurgery for Stroke, edited by Schmiedeck P, New York, Springer Verlag:91-97

Fein JM, Molinari G (1976) Hemodynamic evaluation of superficial temporal cortical artery microanastomosis in the dog. Microneurosurgical Anastomosis for Cerebral Ischemia, edited by Austin GM, Springfield, Illinois, Charles C. Thomas:5-14

Hartmann A, Menzel J, Buttinger C, Lange D, Alberti E (1981) Die regionale Gehirndurchblutung des Pavians beim ischämischen Hirninfarkt unter Dexamethasonbehandlung (1981). Fortschr. Neurol. Psychiat. 10:380-392

Hartmann A, Menzel J, Lange D, Buttinger C (1983) An experimental primate stroke model to study cerebrovascular responses to chronic cerebral ischemia. Advances Biosciences 43:167-183

Hayakawa T, Waltz AG (1975) Changes of epidural pressures after experimental occlusion of one middle cerebral artery in cats. J. Neurol. Sci. 26:319-333

Hayakawa T, Waltz AG (1975) Immediate effects of cerebral ischemia: Evoluation and resolution of neurological deficits after experimental occlusion of one middle cerebral artery in conscious cats. Stroke 6:321-327

Hudgins WR, Garcia JH (1970) Transorbital approach to the middle cerebral artery of the squirrel monkey. A technique for experimental cerebral infarction applicable to ultrastructural studies. Stroke 1:107-111

Levinthal R, Moseley JI, Brown WF, Stern WE (1979) Effect of STA-MCA anastomosis on the course of experimental acute MCA embolic occlusions. Stroke 10 371-375

Molinari GF, Moseley JI, Laurent JP (1974) Segmental middle cerebral artery occlusion in primates. An experimental method requiring minimal surgery and anesthesia. Stroke 5:334-339

Molinari GF, Laurent JP (1976) A classification of experimental models of brain ischemia. Stroke 7:14-17

O'Brien M, Waltz AG (1972) Changes of intracranial pressure during experimental cerebral infarction. Proc. 1st Int. Symp. on Intracranial Pressure Hannover

O'Brien M, Waltz AG (1973) Transorbital approach for occluding the middle cerebral artery without craniotomy. Stroke 4:201-296

Osgood CP, Dujovny M, Barrionuevo PJ, Weir VK, Laha R (1976) Staged middle cerebral artery embolectomy. J. Surg. Res. 20:395-399

Rosner G, Graf R, Kataoka K, Heiss WD (1986) Selective functional vulnerability of cortical neurons following transient MCA-occlusion in the cat. Stroke 17:76-82

Shigeno S, Fritschka E, Shigeno T, Brock M (1985) Effects of indomethacin on rCBF during and after focal cerebral ischemia in the cat. Stroke 16 235-240

Spetzler RF, Selman WR, Weinstein R, Townsend J, Mehdorn M, Telles D, Crumric RC, Macko R (1980) Chronic reversible cerebral ischemia. Evaluation of a new baboon model. Neurosurgery 7:257-261

Sundt TM, Waltz AG (1966) Experimental infarction:Retroorbital, extradural approach for occluding the middle cerebral artery. Proc. Mayo Clin 41:159-168

Symon L, Pasztor E, Branston NM (1974) The distribution and density of reduced cerebral blood flow following acute middle cerebral artery occlusion. An experimental study by the technique of hydrogen clearance in baboons. Stroke 5:355-364

Symon L, Branston NM, Chikovani O (1979) Ischemic brain edema following middle cerebral artery occlusion in baboons. Relationship between regional, cerebral water content and blood flow at 1 to 2 hours. Stroke 10:184-191

Waltz AG, Owen CA jr., Shaw DA (1965) Experimental occlusion of the middle cerebral artery: Its determination using phosphorus[32]-labeled erythrocytes. Neurology (minneap.) 15:491-498

Design of a New Four-Chambered Balloon Catheter for Supraaortic Angioplasty

S. Bockenheimer (Frankfurt/M., FRG)

Percutaneous transluminal angioplasty (PTA) in supra-aortic artery disease is still considered as dangerous procedure, because of fear for brain embolising particles torn off by the dilational balloon. I present the design of a new catheter, which allows to occlude the vessel during PTA and to aspirate broken-off particles.

The catheter has a size of 7 French. It contains four chambers: (1) guide-wire conduit; (2) aspiration and rinsing channel of 1.1 mm diameter; (3) tip occlusion and (4) PTA balloon access.

The catheter is easy to handle. The prototypes have been manufactured.

Non-superselective Intraarterial Chemotherapy with HECNU. Followed by Radiotherapy in the Treatment of Unoperable Malignant Gliomas

D. Dormont, J. Chiras, F. Fauchon, C. Debussche, M. Poisson, and J. Bories (Paris, France)

Between December 1984 and December 1986, 46 patients suffering from malignant gliomas were considered as unoperable because of tumor location or extent. These patients were treated by 4 courses of intra-arterial chemotherapy followed by conventional radiotherapy (50 grays). The response rate after IAC was 49%. The responders had in almost cases good clinical improvement, a median duration of response of 15 months and a median survival of 19 months (median survival of all the patients = 8.5 months). The complication rate is low: major visual loss occurred in 3 cases and neurological complications occurred, always after radiotherapy, in 5 cases.

In conclusion, this treatment protocol gives a good quality of life for more than 1 year in patients who respond to the drug but does not change the prognoses for other patients.

Transcranial Doppler Sonography in Interventional Neuroradiology

S. Bien, A. Laurent, and J. J. Merland (Paris, France)

The development of transcranial Doppler sonography allows noninvasive, continous examination of the arteries at the base of the brain. This method is of particular interest in interventional neuroradiology. In the endovascular treatment of angiomas the effects of embolisation can be continuously monitored with a small probe during and after the treatment. The elevation of peripheral resistance, which results in increased incidence of complications, can be seen early on. In the endovascular treatment of aneurysms and AV fistulas, transcranial Doppler sonography permits to control the blood flow velocity in the parent vessel and allows us to know if the balloon i or is not compromising the flow of the latter.

Hemodynamic changes after treatment can be followed up.

Significance of Intraoperative Cerebral Blood Flow Measurements in Endovascular Occlusion of the Internal Carotid and Middle Cerebral Arteries

I. Weitzner, A. Laurent, A. Luft, and J. J. Merland (Paris, France)

Cerebral blood flow measurements using intraarterial injection of xenon 133 were carried out in ten patients during temporary occlusion of the internal carotid arteries and in two patients in the middle cerebral arteries. This test was more reliable as a predictor of patient tolerence for permanent therapeutic occlusion than clinical or aniographic methods. The criteria for excluding a patient from permanent occlusion are discussed and may indicate the need for EC-IC bypass better than other tolerance tests.

The Present Role of ADSA in Diagnostic and Interventional Neuroradiology

T. G. Tjan and G. Winkel

Introduction

After the introduction of CT scanning, the demands on angiographic evaluation have changed, from a primary diagnostic procedure to a specific and high precision examination. Angiography has been and remains the definitive method of diagnosing vascular abnormalities. It is still needed for detailed information as a roadmap for surgical approach, and to verify the diagnosis obtained with a CT scan.
Recently this method has also expanded from the specific diagnostic into therapeutic application.

Due to the disadvantages of Venous DSA, ADSA has been introduced as a new diagnostic vascular imaging technique to improve the digital images and the diagnostic quality.

The purpose of our study was to review all our intracranial ADSA examinations in diagnostic neuroradiology and emphasis was put on diagnostic accuracy and image quality. We also like to determine the value of this technique in interventional procedure.

Materials

Since April 1984 ADSA was performed in 2630 patients with a variety of brain abnormalities. In 136 cases we compared the value of ADSA with conventional magnification angiography.
326 DSA-assisted interventional procedures were performed in embolization of brain AVMs, detachable balloon treatment of inoperable aneurysms, carotid cavernous or vertebro-vertebral fistula, PTA of the supra-aortic arteries and embolization of hypervascular lesions in the head and neck region. The last 214 procedures have been monitored using a prototype DVI S.

Equipment and technique

Our neuroangiographic suite has Philips Poly I angiographic unit, which is interfaced with the Philips DVI V system. This system was used for all the ADSA examinations, and provides up to three digital images per second for a total of 20 summed images, using a 512x512 matrix, geometrical magnification (1.6-2.2x) and a 0.2 mm focal spot.

Examinations were performed using two monitors allowing simultaneous display of either fluoroscopic or DSA "road-mapping" and previously obtained images. Reference between the two monitors aids rapid and accurate positioning of the catheter and detailed analysis of the images.

All studies were performed with the Seldinger
technique using a 4 or 5 French catheter. Contrast
material was injected selectively at volume and rates
comparable to those used for conventional magnification
angiography, but lowered iodine concentrations (200 mg/ml
iodine).

RESULTS
At the beginning of the study, when we were using
the large 1.0 mm/0.6 mm focal spot and injecting diluted
contrast medium (100 mgI/ml), the image quality was not
very impressive. The pictures were not sharp, blurring of
the vessel margins caused by pulsation was noticed. The
ability to visualize smaller vessels was limited. The
cause of it was the lower spatial resolution and this is
strongly influenced by combination of image intensifier
mode, matrix size, geometrical magnification and size of
the focal spot (Kruger RA and Riederer SJ,1984). (1,5
lp/mm using a large focal spot tube of 1.0 mm, compared
to 6 lp/mm of the conventional technique).

High quality DSA images were obtained with small
focal spot (0.2mm), geometrical magnification technique
(1.6-2.0x) and injecting contrast material selectively
with higher iodine concentration (200mgI/ml). This will
compensate the decreased spatial resolution and improve
the image quality until the limits of the DSA system are
reached (small vessels require higher iodine
concentration for satisfactory definition, maximal 10%
Iodine concentration. Takahashi 1984).

After this technical improvement and upgrading of
the system, the limiting spatial resolution has been
increased to 3.0-3.5 lp/mm, resulting in maximum
opacification and sharpness of almost all vessels and
providing maximum accuracy of information.
Vessels smaller than 1 mm e.g. the distal cortical
branches, the choroidal, the lenticulostriate and
perforating arteries were sufficiently shown or sharply
defined. Although this is of importance in a limited
number of cases only, we still emphasize their
visualization as a criterion for high quality angiogram.
The display of tumor stain and definition of very fine
vascular architecture are excellent.

The diagnostic accuracy is comparable to
conventional magnification angiography. All abnormalities
were identified by both methods. Our DSA images was
believed to be slightly superior to the high quality
images of conventional technique.
There were no pitfalls in the interpretation of the
images and the information obtained by ADSA study is
sufficient for planning surgery.

We still use conventional magnification angiography
with additional stereoscopic or tomographic images in
selected cases to overcome the problem of overlapping
vessels. This is particularly useful for detailed
analysis of individual vessel or to improve detailed
anatomy of an aneurysm.

Interventional Procedure
The optimal performance of interventional procedure
needs sophisticated equipments. High quality diagnostic
images and continuous imaging during the procedure are
necessary for detail analysis and to evaluate the effect
of the maneuvers and the procedure progress. DSA
satisfactorily fulfills this need.

To optimize the use of DSA, our DVI system has been upgraded to a prototype DVI S, designed for therapeutic angiography.

DVI S features includes: improved fluoroscopy, an image processing system with digital subtraction fluoroscopy and road-mapping, variable framerate etc.

The real-time display of DSA permits rapid viewing and evaluation of the subtracted images, so that important decision can be made without any delay to avoid complications. Reduction in procedure time is another benefit of this system.

Real time digital subtraction fluoroscopy and real-time DSA "road mapping" are extremely valuable tools which enhance the clinical value of DSA. By using a contrast filled mask, road mapping provides a static and subtracted image of the vessel(s) in the area of interest. This is very helpful in selective or superselective catheterization, navigation and placement of microballoon catheter, or selective positioning of a detachable/dilatation balloon at the site of the lesion. Unfortunately this technique is limited by motion.

Its superior contrast resolution affords excellent visualization of very small vessels or dangerous anastomoses by injecting a small amount of contrast medium, which may not be visible on conventional angiography.

In this present stage the DVI system has the capability in making the procedure both safe and simpler resulting in increased patient comfort and safety.

Limitations

Limitations of the current DSA system and technique are:
- the spatial resolution is still inferior than in conventional technique but visibly the image quality, opacification and sharpness of the vessels (vessel edge definition) are quite comparable and did not impair the diagnostic results.
- the limited field of view
- the small film size of ADSA hard copy images is considered to be a disadvantage.
- motion and subtraction artefacts which can impair the results of ADSA examinations.

Conclusion

Our experience over the past 4 years with a continuously upgraded system indicate that ADSA is the best examination method, combines the advantages of digital image processing with all the advantages of selective angiography producing high quality diagnostic images. Conventional magnification angiography with additional stereoscopic or tomographic images should be performed when detailed analysis is needed.
Application of DSA in interventional procedure is mandatory.

References
]
1. Brant-Zawadzki M., Gould R., Norman D., et al.: Digital subtraction cerebral angiography by intra-arterial injection: Comparison with conventional angiography. AJNR, 3:593-599,1982
2. Braun IF, Aiken RE, Spalding WW et all.: Real-time fluoroscopic digital subtraction. AJNR 5:214-215, March-April 1984.

3. Foley W.D. and Milde M.W.: Intra-arterial Digital
Subtraction Angiography. Radiologic Clinics of North
America-23:2,293-319, June 1985.
4. Kelly WM., Brant Zawadzki M., Schardt M.A.,
Carrol C.L.: Intra-arterial DSA: early experience with a
1024^2 matrix. Neuroradiology 27: 70-76, 1985.
5. Takahashi M., Bussaka H., Nakagawa N.: Evaluation of
the cerebral vasculature by intraarterial DSA with
emphasis on in vivo resolution. Neuroradiology 26: 253-
259, 1984.
6. Takahashi M, Bussaka H., Miyawaki M.: Stereoscopic DSA
of the central nervous system. Neuroradiology 28:105-108,
1986

M. Bettag, E. Ulrich, E. Lins, W. J. Bock, G. Reifenberger, and R. Schober

Introduction

The reduction of tumor vascularity and the use of surgical techniques
to achieve hemostasis are necessary to decrease risks for patients
with highly vascular tumors. In our study we present a combined management of preoperative embolization and laser-assisted microsurgery in patients with intracranial meningiomas. This treatment was
performed in 12 hypervasculaized meningiomas with a dual arterial
supply of meningeal and cortical or pial vessels. Six tumors were
meningiomas of convexity, four of the sphenoid wing, and two were
located parasagittally. On histological examination, eight meningiomas were classified as endotheliomatous, two as angioblastic, and
two as mainly fibromatous.

As pretherapeutic evaluations, computed tomography and MRI scanning
are most useful. Whereas CT scan provides information about tumor
location and size, MRI scan often demonstrates additionally the
vascular supply of the tumor.

Preoperative Embolization

Embolization of the external carotid artery was performed at the
same session as diagnostic angiography. We used absorbable and nonabsorbable particles as embolic agents. While Felfoam was our absorbable particle of choice, we supplementarily injected lyophilized dura mater as nonabsorbable particulate material. The emboli
were injected slowly so that the higher blood flow of the feeding
vessels would carry the particles into the tumor bed (Fig.1). The
goal of this endovascular approach was to produce tumor necrosis
and to dearterialize the region while preserving normal arteries
(Kerber 1980).

Computed tomography was performed after embolization in seven patients. The appearance of new low-density areas within previously
homogeneous tumors was accepted as evidence of necrosis (Teasdale
et al. 1984). These areas were found in three patients (Fig.2). In

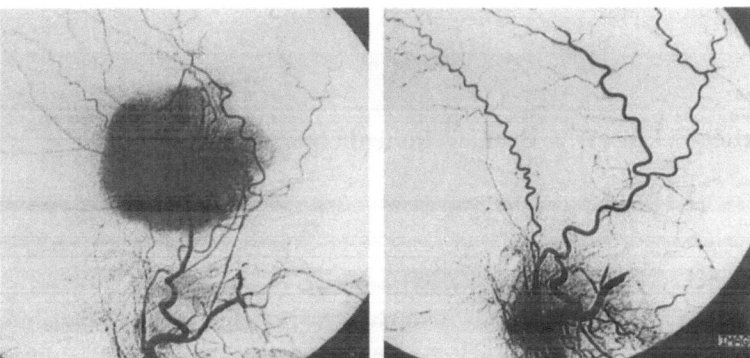

Fig.1a,b. Left temporal convexity meningioma. a: Selective external carotid angiogram demonstrates the arterial supply by the middle meningeal artery. b: After embolization with lyophilized dura mater and
Gelfoam tumor blush disappears, with preservation of superficial
temporal and maxillary artery branches. Note that the main trunk of
the middle meningeal artery is occluded to prevent bleeding during
subsequent craniotomy

the remaining four patients, there was no change in the density of
the tumor.

Histologically, the specimens were examined for microscopic evidence of fresh or recent ischemic and/or hemorrhagic necrosis and
for the presence of embolic agents. Necrotic areas in the tumor bed
were found in nine cases, and embolic amterial could be detected in

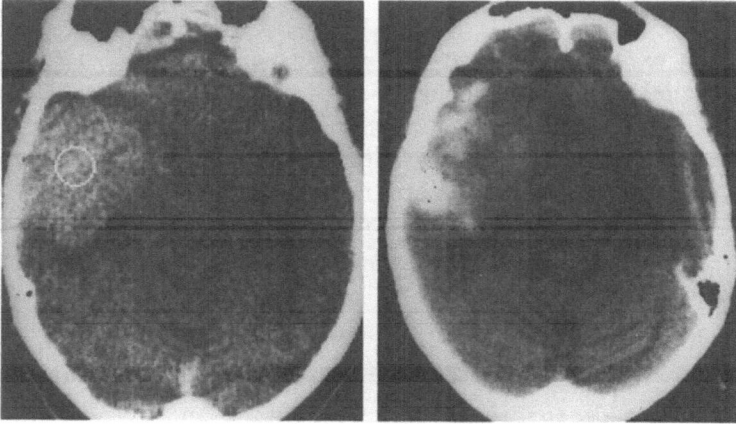

Fig.2. Enhanced computed tomography scans of the same tumor (a) before and 8 h after embolization (b). A large low-density area within
the previously homogeneous tumor has developed

four cases. Although no proper studies have been done to determine the best timing for surgical removal of meningiomas following embolization, it appears advisable to wait at least 24 h, as further thrombosis of the embolized areas may occur. Surgery more than five days after embolization may be disadvantageous as some recanalization occurs during this time (Manelfe et al. 1986; Lasjaunias and Berenstein 1987).

Laser-Assisted Microsurgery

With distal embolization of the meningeal source, we intraoperatively achieved a reduced blood loss at the dural base and the center of the tumor. But the capsular supply by cortical and pial vessels may still be a surgical problem. In meningiomas with a significant arterial supply from internal carotid artery branches we used laser-assisted microsurgery.

The Nd-YAG laser is of particular value in the resection of vascular tumors such as meningiomas because of its excellent coagulation and tumor-shrinking properties (Beck 1984). The Nd-YAG laser causes construction of vessels and coagulation beyond the exposed areas. Thus, arteries of up to 2 mm in diameter and veins of up to 3 mm in diameter can be closed rapidly and reliably (Frank 1984). The depth of coagulation depends on the energy applied so that predefined areas can be thermally destroyed precisely and to a depth that can be predicted with sufficient accuracy.

On pathological examination typical tissue changes following application of Nd-YAG laser could be demonstrated (Beck et al. 1979). A defocused beam produces uniform superficial coagulation. With correct dosage, the damage can be kept within an area of less than 0.2 mm across. Use of a focused Nd-YAG laser beam results in a deeper coagulation zone with a narrow edematous boundary (Frank 1984).

The surgical procedure was always similar. While anatomical structures were kept intact, the tumor capsule was irradiated by laser beam (Fig.3). After coagulation and shrinkage of the capsule the tumor could be excised completely. If short, intermittent pulses of light focused on blood vessels are used, damage to the surrounding tissue is minimized. This makes the Nd-YAG laser a safe and important surgical tool whenever the location and vascularity of a tumor make its removal difficult.

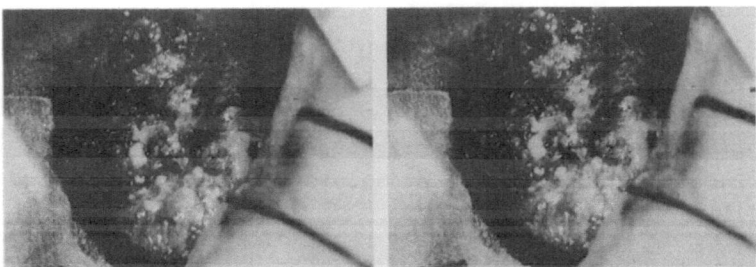

Fig.3a,b. There is a superficial coagulation zone at the peripheral portion of the meningioma after defocused irradiation with Nd-YAG laser. Note also recent tumor necrosis in the center as a result of successful embolization

Conclusion

We consider preoperative embolization and laser-assisted microsurgery to be supplementary methods to reduce blood loss in highly vascular meningiomas. When successful embolization of the meningeal source of arterial supply was performed, we noted intraoperatively a remarkable loss of bleeding at the dural base and the center of the tumor. The use of the Nd-YAG laser is important to control diffuse bleeding from major cortical vessels supplying the peripheral portion of hypervascu-larized meningiomas. Objective evidence of improved operative condi-tions was difficult to obtain. Surgeons' opinions were naturally sub-jective, nevertheless in most patients we noted a decrease in blood loss.

References

[1] Beck OJ, Wilske J, Schönberger J, et al. (1979) Tissue changes following application of lasers to the rabbit brain. Neurosurg Rev 2: 31-36
[2] Beck OJ (1984) Use of the Nd-YAG laser in neurosurgery. Neuro-surg Rev 7: 151-158
[3] Frank F (1984) Biophysical basis and technical requisites for the use of Nd-YAG laser in neurosurgery. Neurosurg Rev 7: 145-150
[4] Kerber CW (1980) Flow controlled therapeutic embolization: Phy-siologic and safe technique. Am J Roentgenol 134: 557-561
[5] Lasjaunias P, Berenstein A (1987) Endovascular treatment of craniofacial lesions. Springer, Berlin Heidelberg New York, p 93 (Surgical neuroangiography, vol 2)
[6] Manelfe C, Lasjaunias P, Ruscalleda J (1986) Preoperative em-bolization of intracranial meningiomas. AJNR 7: 963-972
[7] Teasdale E, Patterson J, McLellan D, MacPherson P (1984) Sub-selective preoperative embolization for meningiomas. J Neuro-surg 60: 506-511

Critical Evaluation of MRI and Percutaneous Ultrasound Following Spinal Intra- and Extramedullary Shunting: Long-term Results After Drainage Procedure of Syringomyella and Cystic Lesions in 21 Patients

A. Aschoff, A. Löhlein, U. Mende, and H. Betz

In 1891 Abbé and Coley were the first to treat syringomyelia by surgery, and in 1926 Puusepp published the first report on a series with surgical interventions in syringomyelia (Table 1). The results were encouraging. Nevertheless, until the 1970s, surgical procedures in syringomyelia were rarely performed. The syringomyelia in Arnold-Chiari malformation was one of the classic indications for operation. However, surgeons discussed for many years whether syringomyelia may be associated with trauma or not. The diagnostic revolution of CT-assisted myelography and even more so that of MRI provided reliability in the diagnosis of syringomyelia. A fair number of posttraumatic intramedullary cysts were thus diagnosed, and the number of surgical interventions consequently increased. In a total of 350 publications, 3591 cases of syringomyelia have been reported, and 1803 of

Table 1. Neurosurgical treatment of syringomyelia over 97 years

1891 Abbé and Coley: First myelotomia and evacuation of a syrinx
During next 35 years only three other operative cases (Elsberg 1916; Sharpe 1917)
1926 Puusepp: First systematic operation series (at least eight cases)
1931 Peiper: Review of 44 cases
1938 Adelstein: Review of 120 cases
1971 Ballantine: Review of 355 cases
1983 Levy: Review of 648 cases
1986 Aschoff and Löhlein: Review of 1005 cases
1988 Aschoff and Löhlein: Review of 1803 cases in literature on the basic of 350 references (including 21 own operations)

these patients underwent a surgical procedure. Therefore, the number of operated cases has increased threefold since Levy's publication in 1983.

In a multicentric study in West Germany, Hertel could demonstrate that the frequency of junctional-malformed and idiopathic syringomyelia has been continuously decreasing, to one-third the previous rate. He found this confirmed even in endemic regions such as Würzburg and Heidelberg, where in the first half of the twentieth century the incidence was 1 in 100 000. The prolongation of life expectancy in tetra- and paraplegic patients allows experience of late complications, including late myelopathy caused by syringomyelia, microcystic lesions, and posttraumatic arachnoid cysts. Among a total of 3591 patients, 633 (18.7%) suffered from posttraumatic syringomyelia; the numbers are steadily increasing.

Surgery in syringomyelia has been performed since 1930 in Heidelberg (Table 2). The lack of complete records does not allow evaluation of this whole period. Therefore, our data are based on records from 1982 to date. In this period 21 patients have received spinal drainage. The etiology of the syringes was as follows. In 12 cases a trauma was evident. One patient had suffered meningeal tuberculosis, one child lumbar meningocele (Arnold-Chiari 1), three patients idiopathic syringomyelia, and three syringes were tumor associated. In three cases a spinal arachnoid cyst was diagnosed and had to be drained. In three cases the preoperative diagnosis was based on CT-assisted myelography and in 18 cases on MRI. In five cases (28%) the MRI diagnosis led unexpectedly to misinterpretation of the scan: one syrinx was mistaken for a cystic tumor; a low-grade ependymoma was mistaken for a syrinx; a technical error concerning the repetition time was the reason for the failure to diagnose an existing syrinx; a very big cyst in a holocord astrocytoma was partially misinterpreted - the cyst was much smaller, as we could confirm sonographically during operation; and in one case we found tissue with very small cysts intraoperatively, whereas syringomyelia had been expected (MacDonald 1988: "microcystic spinal cord degeneration").

According to the literature, there have been only 11 cases of false diagnosis of syringomyelias on MRI. Our experience demonstrates that lack of knowledge by the examiner, technical faults, and insufficient amounts of contrast medium significantly increase the number of wrong diagnoses. In addition, the differential diagnosis of myelomalacia and microcystic degeneration makes it even more difficult to avoid misinterpretation.

Table 2. Clinical results

Condition	Early results: 3 months (n = 21)	Results after 1-2 years (n = 15)	Long-term results: 2-6.3 years[a] (n = 13)
1 Posttraumatic syringomyelias; 1 microcystic myelopathia	10 Improved 1 Stable 1 Deteriored[b]	6 Improved 1 Stable 1 Progressive	5 Improved (two full remission) 1 Stable 2 Progressive (very slow)
3 Idiopathic, 1 postmeningitic, 1 postmyelocelic syringomyelia	4 Improved 1 Stable	1 Improved 2 Stable	1 Stable 1 Progressive
3 Posttumorous cysts; 1 cyst in a holocord astrocytoma	4 Slightly improved	1 Stabile 2 Progressive	1 Stabile 2 Progressive
	18 (85.7%) Improved 2 (9.5%) Stable 1 (4.8%) Progressive	8 (53.3%) Improved 4 (16.7%) Stable 3 (20%) Progressive	5 (38.5%) Improved [5 (50%)][c] 3 (23%) Stable [2 (20%)][c] 5 (38.5%) Progressive [3 (30%)][c]

[a] Mean, 3.4 years.
[b] Additionally substantial arachnoiditis, improved after 1 year.
[c] Tumor patients excluded, in brackets.

Surgery is indicated exclusively in cases of significantly progressive neurological deficits or in cases of therapy-resistant pain. We favor the surgical procedure of a small hemilaminectomy, done at the site of major neurological deficits. If possible, we choose the upper thoracic segments.

Since 1986, we have used ultrasound intraoperatively, in nine cases before we opened the dura mater and in two cases afterwards. The purpose was to confirm the diagnosis and to determine the optimal location for myelotomy. Interestingly, in at least two cases sonography prevented a wrong approach by misinterpretation of the MRI scan. Therefore, the intraoperatively used sonography is not only a helpful adjuvant but an essential feature of intramedullary surgery. The surgical approach we favor is based on drainage of the syrinx into the subarachnoid space by use of a soft Silastic catheter (1.3 mm). Since in one patient a strong cough caused dislocation of the catheter and therefore a recurrence of the syrinx, we decided to use the Shilito's T catheter.

The high concentration of protein in tumor cysts causes other problems. In two cases the shunts were blocked, and follow-up surgery had to be performed. The intraperitoneal implantation of the shunt solved this problem. We used catheters 2.5 mm in width and interposed a low-pressure valve. In three cases of arachnoid cyst the catheters were also implanted intraperitoneally. One cyst had developed after a trauma, and two others were tumor associated.

At first, the results were encouraging: 18 patients improved, two of them with complete remission. Neurological deterioration was noticed in one patient with simultaneous arachnoiditis. In the 1st year the symptoms were reversible. Gradual worsening of the symptoms was evident on long-term supervision of patients. In 1936, Frazier criticized the lack of long-term examinations. It is remarkable that during the past 50 years, there has been only one major study concerning long-term results in syringomyelia (Alvisi 1984).

Data from two studies in the 1930s (Peiper 1931; Adelstein 1938) and those concerning 264 surgical interventions in the 1980s are not sufficient with respect to the described surgical approach (Table 3). Although microsurgery was performed routinely, the neurological outcome of the patients had not improved over this period of 50 years. In postoperative follow-ups 17 patients were examined by the use of MRI and 8 by percutaneous sonography performed through the acoustic window of laminectomy. The most important obser-

Table 3. Results of operation for syringomyelia

Author	Operated cases useful for comparison (total cases)	Results		
		Improvement	Stabilization	Progression
Peiper (1931)	29 (44)	72.4%	24%	3.5%
Adelstein (1938)	86 (120)	76%	12%	12%
Eighteen Authors (1981-1988) [a]	264 (278)	60%	23%	16.3%

[a] Williams 1981; Philips 1981; Schlesinger 1981; Shannon 1981; Tator 1982; Quencer 1983; Pecker 1983; Vernon 1983; Alvisi 1984; Barbaro 1985; Steven 1985; Dworkin 1985; Rossier 1985; Suzuki 1985; Lesoin 1986; Roosen 1987; Calbucci 1987; Vaquero 1987. These were predominantly on syringo-subarach-noidal or -peritoneal shunts.

vation was that four patients were suffering dorsal adhesions of the spinal cord subsequent to surgical fixation of the catheter to the spinal dura mater. The initially good results were overshadowed by iatrogenic cord tethering. In one of these patients the neurological symptoms did not improve; three others suffered from progressive neurological deficits, although the syringes were collapsed.

The most importance advance in the past 10 years has been the application of shunt methods and shunt materials - used for hydrocephalus - in the treatment of syringomyelia. Comparing the cerebrum and the cervical spinal cord with respect to motility, it is obvious that implanted catheters are involved in very different conditions. Whereas the cerebrum is mostly immobile, the cervical spinal cord must compensate a 28-mm difference in length in flexion movements (Breig) and is therefore extremely mobile. It is obvious that relatively rigid catheters fixed to the spinal dura cause rubbing and Bougir movements. Fischer (1977), Welch (1981), and Sullivan (1988) have reported on acquired Arnold-Chiari malformations after lumbar shunting which were caused by overdrainage and arachnoiditis. They concluded that there is an enormous irritability of the spinal subarachnoid space.

The results of surgical interventions with the use of shunt material are not satisfying. With iatrogenic cord tethering in mind, we must critically ask whether methods of hydrocephalus surgery can be applied to the spinal cord.

References

[1] Abbe R, Coley W B (1892) Syringomyelia. Operation exploration of cord, withdrawal of fluid, exhibition of patient. J Nerv Ment Dis 19: 512-520
[2] Adelstein L J (1938) The surgical treatment of syringomyelia. Amer J Surg 40: 384-395
[3] Alvisi C, Cerisoli M (1984) Long-term results of the surgical treatment of syringohydromyelia. Acta Neurochir 71: 133-140
[4] Aschoff A, Löhlein A, Kunze S (1986) Die posttraumatische Syringomyelie - Behandlungsergebnisse von sechs Drainageoperationen mit besonderer Berücksichtigung von prä- und postoperativen NMR-Befunden. Vortrag 37. Jahrestagung der Dt. Gesellschaft für Neurochirurgie 1986
[5] Barbaro N M, Wilson Ch B, Gutin Ph H, Edwards M S B (1984) Surgical treatment of syringomyelia. Favorable results with syringoperitoneal shunting. J Neurosurg 61: 531-538
[6] Ballantine H T, Ojemann R G, Drew J H (1971) Syringohydromyelia. Prog Neurol Surg 4: 227-245
[7] Breig A (1960) Biomechanics of the central nervous system. Almquist and Wiksell, Stockholm
[8] Calbucci F, Andreoli A, Bollini C, Tognetti F, Godano U, Testa C (1987) Surgical treatment of syringomyelia. Clinical results

and post-operative M.R.I. controls. Lecture, 8th European Congress of Neurosurgery

[9] Dworkin G E, Staas W E (1985) Posttraumatic syringomyelia. Arch Phys Med Rehabil 66: 329-331

[10] Elsberg C A (1916) Diseases of the spinal cord and its membranes. Saunders, Philadelphia

[11] Fischer E G, Welch K, Shillito J (1977): Syringomyelia following lumbouretral shunting for communicating hydrocephalus. Report of three cases. J Neurosurg 47: 96-100

[12] Frazier Ch H, Rowe S N (1936) The surgical treatment of syringomyelia. Annals of Surgery 103: 481-497

[13] Hertel G, Ricker K (1977) A geomedical study of the distribution of syringomyelia in Germany. Proceedings of the 11th Worlds Congress of Neurology. Excerpta Medica Congress Series No 434 Neurology 353-365

[14] Lesoin F, Petit H, Thomas C E, Viaud C, Baleriaux D, Jomin M (1986) Use of the syringoperitoneal shunt in the treatment of syringomyelia. Surg Neurol 25: 131-136

[15] Levy W J, Mason L, Hahn J F (1983) Chiari malformation presenting in adults: A surgical experience in 127 cases. Neurosurgery 12: 377-390

[16] MacDonald R L, Findlay J M, Tator Ch H (1988) Microcystic spinal cord degeneration causing posttraumatic myelopathia. J Neurosurg 68: 466-471

[17] Pecker J (1983) La derivation syringoperitonéale. Neurochirurgie (F) 29: 171-173

[18] Peiper H (1931) Die operative Behandlung der Syringomyelie. Nervenarzt 4: 436-453

[19] Phillips T W, Kindt G W (1981) Syringoperitoneal shunt for syringomyelia: A preliminary report. Surg Neurol 16: 462-466

[20] Puusepp L (1926) Traitement and operatoire de la syringomyélie Rev Neurolog 1: 1171-1179

[21] Quencer R M, Green B A, Eismont F J (1983): Posttraumatic spinal cord cysts. Clinical features and characterisation with metrizamide computed tomography. Radiology 146: 415-423

[22] Roosen N, Lumenta C B, Lins E, Stork W, Gahlen D, Bock W J (1987) Magnetic resonance imaging in the management of syringomyelia: Diagnosis and postoperative results. Lecture on 8th European Congress of Neurosurgery

[23] Rossier A B, Foo D, Shillito J, Dyro F M (1985) Posttraumatic cervical syringomyelia. Brain 108: 439-461

[24] Schlesinger E B, Antunes J L, Michelsen W J, Louis K M (1981) Hydromyelia: Clinical presentation and comparison of modalities of treatment. Neurosurgery 9: 356-365

[25] Shannon N, Symon L, Logue V, Cull D, Kang J, Kendall B (1981) Clinical features, investigation and treatment of posttraumatic syringomyelia. J Neurol Neurosurg Psych 44: 35-42

[26] Shillito J (1978) The treatment of intramedullary syrinx of the cervical cord by T-tube drainage. Neurosurgery 2: 171-172

[27] Stevens J M, Olney J S, Kendall B E (1985) Post-traumatic cystic and non-cystic myelopathy. Neuroradiology 27: 48-56

[28] Sullivan L P, Stears J C, Ringel S P (1988): Resolution of syringomyelia and Chiari I malformation by ventriculoatrial shunting in a patient with pseudotumor cerebri and a lumboperitoneal shunt. Neurosurg 22: 744-747

[29] Suzuki M, Davis Ch, Symon L, Gentili F (1985) Syringoperitoneal shunt for treatment of cord cavitation. J Neurol Neurosurg Psychiat 48: 620-627

[30] Tator C H, Meguro K, Rowed D W (1982) Favourable results with syringosubarachnoid shunts for treatment of syringomyelia. J Neurosurg 56: 517-523

[31] Vaquero J, Martinez R, Salazar J, Santos H (1987) Syringosub-

arachnoid shunt for treatment of syringomyelia. Acta Neurochir
84: 105-109

[32] Vernon J D, Silver J R, Symon L (1983) Post-traumatic syringomyelia: The results of surgery. Paraplegia 21: 37-46

[33] Welch K, Shillito J, Strand R, Fischer E G, Winston K R (1981)
Chiari I "malformation" - an acquired disorder? J Neurosurg 55:
604-609

[34] Williams B, Terry A F, Jones F, McSweeney T (1981) Syringomyelia
as a sequel to traumatic paraplegia. Paraplegia 19: 67-80

Haemodynamics in Interventional Neuroradiology

D. de Silva and D. Kühne (Essen, FRG)

The importance of this subject is discussed and illustrated using four examples. These include:

- the management by balloon embolisation of multiple giant intra-cranial aneurysms,
- the successful closure of a sinus-cavernous fistula caused by altering the haemodynamics by partial particle embolisation,
- treatment of an extensive dural and neck angioma involving ver-tebral and carotid arteries by judicious balloon and particle embolisation
- successful selective catheterisation of part of the previously non-catheterizable supply of an intracerebral AVM using the haemo-dynamics of its blood supply.

Radiological and CT Features of Secondary Amyloid Arthropathy as a Frequent Complication of Chronic Hemodyalysis: Spinal Localisation

L. Ticket and R. Potvliege (Brussels, Belgium)

Secondary amyloidosis is currently more readily recognised as a very frequent complication of the use of cellulose membranes during hemodialysis. It usually appears after 10 years of dialysis and is highly destructive.

The radiological features are discussed, mainly through a case report, in which the location is mainly in the cervical spine and the skull base, over a period of 10 years. It appears that the radiological features are not entirely specific and that bone biopsy is often required to make the diagnosis. However, the radiologist can often suggest the diagnosis, and hereby orient such a biopsy.

Amyloidosis secondary to long term dialysis is expected to diminish in the future, with the use of new types of dialysis membranes. However the recognition of these lesions is still very important, since there is a huge number of patients suffering from the disease, which is directly linked to the worldwide use of the cellulose hemodialysis membrane.

Multiple Sclerosis

Magnetic Resonance Imaging in Isolated Optic Neuritis

D. Städt, L. Kappos, E. Rohrbach, R. Heun, and M. Ratzka

I. Introduction

Optic neuritis (ON) is known as a symptom of a number of diseases (see table 1), but is most frequently seen in patients with multiple sclerosis (MS). If ON of unknown origin (see table 2) occurs isolated without any other clinical abnormality, the question arises as to if it represents a disease entity for itself or is the initial symptom of MS. In literature, the percentage of patients developing MS after one or more episodes of isolated ON ranges from 11.5% to 85% (1). This information is mainly based on clinical long term follow-up and sometimes supplemented by computerized tomography.

We examined whether cerebral MRI could provide evidence for dissemination in space by revealing clinically silent lesions and thus contribute defining the risk and perhaps even establishing the diagnosis of MS.

II a. Patients

We examined 24 patients with isolated optic neuritis:
17 females, 7 males, age range 18 - 51 years, median age 26 years,
17 with symptoms on left eye, 6 on right eye, 1 on both eyes.
All patients satisfied the criteria shown in table 2. In each case it was the first episode of ON. The delay time between onset of symptoms and MRI examination ranged from 0 to 176 weeks (median 5 weeks).

Table 1: Possible causes of optic neuritis other than MS

- meningitis, encephalitis
- infectious diseases
- focal diseases (e. g. infection of paranasal sinus), leukemic infiltration etc.
- intoxications, tobacco-alcohol-amblyopia, wood alcohol, quinine, tuberculostatic agents, drugs
- endogenic toxicosis
- chorioretinitis, iridocyclitis
- Leber's optic atrophy
- vascular papillitis, arteriitis temporalis, arteriosclerosis

Table 2: Definition "isolated optic neuritis of unknown origin"

1. One or more of the following symptoms:
   - acute visual loss
   - scotoma
   - blurring of vision
   - retrobulbar pain
   - color vision disturbances
2. Pathological VEP
3. Both history and neurological examination not suggestive for lesions outside the optic nerve or the optical pathways.
4. Exclusion of other possible causes (see table 1)

II b. Methods

The CSF examination included cells, total protein, IgG and isoelectric focussing (oligoclonal bands). The results were regarded as being abnormal when cell count and relative IgG were increased or oligoclonal bands were present.

VEP examinations were done with a black-white pattern-reversal checkerboard. P_{100}-latency and amplitude were measured.

MRI examinations were performed using a Siemens Magnetom 1.0 Tesla (axial slicing, thickness 6 mm, 10% overlap, TR 2900 ms, TE 40 and 120 ms). Only lesions with high intensity in proton density and T2-weighted images and a diameter greater than 2 mm were considered, if two investigators agreed.

III. Results

CSF examinations were pathological in 19 patients (79.1%), 4 patients (16.6%) had normal CSF findings (1 patient refused lumbar puncture).

MRI showed lesions in 19 of 24 patients (79.1%). Only 5 patients (22.9%) had a normal MRI. The number of lesions ranged from 0 to 38 (median 2). Only 1 lesion could be demonstrated in 5 patients, 2 patients had 2 lesions and in 12 patients 3 and more lesions could be seen (figure 3). Most lesions were located in the frontal and parietal white matter.

Patients with positive MRI tended to show pathological findings in the CSF-examination and vice versa (table 3). There was only 1 patient with pathological MRI and normal CSF. All patients with more than 2 lesions in MRI had pathological CSF-findings.

By splitting the number of lesions into three groups (normal = no lesion, possible MS = 1 - 2 lesions, strongly suggestive for MS = 3 and more lesions), the grouped number of lesions correlated with the CSF findings ($p(X^2) < 2\%$).

The location and number of lesions did not correlate with sex and age at onset of ON.

Table 3: Comparison of CSF and MRI-findings

		number of lesions in MRI		
		0	1 or 2	> 2
CSF	normal	3	1	0
	pathological	2	5	12

IV. Discussion

The diagnosis of MS depends on both dissemination in space and dissemination in time (8,9).

As to dissemination in space, our study shows, that nearly 80% of patients with clinically isolated ON have further lesions in the cerebrum. Our findings are within the range of 11.5% to 85% of MS-risk after ON given in the literature (1). These studies were mainly based on laboratory investigations, CT and long term follow-up. MRI-investigations in patients with isolated ON found lesions in 40% to 70% (2,3,5-7,11). Studies including MRI-investigations and long term follow-up to our knowledge do not exist at present.

Evaluating our results, a possible conclusion is, that isolated ON does not really exist as a clinical entity because of the high rate of (clinically silent) abnormalities.

On the other hand, MRI is known to be sensitive but not specific. Lesions, although seeming typical for MS, can have various causes, even without pathological background. With increasing age, the evidence of lesions in MRI rises (10). The low age in our group doesn't exclude possible errors but makes them less probable.

MRI is the best "paraclinical" method to prove dissemination in space (5,7,11), but dissemination in time is the second main preacquisite of a definite MS diagnosis (8,9).

Therefore, contrast agents like Gadolinium, which can help to distinguish between chronic and acute lesions at one certain time point (4,12), may be of special interest in studying optic neuritis in the future.

Systematic clinical follow-up will be necessary for the assessment of the appropriate value of MRI in isolated ON.

References

1. Cohen M, Lessell S, Wolf PA: A prospective study of the risk of developing multiple sclerosis in uncomplicated optic neuritis. Neurology 29:208-213, 1979
2. Jacobs L, Kinkel PR, Kinkel WR: Silent brain lesions in patients with isolated idiopathic optic neuritis. Arch Neurol 3:52-55, 1986
3. Johns K, Lavin P, Elliot JH, Partain L: Magnetic resonance imaging of the brain in isolated optic neuritis. Arch Ophthalmol 104:1486-1488, 1986
4. Kappos L, Städt D, Keil W: Magnetische Resonanztomographie mit Gadolinium. Eine Möglichkeit zur Erkennung aktiver Plaques bei Multipler Sklerose. Psycho 13:386-387, 1987
5. Kinnunen E, Larsen A, Ketonen L, Koskimies S, Sandström A: Evaluation of central nervous system involvement in uncomplicated optic neuritis after prolonged follow-up. Acta Neurol Scand 76:147-151, 1987
6. Ormerod IEC, McDonald WI, Du Boulay GH, Kendall BE, Moseley IF, Halliday AM, Kakigi R, Kriss A, Peringer E: Disseminated lesions at presentation in patients with optic neuritis. Neurol Neurosurg Psychiat 49:124-127, 1986
7. Paty DW, Oger JJF, Kastrukoff LF, Hashimoto SA, Hooge JP, Eisen AA, Eisen RN, Purves SJ, Low MD, Brandejs V, Robertson WD, Li DKB: MRI in the diagnosis of MS: A prospective study with comparison of clinical evaluation, evoked potentials, oligoclonal banding, and CT. Neurology 38:180-185, 1988
8. Poser CM, Paty DW, Scheinberg L, McDonald WI, Davis FA, Ebers GC, Johnsen KP, Sibley WA, Silberberg DH, Tourtelotte WW: Immune diagnostic criteria for multiple sclerosis: guidelines for research protocols. Ann Neurol 13:227-231, 1983
9. Schumacher GA, Beebe G, Kibler RF, Kurland LT et al.: Problems of experimental trials of therapy in multiple sclerosis: report by the panel on the evaluation of experimental trials of therapy in multiple sclerosis. Ann NY Acad Sci 122:552-568, 1965
10. Sarpel G, Chaudry F, Hindo W: Magnetic Resonance Imaging of Periventricular Hyperintensity in a Veterans Administration Hospital Population. Arch Neurol 44:725-728, 1987
11. Shabas D, Gerard G, Slavin M: MRI in optic neuritis. Neuro Ophthalmol 7:267-272, 1987
12. Gonzales-Scarano F, Grossman RI, Galetta S, Atlas SW, Silberberg DH: Multiple Sclerosis Disease Activity Correlates with Gadolinium-Enhanced Magnetic Resonance Imaging. Ann Neurol 21:300-307, 1987

Multiple Sclerosis and Corpus Callosum Atrophy: Relationship of MRI Findings to Clinical Data

J. L. Dietemann, C. Beigelmann, M. Vouge, L. Rumbach, T. Tajahmady, C. Faubert, M. Y. Jeung, and A. Wackenheim

Involvement of the corpus callosum (CC) in multiple sclerosis (MS) appears common and includes areas of demyelination and gliosis on one hand,and loss of callosal axons on the other hand,resulting in CC atrophy [1-4].MRI makes visualisation of CC particularly easy.

We reviewed MR studies in patients with MS in order to determine whether or not CC atrophy correlates with clinical data and other MR findings.

MATERIALS AND METHODS

This study includes 110 patients (45 men,65 women) aged 15 to 66,with clinical and/or biological diagnosis of MS.Severe to moderate corpus callosum atrophy was observed in 67 (60%) patients.

Correlation between corpus callosum atrophy,brain atrophy, duration and severity of clinical symptoms,and high signal white matter areas,was carried out in 90 patients.

All MR studies were performed on a 0,5T superconducting system (GE-CGR Magniscan) with a standard head coil.All study included T1-weighted sagittal sections (TR=300-500 msec,TE=14 msec,4 excitations) and T2-weighted sections (TR=2000 msec,TE=60 and 120 msec,2 excitations).The matrix was 256x256;the field of view was 230 mm.Contiguous T1-weighted sagittal 7 mm thick slices,and noncontiguous T2-weighted 4 mm thick axial slices were obtained with a gap of 4 mm.

Atrophy of the corpus callosum was visually determined on midsagittal T1-weighted images.Patients were classified into 3 categories:normal CC,moderate and severe CC atrophy.We only considered patients with normal CC and with severe CC atrophy,thus excluding those with mild atrophy.

Severity of brain atrophy was also visually determined on both axial and sagittal MR images,according to enlargement of basal cisterns,cortical sulci and ventricles.We distinguished 4 degrees of brain atrophy from absent (0) to severe (3+).

White matter abnormalities were also classified into 3 groups of severity (1+ to 3+),according to the number and size of high signal areas on T2-weighted images.

For clinical symptoms we considered (1) the duration of the disease and (2) the severity of the disease classified into 3 degrees (1+ to 3+).

RESULTS

Results are summarized in the following table:

90 patients	16 with severe CC atrophy	36 without CC atrophy
Mean age (years)	46	33
Mean duration of MS (years)	14	5
Clinical symptoms		
1+	2(14%)	28(78%)
2+	7(43%)	5(14%)
3+	7(43%)	3(8%)
Severity of brain atrophy		
0	4(25%)	33(92%)
1+	4(25%)	3(8%)
2+	6(38%)	0
3+	2(12%)	0
White matter abnormalities		
1+	0	19(53%)
2+	7(43%)	16(44%)
3+	9(57%)	1(3%)

DISCUSSION

It results from our series that severe atrophy of CC in patients with MS correlates well with the long duration of the disease.Relationship between atrophy of CC and intensity of symptoms is also obvious,as 96% of patients with severe atrophy presented moderate to very severe clinical manifestations,while 78% of patients with normal CC presented only mild symptoms.

CC atrophy correlates also well with white matter abormalities.Indeed 57% of patients with severe CC atrophy presented large and numerous high signal areas within white matter,while 53% of patients with normal CC had only few white matter abnormalities.It must yet be noted that moderately severe white matter abnormalities were found both in 43% of patients with severe CC atrophy and in 44% of patients without CC atrophy.

Brain atrophy was absent in 92% of patients without CC atrophy,mild in the remaining 8%.It was absent in 25% of patients with severe CC atrophy,mild in 25% and severe (2+ and 3+) in 50% of them.Thus patients with MS seldom present brain atrophy without CC atrophy,while CC atrophy may exist with mild or absent brain atrophy.This shows that the atrophy of the CC in MS is not simply an element of diffuse brain atrophy which occurs as a consequence of a longstanding disease,but it is due to involvement of the CC by the demyelinating and destructive process itself.

In conclusion it can be said that (1) severe atrophy of the CC occurs in longstanding MS;(2) patients with severe CC atrophy present severe clinical symptoms;(3) there is no close relationship between CC atrophy and white matter abnormalities;this is shown by the fact that nearly 50% of patients without CC atrophy and 50% of patients with severe CC atrophy have the same degree of white matter abormalities;and (4) CC atrophy occurs earlier than brain atrophy in the course of the disease.

REFERENCES

1   BARNARD,RO,TRIGGS,M (1974)
    Corpus callosum in multiple sclerosis
    J Neurol Neurosurg Psychiatr,37:1259-1264

2   DAVIS,RL,ROBERTSON,DM (1985)
    Textbook of neuropathology
    Williams and Wilkins,Baltimore

3   DIETEMANN,JL,RUMBACH,L,BEAUJEUX,R,ROY,C,KASTLER,B,
    ZÖLLNER,G,MARESCAUX,C,BOURJAT,P,WACKENHEIM,A (1988)
    IRM et sclérose en plaques
    In:IRM corps entier
    Eds: JL LAMARQUE, MY MOUROU, J PUJOL, JP ROUANET
    Axone,Montpellier

4   SIMON,JH,HOLTAS,SL,SCHIFFER,RB,RUDICK,RA,HERNDON,RM
    KIDO,DK,UTZ,R (1986)
    Corpus callosum and subcallosum-periventricular lesions in multiple sclerosis:detection with MR
    Radiology,160:363-367

Gadolinium-DTPA Enhanced MRI in Multiple Sclerosis: A New Method to Monitor Disease Activity and Treatment Efficacy

L. Kappos, D. Städt, E. Rohrbach, R. Heun, W. Keil, and M. Ratzka

Introduction:

There is no doubt that MRI is the best imaging modality in the diagnosis of multiple sclerosis. As a result of its high sensitivity in the depiction of clinically silent lesions in the brain and the spinal cord it can help to fulfil the criterion of dissemination in space and to establish a definite diagnosis of MS in patients with clinical signs and symptoms pointing at only one location in the CNS. While this diagnostic support provided by MRI is only needed in a minority of MS patients, the possibility of monitoring disease evolution by MRI is becoming increasingly important. Especially in therapeutic studies the use of serial MRI is going to become an indispensable addition to thorough clinical monitoring. But serial MRI scans have also shown that lesions, once appearing, tend to remain rather stable over time with only minor fluctuations in size. Lesions which have not changed in serial MRI, have no specific features which clearly differentiates them from other lesions which have just appeared. Thus, conventional unenhanced MRI gives us a reliable information about the "plaque burden" which has accumulated in MS patients over the years but is not able to show us the degree of actual disease activity. From neuropathological observations and the data available from acute and chronic experimental autoimmune encephalomyelitis we know that a local disruption of the blood brain barrier occurs at an early stage in the development of new lesions. Like CT contrast agents, Gadolinium DTPA accumulates temporarily only in regions with disturbed blood brain barrier. Its use enables us to depict blood brain barrier disturbances and to visualize a certain phase in the evolution of MS-lesions.

Methods:

All examinations were performed with a Siemens 1.0 Tesla Magnetom. Axial images were obtained in two interlaced sets of 12 slices, 6 mm thick with 0.6 mm overlap. We used a heart rate gated spin echo acquisition sequence of TR=2800-3200 ms with dual echo delays of TE=40 and 120 ms. 5 min. after the i.v. bolus injection of 0.4 ml/kg bw a T1-weighted sequence was performed (TR=650-700, TE=30-40). The images obtained were independently reviewed by two observers without knowledge of the patients' clinical classification. The number of Gd enhancing lesions their localization, signal intensity and size were assessed. In repeat examinations special attention was paid to good reproducibility of the scans. The intervals between the scans ranged between 3 days and 9 months. The patient's clinical status was assessed by Kurtzke's Expanded Disability Status Scale (EDSS, 5) and a quantified neurological examination. Patients were assessed according to disease activity at the time of examination. The label "active" was applied if new clinical signs and/or complaints had occurred or older signs had deteriorated within the last 10 days before the MRI was performed, and the label "not active" for those patients who had experienced either an amelioration or at least a stability of signs and complaints during the last eight weeks before the MRI examination. In the category "probably active" were included all patients with some indication of disease activity in the last few weeks who did not fulfil the criteria for "active disease". The patients were categorized according to the course of their disease as relapsing with complete remissions (EDSS lower than 2.0 between the relapses), relapsing with incomplete remissions (EDSS 2.0 or more between the relapses), relapsing progressive, secondary chronic progressive and primary chronic progressive (from the first signs of the disease up to now a steady progression without relapses and phases of remission). 16 patients were examined immediately before and on average 10 days after starting steroid treatment. Two schedules were used for the steroid treatment: "Normal dose" starting with 100mg prednisone per day and tapering off within 6-8 weeks; and "high dose", starting with 500-1000mg prednisolone i.v. per day for 5 days and tapering off within 6-8 weeks.

Results:
Seventy-six patients with clinically definite diagnosis of MS (7) were included in this evaluation. Table 1 shows the mean numbers of lesions in various groups according to clinically assessed disease activity. Patients with active disease show the highest number of lesions with Gd enhancement. But patients with probable activity and even 9 of 17 of those without clinically detectable activity also showed some Gd enhancement (Table 2). If the patients are divided according to the various disease courses (Table 3) there are also significant differences in the number of enhancing lesions. Only one patient with primary chronic progressive disease showed enhancement and only one single small lesion. Patients with relapsing disease and complete remissions also tended to have only very few enhancing lesions as compared with relapsing progressive or relapsing with incomplete remissions.

Table 1: Number of Gd-enhancing lesions

clinically assessed disease activity	n	mean	SD
"active"	27	9.5	13.7
"probably active"	32	1.9	5.0
"not active"	17	2.2	4.4

p(Kruskal-Wallis) = 0.003

Table 2: Occurence of lesions with Gd-enhancement

clinically assessed disease activity	Gd-enhancing lesions		
	no	1-2	>2
"active"	9	0	18
"probably active"	20	7	5
"not active"	8	4	5

p(chi^2) = 0.0007

Table 3: Occurence of lesions with Gd-enhancement

disease course	Gd-enhancing lesions		
	no	1-2	>2
relapsing with complete remissions	6	3	1
relapsing with in-complete remissions	14	3	14
progressive/relapsing	5	2	10
sec.chronic progr.	3	2	3
prim.chronic progr.	9	1	0
all	37	11	28

p(chi^2) = 0.03

Serial examinations:
26 of the patients underwent repeated (2 to 10) Gd-enhanced MRI evaluations. In untreated patients enhancement was only visible for a few weeks (a maximum of 3 months) in the same location but new lesions appeared in other places. 16 patients were scanned before and after steroid treatment. Although clinically active one of these patients did not show any enhancement in either examination. In all others we observed the disappearance or at least a significant decrease in the number and intensity of enhancing lesions. Table 4 shows a major change in the number of enhancing lesions after steroid treatment while the change in the clinical evaluation with Kurtzke's EDSS is only minor.

Table 4: Number of Gd-enhancing lesions and clinical status
        before and after steroid treatment (n=16)

	mean number of lesions	mean EDSS score
before treatment	10,8	4.3
after treatment	3.4	4.1
	(p=0.001)	(p=0.04)

Wilcoxon matched-pairs signed rank test

Conclusions:
1. Only in rare cases have we been able to see lesions in Gd scans which had not been detectable in unenhanced proton density and T2 scans.This was mainly the case in areas adjacent to the CSF space or in the grey matter and could also be true for spinal lesions. From the diagnostic point of view Gd-scans could help to satisfy the criterion of disse-mination in time (7) at the first presentation of patients with possible MS, if both lesions with and without Gd-enhancement could be detected.
2. At present Gd-enhanced T1 scans seem to provide the most reliable paraclinical evidence in the assessment of disease activity in MS.
3. Patients with primary chronic progressive disease show no or only minimal Gd enhancement. This could point at a different pathogenesis.
4. Relapsing-remitting patients with complete remissions also fail to show - even if clinically active - a significant Gd-enhancement. This finding, if confirmed in larger series, could be of value for the assessment of prognosis and possible therapeutic decisions.

412

5. The prognostic value of Gd MRI as well as its usefulness in directing therapeutic decisions should be the subject of future longitudinal investigations.

Gadolinium enhanced MRI allows the in vivo observation of one certain phase in the evolution of acute MS lesions. This has important implications for our understanding of the disease and possible immunologic correlations. But serial enhanced MRI scans could also enable us to apply more sophisticated, phase-adapted therapeutic strategies.

References:
1. Grossman RI, Gonzalez-Scarano F, Atlas SW, Galetta S, Silberberg DH. (1986) Multiple sclerosis: gadolinium enhancement in MR imaging. Radiology 161:721-725
2. Kappos L, Städt D, Keil W. (1987) Magnetische Resonanztomographie mit Gadolinium - eine Möglichkeit zur Erkennung aktiver Plaques bei Multipler Sklerose. Psycho. 13:386-389
3. Kappos L, Städt D, Ratzka M, Keil W, Schneiderbanger-Grygier S, Heitzer T, Poser S, Nadjmi M. (1988) Magnetic resonance imaging in the evaluation of treatment in multiple sclerosis. Neuroradiology 30:299-302,1988
4. Kilgore DP, Breger RK, Daniels DL, Pojunas KW, Williams AL, Haughton VM. (1986) Cranial tissues: normal MR appearance after intravenous injection of GD-DTPA. Radiology 160:757-761
5. Kurtzke JF. (1983) Rating neurologic impairment in multiple sclerosis: an expanded disability status scale (EDSS) Neurology 33:1444-1452
6. Paty DW. (1988) Magnetic resonance imaging (MRI) in the assessment of disease activity in multiple sclerosis (MS). Can J Neurol Sci (in press)
7. Schumacher GA, Beebe G, Kibler RF, Kurland LT, (1965) Problems of experimental trials of therapy in multiple sclerosis: report by the panel of the evaluation of experimental trials of therapy in multiple sclerosis. Ann NY Acad Sci 552-268

Clinical and MRI Study of Unilateral Thalamic Lesions in Multiple Sclerosis

M. Brainin, G. Goldenberg, A. Eisenstadter, and A. Neuhold

Introduction:

Anatomical and neuroradiological studies of patients with lacunar stroke have shown that a large spectrum of different clinical syndromes results from thalamic lesions. According to their localization and clinical presentation they have been classified as distinct syndromes (Bogousslavsky et.al. 1988). It therefore seemed of interest to find out, whether lesions with a similar anatomical distribution result in similar syndromes in patients with multiple sclerosis (MS). The aim of this study was also to determine the possible significance of thalamic lesions for the cognitive impairment frequently seen in MS-patients.

Methods and results:

The MR-scans (0.5 Tesla) of 40 patients with a clinically definite diagnosis of chronic MS (Poser Criteria) were retrospectively reviewed. All patients with one or more lesion within the thalamus were included into the study. All visible thalamic lesions were schematically correlated with the Schaltenbrand-Wahren Atlas in order to define the anatomic regions involved. The patients's charts were studied for signs and symptoms thought to be relevant for a thalamic lesion. The results of standard neuropsychological testing were also included into the evaluation (Mini-Mental-State Examination, WIP: a standardized German version of the Wechsler Adult Intelligence Test, WMS: subtests from the Wechsler Memory Scale including paired associate learning, logical memory, and digit span). In addition, calculated images of the thalamic region were evaluated from 37 of the 40 patients and compared to a control group of 18 healthy volunteers. Five different regions within the thalamus were chosen for measurements using a ROI device of 0.2 square centimeters. The regions 1-5 were also defined according to the Schaltenbrand -Wahren Atlas (ranging from region 1: thalamopolar to region 5: lateral pulvinar). Statistical evaluation was performed by means of analysis of variance.

Six patients with unilateral thalamic lesions were found. The main clinical data and the thalamic nuclei most probably involved are shown in Table 1 and in Fig.1-6. In five cases the visible lesions were small and not thought to be of detectable clinical relevance. Four lesions were rightsided and two on the left. One patient showed a large rightsided lesion involving the thalamopolar and the thalamocentral region. In this one patient an HMPAO- SPECT examination performed within two days after the MR-exam showed a marked decrease of tracer activity on the right temporal and lower temporoparietal region.

Quantitative T2 measurements of the thalamic regions showed no significant difference between MS patients and normal controls. From this we conclude that at the field strength of 0.5 Tesla the findings of Drayer et.al.(1987) can not be reproduced.

Discussion:

Thalamic lesions were found in 6 out of 40 cases with chronic MS and all lesions were unilateral. In two cases the involved region was thalamopolar, in two cases inferolateral, in one further case paramedian, and in one case median. With the exception of one patient (case 3) no distinct clinical syndrome could be ascribed to any of the lesions.. The one symptomatic case was the only one with an exceptionally large lesion. This lesion involved the entire thalamopolar and thalamocentral region on the right and was thought to be the cause of a leftsided spatial neglect syndrome as well as a decrease of verbal fluency. The HMPAO-Spect examination confirmed the thalamic lesion and additionally showed a deactivation on the right temporal and temporoparietal cortex.

Single case reports of vascular lacunes in the thalamus have also shown that very small lesions can be asymptomatic (Kritchevsky et. al.1987). MRI now has the capability of detecting such small lesions and has been shown to be superior in the detection of small lacunes when compared to CT (Brown et.al. 1988). We therefore also conclude from our series of MS patients that not only the location but also the size of a thalamic lesion determine whether a symptom can be ascribed to this lesion.

Neuropsychological deficits, mostly impairment of learning and of information retrieval have been shown to be a frequent finding in MS patients, also in those with a short clinical course and a relatively mild grade of physical disability. Anterograde amnesia might be caused by thalamic lesions, which are almost always bilateral. One patient showed marked dementia (case 1), which evolved during the past two years of her illness. In this case we do not assume that the small unilateral inferothalamic lesion contributes essentially to the cognitive decline in this patient. In addition, it has been shown in another study that impairment of memory in chronic MS seems to be regularly associated with demyelination in both hippocampal regions (Brainin et.al. 1988). The decline of general cognitive measures may also be related to the total number of brain lesions, as seen on MRI, rather than being linked to the demyelination of specific brain structures (Medaer et.al. 1987).

There are several important limitations to our observations: Thalamic lesions have in our study mostly been found in patients with a longstanding course of the disease and with a high level of disability. Such patients usually show many disseminated lesions and it is therefore difficult to ascribe a clinical sign or symptom to a single lesion. It is therefore likely, that some symptoms that could have been caused by a thalamic lesion, may have been overlooked, especially in those patients with extensive involvement of the brainstem.

A general limitation of studying the clinical manifestations of circumscribed damage to the thalamus results from the fact that such thalamic lesions tend to depress ipsilateral cortical metabolic activity and it has therefore been suggested that a number of symptoms thought to be caused directly by the thalamic lesion are in fact cortical symptoms resulting from metabolic depression (Baron et.al. 1986, Perani et.al. 1987). That a demyelinating lesion in the thalamus can also have such farreaching effects on the ipsilateral cortex certainly deserves further investigation.

Figure 1-6:Inversion-recovery scans through the thalamus.For description of the lesions see Table 1. In case 3 an SE-scan was performed as well as an HMPAO-SPECT examination (courtesy of Doz.Dr.Ivo Podreka),showing the thalamic lesion as well as a cortical deactivation on the right (MR-scans: the viewers right is the left; SPECT: the viewers right is the right).

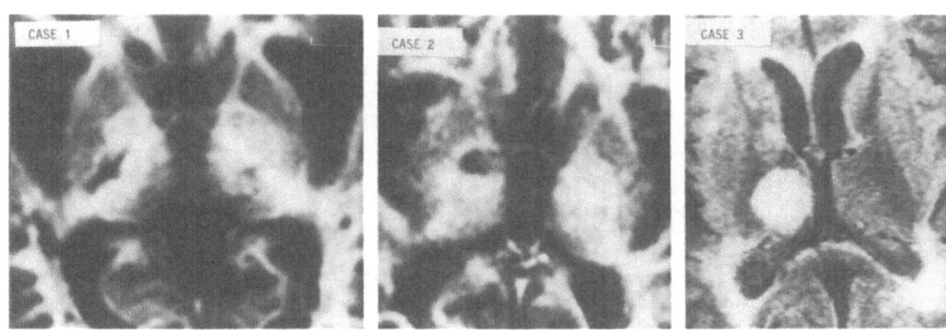

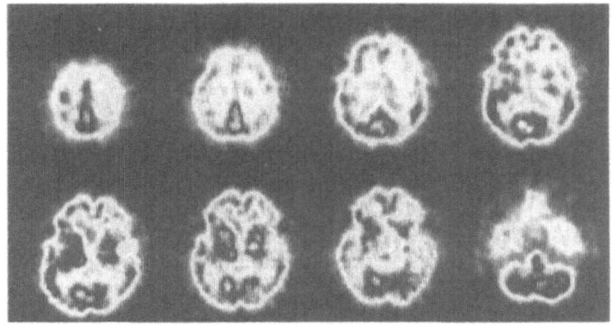

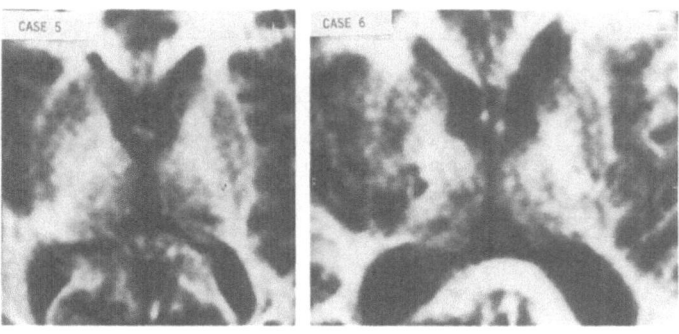

Nr	Pat	age /y	m/f	DD /y	EDSS	Neuropsychology	Clinical syndromes	Thalamic lesions
1	JB	39	f	7	7.5	MMS:24/32 WIP:76 WMS/LM:0 PAL:57 DS:73	Dementia, spastic quadru- paresis, pseudobulbar palsy,	left ventral intermediate nucleus (T2:103)
2	KS	45	m	13	6.5	WIP:97 WMS/LM:100 PAL:95 DS:92	Paraparesis	right medullary lamina, mamillothalamic tract,lateropolar and fascicular nucleus (T2:101)
3	RW	38	m	16	4.0	WIP:97 Rey-Osterrieth and crossing-out test:misses elements on the left,facial recognition and Wisconsin Card Sorting:normal DS:92, verbal fluency:dimin- ished	left sensorimotor syndrome left spatial neclect, episodic dizziness	right ventrooral nucleus mamillothalamic tract, central and dorsomedial nucleus
4	MP	34	f	8	4.5	WIP:94 WMS/LM:100 PAL:92 DS:100	spastic quadru- paresis, cerebellar ataxia, right hemisensory loss, vertical gaze paralysis	right commissural nucleus (T2:111)
5	HJ	57	f	13	7.0	MMS:29/32	spastic paraparesis cerebellar tremor and nystagmus	left ventrocaudal nucleus (T2:107)
6	FS	68	m	17	4.5	MMS:30/32	spastic quadru- paresis,cerebellar limb ataxia, diminished opto- kinetic response bilaterally	right central nucleus (T2:126) right pulvinar (T2:115)

Table 1: Clinical data and thalamic regions involved in six
patients with multiple sclerosis.
(Abbreviations: age/y : age in years; m/f : male/female;
DD/y:disease duration in years; EDSS: Score on the 10
grade Kurtzke Expanded Disability Status Scale; MMS:
Mini-Mental-State Examination (the correct answers in
relation to the total score possible), in this
slightly modified MMS a score below 25 is considered to
be in the dementia range; WIP: standardized German version
of the WAIS (scores in relation to 100); WMS: Wechsler
Memory Scale with the subtests LM: Logical Memory; PAL:
Paired Associate Learning; DS: Digit Span; the raw
scores on the WMS are expressed in relation to age-matched
normal values; T2: measurements of the thalamic lesions
from calculated images)

References:

Baron JC, Antona RD,Pantano P, Serdaru M, Samson Y, Bousser MG
(1986) Effects of thalamic stroke on the energy metabolism
of the cerebral cortex. Brain 109:1243-1259
Bogousslavsky J, Regli F, Uske A (1988) Thalamic infarcts: Clinical
syndromes, etiology, and prognosis. Neurology 38: 837-848
Brainin M, Goldenberg G, Ahlers C, Reisner T, Neuhold A, Deecke L
(1988) Structural brain correlates of anterograde memory
deficits in multiple sclerosis. J Neurol 235:362-365
Brown JJ, Hesselink JR, Rothrock JF (1988) MR and CT of lacunar
infarcts. AJNR 9:477-482
Drayer B, Burger P, Hurwitz B, Dawson D, Cain J (1987) Reduced
signal intensity on MR images of the thalamus and putamen
in multiple sclerosis: Increased iron content? AJNR 8:413-
419
Kritchevsky M, Graff-Radford NR, Damasio AR (1987) Normal memory
after damage to medial thalamus. Arch Neurol 44: 959-962
Medaer R, Nelissen E, Appel B, Swerts M, Geutsen J, Callaert H
(1987) Magnetic resonance imaging and cognitive
functioning in multiple sclerosis. J Neurol 235: 86-89
Perani D, Vallar G, Cappa S, Messa C, Fazio F (1987) Aphasia and
neglect after subcortical stroke: a clinical/cerebral
perfusion study. Brain 110:1211-1229
Schaltenbrand G and Wahren W (1977) Atlas for stereotaxy of the
human brain.Stuttgart Thieme

Serial Clinical and MRI Study of Diffuse Cerebral White Matter Changes in Multiple Sclerosis

M. Brainin, Th. Reisner, E. Maida, A. Neuhold, L. Wicke, S. Lang, and L. Deecke

Introduction:

The measurement of the relaxation times T1 and T2 within the normally appearing cerebral white matter in cases of multiple sclerosis (MS) has yielded some interesting results in a number of studies (Ormerod et.al.1986, Lacomis et.al.1986). They have unequivocally shown that the apparently normally appearing cerebral white matter has longer T1 and T2 relaxation times when compared to normal controls. This finding demonstrates in vivo what has been concluded from earlier neuropathological reports (Allen 1983) that MS is not a disease which is restricted to focal areas of demyelination but rather involves the entire cerebral white matter.

Both clinical significance and biophysical nature of this finding have remained mostly unclear to date. In another study (Brainin et.al.,in press), the normal cerebral white matter of two groups of MS patients differing only in respect to their disease duration were investigated by means of quantitative MRI. Only patients with a longstanding course of the disease (> 5 years) showed a T2 prolongation in the normally appearing periventricular white matter as compared to the group with a shorter disease duration (< 5 years) or with another group of healthy controls. This finding has shown that the prolongation of T2 eventually develops with the further course of the disease and is more pronounced in the later stages.

The purpose of this study was to find out whether such changes of relaxation times of the normally appearing cerebral white matter occur during an acute relapse of the disease and whether these measurements are subject to changes during cortison therapy.

Patients and methods:

13 patients with a clinically definite diagnosis of MS (Poser Criteria) and a recent onset of the disease (less than one year) consented to cooperate in forming a data base and to be rescanned immediately after the onset of a bout. All patients were regularly seen in the MS-outpatient service of the Vienna Neurological University Clinic. All patients showed no or only very mild physical impairment (EDSS Scale: 0-1). Only patients without long-time medication were accepted. All bouts were diagnosed by unequivocal clinical signs. Within one year seven patients had had bouts, one of them a second bout. After the base examination, another scan was taken within three days after the onset of the bout before therapy, the third examination was performed on the 10th day of high-dose cortison therapy (1g of cortison over five days, 500mg to the seventh day, and 250 mg to the ninth day) and

the final fourth examination was perfomed four weeks after the onset of the bout. A control group consisted out of 18 healthy normal volunteers.
In all serial examinations care was taken to achieve exact repositioning with reference to the bicommissural plane. All exams were performed on a 0.5 Tesla unit (Gyroscan) with a standard head coil, using spin-echo sequences (TR 2000ms, TE 50/100ms) with contiguous slices ,a slice factor of 1.1, and a slice thickness of 8mm. Routine scans were displayed on a 256 x 256 matrix. In addition, calculated images were obtained in two different planes, one directed through the bicommissural plane, the second immediately above the corpus callosum parallel to the bicommissural plane through the upper frontal and upper parietal lobe. In the chosen planes IR and SE-sequences were obtained as well as a mixed mode sequence with the chosen parameters: SE repetition time 710ms, IR repetition time 2290ms, inversion delay 310ms, echo time 50ms, slice thickness 8.0mm, number of measurments 2, scan resolution 128. The calculated images were stored on magnetic tape for off-line measurements.
Measurements were performed with a standard cursor device (0.2 square centimeter). The region of interest was always chosen on the IR scan, which is thought to be most sensitive for showing plaques. Care was taken to clearly place the ROI outside a plaque region within the normally appearing white matter. The ROI was then kept constant for the measurments. No measurement was rejected due to a standard deviation considered too large, though it usually did not exceed 10%. T1 and T2 measurements were taken from the upper parietal lobe, the upper frontal lobe, the temporoparietal region, the temporal lobe, and the frontobasal lobe.For each patient or control a total of 20 measurements were taken. Statistical evaluation was performed by means of analysis of variance.

Results:

One patient had to be excluded from this study due to limited availability of the MR-scan. In one patient the quantitative follow-up data could not be evaluated out of technical reasons. Threfore, a total of six patients with seven bouts could be evaluated.
Quantitatively, the base examinations all showed elevated T1 and T2 values of the normally appearing white matter when compared to the control group. During the series of clinical and therapeutic events (base exam, relapse, treatment phase, follow-up) the patient group as a whole did not show a significant change for either T1 or T2 values. This was true for all brain regions measured (upper frontal, upper parietal, temporoparietal, parietal, or frontobasal).
Nevertheless, individual patients did show T2 changes compared to their values obtained at the base examination. Two out of six patients showed a significant T2 elevation during the bout. One of them showed a return to the base value after therapy with a a second elevation at the follow-up examination. One patient showed an elevated T2 throughout the serial study following the base exam which did not change during therapy or four weeks thereafter. In the other four patients the onset of a bout did not significantly affect the T2 value compared to the base value. In two cases no T2 changes were measured throughout the serial study, in one further patient there was a significant T2 prolongation after therapy and in still another patient the only significant change measured was a T2 decrease following the second bout at the time of the second follow-up examination.

Fig.1: T2-values of six patients (serial examinations of the normal white cerebral white matter).

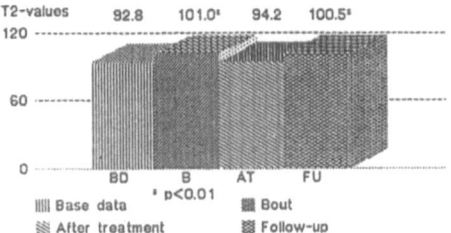

Case 1 (HE)

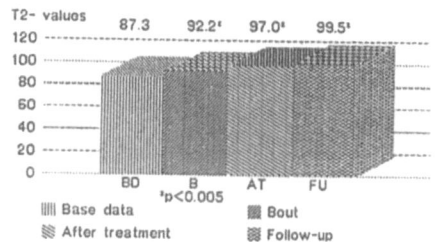

Case 2 (OK)

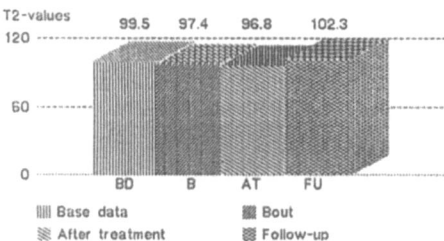

Case 3 (MS)

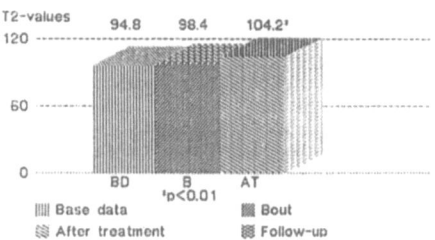

Case 4 (SK)

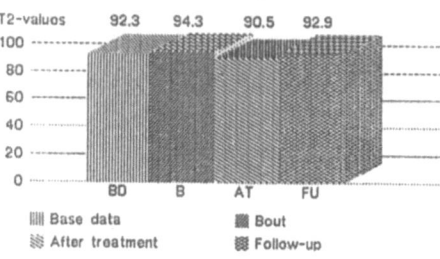

Case 5 (CD)

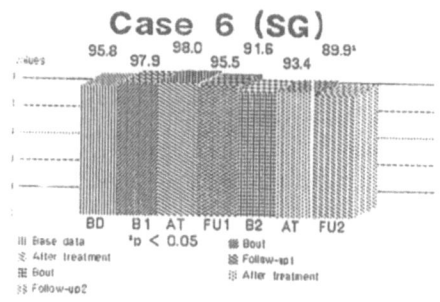

Case 6 (SG)

422

Discussion:

This study shows that T1 and T2 measurements of the visually normal cerebral white matter of MS patients do not change in a uniform way during a clinical relapse. In addition, such measurements do not predictably change as a response to high-dose cortison therapy. Although it could not be shown in all patients, one might speculate that such measurements might reflect discrete changes of the macromolecular environment in single cases. In one patient (case 1) an increase of T2 in the normal white matter could possibly indicate an increase of intercellular water, which was shown to be reversible by cortison. In the further course a second increase of T2 was shown four weeks after therapy which might reflect the beginning of astroglial proliferation within the entire white matter of the brain. But in other patients such measurements were totally unpredictable or did not change at all. Besides, the failure to document changes of T1 during a clinical relapse weighs against the assumption that an increase in the concentration of extracellular water is the main biochemical factor contributing to the change of T2. It has been argued that the degree of elevation of T1 is positively correlated with the total amount of water in a lesion, whereas the degree of T2 elevation also depends on the total amount of water as well as on the macromolecular environment of the water (D.H.Miller 1988). The macromolecular changes within the normally appearing white matter, though, are not well known. One quantitative neuropathological study has shown, however, that the main fragments of demyelination - myelin-associated glycoprotein, basic myeloprotein, and proteolipoprotein - can not be traced within the normally appearing white matter of MS brains, whereas within the plaque- and periplaque area they can be found in abnormal high amounts (Moller et.al. 1987).

Also measurements of T1 and T2 within the plaque areas have shown that neither age nor activity of the plaque can be reliably predicted, although a prolongation of T1 and T2 is frequently noted within an active plaque (Ormerod et.al. 1987; HBW Larsson et.al. 1988). But the measured values are strongly overlapping, so that no conclusive evidence can be derived from single measurements. Therefore, serial measurements of plaque areas with application of Ga-DTPA can today be considered the most reliable biological marker reflecting the activity of the disease (R.I.Grossman et.al. 1986; D.H.Miller et.al. 1988).

References:
Allen IV (1983)Hydrolytic enzymes in multiple sclerosis. In:Zimmerman HR (ed) Progress in Neuropathology, Raven Press New York, 1-17
Brainin M, Reisner T, Neuhold A, Lang S (in press) Mitbeteiligung der scheinbar normalen weissen Hirnsubstanz am Krankheitsprozess der multiplen Sklerose
Grossman RI, Gonzalez-Scarano F, Atlas SW, Galetta S, Silberberg DH (1986) Multiple sclerosis: gadolinium enhancement in MR imaging. Radiology 161,721-725
Lacomis D, Osbakken M, Gross G (1986) Spin-lattice relaxation (T1) times of cerebral white matter in multiple sclerosis. Magn Res Med 3: 194-202
Larsson HBW, Frediksen JL, Oleson J, Henriksen O (1988) Assessment of demyelination, edema, and gliosis by in vivo determination of T1 and T2 in the brain of patients with an acute attack of multiple sclerosis. Soc.Magn.Res.Med. August 20-26, San Francisco, 764 (abstr)

Miller DH, Rudge P, Johnson G, Kendall BE, MacManus DG, Moseley IF, Barnes D, McDonald WI (1988) Serial gadolinium enhanced magnetic resonance imaging in multiple sclerosis. Brain 111:927-939

Moller JR, Yanagisawa K, Brady RO (1987) Myelin-associated glycoprotein in multiple sclerosis lesions: a quantitative and qualitative analysis. Ann Neurol 22: 469-474

Ormerod IEC, Johnson G, MacManus D, du Boulay EPGH, McDonald WI (1986) Relaxation times of apparently normal cerebral white matter in multiple sclerosis. Acta radiol Suppl 1:382-384

Ormerod IEC, Miller DH, McDonald WI, du Boulay EPGH, Rudge P,Kendall BE, Moseley IF, Johnson G, Tofts PS, Halliday AM, Bronstein AM, Scaravilli F, Harding AE, Barnes D, Zihlka KJ (1987) The role of NMR imaging of multiple sclerosis and isolated lesions: a quantitative study. Brain 110: 1579-1616

MR and CSF Findings in the Differentiation Between Optic Neuritis and Multiple Sclerosis

S. Cronqvist, M. Sandberg, and S. Holtås (Lund, Sweden)

Out of a series of 110 patients with unilateral optic neuritis, 26 patients with no neurological deficit symptoms were matched with regard to sex, age and observation time (7-12 years). These patients were further separated into two equally large groups: one with normal and one with abnormal CSF at the onset of the neuritis. MR was performed in 25 of these 26 patients. The examination showed parenchymal lesions compatible with MS plaques in 11 patients. Nine of these 11 belonged to the group with an abnormal CSF, only two to the one with normal CSF findings.

Using MR as an objective method to demonstrate MS lesions, the present study indicates that normal CSF at the onset of optic neuritis is a favourable prognostic sign.

AIDS

Neuroradiological Evaluation of AIDS Patients: A Prospective Study

S. Livian, G. Scotti, S. Pieralli, F. Triulzi, A. Visciani, G. Righi, M. Majno, A. Lazzarin, and A. Castagna

INTRODUCTION

Patients with Acquired Immunodeficiency Syndrome (AIDS) show a high frequency of neurological complications (up to 40%) (Rosenblum et al. 1988), caused by infective and/or neoplastic involvement of the Central Nervous System (CNS).
The role of cranial Computed Tomography (CT) in the diagnosis of CNS involvement in AIDS patients with neurological symptoms has been well established (Post et al. 1985; Levy et al. 1986). A few reports have also examined the effectiveness of Magnetic Resonance (MR) and compared CT and MR studies (Post et al. 1986, 1988). This work was undertaken to evaluate the neuroradiological findings in AIDS patients, to compare CT and MR studies and to correlate neuroradiological images with pathologic data.

MATERIALS AND METHODS

Between January and June 1988 72 neurologically symptomatic patients who fit the criteria for AIDS established by the Centers for Disease Control (CDC) were evaluated. There were 67 men and 5 women; the mean age was 31 years (range 21-65). Forty-two patients were drug abusers (58%),9 were homosexual-bisexual men (13%), 1 was an hemophiliac man; in 20 cases the risk factor was unknown.
Forty-nine patients were evaluated by CT only, 10 by MR only, 13 by both CT and MR. Sixteen patients were evaluated with follow-up CT.
CT examinations were performed on a TCT-60A Toshiba scanner, with plain and enhanced scans (intravenous injection of 30.6 g of iodine).The slice thickness was 5-10 mm. MR Images were obtained on a 1.5 T Siemens Magnetom MR imager, using Spin-Echo T1 (TR 600, TE 28) and T2 (TR 2000, TE 35-90) weighted sequences, with axial, coronal and sagittal sections with a slice thickness of 8 mm.
CT and/or MR images of 15 patients were compared with autoptic data.

RESULTS

CT: CT showed pathological findings in 49 out of 62 patients (78%). Atrophy was found in 20 patients (32%), multiple focal lesions in 12 (19%), single focal lesion in 11 (18%), diffuse white matter abnormalities in 6 (9%).
MR: MR examination was pathological in 20 out of 23 cases (87%). Diffuse white matter abnormalities was found in 8 patients (35%), atrophy in 6 (26%), single focal lesion in 4 (17%), multiple focal lesions in 2 (9%).

CT-MR: in 13 cases TC and MR examinations were compared. In 7 cases no diagnostic difference was found between CT and MR images (3 patients had a single focal lesion, 2 had atrophy and 2 had diffuse white matter abnormality). In 6 cases MR was superior to CT: in 2 cases MR showed white matter abnormalities not detectable by CT (CT was normal in one case and showed atrophy in one); in one case white matter abnormalities were more extensive on MR than on CT. In one case in which CT detected one focal lesion MR showed to more lesions (one in the basal ganglia and one in the white matter of the frontal lobe); in another patient MR showed multiple focal lesions also detected by CT, but in association with bilateral igromas not evident on CT (in this patient, however, MR examination was performed 39 days after the CT study). Another patient had on CT a diffuse white matter hypodensity and an isodense lesion in the head of the right caudate nucleus, in association with bilateral frontal hypodense subdural effusion. MR showed not only the diffuse white matter abnormality but also bilateral inhomogeneous abnormal signal at the level of the basal ganglia bilaterally, and extensive subdural effusion that was isointense in T1 weighted images and hyperintense in T2 weighted images (Fig. 1).
The results of autoptic examination of 15 patients are reported in table I. Eight patients had been evaluated with CT, 3 with MR, 4 with both CT and MR.
In the 6 patients with HIV encephalitis CT and MR showed atrophy and/or white matter abnormalities. In the 5 patients with toxoplasma encephalitis (of whom one had also a concomitant cryptococcal meningitis) multiple focal lesions were demonstrated by neuroradiological studies. The same findings were observed in one patient with Cytomegalovirus (CMV) encephalitis with concomitant HIV infection. Atrophy was found in the patient with CMV encephalitis and a single focal lesion in the patient with a diffuse malignant astrocytoma.

Table 1. Autoptic findings in 15 AIDS patients with neurological symptoms

HIV encephalitis: 6
Toxoplasma encephalitis: 4
CMV encephalitis: 1
Cryptococcal meningo-encephalitis: 1
Diffuse malignant astrocytoma: 1
CMV encephalitis + HIV infection : 1
Cryptococcal meningitis + Toxoplasma encephalitis : 1

DISCUSSION

Neuroradiological examinations of AIDS patients with neurological symptoms showed a wide range of abnormalities. With CT the most common finding was atrophy (32%). Other findings were focal lesions (multiple or single) and white matter abnormalities. In 22% of cases CT was normal.
The most common finding with MR was white matter abnormality (35%). In 13% of patients MR was normal.
MR was superior to CT in detecting white matter abnormalities, small focal lesions, and subdural effusions.
The most common autoptic diagnosis was HIV encephalitis. This encephalitis, previously called subacute encephalitis or AIDS encephalopathy, is almost certainly due to the direct infection of the brain by the virus HTLV-III (Shaw et al. 1985). Clinically HIV encephalitis often determines a characteristic demential syndrome (AIDS Dementia Complex) (Navia et al. 1986). Pathologically HIV encephalitis is characterized by microscopic microglial nodules associated with multinucleated giant

cells. The white matter shows areas of demyelination that can range from small foci to huge, confluent areas.

The CT and MR examinations of patients with HIV encephalitis showed atrophy in all the cases, sometimes associated with white matter abnormalities.

The white matter abnormalities, like those seen in patients with multiple sclerosis are best detected by MR examination than by CT, and may represent the areas of de-myelination seen microscopically.

This white matter abnormality is not, however, specific. Similar findings may, in fact, be also due to CMV encephalitis and Progressive Multifocal Leucoencephalo-pathy.

Multiple enhancing focal lesions are mainly due to Toxoplasma encephalitis, but other infective lesions or neoplastic diseases cannot be ruled out. Toxoplasma le-sions are preferentially localized in the basal ganglia region and at the cortico-medullary junction, and often show a good response to antitoxoplasma drugs.

Patients with cryptococcal infection may show signs of meningitis (ventricular and subarachnoidal spaces dilatation) or meningo-encephalitis (diffuse lesions in both white and gray matter). The diagnosis is confirmed by CSF examination.

In conclusion, MR seems to be the first choice examination in AIDS patients with neurological symptoms. Neither MR nor CT are, unfortunatelly, specific; other means such as CSF examination, response to therapy, and biopsy, are often required for a correct diagnosis.

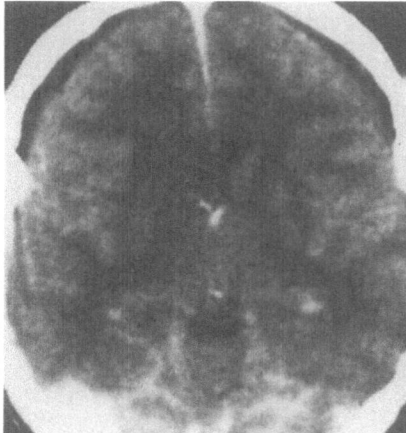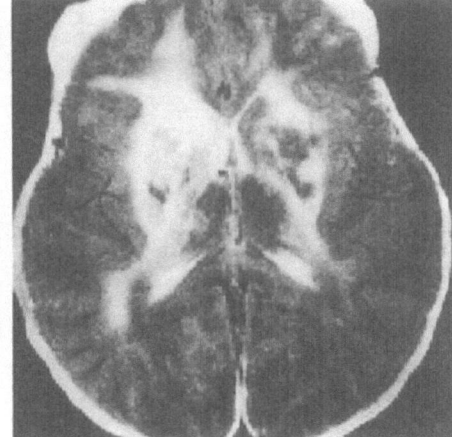

Fig 1 a,b. AIDS patient with cryptococcal meningo-encephalitis (autoptic diagnosis). CT (a) shows diffuse white matter hypodensity and a hypodense lesion in the head of the right caudate nucleus. Frontal subdural effusions are also present. MR (b:T2 weighted image) confirmes the white matter abnormality and shows bilateral inhomo-geneous signal alteration of the basal ganglia. The subdural effusion appears more extensive than on CT.

REFERENCES

Levy RM, Rosenblum S, Perret LV (1986) Neuroradiological findings in AIDS : a re-
    view of 200 cases. AJR 147:977–983
Navia BA, Jordan BD, Price RW (1986) The AIDS Dementia Complex:I. Clinical featu-
    res. Ann Neurol 19:517–524
Post MJD, Kursunoglu SJ, Hensley GT et al.(1985) Cranial CT in Acquired Immunodefi-
    ciency Syndrome: spectrum of disease and optimal contrast enhancement technique.
    AJR 145:929–940
Post MJD, Sheldon JJ, Hensley GT et al.(1986) Central Nervous System disease in Ac-
    quired Immunodeficiency Syndrome: prospective correlation using CT, MR imaging
    and pathologic studies. Radiology 158:141–148
Post MJD, Tate LG, Quencer RM (1988) CT, MR, and Pathology in HIV Encephalitis and
    Meningitis. AJNR 9:469–476
Rosenblum ML, Levy RM, Bredesen DE (1988) AIDS and the Nervous System. Raven Press,
    New York, p121
Shaw GM, Harper ME, Hahn BH et al.(1985) HTLV-III infection in brains of children
    and adults with AIDS encephalopathy. Science 227:177–182

Radiological Findings in HIV-Infected Patients in Relation to Neuropsychological Dysfunction and Immunological CSF Findings

R. Rainiko, I. Elovaara, E. Poutiainen, L. Valanne, and A. Virta

INTRODUCTION

Cerebral infection caused by the human immunodeficiency virus (HIV-1) itself, called HIV encephalopathy, is the most common neurological manifestation in the acquired immunodeficiency syndrome (AIDS). Cortical and central atrophy and white matter changes are common in AIDS patients (de la Paz and Enzmann 1988, Jarvik et al. 1988); yet data about the systematic neuroradiological evaluation of HIV-infected patients, especially in early infection, are scarce (Grant et al. 1987).

The present study was undertaken to evaluate MRI and CT findings in HIV-infected patients' having various stages of the infection, and to relate the results to cognitive abnormalities and to intrathecal humoral immune response.

PATIENTS AND METHODS

Fifty-one HIV-infected patients (49 men and two women, aged 18 to 62 years, median 35 years) were examined. Thirty-one patients had early stages of infection (ASX, LAS), and 20 had advanced stages (ARC, AIDS).

The evaluation comprised historical data, physical examination, determination of HIV antibodies and other relevant laboratory tests for each patient.

Forty-nine patients underwent a brain MRI and 48 a brain CT; most patients thus had both examinations. The MRI examinations were performed with an MR imager operating at 0.02 T. T_2 weighted axial slices using a pulse sequence of SE 2000/150 with four averages were routinely obtained. Other pulse sequences and sagittal slices were used in selected cases. The CT examinations were routinely performed without contrast enhancement. The MRI/CT findings were scored as 0 for normal and 1 for mild, 2 for moderate and 3 for severe atrophic changes.

Forty-eight patients underwent a neuropsychological examination. Intrathecal immune response was evaluated in 47 patients using cerebrospinal fluid (CSF) and blood samples. The parameters used in the study were intrathecal HIV antibody synthesis, intrathecal total IgG synthesis, blood-brain-barrier (BBB) impairment and the CSF leukocyte count.

The examinations used for comparisons were performed within two to three weeks.

RESULTS

Radiological findings

Four of the patients exhibited <u>parenchymal changes</u>. Each of them had bilateral lesions in lentiform nuclei, and three had diffuse periventricular white matter lesions in the frontoparietal regions. One patient had enhancing ring-like lesions on CT; toxoplasma infection was confirmed at autopsy. Parenchymal lesions other than toxoplasma abscesses were detected on MRI only.

<u>Atrophic changes</u> were found in 29 patients. They were usually mild, and ventricular enlargement was the most frequent finding (Table 1). Cortical atrophy was the most pronounced, and occurred most often in the temporal lobes. (Table 1 and the further analysis of the material pertain to only 50 patients, as the patient with toxoplasma infection was excluded from the analysis.)

Patients with advanced stages of infection (AIDS, ARC) had more severe central, cortical, and cerebellar atrophy than patients having early stages (LAS, ASX) (Table 2).

Table 1. Type of brain atrophy in 50 HIV-infected patients. The figures indicate numbers of patients. One patient may have more than one type of atrophy.

| | Scores for the severity of atrophy | | | |
	1	2	3	Total
Central	10	7	2	19
Cortical	9	5	1	15
Brain stem	10	1	1	12
Cerebellar	12	2	1	15

Table 2. Scores of atrophy (mean$\pm$SEM) in early and late stages of HIV infection.

Type of atrophy	Early N=31	Late N=19	p value
Central	0.3 ± 0.1	1.2 ± 0.3	<0.002
Cortical	0.4 ± 0.1	1.0 ± 0.3	<0.05
Brain stem	0.4 ± 0.1	0.7 ± 0.2	ns
Cerebellar	0.3 ± 0.1	0.8 ± 0.2	<0.05

Relation to cognitive dysfunction

Thirty-one patients, aged 26 to 62 years, had variable cognitive deficits whereas 17 patients, aged 18 to 61 years, were cognitively intact. The group with cognitive impairments comprised 16 patients with an advanced stage of infection and 15 with an early stage of infection. The group with intact cognitive functions consisted of three patients with an advanced stage of infection and 14 patients with an early stage of infection.

Atrophic changes were more frequent and more severe among patients with cognitive deficits than among cognitively intact HIV-infected individuals (Table 3).

The severity of cognitive decline correlated positively with the degree of central atrophy, brain stem atrophy, and cortical atrophy (r=0.68, r=0.54, r=0.51, p<0.001, respectively).

Two of the three patients with white matter lesions had dementia, and the third one had cognitive deficits, too.

Table 3. Number of patients with atrophic changes, and scores for atrophy in cognitively impaired (N=31) and cognitively intact (N=17) patients.

Type of atrophy	No. of patients with atrophy		Scores for atrophy		p value
	Cognit. impaired	Cognit. intact	Cognit. impaired	Cognit. intact	
Central	16	2	1.4 ± 0.3	0.2 ± 0.1	<0.0001
Cortical	13	1	1.1 ± 0.3	0.4 ± 0.1	<0.05
Brain stem	11	1	1.1 ± 0.3	0.3 ± 0.1	<0.005
Cerebellar	12	3	0.9 ± 0.3	0.2 ± 0.1	<0.05

Relation to intrathecal immune response

Patients with both normal and pathological brain MRI and/or CT findings had abnormal immune response. Each patient group showed intrathecal HIV antibody synthesis, but the difference did not reach statistical significance. Radiologically normal patients had elevated leukocyte count as compared to the radiologically abnormal group.

Immunological CSF abnormalities were found earlier than neuroradiological changes. HIV-associated CSF changes were found in seven neurologically and neuropsychologically intact patients with atrophic changes.

Follow-up results

The follow-up results are summarized in Table 4.

During the follow-up, the brain atrophy of 12 out of 21 patients showed progression, or if the primary examination had been normal, they developed atrophic changes.

Nine of the 17 patients re-evaluated neuropsychologically showed further deteoration of cognitive functions.

DISCUSSION AND CONCLUSIONS

Brain atrophy, which is a progressive process, was common in the HIV-infected patients studied, and it was also detected in patients with

Table 4. Neuroradiological, neuropsychological and CSF follow-up results

Method	No. of patients	Patients with progression
MRI/CT	21	12
Neuropsychological tests	17	9
Intrathecal HIV antibody synthesis	16	5
Intrathecal total IgG synthesis	16	-
Impaired BBB	16	2
CSF leukocyte count	16	-

early stages of infection. Its presence and severity correlated with cognitive dysfunction and the severity of HIV infection. White matter lesions were found in patients with dementia or severe cognitive deficits as has also recently been observed by others (de la Paz and Enzmann 1988, Price et al. 1988).

Mild atrophy and immunological CSF changes were found even in cognitively and neurologically intact patients. However, immunological HIV-associated CSF changes were found in patients without neurological, cognitive or radiological abnormalities.

The results suggest early organic brain involvement in HIV infection. They also indicate that disease of the central nervous system is a chronic process that takes some time to reach a clinical treshold.

REFERENCES

de la Paz R, Enzmann D (1988)Neuroradiology of acquired immunodeficiency syndrome. In: Rosenblum ML, Levy RM, Bredesen DE (eds) AIDS and the nervous system. Raven Press, New York, pp 121-153
Grant I, Atkinson H, Hesselink JR, et al. (1987) Evidence for early central nervous system involvement in the acquired immunodeficiency syndrome (AIDS) and other human immunodeficiency virus (HIV) infection. Ann Intern Med 107:828-836
Jarvik JG, Hesselink JR, Kennedy C, et al. (1988) Acquired immunodeficiency syndrome. Magnetic resonance patterns of brain involvement with pathological correlation. Arch Neurol 45:731-736
Price RW, Sidtis JJ, Navia BA, et al. (1988) The AIDS dementia complex. In: Rosenblum ML, Levy RM, Bredesen DE (eds) AIDS and the nervous system. Raven Press, New York, pp 203-219

Further Experience with the Diagnosis of Brain Diseases in 120 Patients with AIDS

J. Berkefeld, P. Harth, U. Woelki, H. Hacker, W. Schlote,
R. Söder, and W. Enzensberger

Introduction

Since our earlier CT examinations of 31 AIDS patients with central nervous disease (Hacker and Merdes 1986), we have extended our experience to a total of 127 cases. All patients presented with the full clinical picture of AIDS with manifestation of neurological disturbances, beginning with headache and meningitic reactions and extending to severe AIDS encephalopathy with development of progressive dementia. The patients, who suffered from opportunistic infections and lymphomas, often had supplementary focal neurological deficits.

A total of 127 adults aged 20-62 years (mean, 35.8 years) were examined. Only three of them were females. In 35 cases we obtained a histological diagnosis after death. Neuropathological reports (i.e., Gabuzda et al. 1986; Schlote et al. 1987) show that the probability that the HIV itself gives rise to encephalitis is high. Therefore it was our first interest to look for a relationship between suspected HIV encephalitis and CT morphology.

Method

All CT scans were performed on a Siemens Somatom 2N. A nonenhanced scan was followed by a late examination with 30-min delay after the application of a high dose of contrast medium (150 ml 300 mg% iodine). For the enhanced scans we used 4-mm thin slices. In addition to the usual scanning plane, some cuts parallel to the temporal horns were performed to evaluate one of the most common sites of virus encephalitis - the temporal lobes. This cutline also avoids some of the striking artifacts caused by the temporal bone.

Patients with suspected toxoplasmosis or other treatable lesions were followed up several times to control the success of treatment

438

and to confirm the diagnosis. Usually the first control was carried
out after four weeks. Altogether we did 208 examinations. Ten patients had additional MRI studies.

Results

Looking at the material, it does not seem difficult to order the CT
data systematically. Table 1 shows the different types of reaction
in the brain tissue, and Table 2 presents the corresponding clinical
and neuropathological diagnoses.

Table 1. Frequency of CT findings

	n	%
Normal CT	45	35.4
Mild and moderate atrophy	31	24.4
Severe and progressive atrophy	8	6.2
Encephalitic reactions	8	6.2
Granulomas	31	24.4
Tumors (lymphomas)	4	3.1
Cystic defects	10	7.8
Other lesions	3	2.4

Table 2. Clinical diagnosis and neuropathology

	n	%
Toxoplasmosis of CNS	21	16.5
Other granulomas	10	7.9
Aspergillosis	2	1.6
Cryptococcosis	3	2.4
Listeriosis	1	0.8
HSV encephalities	2	1.6
CMV encephalities	5	3.9
HIV encephalities (neuropathological)	12	9.4
CNS lymphoma	8	6.2

We saw normal CT scans in a high percentage of our cases. Most of
these patients suffered from headache or moderate forms of psycho-
organic syndromes. In four cases brainstem or cranical nerve lesions
were suspected which could be detected by MRI but not by CT. Eight

patients had the clinical signs of severe AIDS encephalopathy but showed normal CT scans.

The next largest group with similar but more severe symptoms showed the signs of moderate brain atrophy, with enlargement of the ventricles and widening of the sulci. Focal lesions were not detectable. The evaluation of this common finding is difficult. It may be the symptom of a diffuse chronic encephalopathy, possibly of HIV encephalitis. On the other hand, there are other explanations which do not presume an HIV-induced CNS desease. Most striking is the fact that many patients are in a bad general condition, with signs of cachexia and therefore resemble anorectic patients, where reversible brain atrophy has been shown by CT. Other possibilities are the side effects of corticoid medication, reaction to brain damage in early childhood, and toxic changes.

Only eight cases had severe, progressive atrophy related to the clinical symptoms of rapidly developing dementia. In two of them, diffuse subcortical areas of decreased density could be seen in the CT, and an HIV encephalities was confirmed by histology.

We described as encephalitic or encephalopathic reactions such diffuse or focal areas of decreased density in the white matter: these could be demonstrated in eight patients. This finding was always combined with atrophy. Besides the cases with HIV encephalities we found it in two patients with cytomegaly infection. Two others showed a typical herpes simplex encephalitis. Sometimes it was impossible to distinguish white matter lesions from the edema of a simultaneously existing toxoplasmosis granuloma.

Generally HIV encephalities cannot be detected reliably by CT. The signs of atrophy and white matter lesions are ambiguous and not specific. The detection rate of focal encephalitic lesions is low (in our series, 2 of 12). T2-weighted MRI is probably more sensitive in detecting these changes. In terms of neuropathology, we must remember that the nodules detected in the glial cells are very small. A predominant location is not known.

The diagnosis of granulomatous encephalitis, mostly toxoplasmosis, is easy if there are the typical nodular or ring-enhancing lesions. Toxoplasmosis prefers the basal ganglia area. After successful treatment the enhancing structures disappear, and small cystic defects often remain. In some cases the granulomas are indistinguishable from small compact lymphomas. Depending on the activity of the

440

immune system, toxoplasmosis may present in different, more diffusely growing forms with concentric ring structures. In recent months we have seen several nodular enhancing lesions which did not response to toxoplasmosis therapy and did not change size for many weeks.

Only four of eight lymphomas in autopsy could be detected by CT. There were two patients with diffusely growing CNS lymphomas mimicking encephalitis or malignant glioma. Rarer opportunistic infections (cryptococcosis, aspergillosis, listeriosis) caused a chronic meningitis without morphological changes observable by CT. In two cases (one cryptococcosis and one aspergillosis) granulomas occurred. The fungal infections were a part of the final phases of the disease, and the patients died after a few weeks.

CT and neuropathological examination show the multimorbidity of the brain. In the final stages several opportunistic infections and HIV encephalitis exist simultaneously. In CT the combination of atrophy and granulomas was most common in our series.

Summary

CT examination is still a valuable diagnostic tool for detection of CNS toxoplasmosis and other granulomas and lymphomas in AIDS patients. The diagnosis is not specific, and we must note that there are unusual, diffusely growing forms of granulomas and lymphomas. With the exception of typical HIV encephalitis, CT is less valuable than MRI for the diagnosis of viral CNS lesions or the HIV encephalitis itself. In spite of careful examination, detection rates are low and the findings are ambiguous. It remains to be proven whether MRI is consistently able to detect beginning encephalities or widespread microscopic encephalitis.

References

[1] Gabuzda DH, Ho DD, Monte SM, Hirsch MS, Rota TR, Sobel RA (1986) Immunohistochemical identification of HTLV-III antigen in brains of patients with AIDS. Ann Neurol 20: 289-295
[2] Hacker H, Merdes W (1987) CT-Befunde am Gehirn bei AIDS. In: Fischer PA, Schlote W (eds) AIDS und Nervensystem. Springer, Berlin Heidelberg New York, pp 64-72
[3] Schlote W, Vitzthum H, Thomas E, Hübner K, Stutte HJ, Woelki U, Kauss J (1987) Neuropathologische Beobachtungen in 28 Fällen von erworbenem Immundefektsyndrom (AIDS). In: Fischer PA, Schlote W (eds) AIDS und Nervensystem. Springer, Berlin Heidelberg New York, pp 85-116

Abnormalities of the White Matter Demonstrated by MR in 50 HIV Seropositive and 140 AIDS Patients

M. Boukobza, L. Feldman, P. Rolloy, Y. Michalik, M. Gentilini,
P. Brunet, and J. Metzger (Paris, France)

MR imaging was performed in 50 HIV seropositive and 140 AIDS patients, using T1 and T2 weighted spin-echo sequences. The appearance of the white matter was evaluated in each case. Pathologic changes in CNS white matter are usually due to viral encephalitis, in most cases to HIV, although CMV, herpes and others may be implicated. Areas of hypersignal are demonstrated on T2-weighted sequences, especially in the centrum semiovale, and occasionally in the internal capsules, brain stem and cerebellum.

These abnormalities are also encountered in more than one-third of patients without neurologic findings (AIDS and HIV seropositive asymptomatic).

A follow up is being done in two-thirds of the patients in these groups.

Prospective Study of Neurological Complications in HIV Infections Evaluated by MRI, CT and Clinical Examination

C. Pedersen, C. Thomsen, P. Arlien-Soborg, H. S. Hansen, F. Boesen, L. Kjaer, J. O. Nielsen, and J. Praestholm (Copenhagen, Denmark)

35 patients with AIDS, 15 patients with ARC and 21 asymptomatic anti-HIV positive individuals were enrolled in a prospective study of neurological complications in patients with HIV infections.

The patients were chosen randomly within each diagnostic category. MRI and CT were done every third month in patients with AIDS and every six months in ARC patients and the asymptomatic carriers.

Cerebral lesions were demonstrated on MR in 14/35 patients with AIDS (one tumor, two cysts, two leukencephalopathies, nine small focal lesions), in 5/15 patients with ARC (one cyst, one encephalitis, three small focal lesions), and in 2/21 asymptomatic carriers (one haemotoma and one arachnoid cyst).

At baseline examination CT only revealed lesions in four patients with AIDS, and none of the small focal lesions in the AIDS and ARC groups were revealed.

Neurological complications by HIV infections are common, and MR is a sensitive investigation to reveal lesions in an early stage of HIV infection, and often before neurological manifestations.

The study is still in progress, and the additional results from two further periods of six months' follow-up will be presented.

Veins

The Transcerebral Venous System

P. Lasjaunias

The transcerebral veins have long been known to be vascular channels
anastomosing the cortical veins to the deep venous system. They
have been analyzed and classified by several authors (Duret 1874;
Poirier and Charpy 1921; Testut 1911; Schlesinger 1939; Kaplan 1959;
Goetzen 1961; Huang and Wolf 1964; Jiminez and Lasjaunias 1988) and
considered as normal; they have been linked to developmental venous
anomalies (Lasjanias et al. 1986). The purpose of our work is to
describe this system and provide an approach to its physiological
and pathological significance.

Embryology-Anatomy

The cerebral benous drainage is cerebrofugal at the early stages of
venous development. The constitution of the telencephalon, diencephalon, ventricular system, and choroid plexus, and the thickening
of the ventricular walls, facilitate both the individualization of
the deep drainage and the appearance of a centripetal venous
drainage (Stephens and Stilwell 1969). Due to this, the transcerebral vascularization demonstrates the developmental hemodynamic
equilibrium and a bridging system available for the hemodynamic
changes occurring between the depth and the surface of the brain
(Padget 1957).

Among the cerebral veins, the transcerebral veins (Duvernoy et al.
1981; Hassler 1964; Oka et al. 1985; Ono et al. 1984; Yasargil and
Damur 1974) can be classified as follows:

- superficial medullary veins. These drain the white matter situated
  9.5 cm below the cortex towards the cortical veins; they anasto-
  mose with the deep veins.
- deep medullary veins. These drain the remaining white matter towards the subependymal veins; they are anastomosed with the superficial veins.

- <u>direct</u> <u>anastomotic</u> <u>veins</u>. The fan-shaped aspect of these transcerebral veins (between cortical and subependymal systems) accounts
  for their convergence at the superolateral angle of the lateral
  ventricle. They join either the medial draining system (septal)
  after a right-angle course ventral to the corpus callosum or the
  lateral one (caudate veins).
- <u>Interstriate</u> <u>anastomoses</u>. These join the superior and interior
  striate veins through the cerebral hemisphere at the junction
  between the diencephalon and telencephalon.

Angiographic Aspects

<u>Normal Aspects.</u> Because of their long course and their diameter
visualization of the deep medullary veins is inconstant in vivo
(Wolf and Huang 1964; Stein and Rosenbaum 1974). Only the deep
portion of the paracentricular medullary veins is seen, converging in a fan-shaped manner at the subependymal veins (Huang and
Wolf 1964).

<u>Arteriovenous Malformations (AVM).</u> Most frequently the drainage
of the AVM and that of the healthy brain communicate at a cerebral or sinusal level. In essence, AVMs provoke a venous hyper-
pressure; when they drain into a deep venous system (anatomically
convergent), this may become overloaded with an additional obstacle (acquired thrombosis or congenital agenesis). In this instance a transcerebral venous circulation is seen; it bypasses
the hemodynamic obstacle, usually located on the straight sinus,
to drain the venous system into the superior sagittal sinus.

The visualization of these transcerebral veins corresponds to that
of the early development of an anatomically normal system already
present in the 40-mm embryo and expresses a collateral circulation
capability. Knowledge of this transcerebral venous vascularization
allows a better understanding of the angioarchitecture of some hemispheric AVMs. It is sometimes difficult to differentiate a cortico subcortical AVM from a cortico ventricular one. A cortico subcortical AVM may drain into subependymal veins if a transcerebral
venous circulation develops. The absence of ventricular extension
is confirmed by the pure arterial cortical vascularization of the
lesion. On the other hand, a deeply situated AVM may present a
cortical drainage if the transcerebral venous system is elicited.
The absence of any arterial cortical vasculatization confirms the
deep localization of the lesion.

Developmental Venous Anomalies (DVAs). As described by Lasjaunias et al. (1986), DVAs illustrate the limits of variability of the transcerebral venous system. Superficial DVAs are superficial medullary veins draining deep medullary zones into cortical veins. Deep DVAs drain subcortical areas (normally dependent on superficial medullary veins) into a septal caudate vein or striate vein. In both cases these veins appear unusual but not pathological. They often represent an incidental radiological finding.

Physiology of the Transcerebral Venous System

Two different entities belong to the transcerebral venous system. The first is constituted by capillary venules of the white matter; their walls contain myosin filaments so that they remain patent even in case of zero or negative pressure (Auer and McKenzie 1984). They present the same microscopic characteristics as capillaries (blood-brain barrier). Their role is obviously both drainage and nutrition (exchange). They retain the same caliber throughout their course (blood-brain barrier).

The other one is formed by direct anastomotic channels stretched between cortical and subependymal veins. No obvious oriented flow can be described. They collect almost no afferent venules. They may be part of the cerebrospinal fluid hemodynamics control.

Conclusion

The transcerebral venous vascularization, although only partially understood, shows the exceptional flexibility of the cerebral vascular system. It may be developed in some exceptional cases and may regress secondarily after treatment of the pathology that enlarged it.

References

[1] Auer LM, McKenzie Et (1984) Physiology of the cerebral venous system. In: Kapp JP, Schmidek HH (eds) The cerebral venous system and its disorders. Grune and Stratton, New York
[2] Duret H (1987) Recherches anatomiques sur la circulation de l'encéphale. Arch Physiol Norm Pathol 6: 316-353
[3] Duvernoy H, Delon S, Vannson J (1981) Cortical blood vessels of the human brain. Brain Res Bull 7: 519-579
[4] Goetzen B (1961) Veins internes du cerveau humain. Arch Anat Pathol 12: 126-133

[5] Hassler O (1964) Angioarchitecture in hydrocephalus. An autopsy and experimental study with the aid of microangiography. Acta Neuropathol 4: 65-74

[6] Huang YP, Wolf BS (1964) Veins of the white matter of the cerebral hemispheres (the medullary veins). Diagnostic importance of the carotid angiography. Am J Roentgenol Ther Nucl Med 95: 808-821

[7] Jimenez JL, Lasjaunias P (1988) The transcerebral venous system. Surg Radioo Anat (in press)

[8] Kaplan H (1959) The transcerebral venous system. AMA Arch Neurol 1: 148-152

[9] Lasjaunias P, Burrows P, Planet C (1986) Developmental venous anomalies (DVA). The so-called venous anigoma. Neurosurg Rev. 9: 233-244

[10] Oka K, Rhoton A, Barry M, Rodriguez R (1985) Microsurgical anatomy of the superficial veins of the cerebrum. Neurosurgery 17: 711-748

[11] Ono M, Rhoton A, Peace D, Rodriguez R (1984) Microsurgical anatomy of the deep venous system of the brain. Neurosurgery 15: 621-657

[12] Padget D (1957) The development of the cranial venous system in man from the point of view of comparative anatomy. Contr. Embryol Carnegie Inst 611, 36: 79-140

[13] Schlesinger B (1939) The venous drainage of the brain with special reference to the Galenic system. Brain 62: 274-287

[14] Stein R, Rosenbaum A (1974) Deep supratentorial veins. In: Newton TH, Potis DG (eds) Radiology of the skull and brain, vol 2. Mosby, Saint Louis

[15] Stephens RB, Stilwell DL (1969) Arteries and veins of human brain. Thomas, Springfield, Ill.

[16] Testut L (1911) Traité d'anatomie humaine 6è édition. Vol II Doin, Paris, p 947

[17] Wolf B, Huang YP (1964) The subependymal veins of the lateral ventricle. Am J Roentgenol Radium Ther Nucl Med 91: 406-426

[18] Yasargil MG, Damur M (1974) Thrombosis of the cerebral veins and dural sinuses. In: Newton TH, Potts DG (eds) Radiology of the skull and brain, vol 2. Mosby, Saint Louis

Cerebral Venous Angiomas (CVA)
A Retrospective Study on 16 Patients

G. Huber and C. Piepgras

Venous angiomas consist of thin-walled vessels showing the characteristics of veins. The walls of these veins and the surrounding brain substance quite often show degenerative changes and gliosis (Cushing and Bailey 1928; Newton and Troost 1974).

The clinical significance of CVA is variable – they can be asymptomatic but could also be responsible for severe clinical disturbances: epileptic seizures, local symptoms, subarachnoid and parenchymal bleedings (Fierstien et al. 1979; Sartor et al. 1978; Yuko and Naotoshi 1981).

The aim of our study was to demonstrate the frequency with which CVA is associated with local parenchymal changes i.e. defects and calcifications, and to try and find an explanation for these findings.

MATERIAL AND METHODS

We found 17 cases of CVA in 16 patients amongst 3.249 angiograms performed at our Institute between 1.5.82 – 1.4.88 (Table 1). All patients underwent CT and angiography sometimes with repeat examinations. 12 patients were also examined by NMR and one patient underwent stereotaxic biopsy of the lesion.

RESULTS

Among the 17 examples of CVA (16 patients) we found 8 examples of calcification and 9 perifocal defects. 5 cases showed both defect and calcification, 3 calcification and defect, 5 defect without calcification. Only 4 cases showed no surrounding parenchymal changes (Table 2). In 2 patients a subacute parenchymal bleed was diagnosed. The surrounding parenchymal change of the lesions extended between 2 – 40 mm. The lesions show a predilection for the cerebral hemispheres but no side preference (Table 3).

Angiography revealed no arterial abnormality but demonstrated a leash of abnormal veins (a caput medusa) converging on a central lacuna or on a large central channel which drains into a persisting dysplastic vein. This vessel often shows atypical characteristics of proximal dilatation and distal tapering. Other lesions showed an abnormal reticular venous pattern with an especially intensive blush effect (Table 4).

Haemodynamically, almost all (16 out of 17) showed a definite prolonged perfusion time with prolongation of the venous phase. An early venous filling or large feeding artery typical of an AV-shunt were never evident.
On plain CT the lesions showed up as a hyperdensity; in some cases more morphological details of the lesion were shown after injection of contrast medium.

DISCUSSION

In our experience CVAs show a delayed perfusion as opposed to the high-flow angiomas. This characteristic slow blood flow is often responsible for the hyperdensity seen on plain CT.

We suppose that together, the slow perfusion and the abnormal vessel wall predispose to thrombosis with or without associated small haemorrhagic infarcts. The result of this localized haemodynamic disturbance is that regressive changes such as "defects", calcification and glioses develop in the tissue surrounding the lesion. The size and location of lesions vary and clinical symptoms are unpredictable. There is no direct correlation between the size of the angioma and the severity of the symptoms. Angiodysplasias are frequent associate findings (Table 4). Angiography gives the final diagnoses in cases where CVA is suspected on CT or NMR. CT is the method of choice for assessing the extent of regressive changes surrounding the lesion. Subacute parenchymal bleedings are best demonstrated by NMR.

CONCLUSION

- Definite CVAs are mostly found in combination with neighbouring secondary brain pathology.
- We are convinced that the brain changes and clinical symptoms result from the delayed venous drainage as well as from the insufficiency of the vessel wall of the malformation.
- The severity of the clinical symptoms shows no relation to size and form of the malformation.
- Angiography is the ultimate differentiating investigation. CT and NMR are very efficient pointers and define the extent of the associated brain changes.

Table 1. Case material (1.5.82 - 1.4.88), Institute of Neuroradiology, Homburg

Patients undergoing angiography	Patients with CVA	No of CVA
3.249	16 (6 F, 10 M)	17
	Age: females	13 - 43 ($\bar{x}$ 30.2) years
	males	13 - 54 ($\bar{x}$ 33.8) years

Table 2. CT and NMR results. 16 patients (17 CVA)

Calcifications	8
Perifocal secondary defect	9
Perifocal secondary defect and calcification	5
Calcification, no perifocal secondary defect	3
Perifocal secondary defect, no calcification	4
Neither calcification nor secondary defect	4
Subacute haemorrhage	2
More than one CVA (one supra-, one infra-tentorial)	1
Associated angiodysplasia	3

Table 3. Location of 17 CVA in 16 patients

Cerebral hemispheres (frontal and parietal lobes)		Subcortical nuclei and brain stem		Cerebellum	
Rt.	Lt.	Rt.	Lt.	Rt.	Lt.
4	6	1	2	4	-

Table 4. Angiographic morphology of 17 CVA (16 patients)

Radiating vessels with central lacuna	6
Radiating vessels with central venous channel	1
Reticular network and blush effect	10
Dysplasia of internal cerebral venous system	14

REFERENCES

Cushing H, Bailey P (1978) Tumors arising from the blood vessels
    of the brain: angiomatous malformations and hemangioblastomas.
    Springfield, Illinois, 3-34
Fierstien SB, Pribram HW, Hieshima G (1979) Angiography and
    computed tomography in the evaluation of cerebral venous
    malformations. Neuroradiology 17: 137-148
Newton TH, Troost BT (1974) Arteriovenous malformations and
    fistulae. In: Newton TH, Potts DG (eds) Radiology of the skull
    and brain angiography, vol 2, Book 4. Mosby, Saint Louis,
    p 2490
Sartor K, Fliedner E, Weber K (1978) Venöse Angiome des Gehirns.
    Fortschr.Röntgenstr. 128: 171-176
Yuko S, Naotoshi K (1981) Cerebral venous angiomas. Radiology
    139: 87-94

MR Diagnosis of Cerebral Venous Thrombosis

C. F. Andreula, P. d'Aprile, R. Paladini, and A. Carella

Introduction

The use of MR, independent of the field strength, can solve the problem
of diagnosing cerebral venous thrombosis, avoiding contrast media and/
or vessel pucture. In fact, the easily detectable hyperintense signal
within venous structures, revealed in T1-weighted images and persisting in T2-weighted images, confirms the clinical hypothesis of cerebral venous thrombosis without any further examinations being performed.

The higher sensitivity of MR allows venous infarcts and hemorragic
seffusions, sometimes not detected by CT, to be shown.

Materials and Methods

We used the MR MAX System by General Electrics with a superconductive
magnet operating at 0.5 Tesla. The spin-echo pulse sequence were used
with TR 600 ms and TE 30 ms for T1-weighted images and with TR 2000 ms
and TE 20-100 ms for proton-density images and T2-weighted images.
Images were obtained in the axial, coronal and sagittal planes. The
results of CT, MR, and angiographic studies of two representative patients were examined (Figs.1-8).

Discussion

The vagueness of the neurological symptoms and the suspicion arising
from CT findings in cerebral venous thrombosis mean that an angiographic study must be done. The CT findings ("delta sign," cord sign),
hyperdensity within dural sinuses detected when scanning along the
long axis of the vessels and an even more unspecific cortical gyri
enhancement, and venous infarcts or venous stasis in the watershed
territory between the deep and cortical veins are not strictly patho-

gnomonic. However, MR can play a fundamental role in diagnosis of cerebral venous thrombosis. The presence of a hyperintense signal in cerebral dural sinuses in heavily T1-weighted images (short TR and short
TE), T1-weighted images (long TR and short TE), and T2-weighted images
(long TR and long TE) can be assumed pathognomonic of a thrombosed venous vessel. As is well known, there is no signal from vascular structures with high flow rates because magnetized protons escape from the
voxel examined. The doubts arising because of the so-called paradoxic
effect of the blood flow in slow structures can be removed by doing
examination in several planes and using pulse sequences that allow
complete recovery of the protons.

Conclusions

The easily detectable bright MR signals within thrombosed venous
vessels, in sharp contrast with uninvolved contralateral veins, confirms the diagnosis of venous thrombosis without any need for further
examination, and MR should be the imaging modality of choice in such
a pathology.

References

[1] Bauer WM, Einhaupl K, Heywang SH, Vogl T, Seiderer M, Clados D
    (1987) MR of venous sinus thrombosis: a case report. AJNR 8:
    713-715
[2] Bradley WG, Waluch V (1985) Blood flow: magnetic resonance
    imaging. Radiology 154: 443-450
[3] Erdman WA, Weinreb JC, Cohen JM, MAximilian-Buja L, Chaney C,
    Peshock RM (1986) Venous thrombosis: clinical and experimental
    MR imaging. Radiology 161: 233-238
[4] Howard Lee S, Rao KCVG (1983) Cranial computed tomography.
    McGraw-Hill, New York, 631-640
[5] Macchi PJ, Grossman RI, Gomori JM, Goldberg HI, Zimmerman RA,
    Bilaniuk LT (1986) High field MR imaging of cerebral venous
    thrombosis. J Comput Assist Tomog 10: 10-15
[6] Maursen White E, Edelman RR, Wedeen VJ, Brady TJ (1986) Intra-
    vascular signal in MR imaging: use of phase display for differen-
    tiation of blood-flow signal from intraluminal disease. Radiology
    161: 245-259
[7] McMurdo-SK, Brant-Zawadzki M, Bradley WG, chang GY, Berg BO
    (1986) Dural sinus thrombosis: Study using intermediate field
    strength MR imaging. Radiology 161: 83-86
[8] Mills CM, Brant-Zawadzki M, Crooks LE, Kaufman L, Sheldon P,
    Norman D, Bank W, Newton TH (1983) Nuclear magnetic resonance:
    Principles of blood flow imaging. AJNR 4: 1161-1166

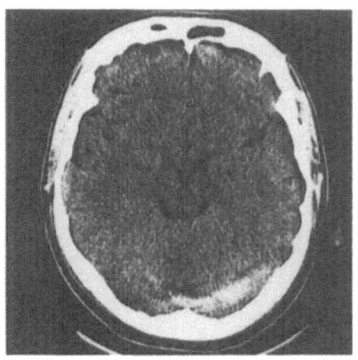 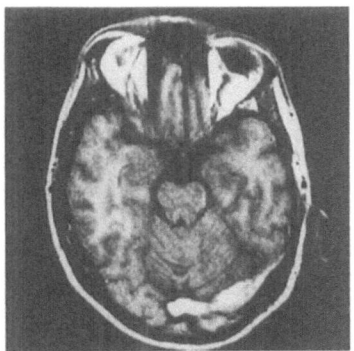

Fig.1. Case 1. CT scan shows hyperdensity along the right transverse sinus

Fig.2. Case 1. MR T1-weighted image shows hyperintense signal in the right transverse sinus and torcular Herophili

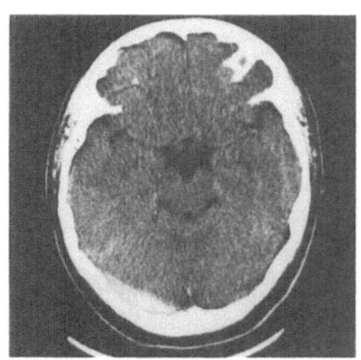 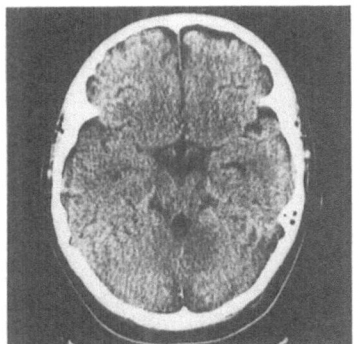

Fig.3. Case 2. CT scan shows hyperdensity along the left transverse sinus

Fig.4. Case 2. CT scan 3 months after thrombotic episode: left transverse sinus completely recanalized

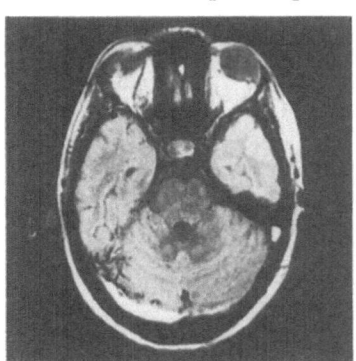 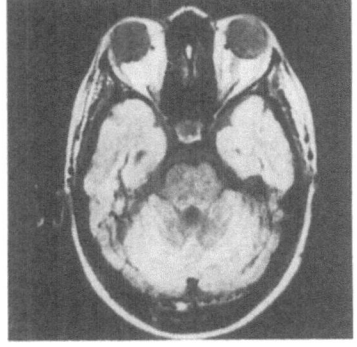

Fig.5. Case 2. MR T1-weighted image shows hyperintense signal in the left transverse sinus

Fig.6. Case 2. MR T1-weighted image shows almost completed recanalization of transverse sinus

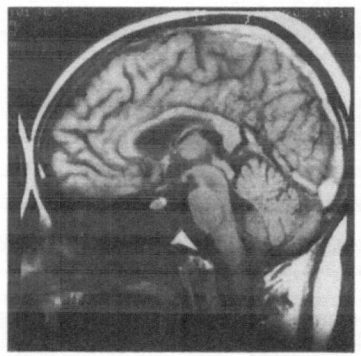 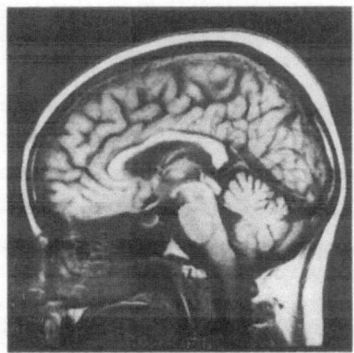

Fig.7. Case 2. MR T1-weighted image shows hyperintense signal in the superior sagittal sinus, torcular Herophili, straight sinus

Fig.8. Case 2. MR T1-weighted image: flow imaging in the sinuses shows complete resolution

Intracranial Medullary Venous Malformations

U. Bergvall, T. Powell, P. S. Dias, and D. M. C. Forster (Sheffield, England)

Intracranial medullary venous malformations (MVM) may be diagnosed by radionuclide brain scanning, angiography, x-ray CT or MRI. A substantial fraction of these malformations present as incidental findings on examinations indicated by symptoms or signs which are not compatible with the site or extension of the MVM.

During the last few years we have been confronted by 14 cases of MVM, some of which have been referred for therapeutic decisions within the framework of stereotaxic irradiation (radiosurgery according to the Leksell technique).

Not enough is known of the natural history of MVM to constitute a rationale for treatment. The purpose of this presentation is threefold:

1) to point to the existence of MVM and the problem of therapeutic decisions;
2) to propose a diagnostic protocol;
3) to invite observations of single cases or small series from other centres, with the aim to elicit characteristics of the natural history of MVM from a larger pooled material and the ultimate goal of creating a basis for choice of therapy.

Evolution of Dural Sinus Thrombosis. A Study with Magnetic Resonance Imaging

D. Dormont, C. Debussche, J. Chiras, M. Dubs, M. G. Bousser, and J. Bories (Paris, France)

The utility of magnetic resonance imaging (MR) for the diagnosis of dural sinus thrombosis (DST) has already been reported. The purpose of our study was to correlate MR findings with angiography, to describe the MR appearance of venous infarctions and to evaluate the ability of MR to follow the evolution of DST.

12 patients with angiographically proven DST were studied with MR at 0.5 T. 20 MR examinations were performed. In all patients, we used sagittal T1 weighted (T1w) and coronal T2 weighted (TR = 2000, TE = 60, 3 echoes) slices. Patients were studied between 9 and 21 days after the onset of symptoms in 7 cases and between 1 and 3 months in 5 cases. MR controls were performed in 8 cases. In all cases, abnormally high signal was observed on all echoes within the affected dural sinus. Hypersignal of dural sinus on T1w images was seen only in cases studied during the first 3 weeks of evolution. Haemorrhagic venous infarctions were observed in 6 cases. They presented a hypersignal both on T1W and T2w slices and were surrounded by a thin region of hyposignal. Partial repermeabilization of dural sinus was seen in 5 cases on follow-up studies, but we never observed a complete normaliyation of dural sinus signal.

In conclusion, we observed that MR findings are well correlated with angiography. MR is highly sensitive to haemorrhagic infarctions. Follow-up studies using MR give important informations about the evolution of DST.

Sella

Correlative Study Between Computed Tomography and Magnetic Resonance Imaging of Pituitary Gland in 80 Patients with Hyperprolactinemia

M. Gallucci, A. Bozzao, A. Splendiani, I. Amicarelli, C. Masciocchi,
B. Beomonte Zobel, and R. Passariello

Introduction

The possibility of studying sellar and parasellar regions with CT
(Brown et al. 1983; Hemminghytt et al. 1983) and MR (Mark et al.
1984; Bilaniuk et al. 1984), taking in consideration both parenchymal
and bone structures, offers a great opportunity for the evaluation
of pituitary neoplasms. Doubts still persist about small ones, particularly under 10 mm in diameter (microadenomas) since recent studies
report possible false-positive CT findings of over 40% (Kendall
1983; Chambers et al. 1982). On the other hand, autopsy series found
a microadenoma in 22.5%-45% of endocrinologically normal patients
(McComb et al. 1982; Parent et al. 1982; Taylor and Jaffe 1983). The
presence of a prolactin (PRL) secreting microadenoma is the most
frequent occurrence. Currently, these tumors are successfully treated
with medical therapy, which is able to avoid surgery in most cases
(McComb et al. 1982; Parent et al. 1982). Therefore, only a strict
clinical correlation can support the radiological evaluation. For
this reason, if the diagnosis of hyperprolactinemia needs laboratory
assay, that of prolactinoma needs the demonstration of morphological
alterations of the pituitary gland. Moreover, since medical therapy
needs a morphological follow-up, MR could be first choice for the
safer ability to investigate the pituitary gland.

In the following study we tried to correlate CT and MR findings in
patients with laboratory-tested hyperprolactinemia.

Subjects and Methods

A total of 80 patients, 71 women and 9 men (age, 12-47 years; mean,
32), with an increased PRL serum level (over 30 ng/ml) were examined.
In order to achieve comparable and homogeneous case histories, we

excluded those with pituitary neoplasms over 10 mm in diameter (macroadenomas) and with other sellar or parasellar pathology. PRL levels were evaluated with radioimmunologic assay (RIA) over three tests performed in 1 h. Patients with PRL serum levels over 30 ng/ml were included in our study and underwent a CT and an MR scan. CT scans were obtained in 50 patients with a Siemens Somatom 2 and in 30 with a Siemens Somatom DRH, performing continguous coronal slices of 2 mm thickness. Postcontrast CT scan was obtained using Iopamiro 370, 100-150 ml, 50-100 ml in rapid infusion.

MR was performed with an Esaote-Biomedica Esatom/5000 unit working at 0.5 T. We performed coronal scans, 3 mm thickness, 1 mm gap, FOV 17.4 cm, matrix 256 × 256, using spin-echo (SE) sequences with a repetition time (TR) of 600 ms and an echo time (TE) of 30 ms and multi-echo (ME) sequences with TR 2000 ms and TE 30/70/120 ms. Sagittal MR scans were acquired with SE technique, TR 350 ms, TE 30 ms, 3 mm thickness, FOV 18.98, matrix 256 × 256. CT scan and MR were evaluated independently and blindly by two different radiologists.

Results

Out of 80 patients, 40 showed a CT scan compatible with the presence of a microadenoma and nine showed only indirect signs of the lesion (two focal convexities, six peduncle displacements, two of which also had convexity of the upper surface, and two exclusively sellar floor ballooning). CT scan findings before and after intravenous contrast enhancement showed the following distribution: in 31 cases the lesion appeared hypodense before and after intravenous injection; in 9, hypodense before and hyperdense after. MR showed a lesion compatible with the presence of a microadenoma in 50/80 patients, and only indirect signs of the pathology in six (three peduncle displacements, in two cases associated with focal convexity of the upper surface, one sellar floor ballooning, and two focal convexities). T1-weighted sequences showed the lesion in all 50 cases mentioned; it appeared to be hypointense in 46 cases and hyperintense in 4. Long TR/TE images showed lesions in 35 cases; they appeared as hyperintense focal areas inside the normal parenchyma.

Thirty-one cases were normal or doubtful at CT examinations, 24 at MR, with an overlapping of results in 10. Out of seven mentioned cases who had a negative CT and a probative MR picture five were less than 6 mm in diameter (6 in two cases, 5 and 3 mm respectively in the others) and two over 8 mm.

Considering both examinations, we were able to detect a pituitary abnormality that could suggest the presence of a microadenoma in 70 patients.

Discussion

In our study, MR seemed to be superior to CT in detecting PRL-secreting pituitary microadenomas. MR showed the lesion directly or with indirect signs in 13 patients in which CT scan was judged negative; on the other hand, in only six cases did CT scan rule out morphological alterations not demonstrated by MR. In eight cases each, MR and CT were considered to offer better diagnostic information than the other.

These data agree with a recent study of Kulkarni et al. (1988) showing MR superior to CT in detecting pituitary microadenoma, even though this author acquired his images with Inversion Recovery sequences and cardiac gating.

In our experience, the most useful sequences were the short TR/TE ones, judged diagnostic in 50/80 cases. This observation is probably due to the unfavorable signal to noise ratio that penalizes thinner long TR/TE scans necessary in this kind of study.

Hypointense lesions in respect to normal parenchyma are typical findings of pituitary microadenomas in short TR/TE sequences (Pojounas et al. 1986). This finding was also confirmed in our study since we found a hypointense lesion in most cases (46/50).

The four hyperintense focal lesions observed with short TR/TE images are probably due to a hemorrhage inside the neoplasm, resulting in blood products like methemoglobin, with its typical paramagnetic effect (Gomori et al. 1985; Fig.1).

It is interesting to notice that in all these patients long-term medical bromocriptine therapy was performed. In these cases, the cellular alteration, probably related to the therapy, could develop (Pojounas et al. 1986) and promote bleeding inside the neoplasm. On long TR/TE images the typical finding we obtained was a focal hyperintensity inside the normal parenchyma (Fig.2.)

The observation of ten patients who did not show morphological alterations of the pituitary gland even in the presence of a PRL serum level over 30 ng/ml is particularly interesting. This again

464

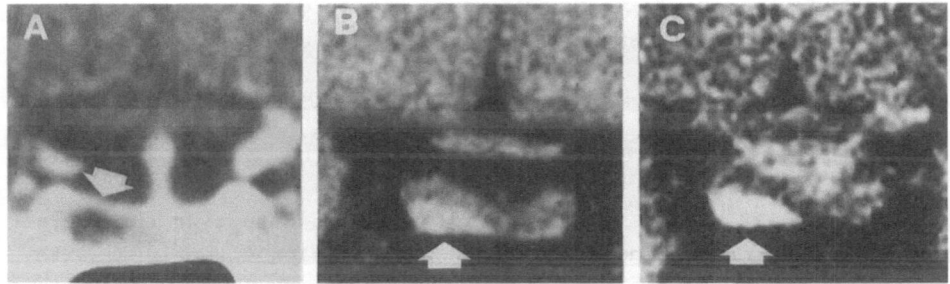

Fig.1. A Postcontrast coronal CT scan shows a well-defined focal
hypodensity (arrow) inside a gland with a slightly abnormal height.
The same lesion has high signal intensity in both T1 (B) and T2 (C)
weighted sequences (arrows). The patient was treated with bromocriptine during the 3 years prior to examination

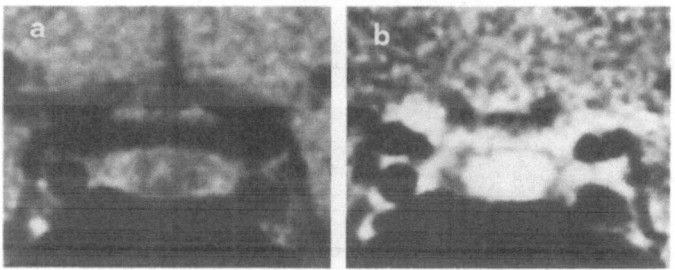

Fig.2a,b. Typical MR findings of a PRL-secreting microadenoma. The
lesion appears as hypointense in short TR/TE SE sequences (a) and
hyperintense in long TR/TE ones (b)

shows that clinical correlation is extremely important in the diagnosis of microadenomas even in the presence of a definite morphological alteration.

In conclusion, our data show that, in patients suspected of harboring prolactinomas, MR must be considered the first-choice examination as well as short TR/TE sequences the best ones (probably
enough to achieve a correct diagnosis in most cases). Moreover, we
underline that MR is an easy and safe examination in the follow-up
of patients treated with medical therapy.

Acknowledgements. We are grateful to the Limmat-Stiftung Foundation
(Zurich, Switzerland) for economical support; many thanks also to
Carmelita Marinelli for help in manuscript preparation.

References

[1]   Bilaniuk LT, Zimmerman RA, Wehrli FW, Snyder PJ, Goldberg HI
      et al. (1984) MRI of pituitary lesions using 1.0 to 1.5 T.
      field strength. Radiology 153: 415-418
[2]   Brown SB, Irwin KM, Enzmann DR (1983) CT characteristics of
      the normal pituitary gland. Neuroradiology 24: 259-262
[3]   Chambers EF, Turski PA, Lamasters D, Newton TH (1982) Regions
      of low density in the contrast enhanced pituitary gland. Ra-
      diology 144: 109-113
[4]   Gomori JM, Grossman RI, Goldberg HI, Zimmerman RA, Bilaniuk LT
      (1985) Intracranial hematomas: imaging by high-field MR. Ra-
      diology 157: 87-93
[5]   Hemminghytt S, Kalkkhoff RK, Daniels DL, Williams AL, Grogan JP,
      Haughton VM (1983) Computed tomography study of hormone-secre-
      ting microadenomas. Radiology 146: 65-69
[6]   Kendall B (1983) Current approaches to hypothalamic-pituitary
      radiology. Clin Endocrinal Metab 12 (3): 535-565
[7]   Kucharczyk W, Davis DO, Kelly WQM, Sze G, Norman D, Newton TH
      (1983) Pituitary adenomas: high-resolution MR imaging at 1.5 T.
      Radiology 161: 761-765
[8]   Mark L, Peach P, Charles C, Williams A, Haughton V (1984) The
      pituitary ossa: a correlative anatomic and MR study. Radiology
      153: 415-418
[9]   McComb DJ, Ryan N, Horvath E, Kovacs K (1982) Subclinical ade-
      nomas of the human pituitary. Arch Pathol Lab Med 107: 488-491
[10] Parent D, Brown B, Smith EE (1982) Incidental pituitary adeno-
      mas: a retrospective study. Surgery 92: 880-883
[11] Pojounas KW, Daniels LD, Williams AL, Haughton VM (1986) MR
      imaging of prolactin-secreting microadenomas. AJNR 7: 209-213
[12] Taylor CR, Jaffe CC (1983) Methodological problems in clinical
      radiology research: pituitary microadenoma detection as a para-
      digm. Radiology 147: 279-283

MRI of Pituitary Adenomas: Comparison with CT

G. C. Dooms, P. Mathurin, G. Cornelis, and R. Demeure (Brussels, Belgium)

A prospective study was performed to compare the results of CT and
MRI for detecting pituitary adenomas. Fifty consecutive unselected
patients (40 females and 10 males, mean age 37 years) were studied
by both modalities, which were always performed within a one week interval. The results were interpreted independently by two different
authors. Findings were confirmed by follow up (clinical data and repeated examination), surgery, or biological data for each patient.
CT exams were performed with state of the art equipment (Philips
Tomoscan 350 mainly) and with IV contrast bolus, at least in the
direct coronal plane. MR was performed with a superconducting magnet
Philips Gyroscan S15 operating at 1.5 Tesla. Coronal and sagittal T1
weighted images (TR = 0.47 sec and TE = 300 msec) were obtained in
every patient (4 averages, field of view = 200 mm, 3 mm slice thickness, with 0.6 mm gap between contiguous sections). Results of both
modalities were identical in all patients with macroadenomas (> 10 mm;
25 patients). However, distinction between empty sella and necrotic
(or cystic) macrodenomas was easier with MRI than with CT (2 patients). Furthermore, the chiasmatic compression by the tumoral process (18 patients) was always better demonstrated by MRI than by CT.

Results of both modalities were identical in 15 out of 25 patients
with microadenomas (< 10 mm). In four patients, MRI detected the microadenomas while CT was considered as negative. The reverse was true
for the six remaining patients. In conclusion, MRI appears to be a
very sensitive modality for detecting pituitary micro- or macroadenomas. It has also many advantages over CT (such as ease of examination in supine position), making it a very good tool for diagnosing
those particular disorders.

MRI of Pituitary Adenomas: Role of Gd-DTPA

G. C. Dooms, P. Mathurin, G. Cornelis, and R. Demeure (Brussels, Belgium)

A prospective study was performed to assess the role of Gd-DTPA in the detection of pituitary adenomas. Fifty consecutive unselected patients (40 females and 10 males, mean age 37 years) were studied by MRI, before and after Gd-DTPA IV injection. The results of both techniques were interpreted independently by two different authors. MR was performed with a superconducting magnet Philips Gyroscan S15 operating at 1.5 Tesla. Coronal and sagittal T1 weighted images (TR = 0.47 sec and TE = 30 msec) were obtained in every patient (4 averages, field of view = 200 mm, 3 mm slice thickness with a 0.6 mm gap between contiguous sections). The same imaging technique was repeated directly after IV injection of Gd-DTPA (0.2 ml/kg body weight). The use of Gd-DTPA did not improve the detection of macroadenomas (25 patients). However, the limits of the tumoral process were better defined after IV injection in 6 patients in which some normal residual pituitary tissue was present. Gd-DTPA did not improve the demonstration of the tumoral extension (either supra- or infrasellar, or laterally into the cavernous sinus). The use of Gd-DTPA masked the microadenoma (which was detected on the precontrast MR study) in 3 out of 19 patients with microadenomas. Conversely, it revealed the microadenomas (which were not detected on the precontrast MR study) in the 6 remaining patients.

In conclusion, the usefulness of Gd-DTPA seems to be relatively limited for macroadenomas. However, it seems to reveal microadenomas which are not detected on the noncontrast MR exams. Therefore, association of pre- and postcontrast MR studies appears to detect nearly all microadenomas, which is essential concerning the sensitivity of the imaging modality.

MR Imaging Detection of Pituitary and Brain Anomalies in Pituitary Dwarfs

F. Triulzi, G. Scotti, S. Pieralli, C. Righi, A. Visciani, and S. Livian

INTRODUCTION

Idiophatic deficiency of growth hormone (IGHD) is the most common cause of pituitary dwarfism. Relationship with birth trauma (Shizume et al. 1977) and radiological pituitary abnormalities were reported, even though a clear syndrome was never demonstrated. In 1964 Fisher and Di Chiro reported a high percentage of small sellae in IGHD patients with onset of hypopituitary symptoms before the age of 6 years. This observation was later supported by CT scan (Stanhope et al. 1986; Inoue et al. 1986) that confirmed the high frequency of both sella and pituitary hypoplasia, also associated with the failure in the detection of the pituitary stalk. 1.5 T MR imaging with thin slice (3 mm) T1-weighted images (T1-WI) technique, is the most accurate diagnostic tool in the depiction of the sellar and parasellar anatomy (Fujisawa et al. 1987a). Moreover it is now confidently proven that MR imaging can differentiate anterior pituitary (adenohypophysis) from posterior pituitary (neurohypophysis) (Colombo et al. 1987). For these reasons it was recently used for a better evaluation of the pituitary anomalies in IGHD patients. The preliminary MR imaging reports (Fujisawa et al. 1987b; Triulzi et al. 1987; di Natale et al. 1987; Kelly et al. 1988) showed a recurrent hypothalamic-hypophyseal abnormality (Fig. 1) that can be summarized as follows: a) severe hypoplasia of both sella and pituitary gland with absence of posterior pituitary hyperintensity; b) absence of the pituitary stalk with evidence of a residual infundibular nodule; c) T1-WI hyperintensity at the level of the residual stalk (posterior pituitary ectopia). In order to evaluate on a large population these preliminary MR findings and to correlate them with the endocrinological data we studied 59 patients with IGHD by MR imaging at 1.5 T.

MATERIALS AND METHODS

Fiftynine patients with growth retardation and IGHD (46 males, 13 females) aged from 4,3 years to 27,6 years, were admitted to the study. Diagnosis of GH deficiency was made with clonidine, arginine or insuline stimulation tests. A TRH test was performed in order to evaluate the tyroid axis; adrenal axis was evaluated by cortisol and ACTH rythm. Gonadotropin response to LHRH was performed only in the eldest patients, because of the non significant response in young children. Fluid balance was normal in all patients. According to the endocrinological evaluation 21 patients had a multiple pituitary hormone deficiency and 38 patients an isolated growth hormone deficiency. Primary hypothalamic or pituitary deficiency was equally distributed in the two groups. Delivery was normal in 33 patients, podalic presentation was reported in 19 patients of whom 4 had perinatal asphyxia. Perinatal asphyxia was reported also in 6 patients with normal presentation. MR imaging studies were undertaken with a 1.5 T unit and spin-echo T1-WI technique (TR 600 ms, TE 28 ms, 4 acquisition). Sagittal and coronal 3 or 4 mm thick sections, with matrix size of 265x256 pixels and field of view of about 20 cm were obtai

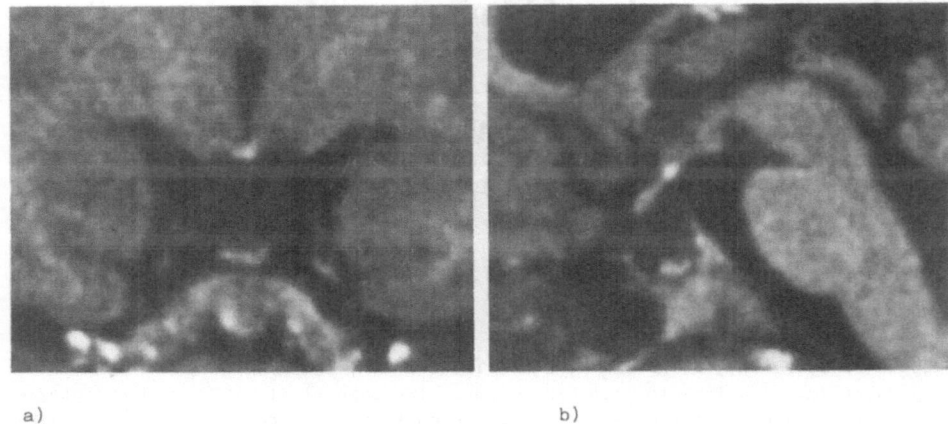

a)   b)

Fig 1. Coronal (a) and sagittal (b), 3 mm thick, T1-WI in a IGHD patient. All MR
typical findings are clearly visible: hypoplasia of the pituitary gland, absence
of the pituitary stalk and posterior pituitary ectopia.

ned. MR imaging studies were qualitatively evaluated in order to assess presence,
size, shape and signal intensity of hypothalamic-pituitary structures. With sagittal and coronal sections it was also possible to evaluate the midline structures
of the brain.

RESULTS

Based on the MR imaging findings two groups of patients can be clearly defined.

Group A – Posterior pituitary ectopia
In 35 out of 59 patients (59%) the posterior pituitary hyperintensity was not detectable in the posterior aspect of the pituitary fossa, while a nodular, 2-3 mm
sized hyperintensity was found at the level of the infundibular recess. In all but
two cases (33 patients) the pituitary stalk was also separate from the gland with
different degrees of length: from the complete absence to a 4-5 mm "drop-shaped"
infundibular prominence. In two cases a very thin stalk connected the hypothalamus
to the hypophysis, but a nodular hyperintensity was detected at the level of the
infundibular recess and not in the pituitary fossa. In all the cases both sella
turcica and pituitary gland were either very small or aplastic. Associated brain a
nomalies were also found at MR imaging examination: one patient showed a septum
pellucidum agenesis, while in two cases a tonsillar ectopia (Chiari I malformation)
was detected. In this group 20 patients had multiple pituitary hormone deficiency
and 15 isolated growth hormone deficiency. In 16 patients podalic delivery was reported of whom 4 had perinatal asphyxia. Two patients had perinatal asphyxia with
cephalic delivery.

Group B – Normal posterior pituitary
In 24 patients the posterior pituitary hyperintensity was normally detected, even
though the sellar and pituitary size was frequently reduced. The pituitary stalk
was detected in all cases; as a rule it was thin or very thin when the gland was
hypoplastic. Also in this group congenital brain anomalies were detected: one ca-

se of septo-optic displasia with hypoplasia of pituitary gland, pituitary stalk
and optic nerves associated with an agenesia of the septum pellucidum and also with
a Chiari I anomaly; one case of partial agenesis of the corpus callosum and one ca
se of agenesis of the septum pellucidum. In this group only one patient, the eldest, had a multiple hormone deficiency while the other 23 patients had isolated gro
wth hormone deficiency. In 3 patients podalic delivery was reported; 4 patients
had perinatal asphyxia with cephalic delivery.

DISCUSSION

The previous preliminary MR imaging findings of morphostructural abnormalities in
the pituitary gland and stalk of IGHD patients are definitely confirmed in a series of 59 patients. About 60% of IGHD patients showed at MR imaging study a nodular
T1-WI infundibular hyperintensity associated with the absence of the normal posterior pituitary hyperintensity. This finding in patients with normal ADH secretion
and high frequency of pituitary stalk anomalies (e.g. the failed connection betwe-
en hypothalamus and pituitary) suggests an ectopic location of the terminal part
of the neurohypophyseal axons that arise from supraoptic and paraventricular hypothalamic nuclei. Fujisawa and coll., that first described this anomaly, stressed
the role that abnormal delivery and/or perinatal asphyxia can play in the damage
of the hypothalamus and of the pituitary portal system. It is well-known that abnor
mal delivery and history of perinatal asphyxia was reported in about 50-60% of
children later shown to have hypopituitarism and our study confirms this high frequency of abnormal birth. However, even though a traumatic perinatal accident cannot be ruled out in a part of IGHD patients, the pathogenesis of posterior pituitary ectopia and stalk abnormalities in patients with normal delivery was, at present, undemonstrated. While adenohypophysis develops from superiorly displaced
cells from the primitive buccal endothelium, the neurohypophysis develops as a down
ward projection of the neuroectoderm from the base of the brain. At the eleventh
week of gestation these two parts are virtually fused in an unique structure. Every pathological stimulus that interfere with this process before the eleventh week
of gestation can cause an anomaly in the formation of the adeno and neurohypophysis: e.g. an incomplete fusion of these two different parts. Also the agenesia of
septum pellucidum and the Chiari anomaly arised from a developmental error that oc
curs before the eleventh week of gestation (van der Knaap and Valk 1988), and their
association with pituitary gland and stalk anomalies could not be casual. On the
other hand the association with brain congenital anomalies was found also in the
group of IGHD patients with normal posterior pituitary and normally connected stalk;
in these cases, however the pituitary gland and the pituitary stalk were both hypo
plastic. On the basis of these findings we suggest that an embriological derangement, that occurred before the eleventh week of gestational age, could explain the
complexity of these anomalies. Like other congenital anomalies that show different
degrees of severity, the developmental derangement that involved the adeno-neuro-
hypophysis complex could damage the fusion of these two parts completely or partially. When a complete damage occurs the pituitary gland is aplastic and the neurohypophysis, both the axonal part with the terminal hyperintensity and the vasculo-
stromal part, do not descend from the base of diencephalon. In these patients the
absence of the pituitary portal system would cause a panhypophytuitarism. When the
damage is only partial the adenohypophysis is hypoplastic and the stalk is thin
but normally connected with the pituitary gland or, as in the two patients of the
group A, only the vasculo-stromal part is normally developed, while the axonal part
remains at the infundibular level. In these patients the pituitary portal system
is preserved, but the hypoplastic gland is probably partially damaged. The GH-cells

of the adenohypophysis are the most sensible to the ischemic damage and a defective development of the pituitary with a reduced trophism to the gland could explain a selective deficit of the cells that produced the growth hormone.

REFERENCES

Colombo N, Berry I, Kucharczyk J, et al. (1987) Posterior pituitary gland: appearance on MR imaging in normal and pathological states. Radiology 165:481-485.
di Natale B, Scotti G, Pellini C, et al. (1987) Empty sella in children with pituitary dwarfism: does it exist? Pediatrician 14:246-252.
Fujisawa I, Asato R, Nishimura K, et al. (1987) Anterior and posterior lobes of the pituitary gland: assessement by 1.5 T MR imaging. J Comput Assist Tomogr 11: 214-220.
Fujisawa I, Kikuchi K, Nishimura K, et al. (1987) Transection of the pituitary stalk: development of an ectopic posterior lobe assessed with MR imaging. Radiology 165:487-489.
Kelly WM, Kucharczyk W, Kucharczyk J, et al (1988) Posterior pituitary ectopia:an MR feature of pituitary dwarfism. AJNR 9:453-460.
Shizume K, Harada Y, Ibavashi Y (1977) Survey studies on pituitary diseases in Japan. Endocrinol Jpn 24:139-147.
Stanhope R, Hindmarsh P, Kendall B, Brook CGD (1986) High resolution CT scanning of the pituitary gland in growth disorders. Acta Paediatr Scand 75:779-786.
Triulzi F, Scotti G, di Natale B, Pellini C, Chiumello G, Del Maschio A (1987) MR imaging of pituitary gland and stalk abnormalities in pituitary dwarfs with idiophatic growth hormone deficiency. Radiology 165(P):350.
van der Knaap MS, Valk J (1988) Classification of congenital abnormalities of the CNS. AJNR 9:315-326.
Inoue Y, Nemoto Y, Fujita K, et al (1986) Pituitary dwarfism:CT evaluation of the pituitary gland. Radiology 159:171-173.

MRI and CT of Sella and Brain in Turner's Syndrom

T. E. Mayer, A. Halbsguth, F. Kollmann, and C. Lorey

INTRODUCTION

These normally female phenotypic patients present multiple organ abnormalities
(e.g. renal in 60%. coarctation of the aorta in 15%) and typical dysmorphias
(webbing of the neck 40%), associated disorders as frequent autoimmune diseases,
most often a gonadal dysgenesis and a short stature.
FSH more than LH serum Levels are high and LRF responses are increased
especially after the 11th year of age. GH levels are in some cases lower than
normal. There are case reports from Nishi et al 1984 and Valenta et al 1984,
which reported 2 cases of pituitary microadenomas and 1 empty sella respectively
two partial empty sellae, discreet pathological sella findings of Samaan et al 1979
and a case of prolactinoma (Gaspar et al 1985); but the rate of sellar pathology
and the pathogenesis of the hormon disorders in this syndrom is unclear.

Turner patients are statistically mentally retarded with a specific pattern of
deficits and have slightly abnormal EEGs. There are almost no neuroradiological
evaluations of their brains recorded, Netley and Rovet, 1982 report from rare
CT scans where abnormalities where found with "no characteristic localizing
features", Diebler and Dulac 1987 mention a personal case of corpus callosum
agenesis. Most of the patients belonging to this study were examined in a
private radiological institute for sella turgica by CT and/or MRI but we also
evaluated the brain and orbitae, where possible.

METHODS

A large variety of techniques were used because the patients were referred to us
from different physicians:
Axial and/or coronal CT, often before and after contrast infusion (one dynamic CT)
with 2 - 4 mm slice thickness, sometimes overlapping. In half of the cases only
or in addition a sagittal and/or coronal MRI with 5 mm thick T1-weighted
spin-echo sequences without the use of paramagnetic substances was carried out.
More than half also had CT's of the head in 8 mm scans.

RESULTS

22 girls aged from 10 to 22 were studied. 11 had a 45 x karyotyp, 9 had structural
x - chromosomal abnormalities and 2 a mosaik. They showed the whole range of
anomalies described above. 2 had epilepsia and one a history of anorexia. The
height of the pituitary was 2.5 to 7.5 mm, mean 4.3 mm, standard deviation 1.5 mm
which is normal (in comparsion: Bonneville et al 1986)
In 12 cases there were no adenomas detected, in 10 only lager microadenomas could
be excluded. One empty sella and two partial empty sellae were found out of 18 in
this question evaluable examinations. That is a bit more than in a normal population
(Busch 1951, 12%).
In 15 of 19 cases cerebral sulci (parietral, parieto-occipital and temporal, in one
case frontal) were from slightly to severely enlarged. Although there is a wide
range of normal external CSF spaces, this sample as a whole was not corresponding

to a normal population of this age. One patient in this group had epilepsia and showed the severest changes (see picture). The cerebral ventricles were normal except in this case of epilepsia with slight asymmetrical enlargement.
The skulls of all patients were thickened and mostly basal pneumatic spaces anlarged. The corpus callosum showed a variety of different forms but no defect. There were only slight enlargements of CSF spaces of the cerebellum in half of the cases. Except for one case of silicon filling of the eye globe because of retinal detachement, normal orbits were seen.

CONCLUSION

No certain increase of sellar pathology was found, i.e. no macroscopic structure as a cause or consequence of the hormonal disorders in this syndrom could be identified.

Alexander et al 1966, Money 1966, 1973, Garron et al 1969, Silbert et al 1977, Ebbin et al 1980, Nettey and Rovet 1982, Lewandowski et al 1985, Bender et al 1986, Mc Cauley et al 1987 and many other authors described the neuropsychological deficits of these patients. In contrast to other chromosomal abnormalities, these patients have less impairment of verbal than of performance IQ.
Visuospatial skills are often affected and described as parietal lobe or right hemisphere syndrom.
Also concerned are neuromotor and sometimes memory function.
Dougherty et al 1983 reported anorexia nervosa in these patients.
In this context it is interesting to note that Artmann et al 1984 reported widening (partially reversible) of cerebral sulci in patients with anorexia nervosa.
Takayuki and Nielson 1976, 1985 found more rapid alpha activity of lower amplitude and amount, slower beta activity of higher amplitude and amount, higher amount of theta activity, asymmetries occipital more than parietal, right more than left and increased paroxysmal slight abnormalities in EEG of Turner patients.
Similar observations were made by Palm et al 1973. There are only a few neuro-pathological examinations recorded. Brun and Sköld 1968, Gulotta et al 1981,and Giustina et al 1985 described cortical and cerebellar hypoplasias, dysplasias and heterotopias in a 16 year old Turner female with medulloblastoma, in 24 cases of XO and XXY fetuses (only 3 pathological findings) respectively in a 2 day old Turner newborn. Inpairment of the late fetal migration process is probable.

Considering that no girl had a history of early acquired brain damages, our neuroradiological findings could be the expression ot this brain pathology.

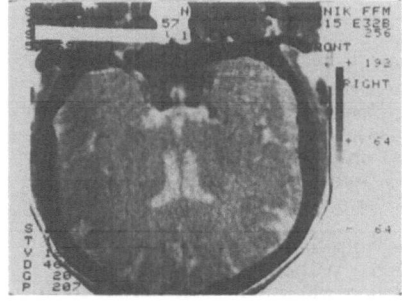

46 X, I (Xq), 20 years, epilepsia.
Enlargement of cerebral sulci, thickened skull, empty sella.

REFERENCES

Alexander D, Erhardt A and Money J (1966) J Nerv Ment Dis 142:161 - 167
    Defective figure drawing, geometric and human, in Turner's syndrome
Artmann H, Grau H, Schleiffer R, Adelmann M Reversible and non reversible
    enlargement of CSF-spaces in anorexia nervosa Neuroradiology 1984
Bender B Puck M Salbenblatt J and Robinson A Cocnitive development of
    children with sex chromosome abnormalities Pediatrics 73 (1984) 175 - 182
Bonneville J.-F. Cattin F, Dietemann J.L Computed tomography of the
    pituitary gland Springer Berlin Heidelber 1986
Brun A, Sköld G CNS malformations in Turner's syndrom Acta Neuropathologica
    1O, 159 - 161 (1986)
Busch W Die Morphologie der Sella turcica und ihre Beziehungen zur
    Hypophyse. Virchows Archiv, Bd. 32O, S. 437-458 ²81951)
Diebler C, Dulac O Pediatric neurology and neuroradiology
    Springer Berlin Heidelberg 1987
Dougherty G, Rockwell K, Sutton and Ellinwood E. Anorexia nervosa
    in treated gonadal dysgenesis: Case report and review. J Clin Psychiatry
    44: 219-221, 1983
Ebbin A, Howell V, Wilson M. Deficits in Space-form perception in patients
    with sex chromosome mosaicism (45,X/46XY) Develop. Med. Child Neurol.
    198o, 22, 352-361
Garron D, Vander Stoep L. Personality and intelligence in Turner's syndrome
    Arch Gen Psychiat - Vol 21 339 - 346 (1969)
Gaspar L, Jolesz J, Kocsis J, Pasztos E, Laszlo F. Mosaik Turner's syndrom
    and pituitary microadenoma Exp.Clin. Endocrinol. Vol 86, No.1, pp87-92 1985
Giustina W, Forabosco A, Botticelli A, Pace P. Neuropatologia della sindrome
    di Turner. Ped. Med. Chir. (Med.Surg.Ped.) 1985,7: 49-56
Gullotta F, Rehder H and Gropp A. Descriptive neuropathology of chromosomal
    disorders in man. Hum Genet 1981 57: 337-344
Lewandowski L, Costenbader V and Richman R. Neuropsychological aspects of
    Turner syndrome. J Clin Neuropsychol 7, 144-147 (1985)
Mc Cauley E, Kay T, Ito J, Treder R. The Turner syndrom: Cognitive Deficits,
    affective discrimination and behavior problems. Child Dev.1987,58, 464-473
Money J, Alexander S, Ehrhardt A. Visual-constructional deficit in Turner's
    syndrom. J. of Ped. 69 (1966) 126-127
Netley C and Rovet J. Atypical hemispheric lateralization in Turner syndrom
    subjects. Cortex 18 (1982) 377-384
Nishi Y, Sakano T, Hyodo S, Masuda H, Kitamura Y, Shindo H, Sakoda K,
    Uozumi T and Usui T. Pituitary abnormalities detected by high resolution
    computed tomography with thin slices in primary hypothyroidism and Turner
    syndrome
Palm D, Pfeiffer A, Ammermann M, Schulte H. EEG-Befunde bei Turner-Syndrom
    Mschr. Kinderheilk.121, 289-292 (1973)
Samaan N, Stepanas A, Danziger J, Trujillo J. Reactive Pituitary abnormalities
    in patients with klinefelter's and Turner's syndromes
    Arch. Intern.Med. 139 (1979) 198-2o1
Silbert A, Wolff P, Lilienthal J. Spatial and temporal processing in patients
    with Turner's syndrom. Behavia Genetics, Vol 7, No.1, 1977
Takayuki Tsuboi and Johannes Nielsen. Electroencephalographic examination of
    64 danish Turner girls . Acta neurolScand,1985:72: 59O-6O1
Valenta L, Elias A, Bocian M. Atypical biochemical findings in Turner's syndrom:
    identification of a possible subset.
    Fertility and Sterility, Vol 42, No.5, Nov.1984

Miscellaneous

MR Angiography of Cerebrovascular Disease

S. Felber, G. Laub, P. Ruggieri, and F. Aichner

Introduction:

Atherosclerotic lesions of the carotid and vertebral arteries are a major
cause of cerebrovascular ischaemic disease. Diagnostic evaluation and
therapeutic considerations require assessment of brain morphology and
vascular supply. Magnetic resonance imaging (MRI) already proved most
sensitive in detection of ischaemic brain lesions (Heiss et al 1986).
Recent developments showed the capability of MR to visualize carotid artery
pathology: Magnetic resonance angiography (MRA). (Masaryk et al 1988;
Felber et al 1988). Our attempt was, to perform MRA as part of a routine
brain examination and to assess the potential of the method in cerebrovascular disease.

Patients:

20 patients with evidence of carotid and vertebral artery disease had
been examined after informed consent was obtained. Age ranged from 32
to 92 years. The external carotid artery was not evaluated in this series,
distribution of artherosclerotic lesions in the CCA, ICA and VA is shown
in table 1.

Table 1

CCA	plaques	n = 1
	occlusion	n = 1
ICA	plaques	n = 3
	stenosis 70 %	n = 8
	stenosis 70 %	n = 5
	occl.	n = 3
VA	occl.	n = 5
		n = 26

Degree and extent of extracranial disease vessel pathology was documented
by Doppler/Duplex sonography (Hennerici and Freund 1984) in all patients,
9 patients had additional X-Ray angiography.

Methods:

MRI (T1 and T2 weighted sequences) and MRA were performed in one session on a 1.5 T Magnetom (Siemens), using the standard head coil (25 cm FOV). Examination time did not exceed 55 min. For MRA a 3D Fisp Sequence was used. Enhancement of flowing blood resulted from inflow of unsaturated spins and compensation of phase-dispersal by 1st-order Gradient-Motion-Refocussing in slice-select and read-out direction (Laub and Kaiser 1988). A set of 64 contiguous,1.2 - 1.4 mm thick slices was obtained in 10.9 minutes (TR 40, TE 12 ms, Flip angle 25°). As tortuous vessels are difficult to follow in 2D images, a ray-tracer algorithm was used to calculate projectional images from the neck vessels only.

Results:

Normal flow within the carotid and vertebral arteries was visualized with high signal intensity, up to the circle of Willis. Turbulent flow and flow reversal, as well as acceleration secondary to vessel pathology resulted in signal void. Plaques without hemodynamic relevance were missed on the MR Angiograms. Stenosis of 40 to 70 % and high grade stenosis were visualized in all cases, but there was a tendency to overestimate the disease, if only the signal pattern within the stenosis was interpreted (fig. 1). The degree of peripheral enhancement proved important for the graduation. No signal enhancement occured in occluded vessels (fig. 2).

Discussion:

MRA was less exact in graduation of stenosis when compared to Doppler/Duplex sonography, but visualizes the carotid and vertebral artery up to the circle of Willis. Signal enhancement of the vascular structure depends on flow velocity and flow dynamics. Signal void caused by turbulent flow, acceleration and flow reversal, indicates vessel pathology.

MRA was sensitive to stenosic and occluded vessels. As MRA reveals functional information about flow dynamics, arteriosclerotic plaque without hemodynamic relevance were not visualized. The limited number of patients in our retrospectively performed study does not allow to draw a conclusion about the specifity of MRA. However, the results show that MRA is sensitive to arteriosclerotic disease of the carotid and vertebral artery. The method can be performed routinely within short examination times, together with conventional MRI of the brain, revealing information about brain morphology and vascular disease in a single examination. Therefore the method shows potential as a new non-invasive screening modality in cerebrovascular disease.

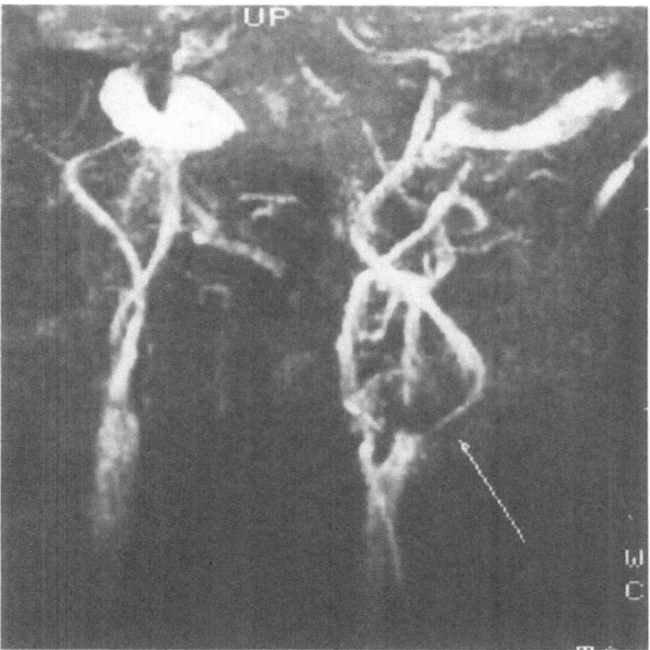

<u>Fig. 1.</u> MR angiography of a 65 year old patient with sonographic proven 75 % stenosis of the left ICA. MRA overestimates the degree of stenosis (arrow). Normal enhancement is present in the peripheral ICA. Occlusion of the right V.A.

482

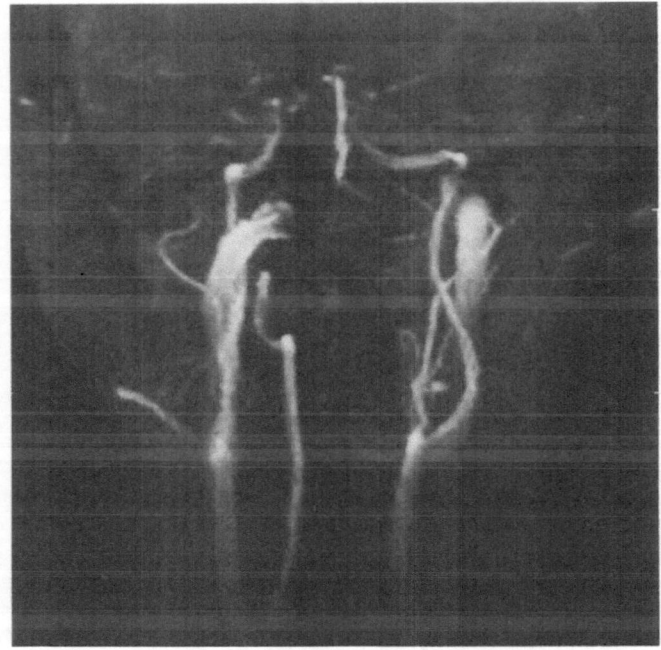

Fig. 2. Occlusion of the left VA in a 32 year old female. Normal
flow enhancement is present in the right VA and the
carotid arteries.

References:
(1) Felber S., Ruggieri P., Magnetic Resonance Imaging
Vol(6), Suppl.(1),46,1988

(2) Heiss,W.D.,Herholz,K.,Böcher-Schwarz,H.G.,Pawlik,G.,
Wienhard,K.,Steinbrich,W.,Friedmann,G.: PET, CT and MR
Imaging in Cerebrovascular Disease (1986) J.of Comp.
Assist.Tomogr. 10(6):903-911

(3) Hennerici,M.,Freund,H.J.: Efficacy of cw-Doppler and
Dupplex-systemexamination for the evaluation of extracranial carotid disease (1984) J.Clin.Ultrasound 12:155-161

(4) Laub G., Kaiser W.: MR-Angiography with Gradient Motion
Refocussing. J.C.A.T. 12(3), 377-382, 1988

(5) Masaryk,T.J.,Ross,J.S.,Modic,M.T.,Lenz,G.W.,Haake,E.M.:
Carotid Bifurcation: MR Imaging (1988) Radiology 166:461-
466

Regional Cerebral Blood Volume and Blood-Brain Barrier Disturbance in Cerebral Infarcts in the Lesion Site and Contralateral

M. H. Adelmann and H. Hacker

Calculated dynamic computed tomography (CDCT) is a simple, non-invasive method to detect physiological and pathophysiological data in vivo in a very easy way. With this method it becomes possible to calculate regional cerebral blood volume (rCBV), extravascular iodine content (EVIC) and blood brain barrier permeability rate (delta) in normal and pathologic brain regions.[2]

When evaluating a cerebral lesion, it is necessary to take care that most lesions are not homogenous so that different regions of interest have to be defined. Usually it is possible to line out a so-called high density region (HDR) and a so-called low density region (LDR).

A series of 1 to 28 days old infarcts was studied by CDCT. Table 1 shows the results for rCBV, EVIC and delta for normal brain tissue (Hildebrandt 1987) and for different infarct areas (LDR,HDR). In normal brain tissue mean rCBV is 2.2% for white matter and 4.5% for gray matter. rCBV in low density infarct regions is nearly the same as in normal white matter (2.48%). Mean blood volume in high density regions increases up to 5.3%.

Table 1. Regional cerebral blood volume, extravascular iodine content and blood brain barrier permeability rate for normal and infarcted brain tissue.

	normal brain tissue		brain infarcts	
	white matter	gray matter	LDR	HDR
rCBV (%)	2.2	4.5	2.48	5.3
EVIC	0.00	0.00	0.11	0.55
delta	0.000	0.000	0.032	0.210

In normal brain tissue blood brain barrier (bbb) is not permeable to contrast medium (Hildebrandt 1987). So no extravasation is detectable and the bbb permeability rate delta is zero. Contrary to these results all evaluated infarct areas show significant extravasation of contrast medium and bbb damage.

It is not only necessary to make sure that the regions of interest are homogenous, but one also has to take care how old the infarct is because rCBV, EVIC and delta show time-dependent changes. Table 2 shows the results summarized.

Table 2. Time-dependent changes of blood volume, extravascular iodine content and bbb permeability rate in brain infarcts.

	BRAIN INFARCTS		
	1-28 d	1-15 d	16-28 d
rCBV (%)	5.29	4.65	6.94
EVIC	0.45	0.16	0.90
delta	0.165	0.047	0.520

Pathologic findings (Spatz 1939), "normal" CT-examinations (Becker et al. 1979) and statistical analysis of the evaluated data indicate that it is important to group the data (group I: 1-15 days old infarcts, group II: 16-28 days old infarcts).

Blood volume rises from 4.6% in the first two weeks up to 6.9% in the second two weeks. More remarkable is the highly significant change of the blood brain barrier permeability rate with time. Also the extravascular iodine content is distinctly increased.

In an infarcted area blood brain barrier is disrupted and an extravasation of contrast medium can be detected by CDCT. In 70% of evaluated examinations extravasation and blood brain barrier disruption can also be detected in the brain hemisphere contralateral to the infarction. The region symmetrical to the lesion shows highest extravascular iodine content. In more frontal or occipital regions (of the non-infarcted hemisphere) extravasation is detectable, too, but not so extensively. The same effect is detectable in 30-40% of evaluated brain tumors.

This effect seems to be time-dependent. In the first days after the stroke no or only little extravasation is detectable in the non-infarcted hemisphere, in the second week extravasation and blood brain barrier permeability are distinctly increased whereas regional cerebral blood volume does not seem to be influenced.

Transhemispheric effects on several physiologic parameters have long been known (Hoedt-Rasmussen and Skinho 1976; Meyer 1964). Interruption of corpus callosum prevents these transhemispheric effects (Kempinsky 1958).

Some toxic agents may be generated in the infarcted area and reach the opposite hemisphere along commissural pathways and induce blood brain barrier disruption directly. Further studies on this effect are in preparation.

REFERENCES

Adelmann MH (1987) Beurteilung der Blut-Hirn Schranke bei Hirntumoren und -infarkten mit Hilfe der dynamischen Computertomographie. Dissertation, Frankfurt

Becker H, Desch H, Hacker H, Pencz A (1979) CT fogging effect with ischemic cerebral infarcts. Neuroradiology 18: 185-192

Hacker H, Becker H (1977) Time-controlled computed tomographic angiography. J Comp Ass Tom 1(4): 405-409

Hacker H (1988) Calculated dynamic CT. XVth Congress of the European Society of Neuroradiology, Würzburg, Sept. 1988

Hildebrandt R (1987) Persönliche Mitteilung

Hoedt-Rasmussen K, Skinhoj E (1964) Transneural depression of the cerebral hemispheric metabolism in man. Acta Neurol Scand 40:41

Kempinsky WH (1958) Experimental study of distant effects of focal brain injury: A study of diaschisis. Arch Neurol Psychiat 79: 376

Meyer JS, Shinohara Y, Kanda T (1970) Diaschisis resulting from acute unilateral cerebral infarction. Arch Neurol 23: 241

Spatz H (1939) Pathologische Anatomie der Kreislaufstörungen des Gehirns. Z Neurol 167: 301-349

The Specific Diagnosis of Enhancing Ring Lesions with Calculated Dynamic CT

J. Berkefeld, H. Rolfes, and H. Hacker

INTRODUCTION

The difficulties in differential diagnosis of enhancing intracerebral mass lesions are well known. Since 1978 our group and other authors (Lewander et al.1978, Lange et al. 1979, Westphal, 1983) tried to use the time-course of contrast enhancement in dynamic CT-scans as an additional parameter for correct diagnosis.

The comparison of only the density-time diagrams of different tumors gives some kind of information, which is not really superior to the visual evaluation of the images. An improvement of the method was the calculation of the regional cerebral blood volume of a lesion by using a simple formula:

$$rCBV = \frac{\mu\ (CL,peak)}{\mu\ (BR,peak)} \times f \times 100\ \%$$

(μ = difference of density-values of enhanced and nonenhanced scans, CL = cerebral lesion, BR = blood reference, f = correction factor)

The next step forward is now the development of a calculation method to separate the extravascular iodine content (EVIC) from the whole regional iodine content (RIC) of an enhancing lesion (Adelmann 1987, Weidauer 1987). Its principle is the subtraction of the rCBV from the RIC:

$$Extravasal\ iodine\ (EVI) = RIC - rCBV$$

$$RIC = \frac{\mu\ (CL,t)}{\mu\ (BR,t)}$$

$$EVI = \frac{\mu\ (CL,t) \times 100 - \mu(BR,t) \times rCBV}{100 - rCBV}$$

For interindividual comparison EVI is divided through the actual density in the superior sagittal sinus (μ BR) and this relationship is called extravascular iodine content:

$$EVIC = \frac{EVI}{\mu\ (BR)}$$

METHOD

The dynamic CT examinations were performed on a Siemens Somatom 2N
with acessory angio-CT unit. After a nonenhanced scan a 100 cc bolus
of contrast medium was injected automatically,and 19 dynamic scans
of the same slice were recorded over a period of 10 minutes.
During the first 2 minutes after bolus injection fast scans with
a frequency of 6/min were used. At the time of maximal intravascular
enhancement (peak) the images were splitted. After the fast series
scans were performed every 30 sec. or every minute in the later phases.

Up to this time we examined 57 patients with different intracranial
tumors:

Table 1:   24 meningeomas
                11 astrocytomas
                 4 malignant astrocytomas
                10 glioblastoma
                 4 metastases
                 4 others

For computer-assisted calculation an evaluation program, which was developed in cooperation with the Siemens Company, was primarily used
in 25 of these cases.
The density values were taken automatically from the regions of interest,
and the computer plotted tables and curves after calculation.

CASE REPORTS

MENINGEOMA

A meningeoma -an extracerebral tumor without blood-brain barrier-
has a high uptake of contrast as the CT and the density-time diagram
show. It is in this special case even similar to the values in the
blood reference. At once after bolus injection there is an extravasation with a very high amount of extravascular iodine (EVIC = 1,15),
while a reference of normal brain tissue (TR) remains low. The regional
blood volume in the meningeoma is 15,5 % in comparison to 2,04 % in
the normal white matter.

GLIOBLASTOMA

An intracerebral lesion, a glioblastoma shows also marked enhancement in CT images and in the density-time diagram.The regional cerebral
blood volume is lower than in the meningeoma (rCBV = 4,34 %). The
curve of the extravascular iodine content increases slower and only
to a level of 0,48.

MALIGNANT ASTROCYTOMA

An astrocytoma grade III with less enhancement and a smaller degree
of pathological vascularisation in the angiogram behaves quite similar
to the more malignant glioblastoma if we look at the curve of EVIC.
The regional blood volume however is only 2,26 % and not different from
the values of normal brain tissue (2,21 %).

METASTASIS

A single metastasis of an adenocarcinoma shows also a very marked
enhancement. In the EVIC curve there is more early extravasation

than in the two gliomas, the maximum values of EVIC are higher (0,73) and a plateau is reached within 10 minutes. The regional blood volume (6,04 %) is not different from the values known from malignant gliomas.

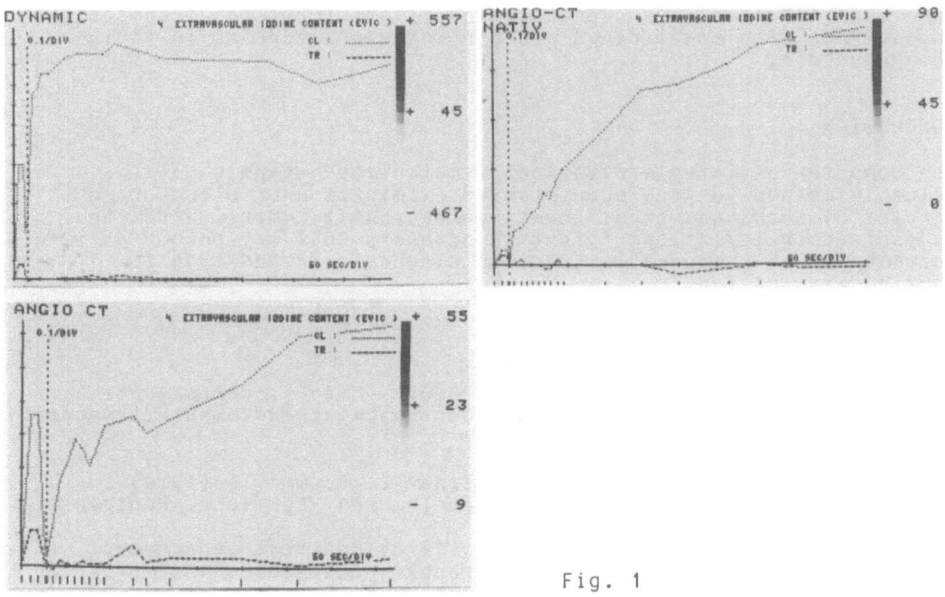

Fig. 1

DISCUSSION

Because of the heterogenous group of tumors our results are not statistically significant, and we can only give a report of representative cases. This case reports however should show some trends in quantitative evaluation of blood-brain barrier disturbances by dynamic CT:

Table 2:   Mean values of rCBV and EVIC (Adelmann, 1987)

	rCBV	EVIC
Meningeoma	14,43 %	0,83
endoth.	17,17 %	0,53
fibrom.	14,82 %	1,37
Glioblastoma	11,29 %	0,32
Astrocytoma	4,41 %	0,04
White matter	2,23 %	0,00
Grey matter	4,59 %	0,00

Generally the meningeomas had a high rCBV and a high degree of extravasation. Possibly a differentiation between variant histological types can be made. The mean values of rCBV of malignant gliomas give a wrong impression. If we look at the single cases, we see a fluctuation of the values from 4 to 15 % depending on the degree of tumor vascularisation. Our experiences in metastases are limited. In the 4 cases we saw a higher degree of early extravasation than in the gliomas. The EVIC curves are similar to the meningeoma curves but the values are on a lower level. The reason for this behavior may also be an absence of blood-brain barrier in metastases.

490

In computer-assisted evaluation we had some problems with movement artifacts. Especially the region within the superior sagittal sinus is very small, and minor head movements during the series can have a great effect. Another problem is the evaluation of thin irregular shaped ring structures. For good results a homogenous region of more than 177 pixels is needed, which is difficult to circumscribe in patients with small rings and CSF space or necrosis in their neighbourhood.

CONCLUSION

The computer-assisted evaluation of calculated dynamic CT is a valuable method for the quantitative examination of blood-brain barrier disturbances in different intracranial tumors. With the widespread installation of fast CT scanners CDCT may become an important part of preoperative specific diagnosis in addition to routine examination.

REFERENCES

Adelmann, M. (1987) Beurteilung der Blut - Hirn - Schranke bei Hirn-tumoren und -infarkten mit Hilfe der dynamischen Computertomographie. Dissertation, Frankfurt, 1987

Lange S , Steinhoff,H, Aviles Ch, Kazner E, Grumme Th (1979) Kontrastmittelkinetik in zerebralen Tumoren. Fortschr. Röntgenstr. 130,6:666-669
Lewander R, Bergström M, Bergvall U (1978) Contrast enhancement of cranial lesions in computed tomography. Acta Radiol 19,4:529-552
Weidauer S (1987) Dynamische Computertomographie Blutvolumen und extravaskuläres Jod in Hirntumoren. Dissertation, Frankfurt, 1987
Westphal M (1983) Dynamische zerebrale Computertomographie Fortschr. Röntgenstr. 139,6:632-639

MR Imaging of Intraventricular Lesions

M. Boukobza, A. Zouaoui, H. Alvarez, V. Vazquez, and J. Metzger (Paris, France)

MR images were obtained in 23 cases of intra-ventricular lesions using T1, T2 spin-echo sequences and gadolinium enhancement: ependymomas (7 cases), colloid cysts (5 cases), meningiomas (5 cases), cysticercosis (2 cases), dermoid cysts (2 cases), glioblastoma (1 case) and choroid papilloma (1 cases). Correlation with enhanced CT was determined. All cases were proven surgically or by autopsy. MR seems the best technique to determine with accuracy the localisation and often the nature of the lesion. In some cases, gadolinium enhancement may be useful.

Idiopathic Cranial Pachymeningitis. Assessment with CT and MR Imaging

N. Martin, C. Masson, D. Hénin, D. Mompoint, C. Marsault, and H. Nahum (Clichy, France)

The authors report three cases of diffuse idiopathic cranial pachy-meningitis. The patients were first examined with a DGR1 Siemens scanner. In two cases, MR studies were performed with a 0.5 T super-conducting magnet (CGR Magniscan 5000): T2-weighted coronal sequences (TR: 1800, TE: 60,120 ms) were obtained, and in one case a T1-weighted sagittal sequence.

Progressively increasing headaches were the usual symptoms, along with ataxia and various cranial nerve palsies. CT in all cases de-tected isolated thickened dura mater, mostly on tentorium with one posterior falx extension. MRI depicted dural involvement as a hypo-intense signal area, and in one particular case there was a very large nodular hypointense area with fine hyperintense edges on these T2-weighted sequences. Dural thickening can be responsible for various occlusions of dural sinuses. Morphological examina-tion of thickened dura revealed extensive fibrotic tissue with a chronic inflammatory infiltrate containing lymphocytes, plasma cells and scattered eosinophils, corresponding closely to MR images.

After discussion of different causes of thickened dura seen in CT, MR, clinical, and microscopic studies, these isolated cases of pa-chymeningitis appear to be unrelated to any known process. Only four previous reports are likely to correspond to similar observa-tions, published before the CT and MR era.

Do Old Patients with Down's Syndrome Develop Premature Brain Atrophy?

P. Stoeter, D. Ehrmann, and N. Prey

A common genetic defect is discussed in trisomy 21 and Alzheimer's disease because of similar degenerative changes on post-mortem brain examinations and a reduced activity of the neurotransmitter systems (Coyle et al. 1986, Oliver and Holland 1986). In a selected group of elderly mongoloids with clinical deterioration, moderate to severe ventricular enlargement and dilatation of the subarachnoid space was found in all cases examined by CT (Lott and Lai 1982). But not every patient with Down's syndrome (DS) becomes demented and CT studies were not able to show significant or increasing cerebral atrophy up to the age of 4o (Ieshima et al. 1984). In the present paper, the degree of cerebral atrophy in DS of older age is reported in correlation to the clinical course.

Patients and CT examinations:

Clinical evaluation and CT examinations are carried out in 2 groups of 1o DS of 4o - 49 and 5o - 63 years of age, who have been hospitalised at 2 centres for mental retardation (Stiftung Liebenau and Anstalt Stetten) for mostly over 3o years. Changes of social behavior and personality, neurological signs, seizures, and deterioration to dementia could be jugded without difficulty. The clinical course is graded into "no changes", "mild deterioration" (e.g. loss of spontaneity, daily living skills), "seizures and/or psychosis" and "severe dementia" and 2 subgroups of 15 non- or moderately and 5 severely affected patients are formed (Table 1).
CT examinations are performed by a Somatom DR (Siemens) in consecutive slices parallel to the orbito-meatal line. Evaluation consists of "first-glance" inspection and measurements of the usual parameters (Fig.1) and the calculation of the CSF-cranial ratio (Nagata et al.1987). The results are compared to 2 age-matched control groups of "normal" patients with minor complaints and without neurological deficits.

Results:

Significant and age dependent differences between patients with DS and the control groups are found only in the temporal lobes (enlargement of temporal horn and Sylvian fissure) whereas other significant differences (size of cisterna magna and cerebral peduncles) were similar in both or found in one age group only (size of the 3rd ventricle and number of the fissures of the superior cerebellar vermis) (Table 2). The frequency of calcifications of the basal ganglia as well as the other parameter show a non-significant trend towards atrophic changes. The subgroup of the 5 more severely affected patients with DS however, has a more pronounced brain atrophy in 4 cases with significant enlargement of the CSF spaces as compared to their non- or mildly affected collegues.

Table 1	Patients and clinical data

M. Down:

2o patients (7 F, 13 M)
4o - 49 y: 1o (mean age: 45,5y)
5o - 63 y: 1o (mean age: 53,9y)

No change	: 6
Slight deterioration	: 9
Severe dementia	: 3
Psychosis/epilepsy	: 2

Control group:

4o patients (15 F, 25 M)
4o - 49 y: 2o (mean age 45,2 y)
5o - 63 y: 2o (mean age 56,8 y)

Minor complaints,
no neurologic deficit

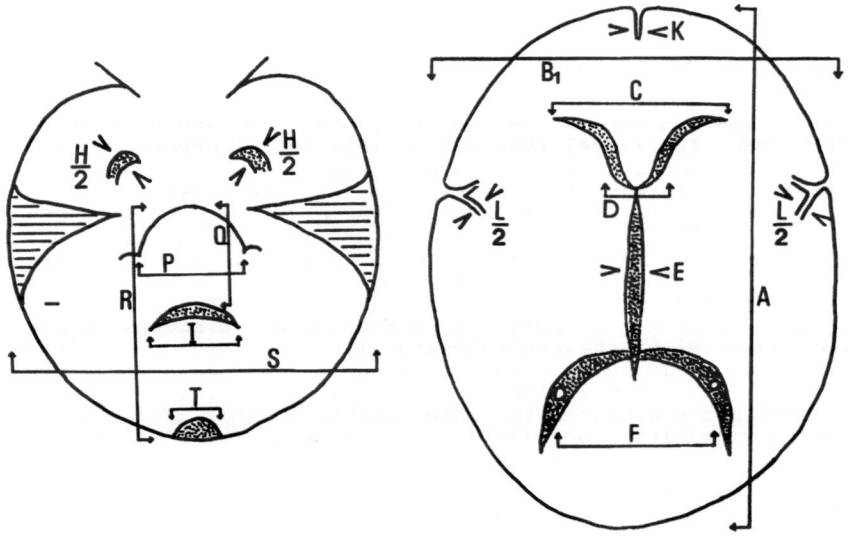

Fig. 1. Schematogram of CT measurements

Table 2: CT findings

	M. Down 40 - 49y n = 1o	50 - 63y n = 1o	CD*** n = 5	Control group 40 - 49y n = 2o	50 - 63y n = 2o
Cer.atrophy("1st glance")	2	2	4**	o	o
Calcif.basal ggl.(No.)	6	3	2	3	2
4th ventricle					
abs.diameter I (mm)	$12.7^\pm 2.8$	$12.9^\pm 3.3$	13.5	$12.7^\pm 2.2$	$13.7^\pm 2.9$
rel.diameter I:S (%)	$12.6^\pm 2.1$	$12.8^\pm 3.3$	13.1	$11.o^\pm 2.2$	$11.9^\pm 2.8$
Cisterna magna					
visible (no.)	1o*	1o*	5	14	11
diameter T 15mm (No.)	4	5	4	8	3
Pons					
rel.sagit.dia. Q:R (%)	$37.9^\pm 3.8$	$36.2^\pm 4.4$	36.7	$33.7^\pm 2.2$	$36.7^\pm 3.7$
rel.lat.dia. P:S (%)	$28.4^\pm 2.3$	$27.8^\pm 1.7$	28.4	$28.o^\pm 2.7$	$27.9^\pm 3.o$
Sulci of sup.vermis					
cerebelli, No.	$2.5^\pm 1.4*$	$2.2^\pm 1.8$	3.2	$o.9^\pm 1.o$	$1.3^\pm 1.1$
Crus cerebri					
abs.diameter N (mm)	$14.9^\pm 1.4*$	$14.o^\pm 2.o*$	13.8	$16.8^\pm 1.3$	$16.6^\pm 1.5$
rel.diameter $N:B_1$ (%)	$11.6^\pm o.8$	$11.o^\pm 1.5$	1o.9	$12.2^\pm 1.3$	$11.9^\pm 1.4$
III. ventricle					
abs.diameter E (mm)	$5.o^\pm 1.8$	$6.5^\pm 3.2*$	8.o	$4.3^\pm 1.3$	$4.2^\pm 1.1$
rel.diameter $E:B_1$ (%)	$3.9^\pm 1.6$	$5.1^\pm 2.5$	6.5	$3.1^\pm 1.o$	$3.o^\pm o.8$
Anterior horn:					
Huckmann No. C+D (mm)	$53.2^\pm 8.7$	$55.3^\pm 17.4$	66.3**	$55.5^\pm 8.3$	$59.5^\pm 5.1$
rel.max.dia.$C:B_1$ (%)	$27.2^\pm 4.2$	$27.7^\pm 8.9$	33.2	$27.6^\pm 3.5$	$28.8^\pm 2.8$
rel.bicaud.dia $D:B_1$(%)	$14.3^\pm 3.7$	$15.8^\pm 5.5$	2o.1**	$12.3^\pm 2.5$	$13.8^\pm 2.7$
Cella media					
rel.dia. $G:B_1$ (%)	$26.9^\pm 4.5$	$28.3^\pm 7.2$	33.7**	$22.1^\pm 7.4$	$25.4^\pm 3.1$
Temporal horn:					
abs.dia. H (mm)	$4.4^\pm 2.9*$	$6.1^\pm 4.2*$	9.1**	$2.2^\pm 1.1$	$2.3^\pm 1.4$
rel.dia. $H:B_1$ (%)	$3.5^\pm 2.6*$	$4.7^\pm 3.5*$	7.5**	$1.6^\pm o.8$	$1.6^\pm o.9$
Anterior IHF K					
width (mm)	$3.3^\pm o.9$	$3.2^\pm 2.o$	4.o	$2.7^\pm 1.3$	$2.3^\pm 1.5$
Cisterna Sylvii L					
width (mm)	$9.1^\pm 3.3$	$1o.2^\pm 2.7$	11.5	$6.6^\pm 2.1$	$6.8^\pm 1.7$
Sulci of convexity, No.	$2.9^\pm 2.4$	$4.7^\pm 2.o$	5.5	$2.3^\pm 1.6$	$3.4^\pm 1.3$
width (mm)	$3.5^\pm 1.2$	$4.1^\pm o.9$	4.3	$2.4^\pm 1.1$	$3.o^\pm 1.6$
CSF cranial ratio (%)	$7.2^\pm 2.6$	$8.5^\pm 3.2$	11.1**	$5.8^\pm 1.8$	$6.8^\pm 1.3$

  * Signif. difference to control group χ^2-test resp. Student's t-test
 ** Signif. difference to other 15 DS patients, α = 99%
*** Subgroup with severe clinical deterioration

Discussion and conclusions:

To which degree the significant differences between the patients
with Down s syndrome and the control groups are due to maldevelopment
or to degeneration cannot be decided. At least in the temporal lobe,
degenerative plaques, tangles and cellular changes are numerous
(Wisniewski et al. 1985). Our CT finding of a (probably) atrophic
temporal lobe with age-dependent progression supports the idea of an
association of M. Down and M. Alzheimer where the histological
changes are similar, but of a slightly different regional distribution
(Ball and Nuttall, 1981). Although a predisposition may exist in
trisomy 21, the process of premature aging results in severe
clinical deterioration only in a subgroup of patients and only
they show marked cerebral atrophy in CT.

REFERENCES

Ball, M.J., Nuttall, K. (1981) Topography of neurofibrilles, tangles,
    and granulovacuoles in hippocampi of patients with Down's syndrome.
    Quantitative comparison with normal aging and Alzheimer's disease.
    Neuropath. Appl. Neurobiol. 7, 21 - 36
Coyle, J.T., Oster-Granite, M.L., Gerhardt, J.D. (1986): The neurobio-
    logic consequences of Down syndrom. Brain Res. Bull. 16: 773 - 787
Ieshima, A., Kisa, T., Yoshino, K., Takashima, S., Takeshita, K. (1984)
    A morphometric CT study of Down's syndrome showing small posterior
    fossa and calcification of basal ganglia. Neuroradiology 26: 493 - 498
Lott, T., Lai, F., (1982) Dementia in Down's syndrome: Observations from
    a neurology clinic. Applied Research in Mental Retardation 3: 233 - 239
Nagata, K., Basugi, N., Fukushima, T., Tango, T., Suzuki, I., Kaminuma, T.
    Kurashina, S. (1987). A quantitative study of physiological cerebral
    atrophy with aging. A statistical analysis of the normal range.
    Neuroradiology 29: 327 - 332
Oliver, C., Holland, A.J., (1986) Down's syndrome and Alzheimer's disease,
    a review. Psychological Medicine 16: 3o7 - 322
Wisniewski, K.E., Wisniewski, H.M., Wen, G.Y., (1985) Occurence of neuro-
    pathological changes and dementia of Alzheimer's disease in Down's
    syndrome. Ann. Neurol. 17: 278 - 282

We thank Dr. S. Letzkus, Anstalt Stetten, for referring 5 patients
into our study.

Radiological and Neuropathological Findings in Gliomatosis Cerebri of Young Age

H. C. Nahser, D. Kühne, and L. Gerhard

Among gliomas, the WHO classification recognizes a group designated as gliomatosis cerebri. In these patients gliomatous neoplastic growth is so diffuse and widespread that both hemispheres, brainstem and cerebellum are involved (Nevin 1938). Most of the glial elements in the type of tumor demonstrate poor differentiation and are fast proliferating, developing multiple areas with accelerated growth (Dunn and Kernohan 1957). By that the rather puzzling type of multifocal clinical symptomatology is explained, which frequently leads to the diagnosis of encephalitis and without brain biopsy is not recognized as a tumour during lifetime.

We have studied 17 autopsy cases, nine of which have been reported in an earlier publication (Nahser et al. 1981). The age of the patients ranges from the first to the sixth decade. Artigas et al. 1985 contributed another 10 cases of their own and compared them with the 48 published cases in 1985. This larger number of cases shows more obviously that the patients belong to two groups regarding their age. The majority of patients are adults with a peak in the fifth decade of life, but a smaller number of patients are children with a peak in the second decade (Fig.1). Our first paper (Nasher et al. 1981) included a 10 year old girl, but recently we observed this tumor in two other children: a 10-year old girl and a 7-year old boy. In all three patients an encephalitis was suspected clinically. This diagnosis was kept up to death in two of our patients. By means of a cortical biopsy in the first a tumor was revealed during lifetime.

The problems of the clinical diagnosis extend to similar difficulties in radiology. Spagnoli et al. (1986) reported the radiological findings in three cases and stated: The diffuse infiltrative nature of this process renders a preoperative diagnosis by classical neuroradiologic studies impossible. The authors believe in a special support of NMR demonstrating a diffuse continuous central high intensity mass demonstrated on T2W1. Our experience in the first nine patients with CT gave a hint only

498

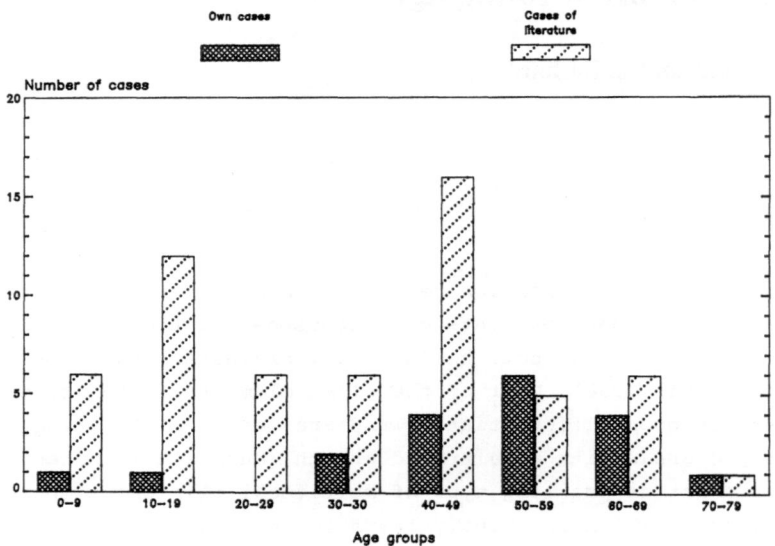

Fig.1. Diagram of own patients and of patients of the literature according to age

in areas with focal mass effect, necrosis or hemorrhage but the field with simple diffuse growth was insignificant. Our recent experience allows the comparison of CT and NMR findings at different stages of the disease and will be reported below.

Case histories

Case 1.

Female, 10 years old (Nahser et al. 1981) (Fig.2). Duration of disease 5 month. The girl first complained about cerebellar symptoms, developed later on focal seizures of Jackson type. To confirm the clinical diagnosis of encephalitis a cortical biopsy was taken according to one of the epileptic foci and the diagnosis of a gliomatosis cerebri was made by microscopical investigation.

The CT, done at that time with a first generation scanner, was totally insignificant.

Histology of the biopsy revealed a widespread glial tumor, characteristic for a diffuse glioma. The girl died with increasing brain stem symptoms 5 months after the onset of first clinical symptoms.

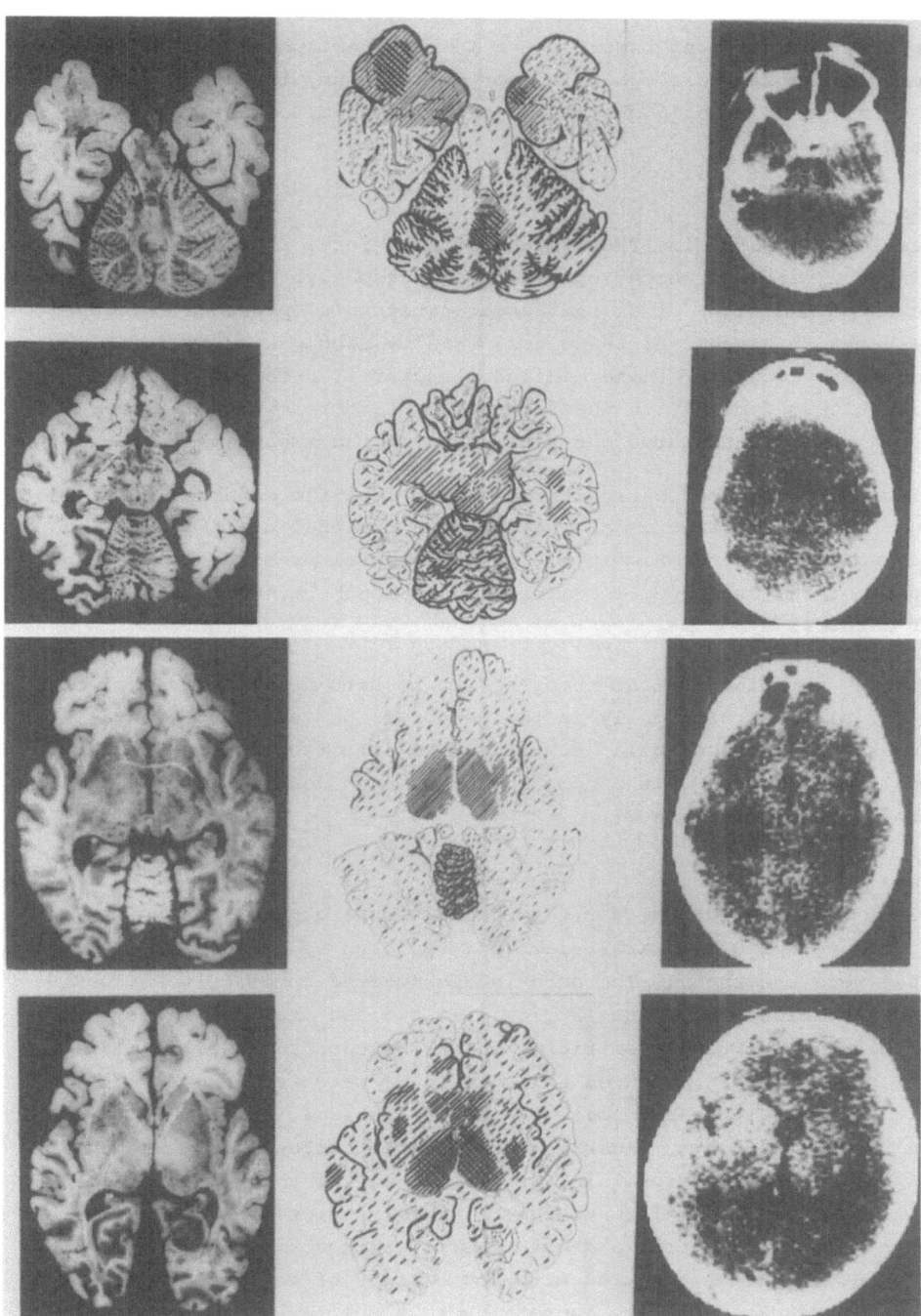

Fig.2. Case 1: Comparison of macroscopic anatomy, distribution pattern of tumor cells and CT at identical levels. The diffuse growth of cells with hyperchromatic nuclei with accentuation in cerebellum, midbrain, temporal lobes and basal ganglia does not lead to pathological changes in the CT (Siretom 1, 1976)

Autopsy demonstrated tumor growth in both hemispheres, especially in temporal lobes, basal ganglia, corpus callosum, thalamus, mesence- phalon, pons, medulla oblongata and cerebellum, especially the white matter.

Case 2.
Female, 10 years old. The disease started for a short phase with vomi- ting and headache which improved sponataneously. After 8 months focal seizures and signs of an increased intracranial pressure developed to- gether with psychic disturbances, finally accompanied by fever. CT demonstrated shift of the midline structures, areas of decreased den- sity situated mainly in the frontal and temporal white matter. An es- pecially hypodense area was recognized in the mesencephalon (Fig.3).

After contrast application there was no specific enhancement besides an attenuation of cortical outlines. An external drainage of liquor was performed by craniotomy, but intracranial pressure increased in- spite of the drainage. The girl died 10 months after the first onset of clinical symptoms.

Autopsy revealed typical tumor growth in both hemispheres including cortical areas especially in the temporal, parietal and frontal lobes, the basal ganglia, central white matter, portions of the thalamus and through the complete brain stem down to the pyramidal crossing (Fig.3,4 and 9).

Case 3.
Male, 7 years old. The first symptoms were a generalized seizure and a fast developing hemiparesis after a few days of headaches. CT find- ings were uneventful. The paresis disappeared completely while NMR investigations were done (Fig.5a). It did not show any shift, but ab- normal small lateral ventricles in the region of the cella media. The basal ganglia appeared enlarged in T1 weighted images while the signal intensity was normal. In T2 both thalami, basal ganglia, dor- sal corpus callosum, midbrain and left temporobasal cortex showed a diffuse increased signal intensity. Because of this peculiar loca- lization herpes simplex encephalitis was suspected and an antiviral therapy started. After a short interval without any symptoms, a sud- den deterioration appeared with acute signs of increased intracra- nial pressure, initially increasing to a complete hemiparesis and later coma. CT scan (Fig.5b) revealed in the left hemisphere a dif- fuse area of low density swelling of both basal ganglia and a small area of increased density at the left temporal pole, where a hemorrhage

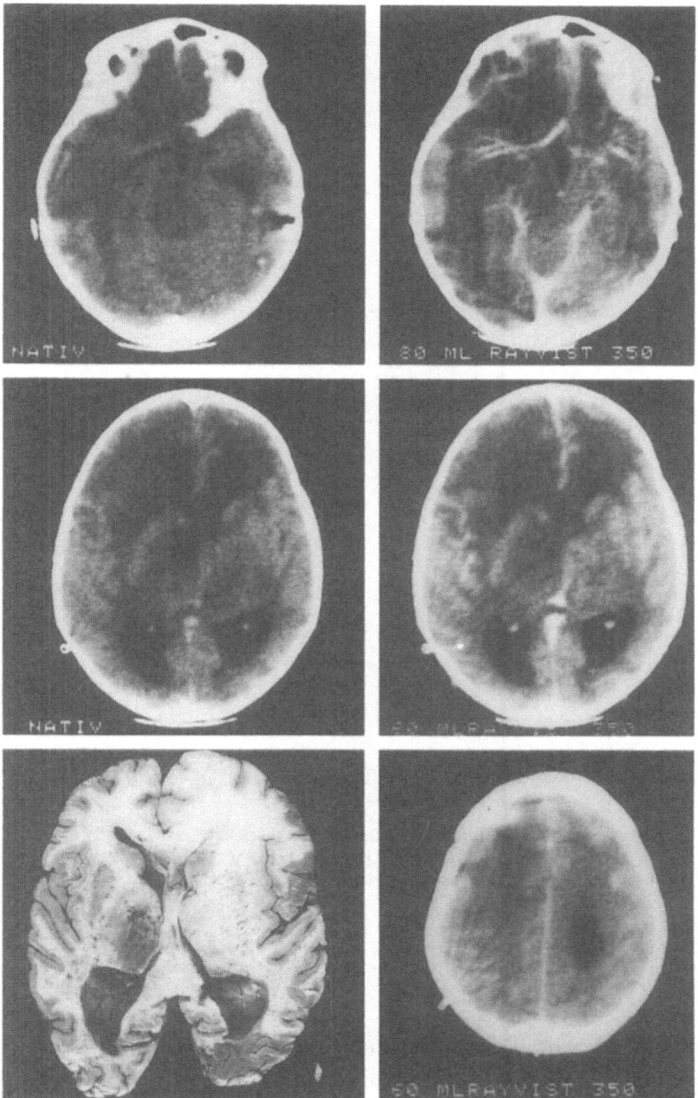

Fig.3. Case 2: CT before and after contrast application reveals decreased density, dilated ventricles and midline shift. No specific enhancement. The anatomic specimen shows the enlargement of corpus callosum and the septum and a focal area of tumor growth with cysts in the left pulvinar

could be discerned. The boy died 24 hours after this event and 2 months after the beginning of the first symptoms.

Autopsy revealed a fresh hemorrhagic necrosis of large parts of the left hemisphere. There was a large hemorrhagic area above the uncus

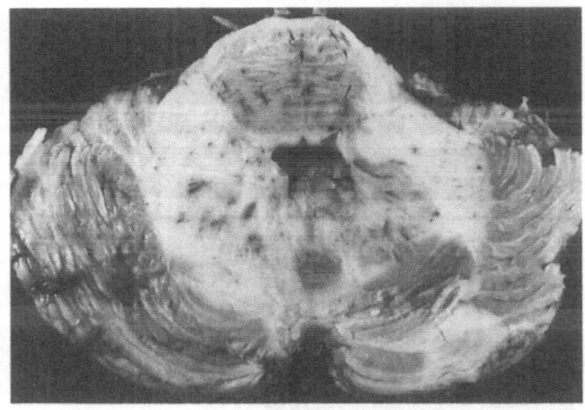

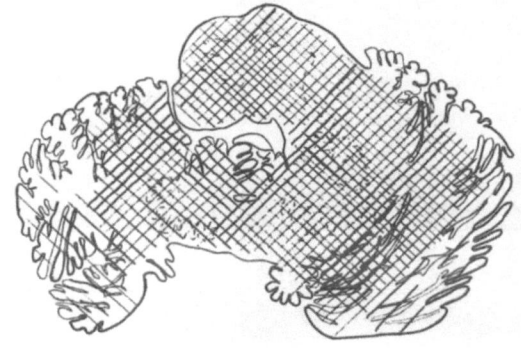

Fig.4. Case 2: Diffuse growth of tumorous cells in pons and white matter of cerebellum as revealed by histology is only suggested by enlargement of the left side of the pons and crus cerebri

herniation in the region of the amygdlum and a midline shift to the right (Fig.6). The tumor extended to both hemispheres concentrating on both temporal lobes with involvement of hippocampal area, both basal ganglia, thalamus, mesencephalon, pons, medulla oblongata and central areas of cerebellum. Tumor cells were still found in the cervical cord in the posterior horn. There was in addition compression of the A. cerebri media on the left side, fresh thrombotic occlusion of the arterial lumina and hemorrhagic hypoxic tissue damage in the left hemisphere (Fig.7). The tumor cells exhibited in some regions characteristic astrocytic differentiation with GFAP-positive cytoplasm, in most of the areas undifferentiated hyperchromatic nuclei with very sparse cytoplasm were found (Fig.8).

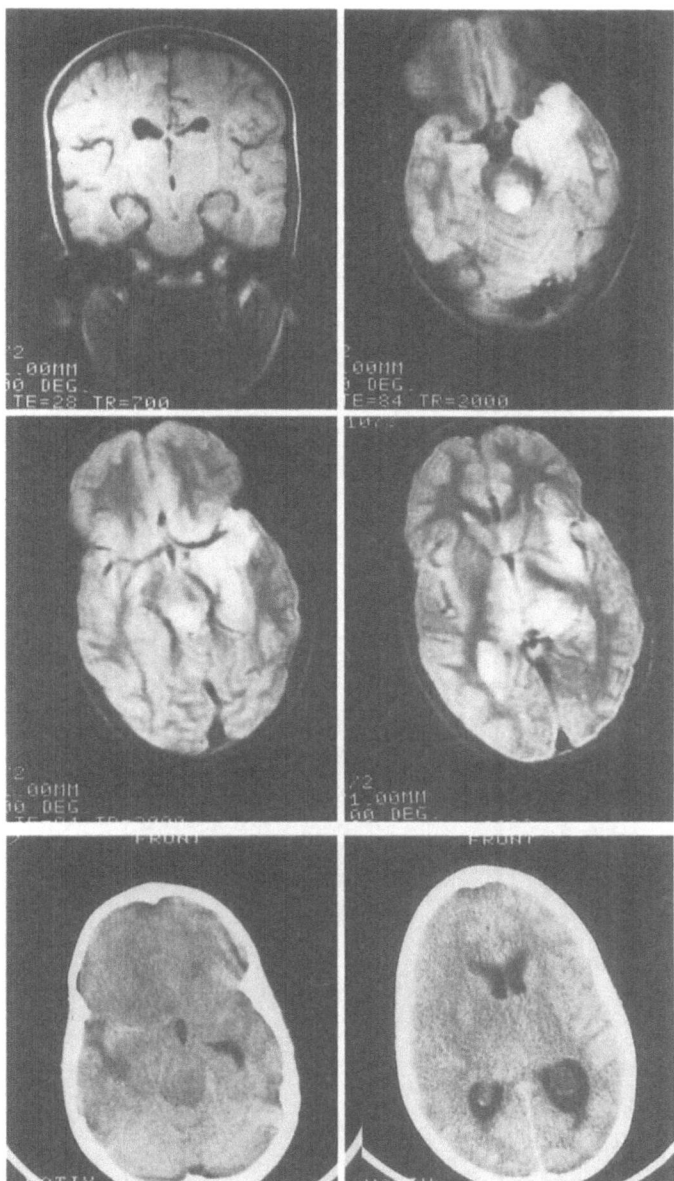

Fig.5. Case 3: a) Abnormal small ventricles and enlarged basal ganglia in T1 weighted images. In T2 WI hyperintensity in a portion of the midbrain, temporal lobe and basal ganglia. b) CT scan performed after clinical deterioration shows a diffuse area of low density in the left hemisphere caused by a pathoanatomically verified compression and thrombosis of the left a. cerebri med.

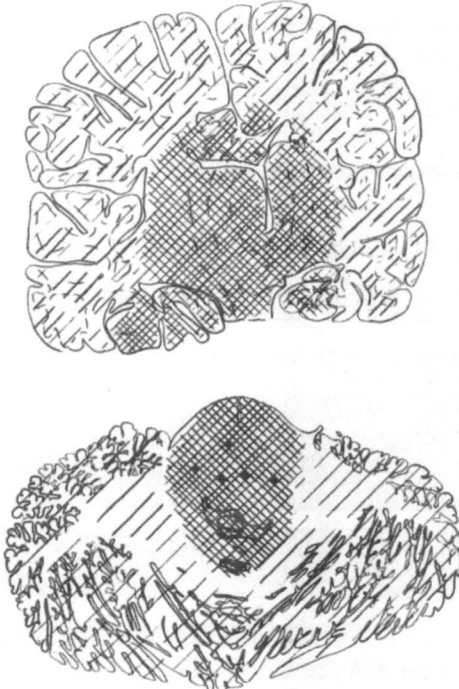

Fig.6. Case 3: Distribution pattern with accentuation of growth of tumor cells in basal ganglia and midbrain while in all other areas the density of tumor cells is lower

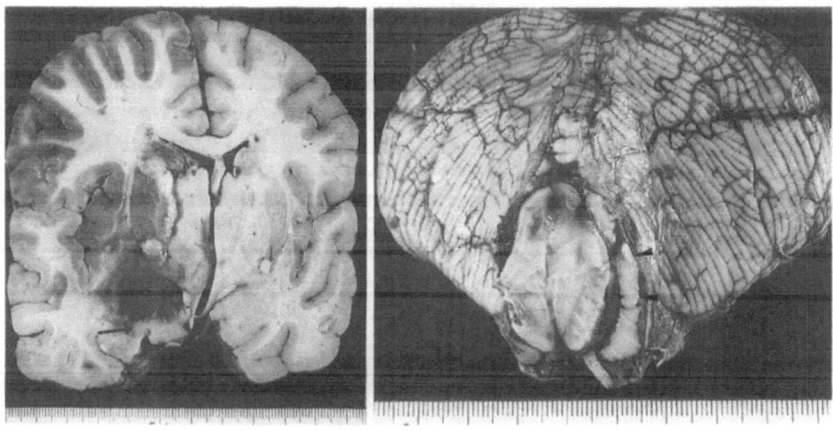

Fig.7. Hemorrhagic necrosis and hemorrhage of the left caused by compression and herniation of the cerebri media. Deep compression (arrow) in the medial region followed by uncus herniation (arrowhead). Considerable shift of the midline. Hemorrhage in the mesencephalon, especially in the corpora quadrigemina with microscopically increased tumor intensity. (Focal accelerated growth with beginning vascular changes and necrosis)

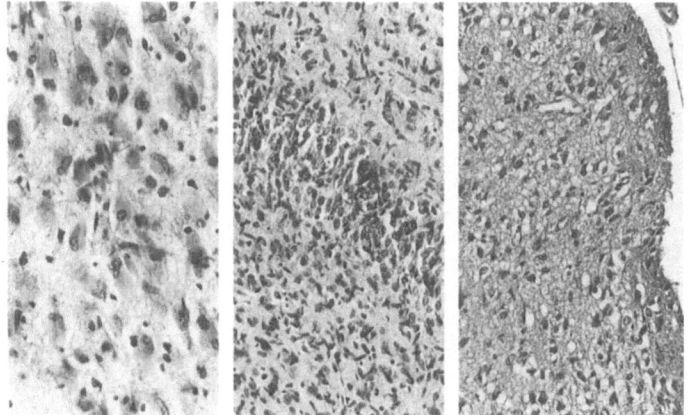

Fig.8. a) Well differentiated GFAP-positive astrocytes in hippocampus and nucleus amygdalae. b) Poorly differentiated cells in
other hippocampal fields with remnants of the fascia dentata. Some
of the tumor cells have irregular and slender nuclei comparable
to active forms of microglia. c) Well differentiated astrocytes
with positive GFAP reaction in the molecular area of cortical layer
leading to an irregular increase of size in the cortical outlines

Discussion

Even today the statement is still justified that with very rare exceptions a diagnosis of gliomatosis cerebri will not be accomplished
during lifetime of adult and of young patients (Nahser et al. 1981,
Artigas et al. 1985, Spagnoli et al. 1987, Dickson et al. 1988). One
exception will be the two cases diagnosed by cortical biopsy (Malamud
et al. 1952, Nahser et al. 1981). The other exceptional case (Miller
et al. 1981) is reported with a suspicious liquor cytology. In adults
the clinical diagnosis may demonstrate a couple of suggested different
diseases including encephalitis, however, in young patients of the
first and second decade of life the clinical diagnosis will be encephalitis in nearly all observed patients.

The microscopic and macroscopic autopsy findings clearly reveal the
reasons for the dilemma of clinical diagnosis. The widespread growth
of tumor has frequently multifocal centers of accelerated growth
leading to necrosis and vascular complications (Fig.9) similar to
glioblastomas or metastasis. The growth in most areas is isomorph,
which means that normal anatomical structures are kept in their outlines but maybe enlarge the structures as in the corpus callosum in
case 1. Liquor cytology will not contribute to the diagnosis since in
most cases no cells or even unspecific changes could be found inspite

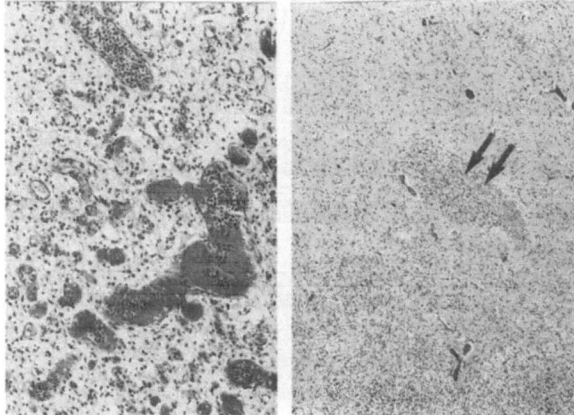

Fig.9. a) Vascular changes in a focal area (Case II) with beginning
necrosis. b) Fiber bundle of the capsula interna demonstrating isomorph growth of tumor cells especially in the white matter (Case II)

of the singular observation of Miller et al. (1981). This is in
contrast to the frequent growth of tumor cells in molecular layer
(Fig.8) and subarachnoidal space. The singular and wide spread growth
will have individual features of the overall pattern and complications
such a hydrocephalus (Dickson et al. 1988) or local compression with
hemorrhagic and hypoxic secondary lesions like in case 3, making the
clinical diagnosis even more difficult. Signs of intracranial pressure
may change during the disease and, in some patients, may sometimes
even be missing. There are only few rather consistent clinical features in gliomatosis cerebri. One is the early appearance of seizures,
frequently of focal seizures. The second fact is the nearly always
present involvement of basal ganglia, temporal lobes with portions of
hippocampal cortex and of the caudal brain stem including the cerebellum. Fever is no symptom in the early stage of the disease, especially at the time when seizures occur, but may appear late in the
disease if intracranial pressure is raised. Haematology will not demonstrate changes pointing to an inflammatory process either inspite
of neurological or psychic symptoms. If focal cortical seizures occur,
cortical biopsy will be of value.

For radiology one important fact is that in large areas with diffuse
tumour growth the disturbance of the blood brain barrier may be slight
or even missing, rendering contrast enhancement not very useful up to
now. If multifocal accelerated growth has led to vascular changes or
necrosis, multifocal lesions may even suggest lymphoma or meta-

stasis. The growth of tumour cells in large areas of the molecular layer of cortical areas may correspond to altered cortical outlines. In NMR the isomorph growth of tumour cells inside normal neuroanatomical borders with slight disturbances of the blood brain barrier may lead to pictures similar to our case 3 with the symmetrically enlarged basal ganglia on both sides exhibiting increased signal intensity which in our case can be contributed to edema. However, in case 2 a considerable involvement of the white central matter had led to loss of myelin. So both interpretations - edema and demyelination - may be true in gliomatosis cerebri in T2 weighted images. As to the special differential diagnosis of herpes simplex encephalitis and gliomatosis cerebri in case 3, one has to keep in mind that temporal lobes and especially the hippocampal areas are frequently and asymmetrically involved in both diseases. Case 3 demonstrates, in addition to this, that even in gliomatosis cerebri vascular complications may occur mimicking hemorrhage necrosis characteristic in herpes simplex encephalitis (Feiden 1986). So only the overall clinical features and the knowledge of the clinical picture of gliomatosis cerebri even in children may lead to a proper diagnosis during lifetime. Case 3 suggests that NMR may support the clinical diagnosis better than CT.

References

[1] Artigas J, Cervos-Navarro J, Iglesias JR, Ebhardt G (1985) Gliomatosis cerebri: clinical and histological findings. Clinical Neuropathology 4: 135-148
[2] Dickson DW, Haroupian DS, Thal LJ, Lantos G (1988) Gliomatosis cerebri presenting with hydrocephalus and dementia. AJNR 9: 200-202
[3] Dunn J, Kernohan JW (1957) Gliomatosis cerebri. AMA Arch Pathol 64: 82-91
[4] Feiden W (1986) Herpes simplex - Encephalitis (HSE). Nervenarzt 57: 19-28
[5] Malamud N, Wise BL, Jones DW (1952) Gliomatosis cerebri. J Neurosurg 9: 409-417
[6] Miller RR, Lin F, Mallone MM (1981) Cytologic diagnosis of gliomatosis cerebri. Acta Cytol 25: 37-39
[7] Nahser HC, Gerhard L, Reinhardt V (1981) Diffuse and multicentric brain tumors: correlation of histological, clinical and CT appearance. Acta Neuropathol (Berl.) 7 (Suppl.): 101-104
[8] Nevin S (1938) Gliomatosis cerebri. Brain 61: 170-191
[9] Scheinker JM, Evans JP (1943) Diffuse cerebral gliomatosis. J Neuropathol Exp Neurol 2: 178-189
[10] Spagnoli MV, Grossman RB, Packer RJ, Hackney DB, Goldberg HB, Zimmerman RA, Bilanivk LT (1987) Magnetic resonance imaging determination of gliomatosis cerebri. Neuroradiology 29: 15-18

Optimized Demonstration of Cerebral Blood Flow with Colour Coded Xenon CT

H. Becker, B. Haubitz, M. Gaab, K. Holl, M.-N. Nemati, and H. Dietz

In the last 18 months we have investigated 250 patients with stable-xenon enhanced x-ray transmission computed tomography (Xe CT) as a noninvasive technique for imaging of cerebral blood flow (CBF). This dynamic Xe CT based on sequential CT scans during inhalation of a mixture of 33 % stable xenon and 67 % oxygen over 5 min. Xe CT may well be suited for diagnostic purposes, especially in patients with cerebrovascular disease. The Xe CT was carried out on a GE 9800 scanner in combination with the commercially available Xenon hard- and software system. Exposure technique at 80 kV and 200 mA, a 256 x 256 matrix, 10 mm slice thickness, and an exposure time of 4 sec was used in all studies. Choosing the level of most significant pathological finding for CBF investigation the scan level was selected from a lateral scout view. Blood flow maps of the Xe-CT studies were calculated by a voxel by voxel evaluation of xenon enhancement over time. The results of data processing are reconstructed on a 128 x 128 matrix. Pre- and postanalysis smoothing routines are used to reduce pixel-to-pixel noise.

At the beginning of our investigations the flow maps were displayed in 16 gray tones from black to white on the monitor and documented on film with a fixed level of +50 HU and a fixed window of 100 HU. In this way the scale ranges from 0 ml/100 g brain tissue/min (black) to 100 ml/100 g brain tissue/min (white). Since October 1987 we have been using a color-coded flow map by transforming the gray tones into different colors. The color scale is according to the natural color spectrum starting with violet and ending with white. The color correlates with the CBF/100 g brain tissue/min, for instance violet (0 ml), blue (25 ml), green (50 ml), red (75 ml) and white (100 ml and more). The color-coded flow maps were displayed on a color screen and then printed with the color hardcopy plotter Delta Scan CH-5301.

These color images offer a diagnostic advantage over the black and white techniques used previously. The color method allows for an improved differentiation especially in regions of extremely low CBF. On the other hand areas of extremely high CBF can be better identified. Small differences in CBF can be easily diagnosed by the increased dynamics of the image. In patients with tumours it will be more easily possible to recognize the vascularisation of the tumour, especially in glioblastomas and meningiomas.

The amount of CBF alterations can be readily determined especially in follow-up studies before and after the administration of acetazol-amide (Diamox[R]). In addition to getting baseline CBF values (resting CBF), this method allows an estimation of cerebrovascular reserve capacity by repeating the CBF study after stimulation with acetazol-amide (Fig. 1).

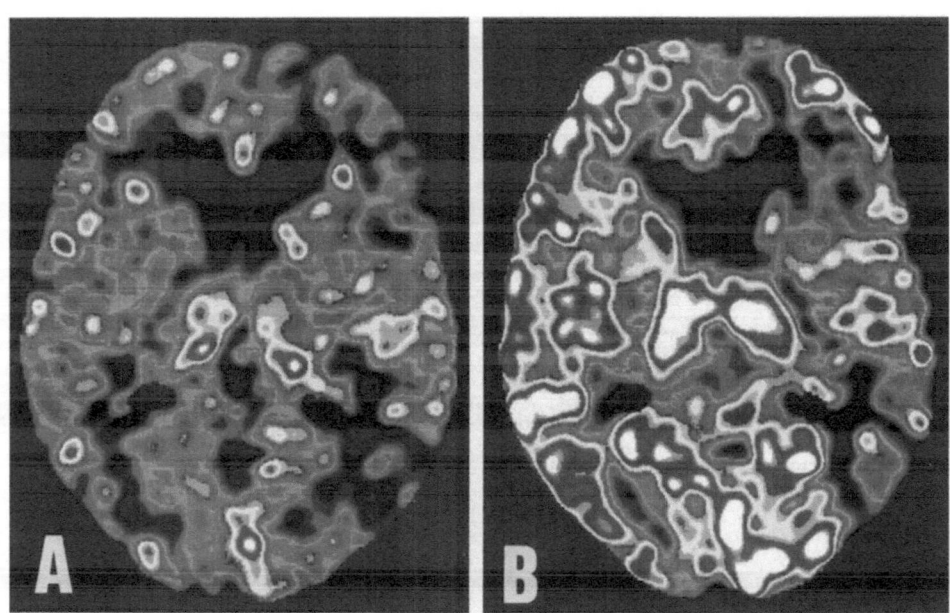

Fig. 1: Xe-CT before (A) and after (B) Diamox[R] in a patient with occlusion of the left internal carotid artery

Unilateral carotid stenoses or occlusion do not usually decrease the resting CBF and differences are missing between the two hemispheres. The cerebrovascular reserve capacity, however, is considerably de-creased by significant extracranial stenoses of occlusion. In patients with unilateral stenosis and contralateral occlusion or bilateral severe stenoses, however, already the resting CBF is decreased and the acetazolamide reaction is often completely missing. In these patients a thrombendarterectomy usually dramatically increases the CBF on both hemispheres and re-establishes a reserve capacity (Fig. 2).

From this point of view color-coded Xe CT is also of value for the approximation of the cerebrovascular reserve capacity as well as in pre- and postoperative studies.

In summary, color-coded Xe CT brings some advantages in comparison to the black and white flow maps. The main point is the improved sensitivity with better differentiation in regions of extremely high or low CBF and improved determination of CBF alterations.

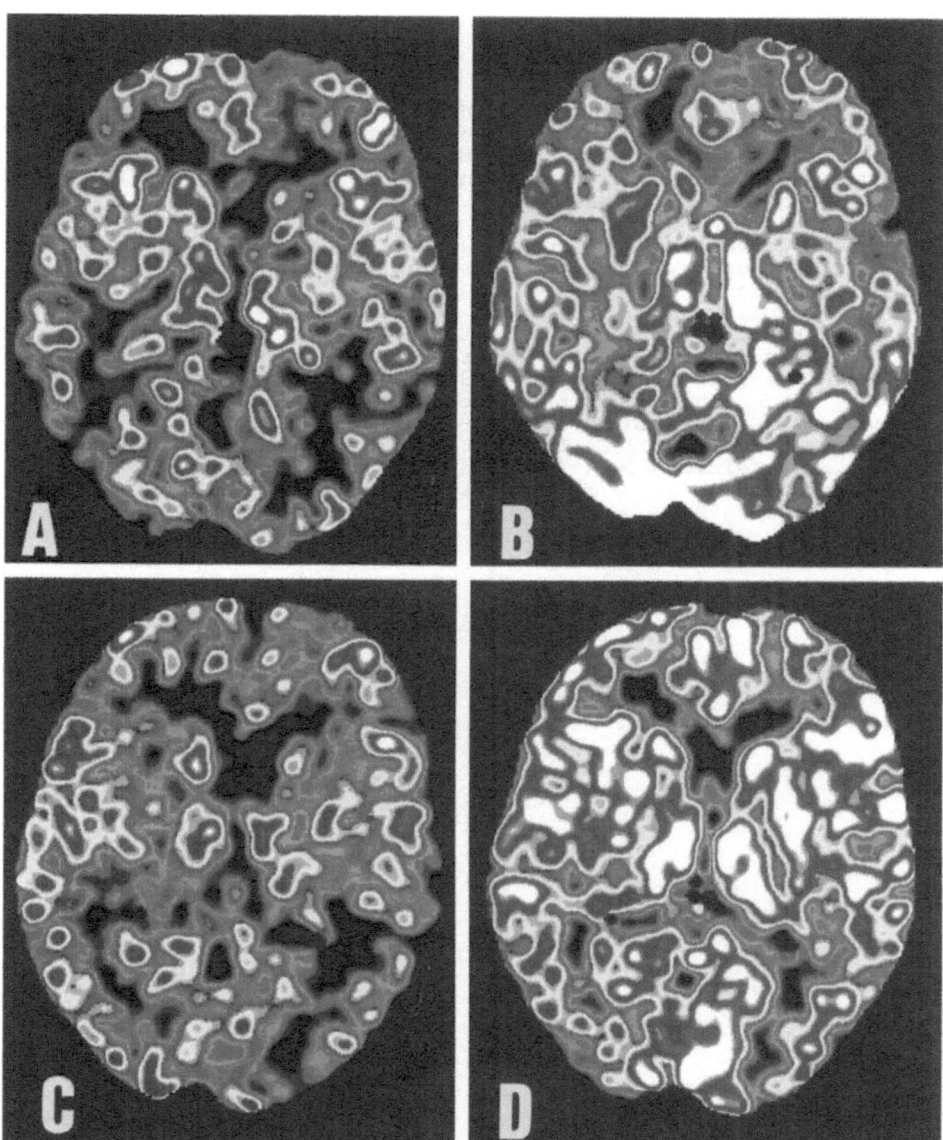

Fig. 2: Preoperative Xe-CT before (A) and after (B) Diamox[R] in a
patient with occlusion of the left internal carotid artery
and highgraded stenosis of the right internal carotid artery.
Control study after thrombendarterectomy on the right side
before (C) and after (D) Diamox[R].

512

REFERENCES

Gaab MR, Schober O, Schwarzrock R, Holl K, Nemati NM, Majewski A,
  Sollmann P, Becker H, Dietz H (1988) Zerebrale Durchblutungsmessung
  bei extra- und intrakraniellen Gefäßerkrankungen: Methoden und Be-
  deutung. In: Supraaortale Arterien, Schütz RM, Schildberg FW (Hrsg.):
  89-109, Hygieneplan Kassel
Majewski A, Holl K, Nemati NM, Gaab MR, Dietz H, Becker H (1988) Xenon-
  CT: Stand der Entwicklung und klinische Einsatzmöglichkeiten. In: Quo
  vadis CT, Claussen C, Felix R (Hrsg.): 320-342, Springer Berlin Hei-
  delberg new York
Majewski A, Holl K, Nemati NM, Gaab MR, Dietz H, Becker H (1988) Die
  Hirndurchblutung im Xenon-CT. Röntgenpraxis 41:311-318
Meyer JS, Shinohara T, Imai A, Kobari M. Sakai F, Hata T, Oravez WT,
  Timpe GM, Deville T, Solomon E (1988) Imaging local cerebral blood
  flow by xenon-enhanced computed tomography - Technical optimization
  procedures. Neuroradiology 30:283-292
Yonas H, Wolfson SK, Gur D, Latchaw RE, Good WF, Leanza R, Jackson DL,
  Jannetta PJ, Reinmuth OM (1984) Clinical experience with the use of
  xenon-enhanced CT blood flow mapping in cerebral vascular disease.
  Stroke 15:443-450

Tissue Characterization by NMR Tissue Parameters Results in 160 Patients with Brain Tumours

M. Just (Mainz, FRG)

In MRI each tissue is characterized by three different parameters: relaxation times T1 and T2, and proton density PD. A reliable tissue characterization is possible if each tissue can be represented by its own region in a three-dimensional space involving the parameters T1, T2, and PD. To evaluate the diagnostic potential of NMR tissue parameters we investigated 160 patients with brain tumors. For simultaneous measurement of T1, T2, and PD we used an interlaced triple CPMG sequence with three different recovery times (320, 640, 1920 ms) and eight echoes/sequences (34 ms < TE < 272 ms). Good agreement with spectrometer measurements of phantoms and small interindividual deviations of tissue parameters of white matter prove the excellent accuracy and reproducibility of the method. In contrast to former clinical studies the simultaneous evaluation of T1, T2, and PD exploits the full quantitative potential of tissue characterization by MRI.

As a result, normal tissues (white and gray matter, fat) are easily separable in a T1,T2,PD space, demonstrating rather narrow distributions. Cystic lesions (craniopharyngiomas) and hematomas are reliably discriminated from other tumors by elevated T2 times and reduced T1 times. Some lesions have a tendency to elevated T1 values (astrocytomas, neuromas) or T2 values (astrocytomas, edemas). However, most distributions demonstrate considerable overlaps, preventing a reliable diagnosis based on tissue parameters alone. One reason might be the varying degree of regressive changes and the different water contents in tumors of identical histology. Close correlations between these changes and the T2 time could be found in meningiomas and neuromas, partly explaining the broad distributions observed.

MR Imaging of Hypothalamic Hamartomas

G. Fahrendorf, J. H. Brämswig, and M. Galanski (Münster, FRG)

Hamartomas of the tuber cinereum are not true tumors but congenital malformations consisting of a tumorlike, ectopic mass of neuronal tissue. The commonest clinical symptom is precocious isosexual puberty.

The diagnosis of hamartoma is most often based on neuroradiologic investigation. CT and cisternography have been the most conclusive radiologic procedures in the majority of cases. With very small lesions and the more diffuse type of hamartoma, CT may, however, be inadequate.

In our series, MRI was performed in six patients with clinical and CT findings suggestive of hamartoma, and showed a highly characteristic appearance of these lesions: a well-circumscribed, more or less pedunculated mass originating from the tuber cinereum, anterior or adherent to the mamillary bodies and extending into the interpeduncular cistern. The lesions were isointense with brain on T1-weighted and hyperintense on T2-weighted images. Due to its capability of multiplanar imaging and optimal delineation of altered morphology, MRI should replace CT and cisternography as a noninvasive method for neuroradiologic evaluation of suspected hamartomas in children with precocious puberty.

Quality Analysis of DSA Equipment

M. A. O. Thijssen, H. O. M. Thijssen, J. L. Merx, and M. P. L. M. van Woensel

INTRODUCTION. In the framework of a quality analysis project the image quality (IQ) and related radiation dose were measured in constructively different DSA equipments in 6 hospitals in the Netherlands. The aim of this work was to develop a simple method for qualification and quantification of image quality, to establish the differences in the equipments and to develop recommandations for improvement. The structure of our investigation was as follows. For dose measurements in the 6 hospitals a human phantom was used to measure the surface dose at the level the thyroid gland using TLD dosimeters. The validity of the use of this phantom was established before in our hospital. We therefore compared the dose measurements on the level of the eye lenses and the thyroid gland on the human phantom with same measurements on 27 patients during a standardized DSA and conventional angiography (CA) of the aortic arch and brachiocephalic arteries. The image quality was measured on a monitor and a hard copy image after optimizing fluoroscopy using a contrast-detail (CD) phantom consisting of a plate of 1 cm of bakelite with dimensions of 26 by 26 cm embedded in 14 cm of perspex. Also the entrance dose on this phantom was measured. In each hospital the IQ parameters of the monitor and hard copy images of the CD phantom were correlated with the entrance dose of the CD phantom and the thyroid dose of the human phantom.

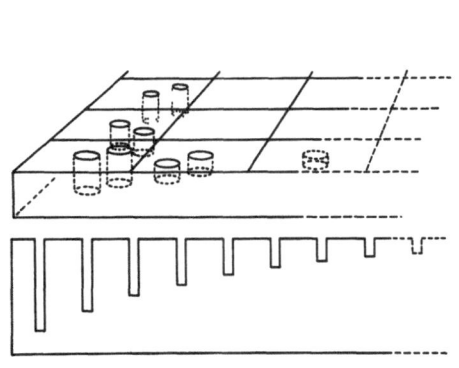

Fig. 1. Schematic drawing of CD phantom

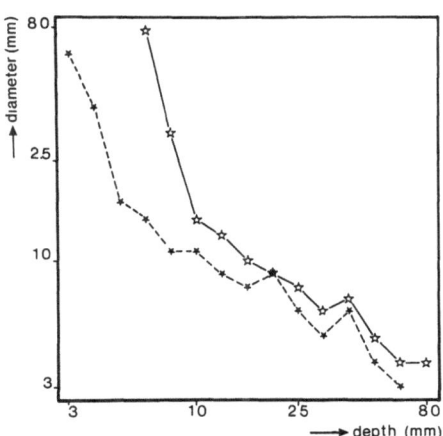

Fig. 2. CD lines of the monitor image (---) and the hard copy image (——) of the DSA equipment in hospital 1

METHOD. For the image quality measurement we use a 1 cm thick plate of bakelite embedded in 14 cm of perspex (fig. 1). It is divided in 225 squares. In the center of each square a hole is drilled varying in diameter and depth in a logarithmic order in 15 steps from 0,3 mm to 8 mm in the vertical and in the horizontal direction, representing contrast and spatial resolution respectively (Ohara et al. 1986; Rose 1974; Starr et al. 1975, 1977; Thijssen 1983). In each square a second hole of the same dimensions is drilled in one of the corners chosen in a randomly manner. In 6 hospitals a monitor and a hard copy image of this phantom was made with the DSA equipment during optimized fluoroscopy at 80 KV and evaluated immediately. Assessment of IQ of the 2 images (monitor and hard copy) of a particular DSA equipment was done by two observers who had to search for the smallest just visible hole for each contrast level. For control they had to agree on the location of the second hole in the square. After the investigation in the 6 hospitals their choice was controlled by comparison with the phantom by a third observer for correctness of the location of the second eccentric hole. The locations of the smallest visible central hole along each of the 15 contraststeps were interconnected to form a contrast-detail (CD) line that represents image quality. However comparison of IQ of 6 hospitals by lines with different slopes and positions is only possible qualitatively. To make a quantitative comparison possible we derived an image quality figure (IQF) from the CD lines. The IQF is defined as the sum of the products of depth (C_i) and diameter (D_i) of the 15 rightly chosen just visible central spots on the CD line. The IQF therefore is described by the formula $IQF = \sum_i C_i D_i$. The lower the IQF the better the IQ.

For the measurement of the radiation dose of the six DSA equipments we used a human phantom. Earlier the validity of this phantom was tested as mentioned before.

Table 1. Some equipment specifications

Equipment DSA/CA DII d/a	IQF monitor image	IQF hard copy image	Image quality ranking	Entrance dose CD phantom	Entrance dose human phantom
1 DSA 28 d	23	33	1	2,16	29,46
2 DSA 23 a	27	34	4	1,77	13,41
3 DSA 20 d	24	39	2	3,30	35,28
4 DSA 18 d	26	26	3	4,93	21,59
5 DSA 23 a	28	32	5	1,04	20,58
6 DSA 33 a	37	54	6	0,23	3,49
7 CA		29*		2,61	25,50

DII: diameter Image Intensifier. d: digital, a: analogue storage.
* IQF of CA measured on serial changer film. Entrance dose in Gy.

It was used for dose measurements at the level of the thyroid gland during a simulated standardized DSA examination of the aortic arch and brachiocephalic arteries in the 6 hospitals. Furthermore in every hospital measurements were carried out of the entrance dose of the bakelite CD phantom for an optimally adjusted image according to local standards at 80 KV.

MATERIAL. The monitor and hard copy images were evaluated for the location of the just visible spot at each contrast (depth) step at the 6 DSA examination-sites. After all investigations in the hospitals the two CD lines of the monitor and hard copy image of each hospital were constructed and the IQF's calculated. The dose measurements of the CD and the human phantoms were correlated to the IQF's of monitor images as determined with the CD phantom.

RESULTS. Concerning image quality there appeared to be large differences in nearly every hospital between monitor and hard copy images as assessed according to the IQF's (table 1 and fig. 2). The IQF of the monitor images is nearly always better. It therefore is advised to use monitor images for the evaluation of clinical DSA examinations.

From the differences in IQF's (table 1) of monitor and hard copy images it can be concluded that much IQ can be gained in hard copy images by using a better or optimized imager (camera).

The difference between the best and the worst IQF of the 6 monitor images indicates that the IQ can be improved in some hospitals.

In table 1 an image quality ranking is given on the basis of the IQF's of monitor images. It is obvious that the equipments with di-

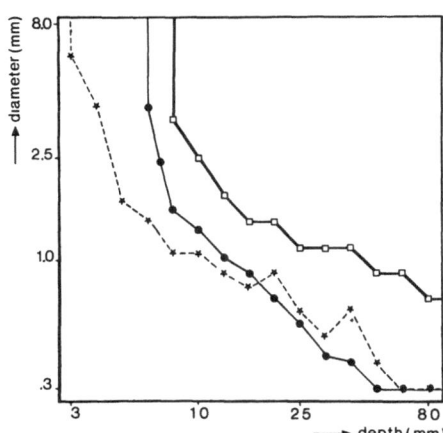

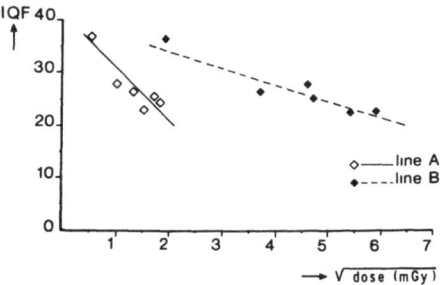

Fig. 3.CD lines of different DSA equipments with the best monitor image (hospital 1): *, the worst hard copy image (hospital 6): □ and of CA equipment (hospital 1): ●

Fig. 4.Correlation between IQF's for monitor images and entrance dose of CD phantom (A) and thyroid dose of human phantom (B)

gital storage of images give the best image quality, another technical factor as image intensifier diameter does not play a significant role.

Comparing the CD line of the best monitor image of DSA equipment and the one of conventional angiography (CA) as visible in fig. 3 it is obvious that CA has the best IQ in the region of the high contrast, in the region of the low contrast however DSA performs better.

There appears to be good correlation (fig. 4) between the IQF's for monitor images and the entrance doses at the CD phantom (correlation coefficient: − 0,92) and the same IQF's for monitor images and the thyroid gland doses of the human phantom (correlation coefficient: − 0,94). The correlation to one another between the entrance doses ($\sqrt{\text{dose}}$) of the CD phantom and the thyroid gland doses ($\sqrt{\text{dose}}$) of the human phantom has a correlation coefficient of + 0,89. On the basis of these correlations it can be pointed out that improvement of IQ of various DSA equipments can be obtained by an increase of radiation dose (dose^2), eventually to the level of the best performing DSA equipment. It is necessary however to define for the future an acceptable minimum IQ (maximum IQF) for DSA equipments.

Our method of IQ measurement as described here is able to assess the performance of any imaging device as is done in ROC analysis. The differences are that in our method only one image is used instead of multiple and that the detection task is not limited to whether an object is seen or not but also evaluates the location where is is seen thereby excluding observer bias. Both methods are similar in that they assess the whole imaging chain including the observer.

CONCLUSIONS. We have developped a method for measurement of IQ of DSA and other imaging equipment. With the resulting CD lines and IQF's it is possible to compare the performance of the DSA-equipments of various manufacturers. Some conclusions can be drawn. Low IQ (high IQF) can be improved by increasing radiation dose and by using the best performing imager (camera). Radiation dose could be increased to the level of the best performing equipment concerning the ALARA-principle. It furthermore is necessary to define a minimum acceptable IQ for DSA and other equipment. Control of performance on a regular base is easy to execute with the method described.

REFERENCES

Ohara K, Chan HP, Doi K (1986) Investigation of basic imaging properties in digital radiography. Detection of simulated low contrast objects in DSA images. Am Assoc Phys Med 13: 304-311

Rose A (1974) Vision, human and electronic. Plenum Press, New York, p 26

Starr JS, Metz CE, Lusted LB, Goodenough DJ (1975) Visual detection and localization of radiographic images. Radiology 116: 533-538

Starr JS, Metz CE, Lusted LB (1977) Comments on the generalization of receiver operating characteristic analysis to detection and localization tasks. Phys Med Biol 22: 376-379

Thijssen MAO (1983) Receiver operating characteristics curves in diagnostic imaging. Diagn Imag Clin Med 52: 163-168

Pattern Recognition in MR Images of Myelin Disorders

J. Valk and M. S. v. d. Knaap

In primary myelin disorders there are two categories of diseases, the hereditary and the acquired myelin disorders. For a new classification based on the cellular substructures, the so-called organelles, of these diseases the reader is referred to [3].

Steps in Pattern Recognition

In pattern recognition of diagnostic images three levels of action can be distinguished [1,2].

Image Formation. The first step is the process by which the image is acquired, dealing with the technical conditions of the equipment and the parameter settings by the operator. Limitations and possibilities of image formation are often the product of factors that cannot be influenced. Quality assessment can guarantee that the machine operates at its optimal level. For a correct setting of the manipulatable parameters, a thorough understanding of the imaging process is a prerequiste.

Image Analysis. Apart from the psychophysiological phenomenon of the human perceptual processes, the second step is the identification and classification of the structural elements of the image. These structural elements should be chosen as possible diagnostic determinants. The knowledge to define these structural elements must be derived from other sources: pathology, biochemistry, and other imaging modalities.

Image Interpretation. To read the image, the above mentioned factors are combined with knowledge of histological entities, clinical course of the relevant diseases, and, of course, the evaluation of the information obtained by the classification of the structural elements.

Here, we will not discuss the first step, image formation, or the physiopsychological perceptual processes involved in the image analysis, but indicate the structural elements as defined by us to recognize the various patterns.

Structural Elements

The structural elements used in pattern analysis are summarized in Table 1. From this table it is clear that the number of structural

Table 1. Structural elements in pattern analysis

Distribution
Involved structures
Pattern of spread
Symmetry
Aspect of the lesion
Isolated - confluent
Demarcation
Extra elements
Calcification
Iron deposition
Gray matter involvement
Enhancement with G-DPTA

Table 2. Preferential sites of diseases

Preferential Site	F	P	O	T	CC	BN	PO	C	UF	WM	GM
Adrenoleukodystrophy	±	+	+++	±	++	±	±	±	−	+	−
Metachromatic leukodystrophy	+	+	+	+	±	±	±	±	−	+	−
Multiple sklerosis	+	+	+	±	++	±	+	±	−	+	±
Schilder's desease	±	++	±	±	++	±	+	±	−	+	−
Posthypoxic demiyelination	+	+	+	±	±	++	±	±	−	+	±
Subacute HIV encephalitis	++	++	±	±	±	−	−	−	−	+	−
Leigh's disease	±	±	±	±	±	+++	++	+	−	+	+
Central pontine myelinalysis	−	−	−	−	−	−	++	−	−	+	−

F, Frontal; P, parietal; O, occipital; T, temporal; CC, corpus callosum; BN, basal nuclei; PO, pons; C, cerebellum; UF, arcuate fibers; WM, white matter; GM, gray matter elements considered in this analysis is rather arbitrary. It is possible to calculate the additional percentage of diagnostic accuracy obtained by adding a further dividing criterion. In Table 2 the preferential sites are shown. From this second table it becomes clear that in a number of diseases location alone can suggest a certain diagnosis, e.g., adrenoleukodystrophy, Leigh's disease, central pontine myelinolysis, subacute HIV encephalities. Table 3 shows the importance of the pattern of spread that also can be a helpful indication of the diagnosis.

Table 3. Pattern of spread

Dorsoventral	Alexander's disease
Ventrodorsal	X-Adrenoleukodystrophy
Centrifugal	Most dys- and demyelinating disorders
Centripetal	Canavan's disease
Diffuse	Aminoacidopathies

After defining and classification of the structural elements the next step in the process is estimating what kind of pattern has emerged:

Diagnostic: the diagnosis is certain on the basis of the image.
Highly suggestive: only one piece of clinical or laboratory evidence is necessary to confirm the diagnosis.
Suggestive: the contribution from several other clinical or laboratory tests is necessary to make the diagnosis.
Probable: most of the evidence for the diagnosis must come from other clinical or laboratory investigations.
Atypical: unusual image with definite clinical or laboratory diagnosis.

Diseases for which a pattern can be classified as diagnostic or highly suggestive are listed in Tables 4 and 5 respectively.

Table 4. "Diagnostic" category of diseases

Adrenoleukodystrophy
Zellweger's cerebrohepatorenal syndrome
Cockayne's syndrome
Connatal Pelizaeus-Merzbacher disease
Subacute encephalities (HIV)
Periventricular leukomalacta

Table 5. "Strongly suggestive" category of diseases

Metachromatic leukodystrophy
Krabbe's Globoid cell leukodystrophy
Leigh's disease
Pelizaeus-Merzbacher disease (later forms)
Canavan's disease
Alexander's disease
Fukuyama's disease
Schilder's disease
Central pointine myelinolysis
Posthypoxic demyelination
Postirradiation leukoencephalopathy

Conclusions

In our opinion it obviously does not make sense to discuss in general terms the specificity of MR images for a defined category of disorders. Specificity does not necessarily have to be considered as an "all or nothing" issue. Diagnostic accuracy can be considered as an intensity scale, as described above. Using this kind of image analysis, it is remarkable how many of the myelin disorders can be categorized as diagnostic or highly suggestive. In this way the role of MRI in these disorders becomes apparent.

References

[1] Valk J, MacLean C, Algra PR (1985) Basic principles of nuclear magnetic resonance imaging. Elsevier, Amsterdam, New York, Oxford
[2] Valk J (1987) MRI of the brain, head, neck and spine. A teaching atlas of clinical applications. Martinus Nijhoff, Dordrecht
[3] Valk J, Knaap vd MS (1988) Magnetic resonance of myelin, myelination and myelin disorders. Springer, Berlin Heidelberg New York (in press)

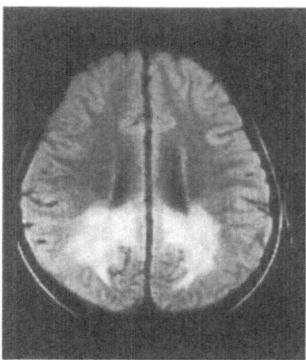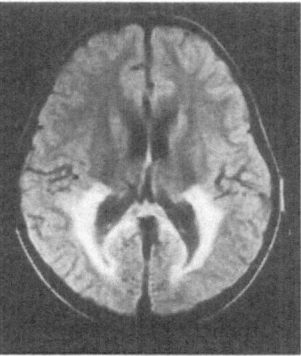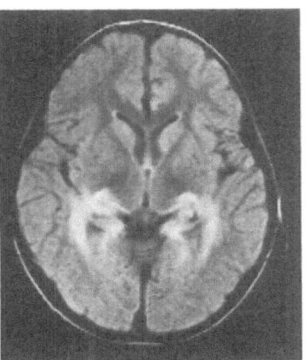

Fig.1. MR image. Pattern of the lesion: normal ventricles, normal cortex; lesions of white matter around the occipital horns, with involvement of the genu corporis callos; sparing of the U fibers. "Diagnostic" of adrenoleukodystrophy

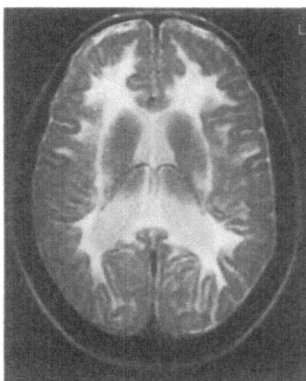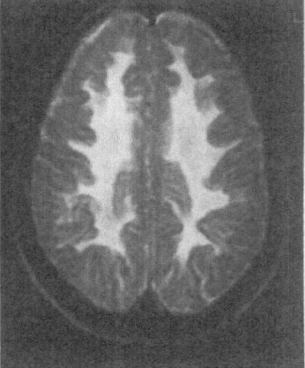

Fig.2. MR image. Pattern of the lesion: normal ventricles, no cortical atrophy; widespread lesion of the central white matter; sparing of U fibers; symmetric; confluent. "Highly suggestive" of metachromatic leukodystrophy. Clinical or laboratory support to confirm diagnos: deficiency of arylsulfatase A

Intraocular Tumours in Adults: MRI versus CT

E. A. Cabanis, M. T. Iba-Zizen, A. Lopez, E. Thervet, J. Tamraz, and J. Haut (Paris, France)

CT has proved useful in diagnosis of intraocular tumours in adults; MR examination seems to verify the importance of the method.

Materials and Methods

Fifteen adults with intraocular melanoma were examined with MRI. All of them had a comparative CT and were histologically proven. T1W and T2W SE (3 echoes) sequences were performed on a 0.15 T (R, prototype) magnet. A double curved elliptic surface coil was used. The neuro-ocular plane (NOP), as well as the transhemispheric oblique NOP (TONOP), were the references. This material was compared to that of previous CT.

Results and Discussion

The signal of the melanoma in T1W sequences appears to have a higher intensity than the vitreous, and a lower one in T2W sequences; the more the sequence is T2 weighted, the weaker is the signal. MR allows positive diagnosis of an intraocular tumoral process and, at the same time, isolates it from all the other reactional phenomena, like hemorragic or serous effusion and retinal detachment. Therapy is becoming more and more conservative (radiotherapy vs. surgery), and MR allows optimal localization of the tumour to reduce the size of the radiotherapy field. A limitation of the method is the small size of the tumour and of its exophytic portion. The follow up examination is not performed in the same way in adults as in children because of the prevalence of metastasis.

Conclusion

After a clinical examination, MR and CT bring complementary information to help determine the therapeutic strategy.

Intraocular Tumours in Children: MRI versus CT?

M. T. Iba-Zizen, E. A. Cabanis, A. Lopez, E. Thervet, J. Tamraz,
and H. Hammard (Paris, France)

The purpose of this work is to compare CT and MR in the initial
diagnosis and follow up of ocular tumours in children, e.g. retinoblastomas.

Materials and Methods

Technical points for pediatric MR are stressed: sedation and ocular
immobility, surface coils and SE sequences at 0.15 T, correct cephalic orientation (neuro-ocular plane (NOP) and trans-hemispheric oblique NOP (TONOP)). All the patients had a preliminary CT. Ten
children with retinoblastomas and twenty others with different ocular
pathologies (Coats' disease, persistent primary vitreous, coloboma)
had an MR examination. This material was compared to fifty retinoblastomas previously diagnosed and followed up with CT only.

Results and Discussion

On T1W and T2W first echo SE sequence, MR fails to identify the calcification of the retinoblastoma, well seen on CT. The T2W third
echo only shows an "intraocular signal defect" corresponding to the
latter. CT seems to be more efficient for the recognition of a trans-
laminar extension. The main MR superiority concerns the lesion homogeneity. Comparison of the signal intensity between T1W and T2W sequences allows solid retinoblastoma to be differentiated from associated retinal detachment. Histological correlations prove the sensitivity of MR with liquid detachment (differential diagnosis). After
surgical or conservative therapy, the follow up examination should
be CT, because of various possible MR artifacts.

In conclusion, modifications of the imaging strategy in ocular
diseases of children are proposed.

MR Findings in Vermian-Cerebellar Hypoplasia

P. M. Parizel, J. van Goethem, E. F. Avni, H. R. Degryse,
A. M. De Schepper, and D. Balériaux

INTRODUCTION

The concept of vermian-cerebellar hypoplasia is a general notion including multiple syndromes (e.g. Joubert syndrome) and posterior fossa malformations resulting in a diminution of cerebellar volume [Sarnat and Alcalá 1980]. The multiplanar imaging capability of MR offers a unique opportunity to study the vermis and cerebellum and has generated a renewed interest in developmental malformations of the posterior fossa [Press et al. 1988]. A relationship between autism and hypoplasia of vermal lobules VI and VII has been suggested in a recent study [Courchesne et al. 1988].

Most malformative syndromes of the posterior fossa are believed to represent abnormalities in structures that are formed simultaneously between the 7 th and 10 th weeks of embryological life [Raybaud 1982], and therefore it is logical to assume that they are the result of an injury occurring during that time period. Further evidence for this hypothesis is provided by their association with the same supratentorial (prosencephalic) malformations [Raybaud 1982].

Because these lesions probably represent a continuum [Barkovich et al. 1988], a precise classification is difficult and is usually only possible by neuropathologic examination. Adding to the problem of classification is the wide range of vocabulary and the plethora of synonyms, used by different authors to indicate similar findings.

Although we are aware that our choice of semantics is open to discussion, we have defined **vermian-cerebellar hypoplasia** as a failure of full development of the vermis or cerebellar hemispheres or both. This definition implies that the vermal lobules are present but hypoplastic. The condition can be subdivided into inferior, complete or superior hypoplasia, depending on whether only the inferior vermis, the entire vermis, or only the upper vermis was affected. Complete **agenesis** of the vermis and cerebellum is only rarely observed.

MATERIAL AND METHODS

The MR examinations of 28 patients with a diminution of the vermian-cerebellar volume and enlargement of the infra- and/or retro-cerebellar cerebrospinal fluid spaces were reviewed.

The MR examinations were performed on a 0.5 Tesla superconducting system (Siemens Magnetom). A 30 cm field of view head coil was used. In all instances, a sagittal T1 weighted spin echo sequence was obtained. In most cases, the MR examination was completed with proton-density and T2 weighted axial, coronal or sagittal images.

In all patients a standardized measurement method was applied on the midsagittal image. The following measurements were obtained: height of the 4th ventricle (AP4V); antero-posterior diameter of the cerebellar vermis (APVER); rostro-caudal diameter of the cerebellar vermis (RCVER); width of the infra-vermian subarachnoid space (INFRA); width of the retro-vermian subarachnoid space (RETRO); largest antero-posterior diameter of the corpus callosum.

On the basis these data, a 'cerebellar vermis index' was calculated; this index was defined as the ratio of height of the 4th ventricle divided by the rostrocaudal diameter of the vermis (AP4V/RCVER). In addition to these measurements, a qualitative analysis was made of the following characteristics: impression on the tentorium cerebelli; position of the torcular; signs of increased intracranial pressure in the posterior fossa (bone erosion); size of the supratentorial ventricular system; width of the 4th ventricular outflow tract; degree of rotation of the cerebellar vermis

The same quantitative (measurements) and qualitative analysis was used in 21 normal controls.

RESULTS

Analysis of the measurement data in Table 1 (all distances represent mean values, expressed in mm) shows that vermian hypoplasia is principally characterized by a decreased rostro-caudal diameter of the vermis. The average

Table 1. Results - cerebellar vermis measurements

MEAN VALUES (in mm)	AP 4V	APVER	RCVER	INFRA	RETRO	INDEX
VERMIAN HYPOPLASIA						
INFERIOR VERMIS (n=11)	13.4	25.2	33.2	15.0	6.2	.42
COMPLETE VERMIS (n=8)	14.9	18.3	25.4	23.9	22.1	.62
SUPERIOR VERMIS HYPOLASIA (n=1)	12	10	29	7	48	.37
VERMIAN-CEREBELLAR ATROPHY (n=1)	15	26	31	4	18	.48
DANDY-WALKER (n=2)	75	22	21	16	56	3.73
BLAKE POUCH CYST (n=3)	9.7	25.7	41.7	6.7	24.7	.23
MEGACISTERNA MAGNA (n=2)	16	25	41	9	14	.24
NORMAL CONTROLS (n=21)	10.2	25.4	43.7	5.5	10.4	.23

rostro-caudal diameters in inferior vermis hypoplasia (11 patients) and hypoplasia of the total vermis (8 patients) were 33.2 mm and 25.4 mm respectively. These values are markedly less than the average measurement of 43.7 mm found in 21 normal controls.

In the patients with complete vermis hypoplasia, the antero-posterior diameter of the vermis was decreased as well (18.3 mm), whereas this measurement was normal in patients within inferior vermis hypoplasia (25.2) when compared to normal controls (25.4 mm).

The 'cerebellar vermis index' (AP4V/RCVER) was 0.42 in patients with inferior vermis hypoplasia and 0.62 in patients with complete vermis hypoplasia. When compared to the index found in normal individuals (0.23), these values reflect the greater size of the fourth ventricle relative to the size of the vermis in cases of hypoplasia.

Associated findings in hypoplasia of the vermis included a cavum septi pellucidi (1 patient), complete agenesis of the corpus callosum (1 patient), and partial agenesis of the corpus callosum (1 patient). In another patient the splenium of the corpus callosum presented an unusually low position, reaching down almost into the posterior fossa.

The degree of rotation of the vermis with respect to the brainstem was not quantified, though it was clear that differences did exist. In 3 instances the vermis appeared almost normal except that it seemed incompletely rotated, resulting in an increased diameter of distance between vermal lobules IX and X and the brain stem (fourth ventricular outflow tract).

It is interesting to note that the sum of the rostrocaudal diameter of the vermis and the width of the infravermian subarachnoid space was virtually identical in patients with inferior vermis hypoplasia (48.2 mm), in patients with complete hypoplasia of the vermis (49.3 mm) and in normal controls (49.2 mm). The similarity of these values indicates that the total height of the posterior fossa does not differ significantly in these groups.

In the 3 patients with a retrocerebellar Blake's pouch cyst, all measurements were within the normal range including the calculated index, except for the width of the retrocerebellar subarachnoid space.

DISCUSSION

In typical cases, vermian-cerebellar hypoplasia is characterized by a small appearance of the vermis and cerebellum, with a prominent folial pattern, a large fourth ventricle, large cisterna magna and wide vallecula. In the complete form, the entire vermis is underdeveloped (Fig. 1), whereas in the partial hypoplasia only the inferior vermis appears too small (Fig. 2). In a patient with hypoplasia of the superior vermis, the superior vermal lobules were grossly abnormal (Fig. 3). This is presumably the result of a secondarily acquired condition.

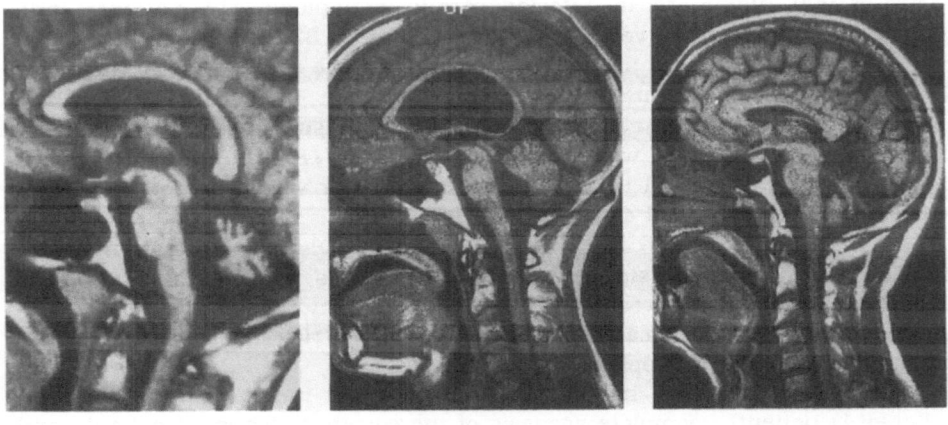

Fig. 1   Fig. 2   Fig. 3

DIFFERENTIAL DIAGNOSIS

Blake's pouch cyst: The classical description defines Blake's pouch cyst as an evagination of the tela choroidea of the 4th ventricle to form a cerebrospinal fluid filled pouch behind an intact vermis and cerebellum. This pouch is easily identified on a midsagittal MR image (Fig. 4). It may present an upward extension between the dural venous sinuses and the tabula interna of the occipital bone, resulting in an elevated position of the torcular. The signal intensities within the pouch are similar to cerebrospinal fluid both on T1 and T2 weighted spin echo sequences. On axial images, a falx cerebelli is often identified within the cyst.

Cerebellar atrophy: In patients with familial heredo-degenerative disorders, cerebellar atrophy is sometimes encountered. It is characterized principally by a dilatation of the vermian sulci, indicating loss of vermal tissue substance (Fig. 5). Similar findings have been extensively described in alcoholics.

Dandy-Walker syndrome and variant: Although hypoplasia of the vermis may be part of the Dandy-Walker syndrome, it must be differentiated from vermian-cerebellar hypoplasia. The Dandy-Walker syndrome is characterized by a malformation of the vermis, a cystic dilatation of the roof of the 4th ventricle, a high insertion of the torcular with 'torcular-lambdoid inversion (Fig. 6). In the Dandy-Walker variant, there is a partial agenesis of the vermis with normal communication between the 4th ventricle and the perimedullary subarachnoid spaces.

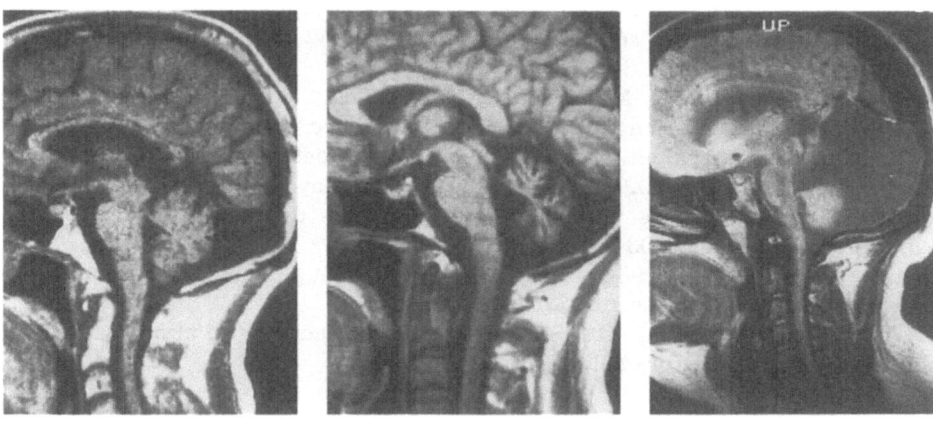

Fig. 4   Fig. 5   Fig. 6

CONCLUSIONS

The multiplanar imaging capability of MR offers a unique opportunity to study the vermis and cerebellum. Our experience appears to indicate that vermian-cerebellar hypoplasia is more common than previously believed. The relatively high frequency of hypoplasia or absence of the inferior vermis supports the hypothesis that the direction of embryological development of the vermis is in a rostrocaudal direction [van der Knaap and Valk 1988].

A precise classification of posterior fossa malformations is difficult, because of the wide range of malformations and the many intermediary types which defy classification. Furthermore, the vocabulary used to describe these lesions is often inconsistent. For these reasons, we have developed a measurement system to describe the various components of the posterior fossa on a midline sagittal MR image. By using this system we were able to define and quantify the characteristics of vermian hypoplasia. Further work needs to be done in this direction to determine whether the patterns we found in a limited number of patients can be confirmed in a larger series.

REFERENCES

Barkovich AJ, Kjos BO, Edwards MS, Norman D (1988) New concepts in posterior fossa cysts in children. Presented at the 26th Annual Meeting of the American Society of Neuroradiology, Scientific Program p. 115, paper #88, Chicago, May 15-20, 1988

532

Courchesne E, Yeung-Courchesne R, Press GA, Hesselink JR, Jernigan TL
(1988)   Hypoplasia of cerebellar vermal lobules VI and VII in autism. New
Engl J Med 318 (21): 1349-1354

Press GA, Courchesne E, Murakami J, Berthoty DP, Wiley CA, Hesselink JR
(1988) The vermis in sagittal plane: MR-pathologic correlation. Presented at
the 26th Annual Meeting of the American Society of Neuroradiology,
Scientific Program p. 192, paper #147, Chicago, May 15-20, 1988

Raybaud C   (1982)   Les malformations kystiques de la fosse postérieure.
J Neuroradiology   9: 103-133

Sarnat HB, Alcalá H   (1980)   Human cerebellar hypoplasia: a syndrome of
diverse causes. Arch Neurol 37: 300-305

van der Knaap MS, Valk J   (1988) Classification of congenital abnormalities of
the CNS. Am J Neuroradiol (AJNR) 9: 315-326

Intraarterial Chemotherapy of WHO Grade IV Cerebral Gliomas with the Nitrosourea Derivate 1-(4-Amino-2-Methyl-5-Pyrimidinyl)-Methyl-(2-Chlorethyl)-3-Nitrosourea (ACNU)

N. Roosen, J. C. W. Kiwit, E. Lins, and T. Kahn

Surgery and radiotherapy are standard therapy for malignant gliomas and have proved efficacity in increasing survival (Walker et al 1980). Other therapeutic approaches have been investigated but their influence on tumor growth remains uncertain; in particular, chemotherapy is judged controversially among clinicians, although some increase in median survival time and in the proportion of longterm survivors has been reported (Kornblith & Walker 1988). Chemotherapy of malignant gliomas may be administered by a locoregional approach via the internal carotid artery (ICA), and this might have a positive influence on the therapeutic efficacity, both on theoretical grounds (Eckman et al 1974) as well as suggested by clinical reports (Greenberg et al 1984; Tyler et al 1986). The hydrophilic nitrosourea ACNU has been shown to achieve high blood and tumor tissue levels after intra-arterial (i.a.) administration (Hori et al 1987) and a preliminary report on i.a. infusion of ACNU (iaACNU) demonstrated a good tumor response with minor side effects (Yamashita et al 1983). Therefore, we initiated a clinical study of adjuvant iaACNU chemotherapy in addition to surgery and irradiation, and present some of our results in patients with WHO grade IV cerebral gliomas.

STUDY POPULATION, TREATMENT PROTOCOL, AND METHODS

During the past 30 months 48 patients with malignant gliomas of the brain were treated according to our protocol of adjuvant iaACNU chemotherapy. Five of these patients had a WHO grade III glioma and are not further considered in this analysis. The remaining patients had WHO grade IV gliomas, either anaplastic gliomas (N=9) or glioblastoma multiforme (N=34). Sex distribution was almost equal ($\female/\male \rightarrow 22/21$). Median age was 45.5 years and mean age 50.5 ± 8.3 years. The frontal and temporal lobes were preferentially involved (76.7%). Thirty-six patients had primarily diagnosed tumors and in 7 cases recurrent neoplasms were treated. Radical surgery was achieved in 24 patients. When this was not feasible due to tumor localization or extent a partial resection (15 cases) or a stereotactic biopsy (4 cases) was performed. Two patients died within 3 weeks after surgery and were excluded from the study population. One of them had a delayed postoperative intracerebral hemorrhage and the other one developed a fulminant pneumonia with S. aureus.

Only patients with histologically verified malignant gliomas were entered into this study. The neuropathological studies were kindly performed by Prof. Wechsler (Institute of Neuropathology, University of Düsseldorf). Malignant gliomas were classified and graded according to the WHO classification of brain tumors (Zülch 1979). We decide not to treat patients <18 years or >70 years. Vascular disease was considered a contraindication, particularly carotid artery disease. Severe neurological or general medical disease were reasons for exclusion. The neurological status and performance were scored according to Duff et al (1986). Patients suffering from a second neoplastic disease were not accepted for iaACNU chemotherapy. Gravidity was excluded in female patients. Within 10 days after surgery the first iaACNU procedure was performed. The ipsilateral ICA was selectively catheterized and an angiograph was obtained. Thereafter 100mg ACNU dissolved in 20ml H_2O were infused: the first 25mg ACNU were given over 3 min as a loading dose, and the remaining 75mg ACNU over 30 min to maintain drug levels. Not later than 7 days after the first iaACNU course, radiotherapy was started with a conventional 2Gy daily dose fractionated irradiation. The goal of radiotherapy was a total tumor dose of 60Gy. A few days after completion of radiotherapy the second iaACNU procedure took place, followed by further iaACNU courses with 6 to 8 weeks interval. After the seventh iaACNU course, therapy was not continued and an expectant attitude was adopted. At regular intervals blood count and clinical laboratory investigations as well as computed tomography (CT) and/or magnetic resonance imaging (MRI) with gadolinium-DTPA were performed. The use of corticoids was kept as low as possible. The tumor volume seen on CT or MRI was determined at every iaACNU course. Responsive disease (RD) or stable disease (SD) was defined as a decrease in tumor volume or a constant tumor volume, and both groups were considered together for this study. Patients with progressive disease (PD) showed evidence of tumor growth on CT or MR. Survival time was the critical factor analyzed for this report. Survival time after diagnosis was evaluated according to Kaplan and Meier (1958). Statistical significance was tested with the Mantel-Haenszel test (Mantel 1966).

RESULTS (Fig. 1)

The median survival time of all malignant gliomas WHO grade IV after diagnosis was 10.2 months, and 21.6% were still living at 18 months. Excluding the recurrent tumors increased both the median survival time and the proportion of longterm survivors (>18 months) resp. 28.5%. This group of primarily diagnosed tumors contained 9 WHO grade IV malignant gliomas and 25 WHO grade IV glioblastomas: a comparative analysis revealed no significant differences between both groups with regard to survival time (p=0.80>0.05); however, a significant difference (p=0.0005) was detected between the patients with primarily diagnosed WHO grade IV gliomas who had PD (N=11) or RD & SD (N=23). The former had a median survival time of 3.3 months and no longterm survivors (>18 months), whereas for the latter the median survival time was 16.2 months and 46.5% were longterm survivors (>18 months). A clear cut difference was also found between both these groups with regard to the neurological status and performance score. The group with PD already scored worse than the RD & SD group at the first iaACNU course, and this finding was accentuated during the course of chemotherapy.

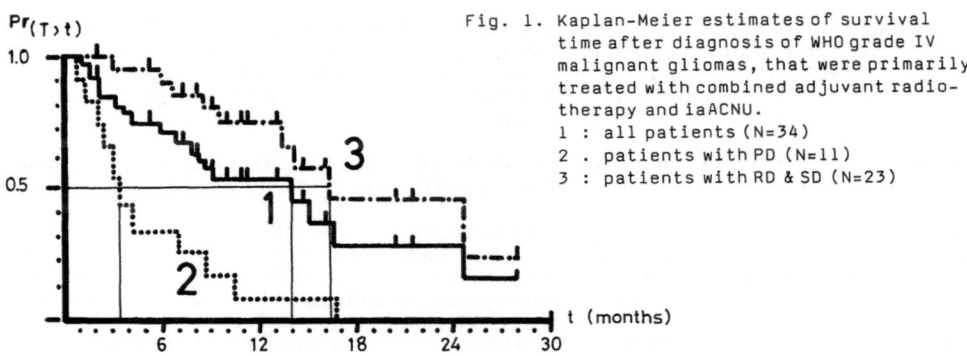

Fig. 1. Kaplan-Meier estimates of survival time after diagnosis of WHO grade IV malignant gliomas, that were primarily treated with combined adjuvant radiotherapy and iaACNU.
1 : all patients (N=34)
2 . patients with PD (N=11)
3 : patients with RD & SD (N=23)

Major complications were found in 17 patients, but fortunately these were reversible or at the least not incapacitating in most instances. They included hemipllegia and transitory ischemic attacks, visual impairment, leuko- and thrombopenia, hepatopathy, and systemic mycosis. Irreversible complications occurred in 4 patients. Minor side effects such as epileptic seizures, anorexia, nausea, and emesis developed in less than 25% of our patients. Side effects and complications were due to the cathetrization procedure, the cytostatic agent, and the use of corticoids in some patients.

DISCUSSION

Although the i.a. approach in chemotherapy of brain tumors has been advocated, there is some concern about its usefulness in human gliomas: e.g. drug streaming by laminar flow during i.a. infusion (Saris et al 1988), penetration of the blood tumor barrier by cytotoxic agents (Blasberg & Groothuis 1986), leukoencephalopathy (Kleinschmidt-DeMasters 1986),etc... In evaluating the results of this kind of therapy, large enough series are needed and the management protocol should be strictly defined. The median survival time should be determined, and the proportion of longterm survivors too. Furthermore, it is important to compare not only the therapeutic effects but also the complications of i.a. vs systemic chemotherapy, bearing in mind that the dose of the cytotoxic agent might be different in both groups.

Comparability of different series should consider the pathology of the tumors treated. Most published series are composed of a more or less larger majority of glioblastomas and a minority of less malignant gliomas (Kornblith & Walker 1988), which are anaplastic gliomas according to the american Brain Tumor Study Group (BTSG) nomenclature (Burger et al 1985), or WHO grade III tumors (Krauseneck 1988). There is an important difference in survival time of both these groups. Combining 3 Phase-III studies of the BTSG a median survival time of ±10 months for glioblastoma and of ±20 months for anaplastic glioma was found (Burger et al 1985). Our own results in WHO grade IV tumors compare favorably (13.9 months median survival time), and no significant difference between WHO grade IV gliomas and WHO IV glioblastomas was detected.

Adjuvant treatment of glioblastomas with intravenous (i.v.) ACNU (2-3mg/kgBW) was performed by Voth et al (1984), and they reported a median survival time of 11.3 months. This is 15% less than our own results, and was obtained with a markedly higher dose causing much more frequently systemic side effects that were more severe with ivACNU than with iaACNU (1.2-1.5mg/kgBW). In addition, this data for iaACNU vs ivACNU demonstrates an interesting difference with regard to the situation with iaBCNU and ivBCNU. The initial iaBCNU dose in a BTSG trial comparing iaBCNU vs ivBCNU, had to be significantly reduced below the systemic dose because of severe complications and side effects (Shapiro & Green 1987). This resulted in inferior survival statistics of iaBCNU compared with ivBCNU, whereas iaACNU results in better survival than ivACNU despite the lower i.v. ACNU dose.

The selection of patients responsive to chemotherapy is essential in order to obtain better results. Reliable chemosensitivity testing will ameliorate patient response and survival by a priori selection of those patients harboring responsive tumors, a group probably analogous to our a posteriori selected RD & SD patients. This can be realized by in vitro tests (Kimmel et al 1987) and possibly by in vivo studies with positron emission tomography, and we address this issue in a separate paper in the Proceedings of XVth Congress of the European Society of Neuroradiology, Würzburg, 1988.

536

REFERENCES

Blasberg RG, Groothuis DR (1986) Chemotherapy of brain tumors: physiological and pharmacokinetic considerations. Semin Oncol 13:70-82
Burger PC, Vogel FS, Green SB, Strike TA (1985) Glioblastoma multiforme and
anaplastic astrocytoma. Pathologic criteria and prognostic implications.
Cancer 56:1106-1111
Duff TA, Borden E, Bay J, et al (1986) Phase II trial of interferon-β for
treatment of recurrent glioblastoma multiforme. J Neurosurg 64:408-413
Eckman WW, Patlak CS, Fenstermacher JD (1974) A critical evaluation of the
principles governing the advantages of intra-arterial infusions.
J Pharmacokinet Biopharmaceut 2:257-285
Greenberg HS, Ensminger WD, Chandler WF, et al (1984) Intra-arterial BCNU
chemotherapy for treatment of malignant gliomas of the central nervous
system. J Neurosurg 61:423-429
Hori T, Muraoka K, Saito Y et al (1987) Influence of modes of ACNU administra-
tion on tissue and blood drug concentration in malignant brain tumors.
J Neurosurg 66:372-378
Kaplan EL, Meier P (1958) Nonparametric estimation from incomplete observa-
tions. J Amer Statist Assoc 53:457-481
Kimmel DW, Shapiro JR, Shapiro WR (1987) In vitro drug sensitivity testing
in human gliomas. J Neurosurg 66:161-171
Kleinschmidt-DeMasters BK (1986) Intracarotid BCNU leukoencephalopathy.
Cancer 57:1276-1280
Kornblith PL, Walker M (1988) Chemotherapy for malignant gliomas.
J Neurosurg 68:1-17
Krauseneck P (1988) Der Stellenwert der Chemotherapie in der Behandlung ma-
ligner Gliome des Erwachsenenalters. In: Bamberg M, Sack H (eds) Therapie
primärer Hirntumoren, pp 83-91. W Zuckschwerdt, München
Mantel N (1966) Evaluation of survival data and two new rank order statistics
arising in its consideration. Cancer Chemother Rep 50:163-170
Saris SC, Wright DC, Oldfield EH, Blasberg RG (1988) Intravascular streaming
and variable delivery to brain following carotid artery infusions in the
Sprague-Dawley rat. J Cereb Blood Flow Metab 8:116-120
Shapiro WR, Green SB (1987) Reevaluating the efficacity of intra-arterial
BCNU. J Neurosurg 66:313-315
Tyler JL, Yamamoto YL, Diksic M, et al (1986) Pharmacokinetics of superselec-
tive intra-arterial and intravenous [^{11}C]BCNU evaluated by PET.
J Nucl Med 27:775-780
Voth D, Hüwel N, Al-Hami S, Kuhnert A (1984) Erste Ergebnisse der Monochemo-
therapie mit ACNU bei der Behandlung maligner Gliome des Menschen. In: Voth
D, Krauseneck P (eds) Chemotherapy of gliomas, pp 361-372. Walter de Gruy-
ter, Berlin
Walker MD, Green SB, Byar DP, et al (1980) Randomized comparisons of radio-
therapy and nitrosoureas for the treatment of malignant glioma after surgery. New Engl J Med 303:1323-1329
Yamashita J, Handa H, Tokuriki Y, et al (1983) Intra-arterial ACNU therapy
for malignant brain tumors. Experimental studies and preliminary clinical
results. J Neurosurg 59:424-430
Zülch KJ (1979) Histological typing of tumours of the central nervous system.
World Health Organization, Geneva

ACKNOWLEDGEMENT

The authors want to express their gratitude to Ms. Dr. H. Hüttmann, ASTA-Degussa Pharma,
D-6000 Frankfurt/Main, for her interest and support with regard to brain tumor therapy at
the University of Düsseldorf.

Dynamic CT Scanning of the Cavernous Sinus

J. F. Bonneville, F. Cattin, Y. S. Tang, M. Abitbol, I. Nouy, and M. Bouchareb

INTRODUCTION

There is controversy about the exact nature of the parasellar extradural venous spaces. The classical description is that of a blood-filled trabeculated channel which completely surrounds the internal carotid artery (Paturet 1964, Rouvière 1985). Others maintain that the plexus is composed of various sized veins (Dolenc 1983, Olivier 1951, Parkinson 1965, Rhoton 1978, Taptas 1982). Dynamic CT is today able to clarify these anatomical conceptions.

MATERIAL AND METHODS

700 patients with suspected tumor of the pituitary region have been specifically examined for demonstrating the cavernous sinus. The technic is slightly modified from our usual technic for demonstrating the pituitary tuft and the pituitary enhancement (Bonneville 1983, 1986). The patients were placed in prone position with the head hyperextended. A preinfusion coronal CT scan at the midsellar level is performed first. 80 ml of 32% iodinated contrast (25g iodine) pushed with 30 cc of saline solution were mechanically injected at 15 ml per sec. through a 16 gauge needle in an arm vein. 8 cuts are carried out at the same level, with the technical parameters mentioned in fig.1. The first three cuts after the bolus injection are reconstructed with special algorithm for bone detail to minimize the partial volume effect and displayed in the black bone mode.

NORMAL RESULTS AND SYSTEMATIZATION OF THE PARASELLAR EXTRADURAL VEINS

Visualization of the veins was obtained in all the patients. The venous asymmetry is the most constant radiological finding. The intracavernous cranial nerves are generally well demonstrated in negative. Apart the "true" cavernous sinus, i.e. a large blood-filled channel totally surrounding the intracavernous internal carotid artery which is rare, we can classify the veins in five groups (fig. 2, 3).

1. The veins of the lateral wall of the cavernous sinus are quite constant and appear as small round, oval or linear vascular structures delineating partially the lateral wall.

2. The inferolateral venous group is also quite constant. It is demonstrated below the internal carotid artery, just below the abducens nerve which is consequently well delineated.

3. The medial vein, situated between the internal carotid artery and the pituitary gland appears as a linear or comma-shape structure and constitutes the medial limit of the cavernous sinus. It is observed in 20-30% of the cases.

4. <u>The vein of the carotid sulcus</u>, located between the internal carotid artery and the carotid sulcus of the sphenoid bone is usually bilateral but asymmetrical. This vein can communicate freely to the inferolateral venous group and the medial vein. The vein of the carotid sulcus is only absent in the 35% of the cases where there is no space between the internal carotid artery and the sphenoid bone.

5. <u>The pericarotid sulcus</u> is generally thin and surrounds more or less completely the internal carotid artery. Its opacification is delayed in relation with the other laterosellar veins.

The intercavernous sinus can be also demonstrated by dynamic CT scan. <u>The anterior intercavernous</u> can be visible when the dynamic CT scan is performed at the tuberculum sellae level as a dense band extending transversely. <u>The inferior intercavernous sinus</u> is only demonstrated when large enough and is seen as a enhanced band doubling the sellar floor.

CONCLUSION

Dynamic CT scanning can routinely demonstrate the parasellar extradural venous spaces and the intracavernous cranial nerves. A systematization of these veins is proposed.

Moreover the demonstration of the parasellar extradural veins can be of interest for early diagnosis of cavernous sinus invasion by pituitary tumors.

It is logical to consider that intracavernous veins, whose walls are easily depressible, are the first structures to be changed in the case of subtle cavernous sinus invasion. The medial vein situated in close contact with the pituitary gland is too inconstant to be of interest. Contrary, the vein of the carotid sulcus which is constant except in the cases where the internal carotid artery is close to the sphenoid bone, is considered as the best landmark : obliteration of the carotid sulcus vein is in favor of a cavernous sinus involvement.

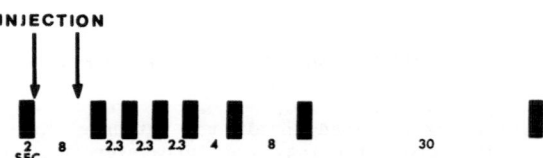

Fig.1. Technic of the dynamic CT scan for demonstrating the parasellar extradural veins. - Injection of 80 ml of 32% iodinated contrast medium (25 g iodine) pushed with 30 ml of saline solution at 15 ml per sec. - Section thickness : 1.5 mm - Scan time : 2 sec. - mA : 200 - KV : 120 - Each scan is represented by a black bar.

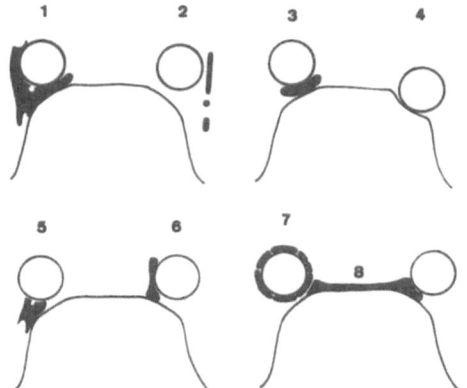

Fig.2. : Schematic drawing of the different patterns of the parasellar extradural venous spaces. 1) True cavernous sinus, 2) Veins of the lateral wall of the cavernous sinus, 3) Vein of the carotid sulcus, situated between the intracavernous internal carotid artery and the sphenoid bone, 4) Absence of vein of the carotid sulcus, when the intracavernous internal carotid artery is in close contact with the sphenoid bone, 5) Inferolateral venous group below the intracavernous internal carotid artery, 6) The medial vein situated between the intracavernous internal carotid artery and the pituitary gland, 7) The pericarotid plexus, 8) The inferior intercavernous sinus.

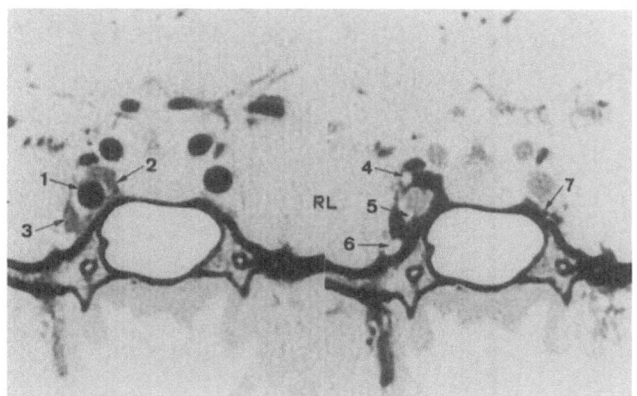

Fig.3. : Coronal dynamic CT scan for demonstration of the cavernous sinus. The parasellar extradural veins are asymmetrical. 1) Internal carotid artery, 2) Medial vein, 3) Inferolateral venous group, 4) Oculomotor nerve, 5) Abducens nerve, 6) Maxillary nerve, 7) Vein of the carotid sulcus.

REFERENCES

Bonneville JF, Cattin F, Moussa-Bacha K, Portha C (1983). Dynamic computed tomo-
    graphy of the pituitary gland : the "tuft sign". Radiology 149 : 145-148.
Bonneville JF, Cattin F, Dietemann JL (1986). Computed tomography of the pituitary
    gland. Springer-Verlag, Berlin, Heidelberg, New York, Tokyo.
Dolenc VV (1983). Direct microsurgical repair of intracavernous vascular lesions.
    J Neurosurg 58 : 824-831.
Olivier E, Papamiltiades M (1951). Le système caverneux veineus de la région latéro-
    sellaire. Bull Ass Anat (Nancy) 36 : 769-773.
Parkinson D (1965). A surgical approach to the cavernous portion of the carotid
    artery. Anatomical studies and case report. J Neurosurg 23 : 474-483.
Paturet G (1964). Traité d'anatomie humaine, vol 4. Système nerveux. Masson, Paris.
Rhoton AL, Harris FS, Reen H (1978). Microsurgical anatomy of the sellar region
    and cavernous sinus. Neurosurgery 8 : 54-58.
Rouvière H, Delmas A (1985). Anatomie humaine, 12è éd., Masson, Paris.
Taptas JN (1982). The so-called cavernous sinus : a review of the controversy and
    its implications for neurosurgeons. Neurosurgery 11 : 712-717.

Color 3-D CT Imaging Reconstruction of Bones, Blood Vessels and Tumors

R. Tadmor, M. Feivel, and D. Dekel

Since 3-dimensional CT reconstruction is easily applied to tissues
of high contrast such as bones, previous publications refer mainly
to osseous reconstruction of the skull, facial bones, pelvis, spine
and others (Burk 1985, Hemmy 1983, Sartoris 1986, Totty 1984, Vannier
1984). Only few reports deal with soft tissues reconstruction (Vannier
1983, Gillespie 1986 and 1987) and the availability of a color display
has also been mentioned (Jaffe 1985, Sartoris 1986). The purpose
of this study is to report on our initial experience using 3-D color
reconstruction for evaluation of bones, soft tissues, tumors and
blood vessels.

Material and Methods

We used a special software imaging processing system running on an
Elscint-Exel 1800-2400 CT scanner's console, which employs special
algorithms.

A series of at least 15 or more CT contiguous thin slices of 2-5
mm thick are acquired using a 2-sec scan time and low patient dose
as in a routine study. Identification of bone details is easily achieved, but for tumor or blood vessels delineation i.v. contrast medium
was injected. This allows to define an enhancing lesion separately
from surrounding soft tissues. The time necessary for the reconstruction varies between several minutes up to 30 minutes, depending on
the method used for surface definition, whether global thresholding
or slice-by-slice identification. The models are displayed together
on a color monitor and can interactively rotated, tilted and zoomed.
The position of a simulated light source can be altered across the
image to enhance details and depth perception. Also tissue sections
can be selectively graphically removed thus allowing inspection of
the deeper structures. More than 20 patients with various bone and
soft tissue pathologies have been evaluated by this method. Two il-
lustrative examples are reported: Case 1 and 2, Fig. 1 and 2.

Results and Discussion

The 3-D program allows to create realistically looking models of any
anatomical feature that can be identified on the slice images. 3-D
reconstruction does not provide additional information than the one
present on each of the CT slices. However it allows a volumetric
display of the findings that can be visualized from any imaginary
angle when rotated and tilted. The contribution of 3-D reconstruction
of bones is already accepted. The optional 3-D reconstruction with
colors is a further step allowing better understanding and a useful
mean to transfer information to the clinician, oncologist and surgeon
when contemplating therapy or surgery. The flexibility of organ definition, display and short processing time make this system highly
promising.

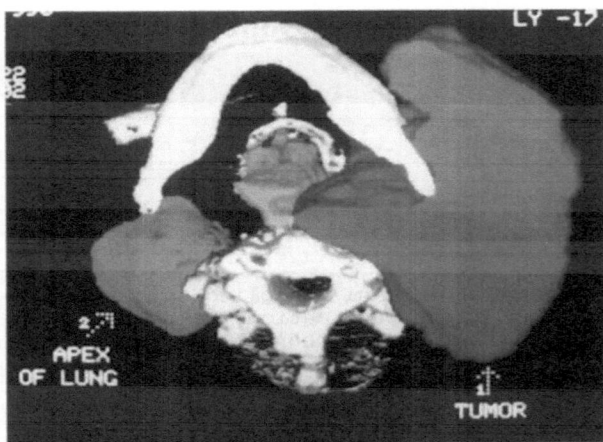

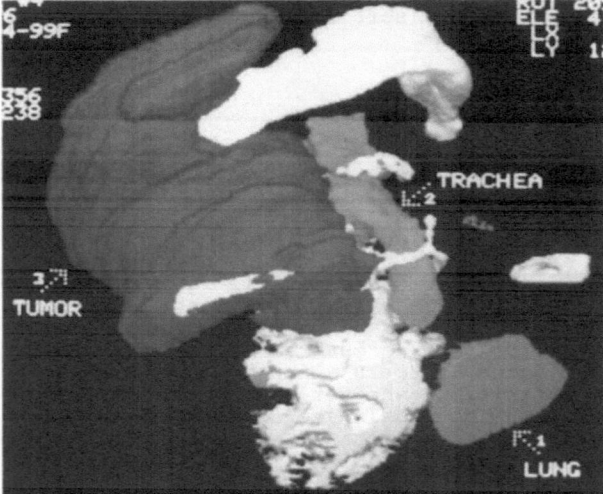

Fig. 1. 3-D reconstruction of bone (mandible, cervical spine, hyoid and partial clavicles) -white, tumor-pink, trachea and apex of lung-blue.

a. A semi-axial view with anterior tilt shows the posterior retro-mandibular- and prevertebral extent of a mass and its relation to the trachea. No bone involvement.

b. Lateral semi-rotated and tilted view, allows appreciation of the entire mass longitudinally as well as its anterior intra-thoracic extent; note deviation of trachea.

Case 1. Lymphoma in a 55 year old man presenting with a large lateral neck mass.

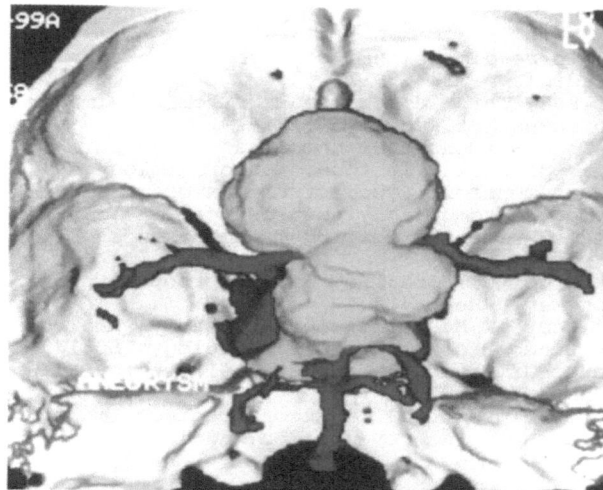

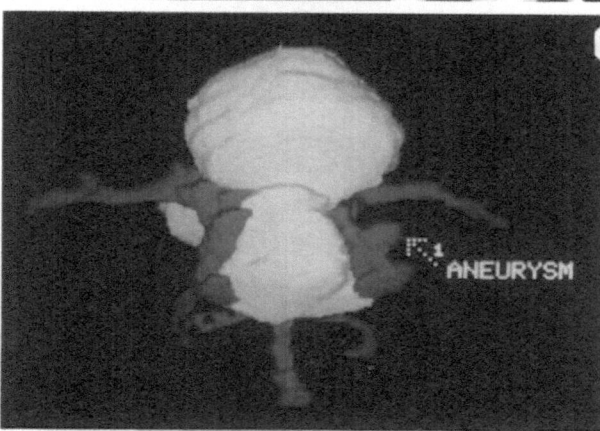

Fig. 2. 3-D color reconstruction of skull (white), tumor (yellow) and blood vessels (red).

a. Vertex view. Large pituitary tumor extending subfrontally. Note unilateral carotid enlargement - aneurysm.

b. 180° rotation with removal of the bone, allows a basal view of the intrasellar portion of tumor and the aneurysm.

Case 2. A 64 year old man presenting with visual field defects. On a dynamic CT study a large pituitary tumor was shown with an intracavernous aneurysm demonstrated by angiography and proven at surgery.

REFERENCES

Burk DL, Jr. et al. (1985). Three-dimensional computed tomography
  of acetabular fractures. Radiology 155:179-184
Gillespie JE, Isherwood I (1986) Three dimensional anatomical images
  from computed tomographic scans. BrJRadiol 59:289-292
Gillespie JE et al. (1987) Three-dimensional computed tomographic
  reformations of sellar and parasellar lesions. Neuroradiology 29:30-35
Hemmy DC et al. (1983) Three-dimensional reconstruction of cranio-
  facial deformity using computed tomography. Neurosurgery 13:534-541
Jaffe CC (1985) Color displays: widening imaging dynamic range. Diagn
  Imag Dec 52-58
Sartoris DJ (1986) 3-D display of CT data: new aid to preop surgical
planning. Diagnostic Imaging May/June:6-32
Totty WG, Vannier MW (1984) Complex Musculoskeletal Anatomy: Analysis
  using three-dimensional surface Reconstruction. Radiology 150:173-177
Vannier MW et al. (1983) Three-dimensional display of intracranial
  soft tissue structure. AJNR 4:520-521
Vannier MW et al. (1984) Three dimensional CT Reconstruction Images
  for Craniofacial Surgical Planning and evaluation. Radiology 150:
  179-184

Calculated Dynamic CT

H. Hacker and M. Adelmann (Frankfurt/M., FRG)

A new approach to gain more quantitative information from dynamic CT than just time-density curves has been developed and tested by us in recent years.

Basic experiments proved that with the injection of 30 g iodine the enhancement in any 300 pixel region is high enough for an exact calculation of the local blood volume (rCBV) and the change of permeability of the blood brain barrier (BBB) should there be any pathology. Likewise under pathological conditions a ratio of extravascular to intravascular iodine is calculated. This ratio can be compared between individuals. A computer program for quick evaluation of a dynamic CT has been developed by us and is now being adapted by Siemens for the Somatom.

The first clinical applications demonstrate that the quantitative knowledge of rCBC, permeability of the BBB and the amount of contrast extravasation are most valuable data in the description of a pathological process. The specific diagnosis of brain disease will be much better using this technique. The further software development strives for parameter images.

Lacunar versus Non-lacunar Stroke: Clinical and Radiological Differentiation

S. Cronqvist, B. Nilsson, and B. Norrving (Lund, Sweden)

In a consecutive series of 122 patients with a first minor ischemic stroke in the carotid vascular territory, the clinical observations and the findings at CT were compared with the angiographic findings. Patients with a cardiac source of embolization were excluded.

Based upon the clinical characteristics and the CT changes, 61 patients were classified as having a lacunar and 53 a non-lacunar infarct. It was not possible to determine type of lesion in eight. In the two groups the angiographic changes differed markedly. Thus, the lacunar group showed no or bilaterally low-grade changes in 90%, while the majority of the non-lacunar patients had marked ipsilateral changes (79%), with similar changes also on the contralateral side (20.5%).

The study confirms the general concept that the main pathogenic mechanism causing a lacunar type of stroke is small vessel disease, while the cause of cerebral ischemia with cortical involvement is "large vessel disease". Acceptance of these facts has important implications with regard to practical management of this type of patient.

Neurofibromatosis Type 2: MR Evaluation and Clinical Correlation

J. L. Sherman, D. M. Parry, R. Eldridge, M. Kaiser-Kupfer, A. Pikus, and C. M. Citrin

INTRODUCTION

The neurofibromatoses consists of at least two distinct autosomal dominant disorders with differing clinical manifestations (Martuza 1988; NIH 1988). Neurofibromatosis 1 (NF-1) was originally described by von Recklinghausen and was previously known as peripheral neurofibromatosis. Recently the gene has been assigned to chromosome 17. Neurofibromatosis 2 (NF-2), also known as central neurofibromatosis, is an autosomal dominant disorder, the hallmark of which is the presence of bilateral acoustic neuromas (AN). NF-2 has recently been assigned to chromosome 22. The affected persons generally become symptomatic in their teens or twenties with hearing loss or tinnitus as a result of the acoustic neuroma.

As part of a screening study, we prospectively evaluated the MR findings in 20 members of one NF-2-afflicted family (ages 19 to 72 years). There were 4 females and 16 males. Four patients had previous cerebellopontine angle (CPA) surgery.

MATERIALS AND PATIENTS

The MR diagnosis of a tumor was based on the observation of a CPA mass, nodularity of the 8th nerve complex, or displacement of CSF from the internal auditory canal. Displacement of CSF resulted in signal intensity that was isointense compared to brain, whereas in the normal auditory canal the partial volume effect of CSF and neuronal tissue together causes decreased intensity compared to brain.

Axial and coronal T1-weighted (T1w) and axial T2-weighted (T2w) images were obtained in all subjects. Section thickness was 3 mm or 4 mm for T1w techniques and 5 mm for T2w images. The magnetic field strength was 0.5 T (n=8) and 1.5 T (n=12). The examinations were graded on a scale of 0-4 (0 = normal; 1 = intracanalicular (IC) only; 2 = IC tumor convex margin at porus acusticus; 3 = CPA tumor less than 5 mm; 4 = CPA tumor larger than 5 mm). The results were then correlated with history, physical findings, audiology, and ophthalmology. All subjects had audiological and auditory brain stem evoked potentials (ABR), and complete ophthalmic examination including iris and lens biomicroscopy and Scheimpflug photography, including lens evaluation for posterior subcapsular opacities or cataracts. MR, audiological testing, and ophthalmological evaluations were blinded to each other.

RESULTS

Twenty-one ears were normal and none of these had hearing loss, but audiological testing was positive in 3.

Nineteen AN were documented by MR in 10 members (bilateral in 9, unilateral in 1). All tumors were isointense compared to brain on T2w and T1w images and were most clearly visible on T1w axial images (Fig. 1).

Four of the 10 subjects with AN had no symptoms, but 3 had positive audiologic and all 4 had positive ophthalmoscopic findings. The smallest tumor was 3-4 mm and unilateral in a 19-year-old asymptomatic male. Of the 9 Grade 1 ears there was hearing loss in 4 (including 1 with previous surgery). There were 2 Grade 2 ears (1 with surgery), both with hearing loss. There were 8 Grade 3 or Grade 4 ears (2 with surgery), 6 with hearing loss; 1 had an abnormal ABR with normal hearing, and 1 had normal audiological and ABR evaluation.

Ophthalmological evaluation for posterior subcapsular lens opacities (PSLO) was positive in 9 of 10 patients with Grade 1-4 MR studies and positive in 1 of 10 patients with Grade 0 MR studies. This 23-year-old asymptomatic patient also had an abnormal ABR but had normal hearing.

CONCLUSIONS

There was 1 patient with a presumed false negative MR examination. This patient does not meet the criteria for the diagnosis of NF-2 but is highly suspect because of positive ophthalmological evaluation (Pearson-Webb et al. 1986). Gadolinium-DTPA enhanced MR has not been performed but is recommended for this patient.

We were able to validate the criteria we used to make an MR diagnosis by retrospectively correlating the MR appearance with clinical data, especially the presence of PSLO. T1w axial images were most useful in the evaluation of intracanalicular neuromas. Recognition of displacement of CSF from the internal auditory canal was particularly useful. These observations should also be valid in the evaluation of patients with sporadic AN.

It should be recognized that patients with acoustic neuromas may be asymptomatic and that a positive MR may be the only indication of the disease. This probably applies to both NF-2 and sporadic AN patients. Ophthalmological and audiological testing and MR are complementary procedures in the evaluation of patients with suspected NF-2.

REFERENCES

Martuza RL, Eldridge R (1988) Neurofibromatosis 2 (bilateral acoustic neurofibromatosis). N Engl J Med 318:684-688
National Institutes of Health consensus development conference statement of neurofibromatosis (1988) Arch Neurol 45:575-580
Pearson-Webb MA, Kaiser-Kupfer MI, Eldridge R (1986) Eye findings in bilateral acoustic (central) neurofibromatosis: association with presenile lens opacities and cataracts but absence of Lisch nodules. N Engl J Med 315:1553-1554

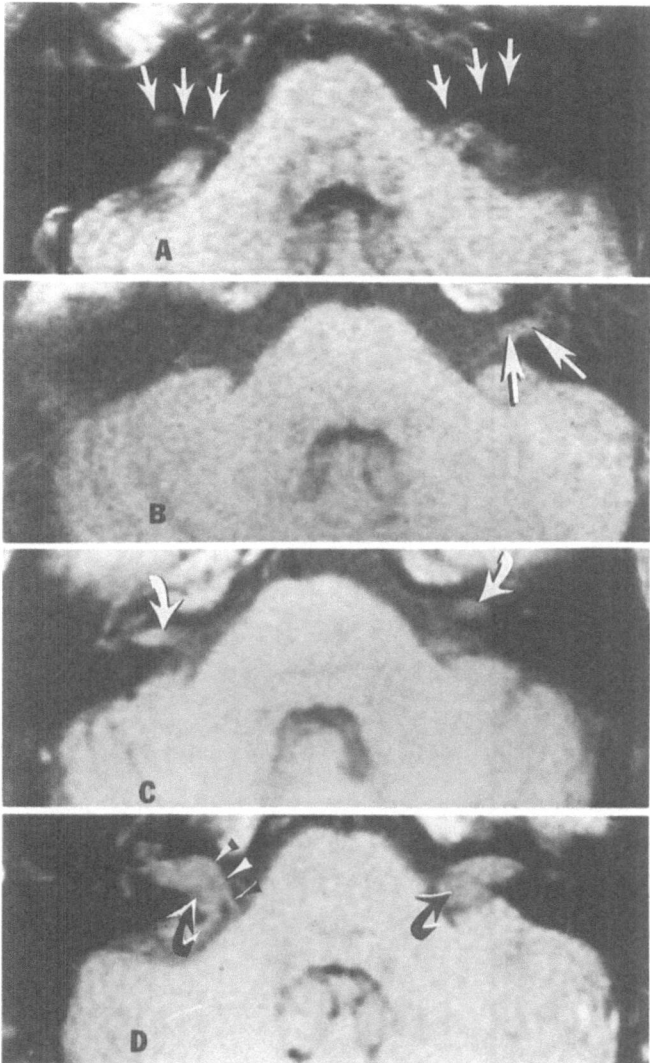

Fig. 1. Axial T1-weighted images of internal auditory canals (IAC) at
0.5 T (A,B) and 1.5 T (C,D).
(A) Normal IAC (arrows). Note low intensity of IAC and neural tissue averaged
     together.
(B) 25-year-old NF-2 female with Grade 1 acoustic neuroma (AN) on left side
     (arrows). Abnormal left acoustic reflex on left and abnormal ABR on right.
     Bilateral posterior subcapsular lens opacities (PSLO).
(C) 33-year-old NF-2 male with bilateral Grade 1 ANs (curved white arrows).
     Normal hearing and ABR but with bilateral PSLO.
(d) 24-year-old NF-2 female with Grade 3 AN on right and Grade 4 AN on left
     (curved arrows). Note displacement of right 7th cranial nerve (arrowheads).
     No facial symptoms. Normal hearing on right, abnormal ABR on left. Patient
     does not have PSLO.

Magnetic Resonance in the Characterization of Vascular Lesions

M. Gallucci, E. Di Cesare, P. Pavone, P. Di Renzi, G. Patrizio,
A. Splendiani, and R. Passariello

INTRODUCTION

Magnetic Resonance (MR) imaging has been proved to be useful in
cardiovascular investigations (Herfkens et al 1983, Soila et al
1986). In atherosclerotic pathology an accurate imaging study is
important for providing opportune surgery or medical therapy
(Higgins et al 1984). Angiography is considered the most sensitive
diagnostic procedure but does not allow the precise characterization
of stenotic lesions and presents some risks.
The vascular wall and small parietal irregularities may be
accurately evaluated with MR (Bradley et al 1985). Moreover,
theoretically it is possible to characterize normal and
atherosclerotic vessels by means of the signal intensity evaluation
of the different components. However, in vivo characterization is
limited by artifacts due to respiratory movements and vessel
pulsatility. Therefore, we tried to characterize in vitro the normal
wall and atherosclerotic lesions using MR imaging and spectroscopy.

MATERIALS AND METHODS

We examined 10 arteries (6 carotids and 4 aortas) removed from 10
cadavers. The subjects ranged in age from 55 to 78 years. The
autopsies and the removals were done between 24 and 48 hours after
death. Death was not caused by cerebrovascular disease in any of the
cases. The arteries removed were frozen in liquid nitrogen and
preserved at - 70 degrees centigrade until 3 hours before MR
examination. MR imaging was performed with a superconductive magnet
operating at 0.5 Tesla (ESAOTE biomedica, Genova, Italy). T1
weighted Spin Echo (SE) sequence (TR 300 msec, TE 30 msec, 2
acquisitions) T2 weighted Multiecho (ME) (TR 1800 msec, TE 70, 120
msec) were used in axial and sagittal planes. Slice tickness was 5-7
mm, and matrix 256x256. A double ellipse coil with a 16 cm diameter
was used. A 5 cm diameter tube containing H_2O_2, was placed inside
the coil, and used as a reference sample. Signal intensities were
measured on normal walls, on atherosclerotic lesions and on the
reference sample utilizing a Region Of Interest (ROI) of less then 8
pixels. Ratios were calculated between the values obtained from the
normal and pathological tissues and those obtained from the sample.
Field of view was of 13.92 cm and resolution was of 0.54 mm. Part of
each autopsy specimen also underwent MR spectroscopy for T1

measurements. A Bruker Spectrometer SXP 2-100 was utilized at
working frequences of 21 MHz (0.5 Tesla) with a 180 -t - 90 - T -
180 sequence. The temperature was 37 , controlled by an Bruker BVT-
1000 air flow temperature control. The specimens, which had a 0.1 cm
volume, were gently packed by centrifugation into a NMR tube with
internal diameter of 6 mm. The T1 measurements began about 1 hour
after defrosting the vessels. After the MR imaging examination, the
material was fixed with 10% formalin. Later, transversal and
longitudinal sections were conducted to evaluate the presence of
plaques and reduction of the vessel intraluminal diameter. Paraffin-
fixed samples were also obtained, and were coloured with
ematossilina-eosina, threcromic of Masson and Wrigert specific for
elastic fibres. The degree of stenosis, the presence and the kind of
plaque and the thickness increase of the intima was evaluated.

RESULTS AND CONCLUSIONS

MR imaging was able to identify the differentiation of 3 layers
inside the wall, related to intima, media and adventitia, which were
mostly evident in the 120 msec T2-weighted Spin-Echo sequences. The
above was attributed to the signal decay of the media. In some
cases, the differentiation was also possible in the T1-weighted
sequences, even though the signal intensities from the 3
different layers always appeared to be very similar. Moreover, the
detection of the stenosis and the evaluation of its entity was
possible according to Higgins et al 1984, Bradley et al 1985,
Hinshaw et al 1987. 16 atherosclerotic lesions have also been well
documented in our study. In 6 cases they appeared as a circular
thickening of the vessel wall, while in the remaining 10 cases,
circumscribed lesions protruding inside the vessel lumen were
evident. One of these was ulcered and 2 had characteristics of
hemorrhagic plaques. In all the lesions a high signal intensity was
observed in the T1-weighted sequences, while a mild decay was
evident in the T2-weighted ones.
However, at least 2 different patterns became evident in the last
sequences: a markedly low signal and a moderately low one. We
hypothesized the mild hypointensity to be due to fatty compounds,
while the marked one due to fibrous compounds. In 3 cases
hyperintense focal areas adjacent to the lesion were evident in both
T1 and T2-weighted sequences. The signal characteristics attributed
these aspects to hemorrhagic components with the presence of
methaemoglobin. The above described findings were compared to the
histological examination, which showed a very close cerrespondence
(Fig.1). In fact, 7 lesions showed fibro-intimal thickening without
intimal interruptions, Ca++ deposits or sub-intimal hemorrhage. The
remaining 9 lesions were typical subintimal plaques, with fatty
deposits, modification of internal elastic membrane and calcific
components in 5 cases.
The spectroscopic measurements performed were obtained from 4 normal
walls, 2 lipid plaques, 2 hemorragic plaques and 2 fibrous plaques.
The signal intensity vs. the interpulse time of the normal walls
showed single exponential behaviour and a T1 of 390 q 40 msec.
The fibro-atherosclerotic plaque was characterized by a typical
multiexponential behaviour. It was possible to calculate the short
component-T1, considered to be due to tissutal fat, equal to 105
q 22 msec, and the long component-T1, attributed to the remaining
components, equal to 676 ± 35. Both fibrous and hemorragic
plaques showed single exponential behaviour and a T1 of 336 ± 29
and 429 ± 18 msec respectively. The T1 values obtained showed a
good correlation with the signal intensities detected by the MR

imaging. In fact, we found high signal intensity from both the normal and the atherosclerotic vessels. In the T1 weighted sequences, the fatty component of the plaque showed a high signal intensity, while the fibro-sclerotic one had a low signal. In the T2 weighted sequences we observed a progressive decay of signals of both the normal wall and the fibrous component, while the fatty one

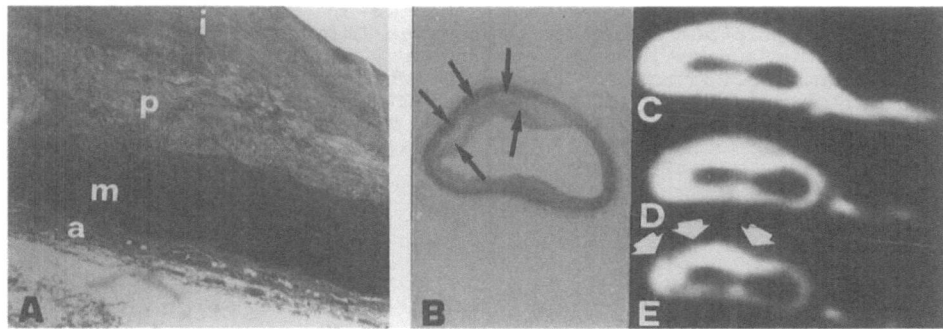

Fig.1: Histological (A) and anatomical (B) sections of an atheromatous carotid. Arrows indicate the fatty deposits inside the tickened wall; i=intima; m=media; a=adventitia; p=sub-intimal plaque. C-D-E MR of the same vessel. The T1-weighted sequence (C) and the Proton Density one (D) show a focalized thickening of the wall. The T2-weigted sequence (E) differntiates the lipid component, which has a moderately higher signal than the rest of the wall (arrows).

showed only a mild decay. The hematic components had high signal in all the sequences utilized, due to the presence of methaemoglobin, while the presence of Ca++ deposits was poorly evidentiated as a lack of signal in all the sequences used. The imaging evaluation also detected little wall irregularities, or ulcers.
The application of these results in "in vivo" studies is nowadays difficult, due to the presence of respiratory movements, vessel pulsatile movements and tortuosity of the vessels. These limits can be partially overcome by using gated sequences and 3D acquisition modality. The introduction of specific surface coils could also improve the spatial resolution.
In conclusion, MR imaging "in vitro" studies are able to detect the presence of minimal differences in the relaxation times of intima, media and adventitia which, respectively, show high, low and high intensity signal in the T2-weighted sequences. The differentiation between atheromatous and fibro-atheromatous lesions also appears to be possible. In fact, while the first ones have high signal intensity in the T1-weighted sequences, with a mild decay in the T2-weighted ones, the fibro-atheromatous plaques show intermediate signal intensity in the T1-weighted sequences and low intensity in the T2-weighted ones. Moreover, the evaluation of the degree of the stenosis is also possible.
The overcoming of some limitations for the "in vivo" application of these results could allow MR to be considered as a safe technique useful mostly to monitor surgically or medically treated patients.

Acknowledgements: we acknowledge Limmat-Stifftung Foundation (Zurich, Switzerland) for the economical support; many thanks also to Carmelita Marinelli for help in manuscript preparation.

REFERENCES

Bradley WG, Waluch V (1985) Blood flow: Magnetic Resonance Imaging. Radiology 154: 443-450.

Herfkens RJ, Higgins CB, Hricak H, Lipton MJ, Crooks LE, Sheldon PE, Kaufman L (1983) NMR Imaging of Atherosclerotic Disease. Radiology 148:161-166.

Higgins CB, Stark B, McNamara M, Lanzer P, Crooks LE, Kaufman L (1984) Multiplane Magnetic Resonance Imaging of the and major vessels: Studies in normal volunteers. AJR 132: 661-667.

Hinshaw DB, Holshouser B, Hasso AN, Thompson JR (1987) MRI of the normal carotid biforcation. Neurorad 29: 7-97.

Soila K, Nummi P, Ekfors T, Viamonte M, Kormano M (1986) Proton relaxion time in arterial wall and atheromatous lesions. Invest Radiol 21: 411-415, 1986.

The Effect of Omnipaque and Hexabrix on the Calibre of Human Cerebral Arteries

P. Nakstad, S. J. Bakke, J. Hald, K. F. Lindegaard, W. Sorteberg, and I. O. Skalpe

INTRODUCTION

Animal and human studies (1,2) have shown a vasodilatator effect of hyperosmolar ionic contrast media, while animal studies with low-osmolar contrast media have shown both vasoconstrictive and vasodilatator effects (3,4,5) on cerebral arteries. The aim of the study was therefore to evaluate a possible vasoconstriction or vasodilatation after injection of low-osmolar contrast media in humans.

MATERIAL and METHODS

The material consists of 100 patients undergoing cerebral angiography performed with iohexol 300 mg I/ml (Omnipaque) and 27 patients with ioxaglate 320 mg I/ml (Hexabrix) in the period from March 1982 to January 1988. The sex and age distribution was similar in the two groups (Table 1). Only patients with migraine and trigeminal neuralgia (6) were excluded from the study.

All angiographies were performed in local anaesthesia. In order to evaluate a possible effect on the arterial calibre the two first successive injections had to be done in the same carotid or vertebral artery with the same contrast medium. Catheter position, injected volume, injection rate and contrast medium concentration was unchanged. Ten ml was injected in the carotid and 7 ml in the vertebral artery and the injection rate was 7 ml and 5 ml per second respectively. Alterations in the projections between the first and the second injection were accepted if the cranial or caudal angulation or the obliquity of the frontal x-ray tube was not altered more than 10 degrees. The time interval between the injections was always recorded (Table 2). Only the frontal angiograms were used for the calibre measurements. All measurements were performed on native angiograms and not on subtracted images that often are less exact because of blurred contours. The angiograms were magnified with a factor of 4 in order to improve the accuracy. All measurements were made by a single observer (PN). Six locations of the carotid and 5 locations of the vertebral arterial region were measured (Figs 1 and 2). The points where the measurements were made on the first angiogram series were carefully adhered to for the second measurement. The most peripheral branches were not evaluated since the possible inaccuracy.

In order to test the reproducability ten angiograms were evaluated with a three days interval.

In 14 patients with Omnipaque and in 4 with Hexabrix an additional third identical injection was done within 22-47 minutes after the first injection.

RESULTS

Increase of the arterial diameter at one or more locations was found in 58% (58/100), decrease in 61% (61/100) and increase as well as decrease in the same arterial region in 27% (27/100) after Omnipaque injections. With Hexabrix the numbers were 51.8% (14/27), 14.8% (4/27) and 4% (1/27) respectively. The number of patients with the same type of changes of the same arterial region was reduced markedly when patients with an increasing number of changes were counted. No case with calibre changes at all evaluated locations of an artery was found. Most changes were slight, that is 1-5%. Changes of more than 20% were not found. The few changes of more than 10% were almost exclusively found at only one location of the arterial region. Statistical evaluation did not show any significant vasoconstrictive or vasodilatator properties of the contrast media used. It had no effect on the degree of changes whether the time interval was short or long. The patients who received 3 injections had similar changes from the first to the second injection as from the first to the third. The reproducabilty of the measurements was excellent.

No difference in the image quality from the first to the following injections was seen. No complications occurred, but in some patients with reduced consciousness this was hard to evaluate.

DISCUSSION

Since du Boulay and Wallis (4) have shown that vasoconstriction appears already after 90 seconds in baboons it is of great concern that our time intervals were not shorter. It seemed, however, impossible to obtain an ethical defendable angiographic study in humans with such short intervals. As du Boulay and Wallis did not evaluate the effect of only one injection after longer intervals, it is not known if that would have given the same results as their repeated injections after 1.5, 6 and 20 minutes. It is possible that we were unable to find shortlasting vasoconstriction. However, sixteen patients with the second injection after 5 minutes did not show any other pattern of calibre changes than those with longer intervals. Furthermore, no patient showed any clinical reaction indicating significant change of the arteries.

The calibre changes seen in our study seemed too irregular to be explained by blood pressure variations. Small drops in the blood pressure would probably have caused slight vasoconstriction while moderate drops (30-50%) would have caused dilatation (3). A proximal vasoconstriction of the artery would by an autoregulatory mechanism have led to a peripheral vasodilatation and a fall of blood pressure if the other parameters had remained unchanged.

Although acute subarachnoid hemorrhage (SAH) was the indication for cerebral angiography in 61% of the patients, no complications

occurred. It is often believed that the arteries are more exposed
to spasm during cerebral angiography in these patients. This
study is in concordance with an earlier study (7) that showed
that cerebral angiography is a safe procedure in patients with
SAH. An impairment of the fluoroscopic and image quality (8)
should be expected concomitant with vasoconstriction, but this
never occurred during fluoroscopy or while reviewing the angiograms.

We conclude from this study that no significant vasoconstrictive
or vasodilatator effects on cerebral arteries were found using
normal doses of the low-osmolar contrast media Omnipaque and
Hexabrix in cerebral angiography performed with adequate injection technique. Reservations are taken with respect to the smaller
peripheral arterial branches and to the possibility of an effect
limited to the first minutes after the injection.

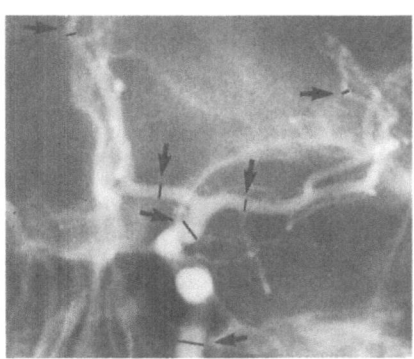

Fig.1. Locations for measurements of the carotid artery.

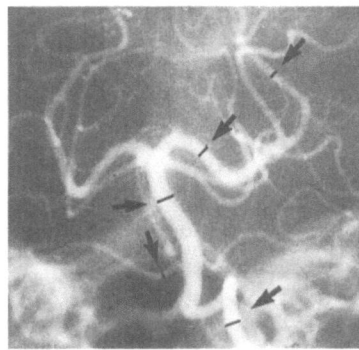

Fig.2. Locations for measurements of the vertebral artery.

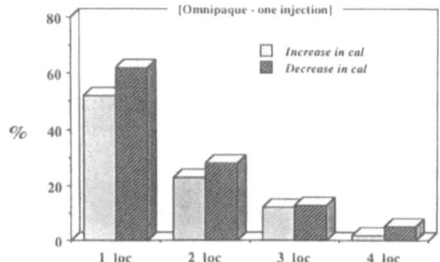

Fig.3. Patients in per cent with
calibre changes at 1, 2, 3 and 4
different locations after
injection of OMNIPAQUE.

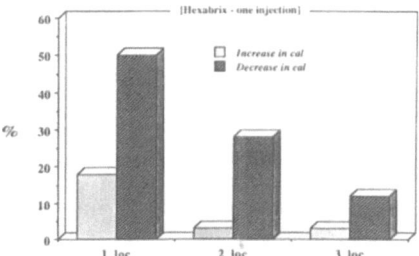

Fig.4. Patients in per cent
with calibre changes at 1, 2
and 3 different locations
after injection of HEXABRIX.

Table 1. Sex and age distribution

	No.of males	No.of females	Total no.	Age (range)
OMNIPAQUE 300 mg I/ml	50	50	100	45 (12-73)
HEXABRIX 320 mg I/ml	14	13	27	48 (10-63)

Table 2. Mean time interval between first and second injection

	Carotid artery	Vertebral artery	Both arteries
OMNIPAQUE	12 min.11 s. (5-45 min.)	18 min.30 s. (5-44 min.)	13 min. 38 s.
HEXABRIX	17 min.06 s. (5-45 min.)	15 min.00 s. (5-30 min.)	16 min. 30 s.

REFERENCES

1. Du Boulay G, Kendall BE, Symon L, Pasztor E, Crocard A, Belloni G, Sage M. (1975) The vasodilatator action of angiography with urografin 60% on basal vessels of the brain of the baboon. Neuroradiology 9:133-137.
2. Huber P, Hand J (1967) Effect of contrast material, hypercapnia, hyperventilation, hypertonic glucose and papaverine on the diameter of the cerebral arteries. Invest Radiol 2:17-32
3. Du Boulay G, Wallis A (1986) The effect of Iohexol and Hexabrix on the calibre of cerebral arteries in baboons during angiography. Radiol Med (Suppl) 2:31-36
4. Du Boulay G, Wallis A (1987) Cerebral arterial constriction due to contrast media. Acta Radiol (Suppl) 369:518-520.
5. Skalpe IO, Aulie Aa (1985) The toxicity of non-ionic water-soluble contrast media in selective vertebral angiography. Neuroradiology 27:77-79.
6. Ericson K (1983) Size of the internal carotid and middle cerebral artery in patients with trigeminal neuralgia. Acta Radiol 24:459-463.
7. Nakstad P, Nornes H, Hauge HN, Kjartansson O (1988) Cerebral panangiography in spontaneous subarachnoid hemorrhage from intracranial aneurysms. Acta Radiol (in press)
8. Doyon D, Ducot B, Halimi PH, Spira A, Noviant Y, Jacolot A, Lopez-Ibor L. (1987) Comparative trial of Hexabrix (320 mg I/ml) and iohexol (300 mg I/ml) and Iopamiron (300 mg I/ml) in cerebral and spinal angiography: a preliminary report. Brit J Radiol 60:671-675.

Initial Clinical Results with the Paramagnetic MR Contrast Agent Gd-DOTA in the Diagnosis of Central Nervous System Lesions

P. M. Parizel, H. R. Degryse, J. Gheuens, J. J. Martin, M. Van Vyve,
C. De la Porte, P. Selosse, P. Van de Heyning, and A. M. De Schepper

INTRODUCTION

Gadolinium tetraazacyclododecane tetraacetic acid (Gd-DOTA) is a new macrocyclic paramagnetic contrast agent. Gd-DOTA is an anionic macrocyclic chelate with a net charge of -1, versus a net charge of -2 for Gd-DTPA [Runge et al. 1988]. The compound is characterized by a very high stability of the Gd^{3+} ligand binding [Bousquet et al. 1988, Caillé et al. 1988]. Gd-DOTA is similar to Gd-DTPA with respect to its effect on tissues: both agents produce a decrease in relaxation times (T1 and T2). After intravenous injection, Gd–DOTA has an extracellular distribution and undergoes renal clearance by glomerular filtration.

In France and Belgium, clinical phase 2 studies with Gd-DOTA were started in 1987 [Berry et al. 1987, Allard et al. 1988, Caillé et al. 1988, Kien et al. 1988, Parizel et al. 1988]. The purpose of the present report was to evaluate the clinical efficacy in magnetic resonance (MR) imaging of central nervous system tumors, and to determine whether the use Gd-DOTA increases MR sensitivity or specificity.

MATERIAL AND METHODS

The paramagnetic contrast agent Gd-DOTA (Laboratoire Guerbet, Aulnay sous Bois) was used in a series of 39 patients with suspected intracranial or spinal tumors. In the initial 25 patients numerous biochemical, hematological and urinary tests were obtained prior to the examination, and at 2 and 24 hours after the intravenous injection of Gd–DOTA.

All patients were examined on a superconductive magnet system (Siemens Magnetom) operating at 0.5 T. Spin echo T1 and T2 weighted images (WI) were obtained before contrast injection. Following slow intravenous injection (injection rate: 3-5 ml/min) of Gd-DOTA in a dosage of 0.1 mmol/kg body weight, additional T1 WI were obtained in at least two imaging planes. All examinations were completed within 5 to 40 minutes of Gd-DOTA injection.

RESULTS

The contrast injection was well tolerated in all subjects. There were no adverse reactions, either during the examination or in the next 24-48 hours.

The clinical usefulness in different types of tumors is summarized in Table 1.

Table 1. Histologic diagnoses in 39 patients

Topography		Diagnosis	n	Enhan-cement
BRAIN	Intraaxial	Low grade glioma	7	-/±
		High grade glioma	3	++
		Metastasis	4	++
		Ischemic lesions	2	±
		Cryptic vascular malformation	1	±
	Extraaxial	Meningioma	8	++
		Hemangiopericytoma	1	++
		Acoustic Schwannoma	1	++
		Trigeminal Schwannoma	1	++
		Pituitary macroadenoma	1	+
		Tumors of the skull base	2	±
SPINE	Intraaxial	Low grade glioma	2	+
		High grade glioma	1	+
	Extraaxial	Schwannoma	2	+
		Meningioma	1	+
		Neurofibroma	1	+
		Metastasis	1	+

DISCUSSION

In *intraaxial tumors*, Gd-DOTA is a marker of blood-brain-barrier (BBB) breakdown and an indicator of tumor vascularity. As a general rule, malignant intraaxial tumors (high grade gliomas, metastases) showed intense contrast enhancement, whereas there was no or minimal contrast uptake in low grade astrocytomas, presumably because in these tumors there is no BBB disruption. The use of Gd-DOTA improved border definition of lesions with heterogeneous signal intensities and tumor versus edema differentiation.

In *extraaxial tumors*, which do not have a BBB, the degree of enhancement after Gd-DOTA presumably indicates tumor vascularity. In our series, all meningiomas and schwannomas (intracranial and spinal), showed immediate, intense and sharply defined contrast enhancement. Small tumors, that were initially overlooked on the precontrast MR study, were correctly diagnosed after Gd-DOTA injection. In this respect, Gd-DOTA increases the sensitivity of the MR examination in some patients, especially when the lesion is small. In some instances, Gd-DOTA increases MR specificity, such as in the demonstration of dural attachment in meningiomas, and intracanalar extension in acoustic schwannomas. Thus the paramagnetic contrast agent may contribute to the presurgical evaluation of certain patients.

CONCLUSIONS

Our findings in a series of 39 patients indicate that Gd-DOTA is an effective and well tolerated paramagnetic contrast agent. Gd-DOTA was useful in the anatomic definition of cerebral and spinal lesions, and increased MR sensitivity and specificity in some instances.

REFERENCES

Allard M, Kien P, Allard M, Lebrun PH, Chastin I, Caillé JM (1988) Efficacy and safety of Gd-DOTA used in neuroradiological MRI: a clinical study. Presented at the 26th Annual Meeting of the American Society of Neuroradiology, Scientific Program, paper #164, p 213, Chicago, May 15–20, 1988

Berry I, Manelfe C, Chastin I, Arrue P, Prere J. Gd-DOTA enhancement of cerebral and spinal tumors on MR imaging. Presented at the 73rd Scientific Assembly and Annual Meeting of the Radiological Society of North America, RSNA Scientific Program, paper #75, p 38, Chicago, November 29–December 4, 1987

Bousquet JC, Saini S, Stark DD, Hahn PF, Nigam M, Wittenberg J, Ferrucci JT (1988) Gd-DOTA: characterization of a new paramagnetic complex. Radiology 166: 693-698

Caillé JM, Kien P, Bonnemain B, Doucet D, Meyer D (1988) Gd^{3+} DOTA: a review of preclinical and clinical experience. Presented at the Second European Congress of NMR in Medicine and Biology, Abstract Book, paper#47, Berlin, June 23-26, 1988

Kien P, Allard M, Bonnemain B, Caillé JM (1988) Efficacy and safety of Gd–DOTA used in neuroradiological MRI. Presented at the Second European Congress of NMR in Medicine and Biology, Abstract Book, paper#123, Berlin, June 23-26, 1988

Runge VM, Jacobson S, Wood ML, Kaufman D, Adelman L (1988) MR Imaging of rat brain glioma: Gd-DTPA versus Gd-DOTA. Radiology 166: 835-838

Ultrasound Imaging of Brain Pathology Through a Skull Defect

B. Góraj and M. Kopytek

Introduction

Actual and detailed information about intracranial conditions in patients with brain pathology is the basic goal of neuroradiological
diagnostics. Neuroradiologists and neurosurgeons expect from it data
about the presence, location, and nature of the pathological process,
and also about intracranial translocations. The most useful in this
field are considered those methods which allow one to evaluate intracranial space in a noninvasive, accurate, and repeatable way. Among
other methods, real-time ultrasonography gains increasing importance.
This results from its high validity in characterization of tissue
morphology (Enzmann et al. 1981, 1985) and noninvasiveness and also
from the fact that there is no exposure to ionizing radiation during
the US examination. Investigations for establishing the US patterns
of different brain lesions have been performed. This paper presents
the brain pathology characterization of various kinds, based on 100 US
examinations.

Materials and Methods

Over a period of 3 years 100 US examinations of the brain were performed in patients aged 14-71. The use of US depended on the presence of an acoustic window, after craniotomy, craniectomy, or enlarged burr hole. In 87 cases the examination was performed through
the skull defect after operation for different brain lesions, such
as brain neoplasm, posttraumatic hemorrhage, abscess, and cyst. The
earliest time of investigation was the 8th day after surgury, with
attention paid to early complications. In patients examined a few
months after operation we looked for late complications and tumor
recurrence. Thirteen of our patients were disqualified from surgery
because of the presence of deep or multilobar neoplasms. These persons were examined through an enlarged threphine hole made as a preparation for US-guided diagnostic biopsy. The minimal diameter of
the skull defect was 3 cm.

Real-time equipment with sector transducers of 3.5 and 5 MHz and
90°-115° field of view was used. The acoustic gel was placed between
the US probe and the head surface. All patients underwent either CT
examination or angiography in the course of the diagnostic process.
In tumors the histopathological diagnosis was obtained from specimens taken intraoperatively or via biopsy. The following features
of the lesions were characterized: location, shape, echogenicity,
dimensions, internal architectural margins, and relations to neighboring structures.

Results

The most numerous group in our study was that of brain neoplasms
(Table 1). There was a variety of images of different tumors, but
all of them contained a hyperechogenic portion, and all produced mass
effect. There occurred a considerable differentiation in internal
structure, echogenicity, margins, and size of surrounding edema in
individual types of neoplasms. Malignant glioma demonstrated the
most inhomogeneous architecture, irregular shape, and ill-defined
margins. The hypoechogenic area within tumors was established as a

Table 1. Distribution of lesions studied with US through skull defect

Type of lesion	–
Brain neoplasm	
Glioma malignum	22
Glioblastoma multiforme	17
Astrocystoma III	2
Astrocystoma IV	1
Digodendroglioma	2
Medulloblastoma	1
Tumor metastaticum clarocellulare	1
Meningioma	1
Brain abscess	4
Brain cyst	8
Intracerebral hemorrhage	27
Ischemic lesions	9
Brain edema (as an isolated change) postoperatively	2
Hydrocephalus	3
Total	100

cystic or necrotic part (Fig.1). Meningioma and tumor metastaticum were characterized as having the most homogeneous, hyperechogenic structure and rather regular shape.

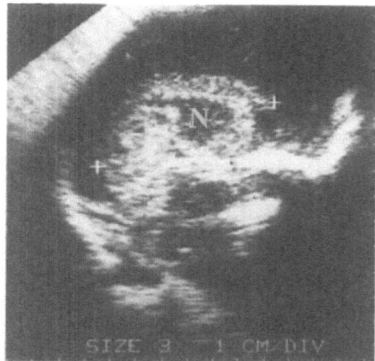

Fig.1. Deep-sited brain tumor, glioblastoma multiform

Among brain abscesses there could be noticed different US images of acute and chronic types. The acute abscesses were sonolucent, of regular shape, with a thin, well-defined wall. In the chronic ones we observed a more polymorphic structure and a thick wall (Fig.2).

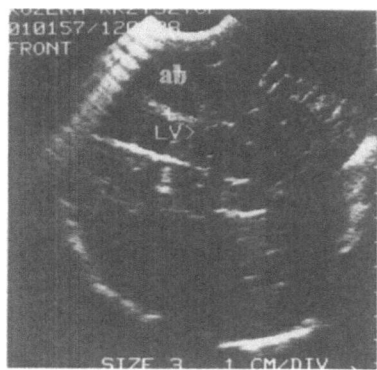

Fig.2. Subacute abscess in left temporal lobe

Brain cysts were seen as a sonolucent, well-defined area with regular shape and margins. In all cases there occurred mass effect. In two cases there were hyperechogenic calcifications in the cyst wall (Fig.3).

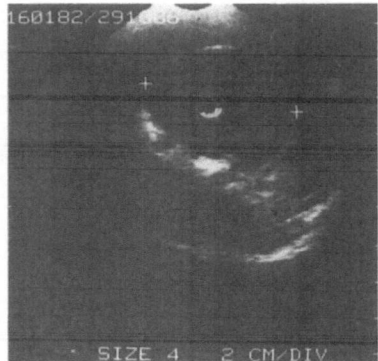

Fig.3. Large brain cyst in right hemisphere

Intracerebral hemorrhage was found in 27 cases. In the first period it was intensely hyperechogenic and well defined (Fig.4). Later its echogenicity became lower from the center. In one case in which the development of this change was observed the features of brain atrophy were noticed in the examination made 6 months after the hemorrhage.

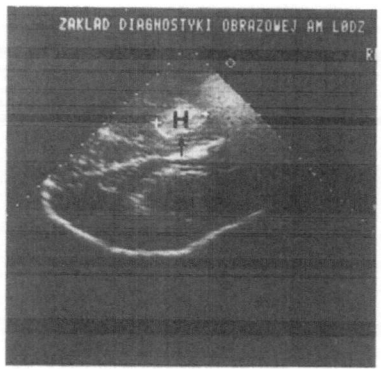

Fig.4. Intracerebral hemorrhage lasting 4 days

The hypoechogenic irregular area was visible in the region surrounding the site of clipping of the aneurysm. After a few weeks there appeared the hypoechogenic field, with a displacement of neighboring structures in the direction of ischemia (Fig.5).

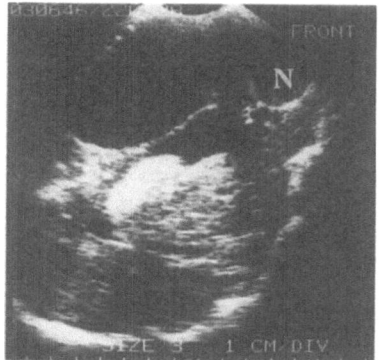

Fig.5. Ischemic lesion after clipping of MCA aneurysm

Regarding edema, in almost all cases there was visible a moderately hyperechogenic region surrounding the main lesion. Based on the results of other verifying tests (such as CT and histopathology), we considered it to be a cerebral edema. It was also present in the early period after lesion removal (Fig.6).

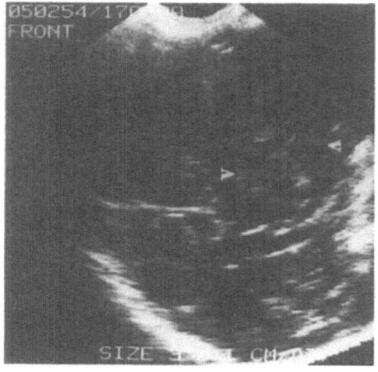

Fig.6. Isolated cerebral edema after removing the tumor

Discussion

In our study all the pathological brain lesions found with other methods (CT, angiography, intraoperatively) were confirmed by US image. This high sensivity of US is also reported by other authors (Merrit et al. 1983; Rubin and Dohrmann 1983). On the other hand, the ability of US to differentiate various changes seems to be lower, especially in establishing the histopathological type of neoplasms, as well as in evaluating hyperechogenic lesions (Enzman et al. 1981, 1985). The problems can arise in characterization of the components of lesion margins. McGahan et al. (1986) state that echogenic margins of the mass may represent active tumor infiltration, tumor necrosis, vascular invasion, or edema, and that biopsy from more than one point can furnish the only way of establishing the histopathological type of tissue changes.

There are different opinions on the US appearance of tumor necrosis. In our studies, and also according to the results of Gooding et al. (1984), it is demonstrated as a mottled, slightly hypoechogenic area in the tumor center (Fig.1). The investigations of McGahan et al. (1986) indicate that tumor necrosis more frequently appears as a hyperechogenic area.

Contrary to hyperechogenic patterns, US seems to be better than other diagnostic methods in evaluation of cystic lesions and cystic portions of them (McGahan et al. 1986; Rubin and Dohrmann 1983).

In conclusion, we consider US to be very helpful for the detection and localization of brain lesions. The US diagnosis value is lower in distinguishing the different types of brain pathology, but in these cases the US-guided biopsy may be useful. US as a noninvasive and easy to perform procedure is a proper method in screening and postoperative follow-up.

References

[1] Enzmann DR, Britt RH, Lyons B, Buxton TL, Wilson DA (1981) Experimental study of high-resolution ultrasound imaging of hemorrhage, bone fragments and foreign bodies in head trauma. J Neurosurg 54: 304-309
[2] Enzmann DR, Wheat R, Marshall WH, Bird R, Irwin KM, Karbon K, Hanbery JW, Silverberg GM, Britt RH (1985) Tumors of the central nervous system studied by CT and ultrasound. Radiology 154: 393-399
[3] Gooding GAW, Boggan JE, Weinstein PR (1984) Characterization of intracranial neoplasms by CT and intraoperative sonography. AJNR 5: 517-520
[4] McGahan JP, Ellis WG, Budenz RW, Walter JP, Boggan J (1986) Brain gliomas: sonographic characterization. Radiology 159: 485-492
[5] Merrit CRB, Coulon R, Connoly E (1983) Intraoperative neurosurgical ultrasound. Transdural and transfontanelle application. Radiology 148: 513-517
[6] Rubin JM, Dohrmann GJ (1983) Intraoperative neurosurgical ultrasound in the localization and characterization of intracranial masses. Radiology 148: 519-524

MRI in Parkinson-Plus Syndromes: Differences Between Progressive Supranuclear Palsy (PSP) and Shy-Drager Syndrome (SDS)

M. Savoiardo, L. Strada, F. Girotti, P. Soliveri, and M. Sberna (Milano, Italy)

In Parkinson-plus syndromes, decreased signal intensity (SI) in the putamen in high-field-strength T2 w.i. has been observed. This finding has been attributed to abnormal distribution of iron or other paramagnetic substances.

We reviewed the 1.5 T MRI studies of 12 patients with Parkinson-plus syndromes: 7 with PSP and 5 with SDS.

In the PSP group, 6 patients had normal iron distribution; only 1 (with somewhat atypical history) had "inversion" of decreased SI between pallidum and putamen. Examination of the substantia nigra, red nucleus and dentate nucleus provided variable results. Questionable increased SI in the periaqueductal region was sometimes observed. The only specific finding was that the atrophy, already known to involve the mesencephalic region, in 5 of 7 cases involved particularly the superior collicular region with flattening of the upper part of the quadrigeminal plate versus the inferior collicular region.

In the SDS group, 4 of 5 cases had markedly decreased SI in the putamen, more evident than in the pallidum in 3, equal in 1. In one atypical case, with features of olivopontocerebellar atrophy, minimal evidence of iron was present in the putamen where high SI was seen in intermediate weighted images. In 2 SDS cases, T2 w.i. obtained with 0.15 and 0.5 T MR demonstrated high SI in the putamen, where 1.5 T T2 w.i. exhibited decreased SI.

PSP appears, therefore, different from other Parkinson-plus syndromes, at least from SDS, regarding iron distribution in the basal ganglia. Focal atrophy of the superior collicular region may be its most specific finding.

MR Imaging of Posterior Fossa Hemangioblastomas

M. Boukobza, A. Villanueva, J. Kardouss, and J. Metzger (Paris, France)

MR images were obtained in 10 cases of posterior fossa hemangioblastomas using T1, T2 weighted spin-echo sequences and gadolinium
enhancement. Although abnormalities could be detected without contrast, gadolinium allows a better delineation of the lesion in demonstrating the nidus of the hemangioblastoma and the exact extent
of the lesion to the medulla.

MR Imaging Evaluation of Intracranial Lesions with Gadolinium Enhancement in 500 Cases. Histopathologic Correlation

P. Rolloy, M. Boukobza, A. Zouaoui, L. Feldman, J. Kardouss,
F. Kikhya, and J. Metzger (Paris, France)

Over 500 intracranial lesions were studied with MR before (T1 and T2
weighted sequences) and after injection of gadolinium. Diseases included primary and metastatic brain tumors, neuromas, meningiomas, infections and vascular malformations of the central nervous system.

In all cases the correlation with histopathologic findings is made.
The enhancement characteristics of these lesions are considered and
the findings are compared with contrast enhanced X-ray CT.

Gadolinium is likely to increase the potential of MR and to refine the
evaluation of these lesions and is vital for proper diagnosis in many
instances.

Magnetic Resonance Appearance of Angiographically Silent Slow Flow Angiomas of the Brain Stem

K. Mathias, H.-O. Lincke, and G. Hoffmann (Dortmund, Germany)

In five patients with the clinical signs of an acute brain stem process magnetic resonance imaging detected the typical pattern of parenchymal hematoma with hyperintensive signals in the lesion and a well defined thin band of low signal intensity. None of the lesions had a surrounding edema.

These lesions could not be revealed by selective angiography, but by computed tomography. In the past, occult vascular malformations were best identified by CT, but the findings were not always specific. MRI reveals the true nature of these brain stem lesions avoiding biopsy procedures.

The typical findings of these vascular malformations and the intensity behavior in T1- and T2-weighted images in the follow-up period are demonstrated together with angiograms and CT studies.

Intracranial Giant Aneurysms Caused by Radiation Damage

F. Thun and H. Lanfermann

Among intracranial vascular malformations, aneurysms have been found
in 2%-4% in general autopsies [1,2] and in up to 9% in brain autopsies alone [3]. In the vast majority of cases, saccular arterial dilatations were involved. The etiological classification of aneurysms
includes the congenital, arteriosclerotic, mycotic, traumatic, and
dissecting forms. A further cause that has not yet been described,
as far as we know, is radiation damage. That this may be a cause of
aneurysms is very probable in view of the case histories of two patients at our hospital. Both were treated with transsphenoidal
yttrium 90 implantation for a pituitary tumor. A vascular malformation had been ruled out by angiography before the operation and was
demonstrated some years later. There is no indication of another etiological factor.

In the first case, that of a female patient, acromegaly occurred for
the first time in the 19th year of life, after a normal youth. Two
years later, visual disturbances developed which were more pronounced
on the left, with upper quadrant anopsia. The neurological findings
were otherwise normal. Cisternography revealed a pituitary tumor which
passed beyond the sellar entrance plane by 14 mm. In the subfrontal
hypophysectomy performed at the age of 21 years, an endocrinologically active adenoma was removed in toto and without complications. The
surgeon did not observe any vascular malformation. Vision improved
postoperatively, but growth hormone values rose again. Two years later, bilateral carotid angiography revealed a suprasellar recurrence;
an aneurysm could not be demonstrated. The immediate transsphenoidal
implantation of eight 4.4 mCi 90Y seeds, i.e., a total of 35 mCi, was
without noteworthy incidents. On X rays of the cranium, the seeds
were located markedly paramedian at the right in the sellar lumen.
During the subsequent 7 years, checks of hormone values and vision
showed a stationary course, but there was then a rapid deterioration
in vision of the right eye. Computed tomography (the first CT to be
performed in the patient) revealed a hyperdense zone the size of a
bean, with enhancement to 100 HU and localized on the right beside
the dorsum sellae. This was interpreted as a fresh recurrence of the

tumor. However, carotid angiography showed an infraclinoid giant aneurysm. After extraintracranial anastomosis and ligation of the internal carotid artery in the neck, this vessel was clipped intra-cranially proximal to the posterior communicating artery. The intra-operative pucture of the aneurysm did not reveal any blood. Later angiographies showed good vascularization of the brain and exclusion of the aneurysm.

In the second patient, a hitherto healthy man, acromegaly appeared at the age of 37 years, and diabetes mellitus occurred 2 years later. The sella turcica was markedly dilated by an intrasellar tumor, but this did not extend to suprasellar on cisternography. Carotid angio-graphy was also normal. In view of a bilateral quadrant anopsia and greatly increased growth hormone values, eight 5.6 mg 90Y seeds (44 mCi in total) were implanted in this patient at the age of 42 years. Tumor tissue from the cannula correspond to a mainly eosino-philic adenoma. As the sole complication of this procedure, there was a nasal CSF fistula, which promptly ceased after stereotactic filling of the sphenoid sinus with Pallacos. Afterwards, the patient no longer had any symptoms, and he presented again only after 11 years because of diffuse headache. In the CT of the head, an intra-sellar tumor extending to suprasellar was to be seen which was diagnosed as an adenoma recurrence. In the subfrontal craniotomy carried out a few days later, the neurosurgeon discovered a black-reddish expansive lesion in front of the chiasm, exploratory puncture of which revealed blood and a dramatic pucture hole hemorrhage from an intrasellar aneurysm. It was imaged postoperatively by angiography and isolated with a Selverstone clamp on the left after extraintra-cranial anastomosis.

Despite the considerable number of pituitary tumors treated by im-plantation of 90Y or other radioisotopes, only Jakubowski and Kendall [4] have reported on two cases of aneurysms adjacent to yttrium im-plants. However, they could not rule out with certainty the preopera-tive presence of an aneurysm for lack of preliminary angiographic in-vestigation. On the other hand, this could be proved in our patients. The effect of the 90Y β-radiation on pituitary tissue is known [5]. At 300 krad, 90% of pituitary tumors could be destroyed as a rule. The threshold dose of β-radiation necessary for necrosis of arterial smooth muscle varies from 32 to 349 krad, with a mean of 146 krad. It is thus conceivable that the local radiation exposure of the siphon wall causes necrotic damage to the internal elastic membrane as well. In veins, fibrosis and a progressive vascular occlusion may develop from such damage. On the other hand, in arteries the high and, moreover, pulsating blood pressure may lead to a local loss of elasticity of the vascular wall at the site affected over a long period, so that a ballooon-like dilatation may ensue.

Further additional factors may possibly play a coadjuvant role: a weakening of the vascular wall of hormonal origin in the context of the pituitary disorder or mechanical factors in terms of traction exerted on the siphon wall by reduction of the pituitary volume in consequence of the radiotherapy. Furthermore, damage may be caused to the vasa vasorum and thus to the microcirculation of siphon wall by excessively lateral localization of an yttrium seed or by encroachment of the intracavernous segments of the carotid arteries up to the midline. There is no indication of direct vascular damage, since both stereotactic operations were completely without complications. The course after implantation did not provide any indication for an inflammatory lesion, arteritis, or an abscess.

Yttrium implantations in the treatment of pituitary tumors have no longer been practiced for about 10 years. Potential patients with radiation-induced aneurysms are thus becoming increasingly rare. Nevertheless, our two cases are likely to prove the possibility of the development of aneurysms in consequence of the direct action of radiation. This aspect may once more be of importance in stereotactic interstitial radioisotope therapy of extrasellar brain tumors, a methods which has been experiencing a fresh impetus, if radioisotope seeds are situated in the immediate proximity of large vessels.

References

[1] Chason JL, Hindman WM (1958) Berry aneurysms of the circle of Willis, results of a planned autopsy study. Neurology 8: 41-44
[2] Housepian EM, Pool JL (1958) A systematic analysis of intracranial aneurysms from the autopsy files of the Presbyterian Hospital - 1914 to 1956. J Neuropathol Exp Neurol 17: 409-423
[3] Alpers BJ (1965) Aneurysms of the circle of Willis. In: Fields WS, Sahs AL (eds) Intracranial aneurysms and subarachnoid hemorrhage, Chapter I. CC Thomas, Springfield
[4] Talbor IC et al. (1980) Pituitary ablation by yttrium-90 implantation: some post mortem and clinical observations. Int J of Applied Radiation and Isotopes 31: 695-701
[5] Jakubowski J, Kendall B (1981) Coincidental aneurysms with tumours of pituitary origin. J Neurol Neurosurg Psychiat 41: 972-797

MRT/CT Correlations in Patients Years After Severe Head Injury Combined with Mid-Brain Syndrome

A. Laun, A. L. Agnoli, and A. Halbsguth

INTRODUCTION

Besides computerised tomography (CT), MRT is a very important tool
of neuroimaging (Spetzler et al. 1985). It is rarely done in acute
severe head injury because of technical problems, for instance
mechanical life support devices (Han et al. 1984). However, it has
been seldom performed years after a severe head injury, probably
because of its financial expenses.
We have done a study on patients who had suffered a severe head
injury with a midbrain syndrome years ago. Aim of the study was to
find out if MRT is of benefit in detecting lesions not visible in
CT.

MATERIAL

36 patients have been reinvestigated, all had suffered a severe
brain lesion with midbrain syndrome of variable duration. In colla-
boration with family doctors, insurances and the patients themselves, we performed neurological, neurophysiological, psychometric
(Laun et al. 1989) and neuroendocrinological (Lenzen et al.1988)
investigations. Besides, CT and MRT were done in 30 patients.
Mean age was 21.7 years (range 8-57 years), mean follow up period
was 5.7 $\pm$ 2.2 years (range 1-9 years).

RESULTS

1. 5 out of 30 patients revealed an atrophy of the corpus callosum
   (Fig. 1) in MRT, which could not be detected in CT, even with
   reformatting techniques.

2. In 2 patients MRT showed an atrophy of a crus cerebri (Fig. 2).
   In one patient an atrophic lesion of the brain stem was visible,
   which could be seen in CT too.

3. Sequelae of small haematomas (up to 1 cm in diameter) might be
   missed as well in CT as in MRT, probably due to present resolution quality.

4. In 3 patients MRT detected additional cortical and subcortical lesions as well as lesions in the white matter.

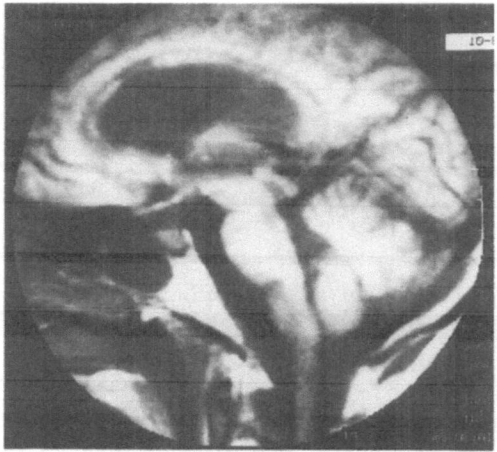

Fig. 1   Atrophy of the corpus callosum

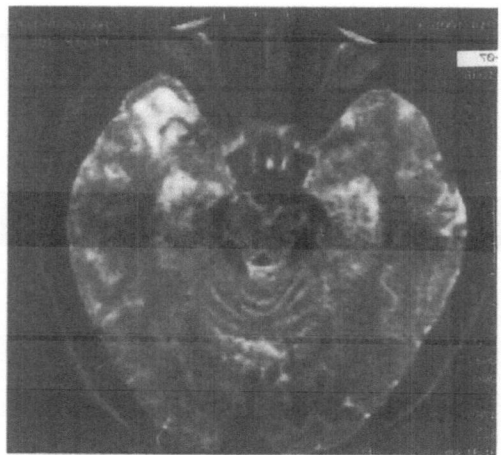

Fig. 2   Atrophy of the crus cerebri

DISCUSSION

Up to now, MRT investigations in head trauma patients are seldom done (Gandy et al. 1984; Snow et al. 1986; Spetzler et al. 1985). They seem to be superior (Mauthner et al. 1987) in comparison to CT at least in the acute stage (Wilberger et al. 1987). Our study

in severely head injured patients years after trauma is to our
knowledge the first systematic study on this subject. The most
striking result is the diffuse or localised atrophy in the corpus
callosum in five of 30 cases, which was not visible in CT. We
could not detect distinct neuropsychological correlations to this
defect (Laun et al. 1989). In one case atrophy of the crus cerebri
correlated to a slight hemiparesis. This atrophy has not been revealed in actual nor in former CT scans. The neurological deficit
of this patient remained unexplained until MRT was done.

In conclusion, MRT investigations seem to be of further value to
detect sequelae of severe head injuries. Therefore, MRT should
have priority to CT because of its higher resolution capacity.

REFERENCES

Gandy SE (1984) Cranial nuclear magnetic resonance imaging in head
    trauma. Ann Neurol 16:254-257
Han JS (1984) Head trauma evaluated by magnetic resonance and
    computed tomography: A comparison. Radiology 150:71-72
Laun A et al. (1989) Outcome after severe head injury with midbrain
    syndrome in the acute stage. In: Advances in Neurosurgery Vol. 17
    Springer, Berlin, Heidelberg, New York, in press
Lenzen J et al. (1988) Endokrinologische Funktionsuntersuchungen
    des hypothalamo-hypophysären Systems nach schwerem Schädelhirn-
    trauma. 39. Jahrestagung der Dt. Ges. für Neurochirurgie, Köln
    8.-11.5.1988
Mauthner VF et al. (1987) Kernspintomographie versus Computertomo-
    graphie in der Initialphase des leichten Schädelhirntraumas.
    Akt Neurol 14:145-148
Snow RB et al. (1986) Comparison of magnetic resonance imaging and
    and computed tomography in the evaluation of head injury. Neuro-
    surgery 18:45-52
Spetzler RF et al. (1985) Clinical role of magnetic resonance
    imaging in the neurosurgical patient. Neurosurgery 16:511-524
Wilberger JE (1987) Magnetic resonance imaging in cases of severe
    head injury. Neurosurg. 20:571-576

Neurophysiologic Assessment of Neural Tolerance of a New Paramagnetic Complex

N. Corsico and P. Tirone

INTRODUCTION

The compound coded B-19036, an octadentate chelate of the paramagnetic ion Gd^{3+} (3,6,9-triaza-12-oxa-3,6,9-tricarboxymethylene -10-carboxy-13-phenyl-tridecanoic acid, gadolinium chelate, Fig. 1), is a new contrast agent for magnetic resonance imaging, developed in our laboratories (Felder et al. 1985). Systemic and neural tolerance for B-19036 was evaluated both after intravenous and intrathecal administration.

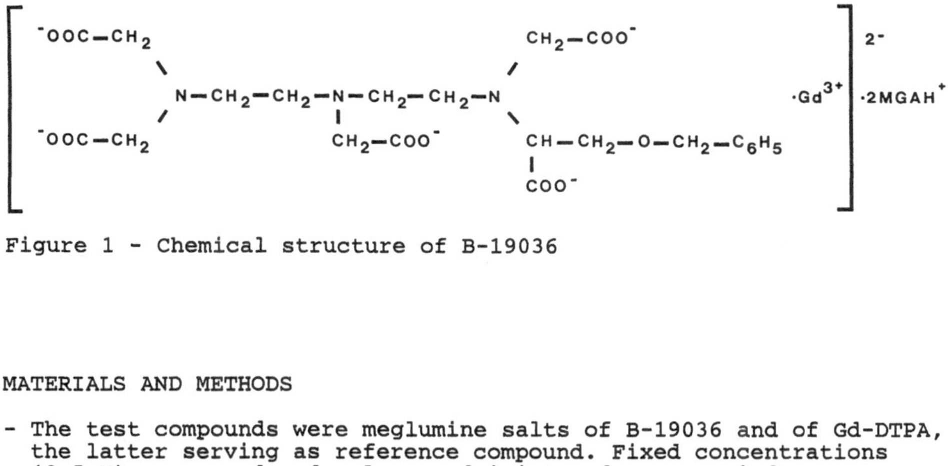

Figure 1 - Chemical structure of B-19036

MATERIALS AND METHODS

- The test compounds were meglumine salts of B-19036 and of Gd-DTPA, the latter serving as reference compound. Fixed concentrations (0.5 M) were used and volumes administered were varied.
- Acute intravenous and intracerebral toxicities were assessed following a single administration of the solutions to CD^R-1 mice and CD^R(SD)BR rats. The LD_{50} was calculated according to Litchfield and Wilcoxon (1949).
- EEG spectral analysis was carried out after intravenous and intraventricular injection of male conscious unrestrained CD^R(SD)BR rats as previously reported (Corsico and Tirone 1987).
- Behavioural studies were performed according to the protocol of Irwin (1968) after intracisternal administration to male CD^R(SD)BR rats.

582

RESULTS

Intravenous route

Acute toxicity

LD_{50} values of B-19036 and Gd-DTPA after intravenous injection to mice and rats are summarized in Table 1. LD_{50} values of the new compound obtained in rodents are more comparable than those of the reference compound Gd-DTPA.

TABLE 1

Compound	LD_{50} mmol/kg	Animal	Admin.
B-19036	5.80	mouse	i.v.
	5.85	rat	i.v.
Gd-DTPA	4.80	mouse	i.v.
	4.96	rat	i.v.

EEG Spectral analysis

B-19036 at an intravenous dose of 2 mmol/kg, about 20 times the anticipated clinical dose, did not cause obvious changes of the EEG pattern. Spectral analysis showed that the total power (0-16Hz) of the signal was slightly increased; the percentage content of the frequency bands 0.25-4Hz, 4.25-8Hz and 8.25-13Hz was not consistently changed.

Intrathecal route

Acute toxicity

In the mouse, the intracerebral LD_{50} of 0.61 mmol/kg, found for B-19036 was comparable to that obtained for Gd-DTPA, i.e. 0.68 mmol/kg.

Behavioural studies

B-19036 caused mainly mydriasis and a decrease in altertness and motor coordination. At the highest injected dose (0.3 mmol/kg) some jerks were also observed. The other behavioural, neurophysiologic and neurovegetative parameters of the protocol of Irwin (1968) were unchanged.
Comparable effects were caused by Gd-DTPA. The minimal dose affecting behaviour was the same for the two compounds (see Table 2).

TABLE 2

Compound	MED mmol/kg	Animal	Admin.
B-19036	0.03	rat	ici
Gd-DTPA	0.03	rat	ici

MED = minimal effective dose
ici = intracisternal

EEG spectral analysis

Injection into the cerebral lateral ventricle of either compounds at the minimal dose affecting behaviour elicited an increase in the total power of the EEG signal (see Fig. 2). No consistent changes in the relative contributions of the frequency bands 0.25-4 Hz, 4.25-8 Hz and 8.25-13 Hz could be identified.

EEG TOTAL POWER (0-16H$_z$)

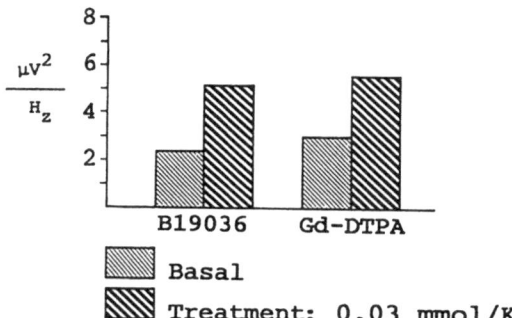

Figure 2

Basal

Treatment: 0.03 mmol/Kg

DISCUSSION

Neural tolerance is an important requirement for the safety of paramagnetic contrast agents since they might penetrate CNS tissues, even in the absence of an intrinsic permeability of the BBB, if the latter is injured. Results of our investigations revealed no signs of neurotoxicity of the new gadolinium complex after systemic administration at a dose-level 10-20 times higher than that foreseen in clinical use. Neural tolerance of B-19036 was good also after direct CNS application. The minimal effective dose of B-19036 on behaviour and EEG spectral pattern in rats was 10 μmol/animal. This amount is about 10-20 times the maximum quantity that might cross an injured BBB after intravascular injection of a clinical dose. These findings indicate that the complex most likely does not cross an intact BBB.

In conclusion, the new complex B-19036 proved to have a satisfactory systemic and neural tolerability and can, therefore, be proposed for intravascular use as a contrast agent for magnetic resonance imaging.

REFERENCES

Corsico N, Tirone P (1987) EEG studies in the conscious unrestrained rat: a tool for the study of immediate and delayed neurotoxicity of contrasts media. In: Calabrò A, Leonardi M (eds) Computer Aided Neuroradiology p 255-258

Felder E et al. (1985) Bracco Industria Chimica EP Patent application n. 230893

Irwin S (1968) Comprehensive observational assessement: Ia-A systematic quantitative procedure for assessing the behavioral and physiologic state of the mouse. Psychopharmacologia 13, 222-236

Litchfield Jr J T, Wilcoxon F (1949) A simplified method of evaluating dose-effect experiments. J Pharmacol Exp Therap 96, 99-113

Tumours of the Brainstem. Clinical and Radiological Aspects and Statistical Evaluation

R. L. Prevo, G. J. Vielvoye, and E. A. van der Velde

INTRODUCTION

In the Netherlands the number of people dying from a brainstem tumour has remained more or less constant and between 1979 and 1985 this averaged 10 patients a year. The number of first admissions on suspicion of a brainstem tumour was also fairly constant. In contrast with the number of people dying of a malignant braintumour, which shows a definite increase.

CLINICAL MATERIAL AND METHODS

In order to get a series of sufficient extent, all major Dutch hospitals were approached for clinical records and radiological material of patients, admitted on suspicion of a brainstem tumour in the period January 1978- January 1984. Totally 112 patients were included, divided in 75 patients with a primary brainstem tumour and 37 patients with a secondary or extra-axial tumour. Clinical and histological data were reviewed and compared with radiological data. The analysis of the following clinical information was performed: age at diagnosis, sex, duration of symptoms before diagnosis, histology, pyramidal tract signs, cerebellar lesions, deficit in sensibility, presence of raised intracranial pressure, presence of cranial nerve palsies at the time of diagnosis and at the end of the observation time. The total material was divided in 7 groups: pontine glioma without radiotherapy, pontine glioma with radiotherapy, metastases, non Hodgkin lymphoma, medulloblastoma, ependymoma and miscellaneous. Totally 99 CT scans, 56 vertebral angiograms and 34 ventriculographies were available. The following CT variables were reviewed: tumour density, tumour localisation, enhancement and presence of ventriculomegaly. In angiography the position of the basilar artery, PICA, AICA and precentral cerebellar vein was reviewed. Statistical analysis was performed using the computer software program SSPS-X 2.1. Standard statistical methods were used, like the chi-square test statistic etc. Survival distributions were compared with the Lee-Desu test.

RESULTS

In the total material of 112 patients with a brainstem tumour is a slight male predominance, caused by the patients in the groups non Hodgkin lymphoma, medulloblastoma and ependymoma. The sex ratio is equal, according to the series of Bray 1958, Panitch and Berg 1970. 51 patients are younger than 15 years and 41 patients older than 35 years. The slight increase in the fourth and fifth decade is according to the series of White 1963, Lassiter et al 1971, Kim et al 1980 and Tokuriki et al 1986. The duration of symptoms and observation time was respectively 9- 12 weeks and 25-52 weeks. Pyramidal tract signs on admission were noticed in 84 patients (75.0%), while no statistical association was found between right- and left sided lesions. Cerebellar symptoms were noticed in 89 patients (79.5%). In 52 patients the symptoms were from the medial cerebellar compartments alone. Sensibility disorders were found only in 11 patients (9.8%). Histology was obtained in 62 patients, while an astrocytoma, varying in degree, was found in 26 patients (23.2%). The incidence of raised intracranial pressure was found in 53 patients (47.3%), confined to the group patients with a pontine glioma this was 33.8%. In this material most frequently cranial nerve palsies of the sixth (56.3%) and seventh (59.8%) cranial nerve happened to occur. There was no significant difference between clinical manifestations on admission and at the end of the observation time. Statistical significant associations were found between tumour density versus tumour localisation, tumour density versus cerebellar lesions and lesions in the combinations of the cranial nerves III-V, VI-VIII, V-VII and VIII-XII. Also significant associations were found between tumour localisation versus hydrocephalus and cerebellar lesions. Median survival time of all patients was 42 weeks (Fig.1).

Survival time after 1 year, 2, 3 and 5 years was respectively 46%, 32%, 27% and 22%. 1-Year survival of the untreated patients with a pontine glioma was 30% and for the treated patients this was 50% (Fig.2).

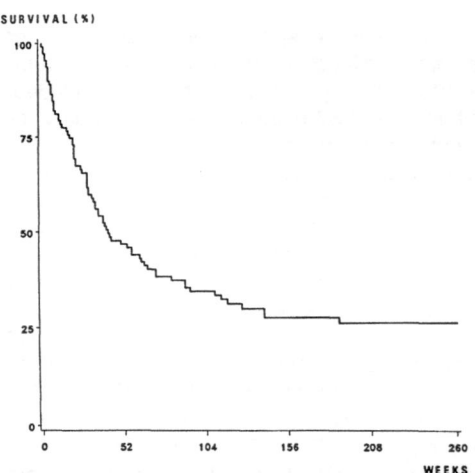

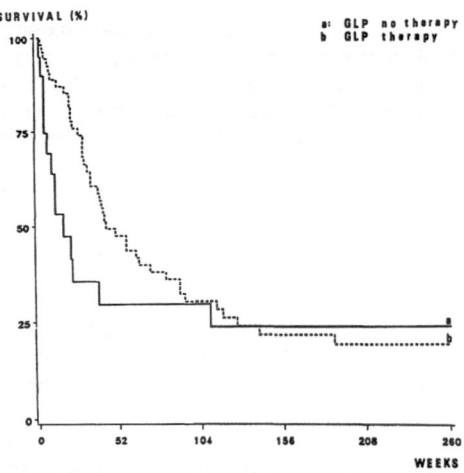

Fig. 1   Actuarial life table for all patients with diagnosis of a brainstemtumour on admission.

Fig. 2   Actuarial life table for 75 patients with a pontine glioma (GLP).
Group a: Pontine glioma without therapy
Group b: Pontine glioma with therapy

The curves are significantly different (P=0.03). If the material is divided into gliomatous brainstem tumours (GLP) and tumours of other kind (non GLP), the pattern of survival of both groups does not differ significantly (P=0.40, Fig.3).

Of all CT variables no significant association with the length of survival could be found. In 62 patients histology was obtained by means of biopsy, surgery or autopsy. The histology (PA) was divided into: 1) Histology unknown (PA unknown) and 2) Histology known (PA known). The latter subdivided in PA stem and PA no stem. The curves, also in comparison in pairs, differ significantly in the length of survival (P<0.01, Fig.4).

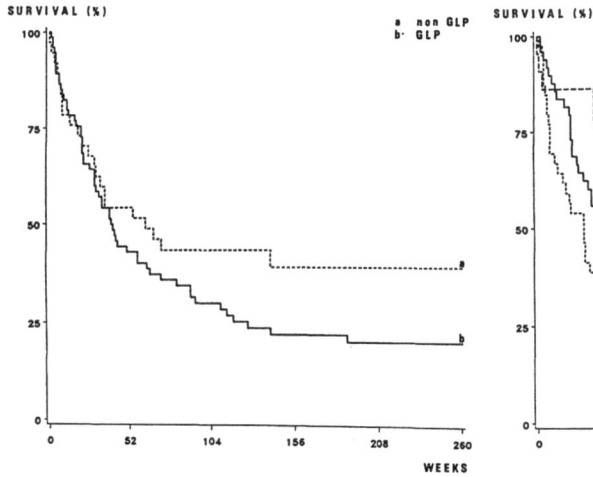

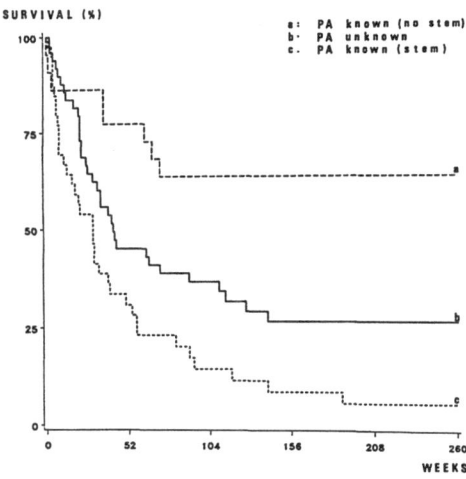

Fig. 3   Actuarial life table for 75 patients with
a pontine glioma (GLP) and 37 patients with
tumours of other kind (non GLP).

Fig. 4   Actuarial life table for all patients,
divided according the histology of the tumour
(PA).
Group a: PA known (no stem)
Group b: PA unknown
Group c: PA known (stem)

According to the aspect of the tumour on CT scanning, a radiological selection was made, which does not confirm the clinical diagnosis in every way. In this selection 2 groups were also made: 1) CT stem   tumour in the brainstem and 2) CT no stem   tumour outside the brainstem (Fig.5).

The variables were significantly associated with the length of survival.

DISCUSSION

All these results indicate that prognosis of people, mostly children, with a brainstem glioma is still worse than patients with a supratentorial localised glioma. In contradiction to the series of Albright et al. 1986 we could not find any association of CT variables with the length of survival. No significant association was found between gliomatous brainstem tumours and tumours of other kind, because the most important selection criterion for this study was "suspicion of a space-occupying lesion in the brainstem. At the end of this series only 33 patients were still alive. Retrospectively we were able to recognize in about 80% the underlying lesion. No additional information was obtained from angiography and ventriculography. Therefore we can consider to examine the other 20% of the patients with a clinical history of a brainstem lesion with NMR. Also in case of a positive CT scan, one should perform a NMR for planning of the radiotherapy.

588

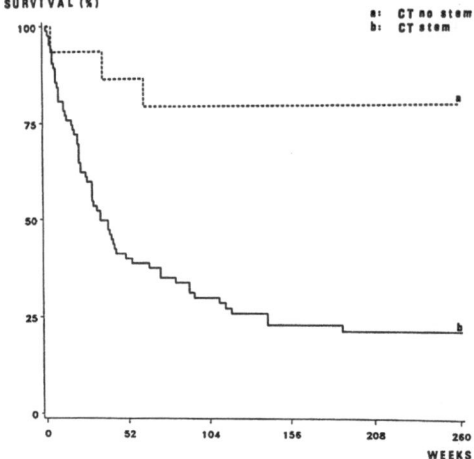

Fig. 5   Actuarial life table for 99 patients,
examined with CT scanning. This radiological
selection is based on the localisation of the
tumour with CT scanning.
Group a: CT no stem
Group b: CT stem

REFERENCES

Albright A.L., Guthkelch A.N., Packer R.J., Price R.A. and Rourke L.B.: *Prognostic factors in pediatric brainstemgliomas* J.Neurosurg. 65:751-755, 1986

Bray P.F., Carter S. and Taveras J.M.: *Pontine gliomas, a pathological study and classification of 25 cases.* Archives of Pathology vol.9, April 1930, no. 4, 799-810.

Kim T.H., Chin Hong W., Pollan S., Hazel J.H. and Webster J.H.: *Radiotherapy of Primary brainstemtumours.* J. Radiation Oncology Biol. Phys. vol.6, 51-57, 1981

Lassiter K.R.L., Alexander E., Davis C.H. and Kelly D.L.: *Surgical treatment of brainstemgliomas* J. Neurosurg. 34: 719-725, 1971

Panitch H.C. and Berg B.O.: *Brainstemtumours of childhood and adolescence* Am. J. Dis. Child 119: 465-472, 1970

Tokuriki Y., Handa H., Yamashita J., Okamura T. and Paine J.T.: *Brainstem Glioma: An Analysis of 85 cases.* Acta Neurochirurgica 79: 67-73, 1986.

White H.H.: *Brainstem tumours occurring in adults.* Neurology 13: 292-300, 1963.

MRI of Callosal Dysgenesis

J. R. Jinkins, A. R. Whittemore, and W. G. Bradley

INTRODUCTION:

The direct multiplanar imaging of MRI lends itself ideally to the evaluation of callosal dysgenesis (CD) together with the important associated hemispheric findings. Older classification systems including only agenesis and partial agenesis were found to be inadequate for a precise description of the spectrum of developmental callosal anomalies. MRI illustrates patterns which allow a categorization of morphologic forms of CD based upon the embryogenesis of the telencephalon.

METHODS:

The study consisted of a retrospective review of 15 subjects with CD. Patterns were sought in the morphology of the corpus callosum (CC) and the cerebral hemispheres which revealed a predictable relationship to embryonic development both in regard to the decussation of the CC as well as the formation of the cortex responsible for projection of the callosal fibers.

RESULTS:

MRI enabled the differentiation of three distinct categories of dysgenesis. In agenesis the CC was completely absent (Fig. 1, 3 subjects). In hypogenesis the CC was variably curtailed in development due to primary factors (Fig. 2, 5 subjects) or factors related to organic obstruction (i.e., lipomatous neural tube inclusion - Fig. 3, 4 subjects). In hypoplasia the CC was completely formed although focally or generally small in size and associated with prominent dysgenesis of the hemispheric cerebral cortex (Fig. 4, 3 subjects). This cortical dysgenesis was invariably attributable to one of the neuronal migration anomalies (i.e., polymicrogyria, heterotopia, etc.).

DISCUSSION:

The normal embryogenesis of the telencephalon dictates the final structural morphology of the CC. This depends upon the uncomplicated closure of the neural tube, the formation and maintenance of the inductive bed of the massa comissuralis throughout decussation, and the proper migration and lamination of the elements of the cerebral cortex. Interference with, or interruption of any one or combination of these parameters may result in CD of varying expression. Thus, the basis of CD reflects its origins in essential failure of decussation induction, interrupted decussation, and/or partial failure of commissural fiber projection secondary to primary cortical dysgenesis.

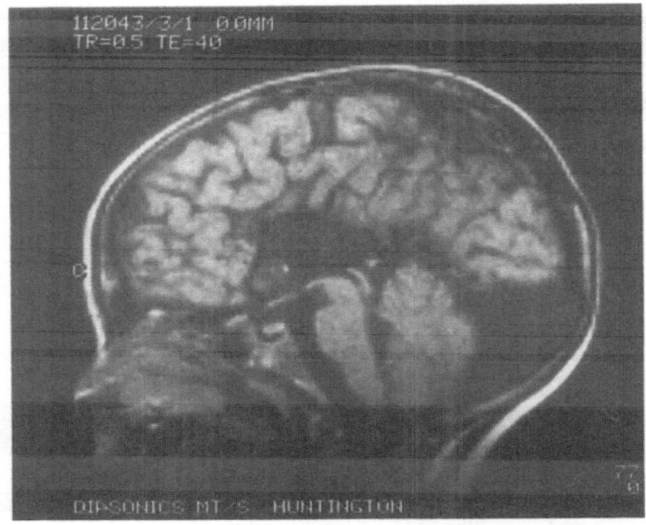

Fig. 1. Sagittal section demonstrating the agenesis of the CC.

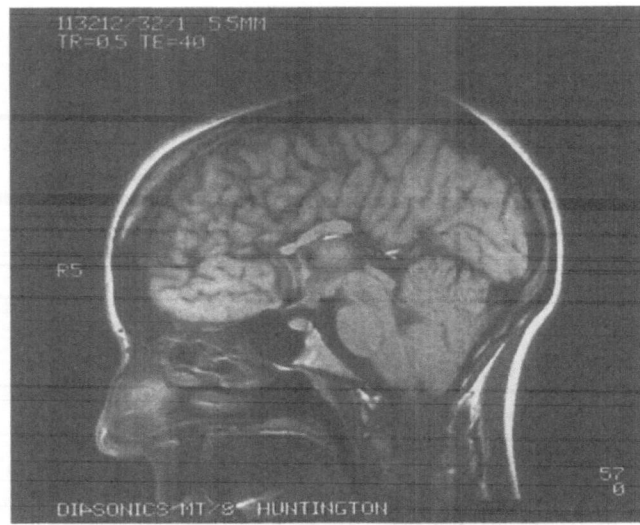

Fig. 2. Sagittal section illustrating the primary hypogenesis of the CC.

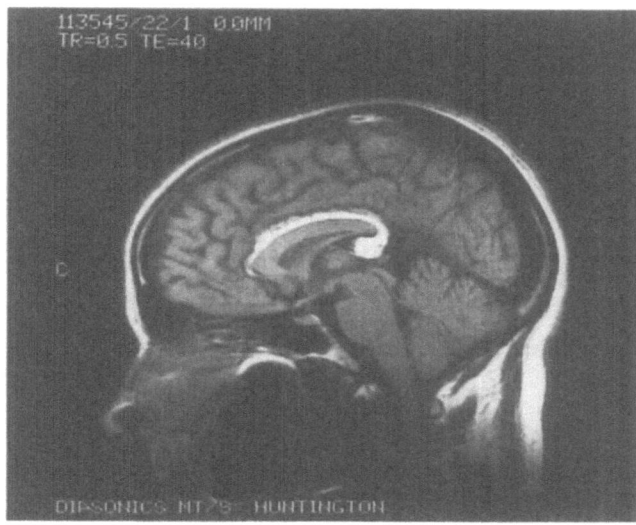

Fig. 3. Sagittal image showing the lipomatous callosal cloaking and minor terminal callosal hypogenesis secondary to the embryonic collision of the developing CC with a lipomatous neural tube inclusion.

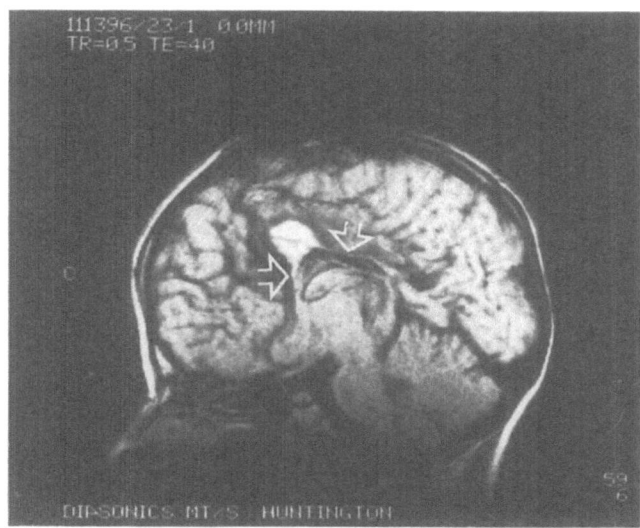

Fig. 4. Sagittal section demonstrating the multifocal hypoplasia of the CC (arrows) secondary to extensive hemispheric polymicrogyria.

REFERENCES

Brun A, Probst F (1973) The influence of associated cerebral lesions on the
  morphology of the acallosal brain: a pathological and encephalographic
  study. Neuroradiology 6:121-131
Curnes, et al. (1986) MRI of corpus callosal syndromes. AJNR 7:617-622
Kendall BE (1983) Dysgenesis of the corpus callosum. Neuroradiology 25:239-256
Larroche J (1984) Malformations of the nervous system. In: Adams HJ, Corsellis J,
  Duchen LW (eds) Greenfield's Neuropathology. John Wiley and Sons, New York,
  pp 385-450
Parrish ML, Roessmann U, Levinsohn MW (1979) Agenesis of the corpus callosum: a
  study of the frequency of associated malformations. Ann Neurol 6:349-354
Rakic P, Yakovlev PI (1986) Development of the corpus callosum and cavum septi in
  man. J Comp Neur 132:45-72
Wallace D (1976) Lipoma of the corpus callosum. Neurol Neurosurg Psych
  39:1179-1185

Clinico-Radiological Aspects of the Hypoplastic Internal Carotid Artery Syndrome

Z. Patay and M. Berky

Introduction

True hypoplasia of one or both internal carotid arteries (ICA) is
a rare clinico-radiological entity. To our knowledge, so far only
31 cases of this syndrome have been reported in the literature. For
different reasons, unfortunately, quite a few of them could not be
verified retrospectively. It has also to be admitted that, there is
some confusion in the literature about the nomenclature concerning
the different aspects of the syndrome. For example the criteria for
certain categories, such as primary and secondary, or absolute and
relative hypoplasia, have not yet been clearly established. Anyway,
we are probably not too far from the truth if we define an internal
carotid artery of small caliber as a hypoplastic one, when its inner
diameter does not exceed 3.5 mm in its whole length or in a major
part of its course, and any other possible etiologies of the narrowness can be excluded.

Case Report

A couple of days before his admission to our department, a 21 year
old male experienced a 10 minute long monocular blindness of the
right eye, which resolved spontaneously and had no recurrence. On
neurological and ophthalmological examinations, no abnormalities
could be found, except for a right-sided, incomplete Horner's syndrome, which had been present through all his life, as told by the
patient and confirmed by a family member. History from the patient,
more over, did not provide evidence for any possible cause, that
could be related in a way or another, to the development of his
clinical signs and symptoms. The most probable diagnosis to be made
on clinical grounds was some sort of lesion or malformation of the
right ICA, presumably below the origin of the ophthalmic artery.

For this reason, catheter angiography of the cerebral vessels was
performed. The branching of the right common carotid artery (Fig. 1)
looked like a trifurcation, giving origin to the external carotid
artery trunk, an independent external occipital artery and a strikingly thin ICA. The narrowness of the ICA extended to its whole
extracranial part. Localized to the bony carotid canal, an even more
severe but circumscribed stenosis could be observed (Fig. 2).

On CT examination, both direct visualization (Fig. 3) and paraxial
reconstruction imaging (Fig. 4) of the carotid canals was possible
and comparative measurements of the canal diameters could be made.

594

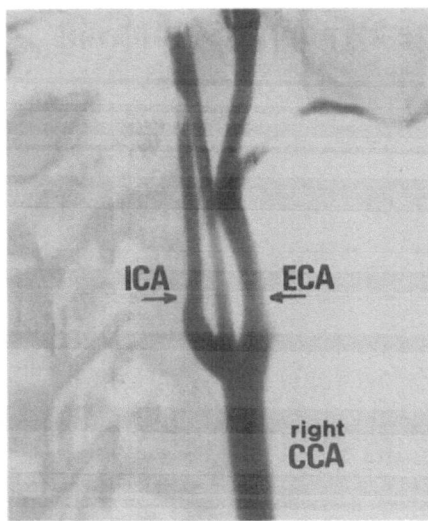

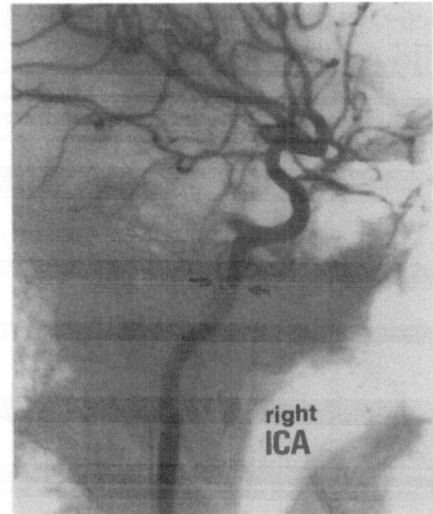

Fig. 1.   Fig. 2.

The diameter of the left carotid canal varied between 7–8 mm, while
the one on the right ranged between 3–4 mm. The difference between
the respective values on all the slices was significant, resulting
in carotid canal diameter ratios of 2.0 and higher, which are much
above the greatest acceptable normal value of 1.4, as determined
originally for artery diameters in fact, on the basis of biostatis-
tical calculations (Lehrner 1968).

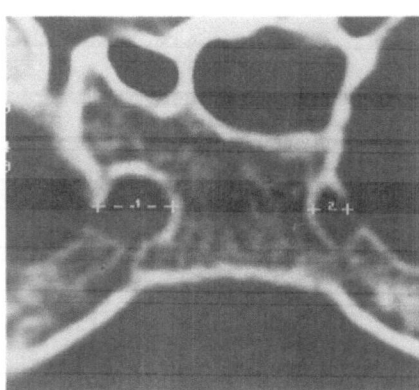

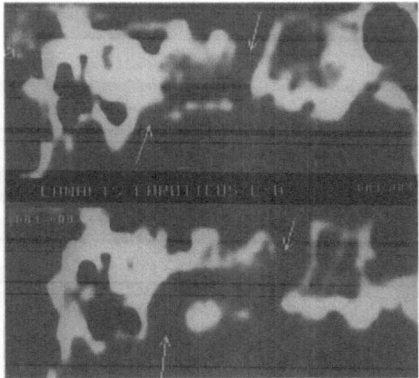

Fig. 3.   Fig. 4.

Comparative measurements of the
carotid canal diameters on a
typical axial slice through the
cranial base. (D_1=8mm, D_2=4mm,
internal carotid canal diameter
ratio=2.0)

Paraxial reconstruction images
of the two carotid canals passing through the cranial base.
The right one (above) is apparently narrower than the left
one (below).

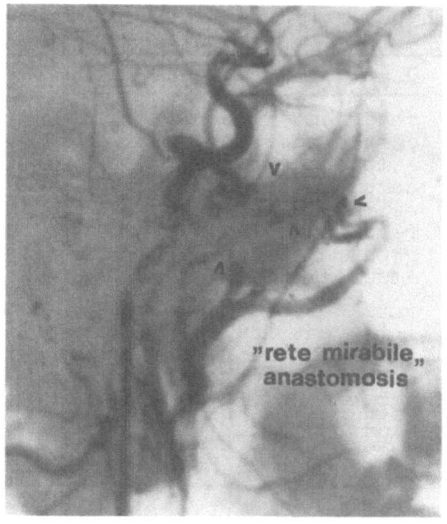

"rete mirabile„ anastomosis

Intracranially, an obviously effective collateral network from the vertebrobasilary and contralateral ICA systems could be observed, including well functioning anterior and posterior communicating arteries and leptomeningeal anastomoses.

Of special interest is the anastomotic network between the internal maxillary artery and the intracavernous portion of the internal carotid artery, on the right side. In a wider sense, this may be regarded as a "rete mirabile"-like vascular pattern, and in our opinion, this is probably the most significant collateral route to the right hemisphere. (Weidner 1965), (Fig. 5.)

Fig. 5.

Discussion

In interpreting the clinico-radiological findings, we presumed, that the clinical syndrome was a typical transient ischemic attack, which manifested itself in the form of an amaurosis fugax. The stenosis of the bony canal suggests, that the original cause of the partial hypoplasia of the right ICA must have been a lesion of unknown origin to the cranial base, which might have prevented the normal development of the ICA, below that level. The longstanding neurological signs, that is the incomplete Horner's syndrome, indicating the malfunction of the sympathetic plexus around the ICA, then the highly extensive intracranial collateral network, but even more, the existence of a natural transcranial bypass system, between the external and internal carotid arteries, all make it likely, that the pathological process of the right petrous bone must have occured in the pre-or early postnatal period of life. Review of the literature also suggests, that some preformed, but normally non-functioning, rare forms of collateral circulatory pathways, such as the what we called, "rete mirabile" in our case, may be characteristic of the true ICA hypoplasia (Weidner 1965, Guy 1974).

On the basis of the review of the clinical data of 15 verified hypoplastic ICA cases, it can be ascertained, that the clinico-pathological manifestations of this syndrome may be of either ischemic or hemorrhagic nature (Table 1). Clinical symptomatology of both is absolutely similar to the various types of other, commonly encountered stroke processes of diverse origin. However, age prevalence data suggest, that the ischemic manifestations are more likely to occur in younger patients, while hemorrhagic manifestations tend to affect older age groups, but this may not hold true, as due to the small number of cases, it cannot be confirmed statistically. The pathomechanism of the ischemic manifestation can sometimes be related to sys-

Table 1. List of verified cases with hypoplastic internal carotid
         artery syndrome.

Author	Age	Sex	Clinical appearence
Austin (1971)	30	male	recurrent TIAs
	33	male	completed stroke
Ebner (1982)	47	male	completed stroke
Gál (1976)	24	male	completed stroke
Jones (1970)	43	male	epileptic seizures
Tharp (1965)	37	female	recurrent TIAs
	37	female	recurrent TIAs
Patay	21	male	amaurosis fugax
Fischer (1959)	17	female	intracerebral hemorrhage
	56	female	intraventricular hemorrhage
Guy (1974)	21	male	subarachnoid hemorrhage
Hawkins (1967)	37	male	subarachnoid hemorrhage
Lagarde (1957)	42	male	subarachnoid hemorrhage
Lhermitte (1968)	63	female	subarachnoid hemorrhage
Occleshaw (1969)	45	female	subarachnoid hemorrhage
Smith (1968)	53	female	intracerebral hemorrhage

temic hemodynamic disturbances, causing symptoms of central nervous
system dysfunction, in that vascular territory, where the compensatory mechanisms lack further reserve capacity. This may be the most
probable explanation for the transient monocular blindness of our
patient, just because there is no other feasible explanation for that.
Hemorrhage on the other hand, is often related to the rupture of
pathologically enlarged and dilated collaterals (Lhermitte 1968) and
if it occurs, it can be intraventricular, subarachnoid or intracerebral, depending on the site of the ruptured vessel segment.

Some neurosurgical implications of the syndrome may theoretically be
determined, as well, concerning the possible therapeutic approach to
it. As the hypoplastic ICA syndrome and the so-called Moyamoya disease show much similarities in their clinico-pathological characteristics, similar therapeutic measures may also be considered. As it
is well known, Moyamoya disease is one of the few remaining, possible
indications of the surgical external-internal carotid anastomosis
(Nyáry 1987). In the same way, hypoplasia of one or both ICAs, especially if clinically symptomatic and recurrent but benign, may also
be suitable for that type of surgery. It could serve basicly as a
preventive method for both ischemic and hemorrhagic complications by
providing further collateral circulation to the affected hemisphere
and by relieving some stress from the other, possibly overloaded
natural collaterals which, as mentioned earlier, are most likely to
become the source of a subsequent disastrous hemorrhage.

References

Guy, G. et al. (1974). Sem. Hop. Paris, 50: 809
Lehrner, H.Z. (1968). Brain, 91: 339
Lhermitte, F. et al. (1968). Neurology, 18: 439
Nyári, I. et al. (1987). Orvosi Hetilap, 128(8): 403
Weidner, W. et al. (1965). Neurology, 15: 39

Information System for Radiologists

H. Traupe and S. Purgold

Introduction

The medical information system introduced here was not planned to be universal or an expert system. Our primary intention was to create a tool for collecting data, literature and images, gather them in a consistent form for interindividual exchange and use them as a help in comparing radiological data of all provenience. The information system was created by a medical doctor and a mathematician in strict division of tasks. The physician defined the problems, the mathematician managed to make the problems understandable to the computer and resolved the difficulties involved in how a computer system could come along with common medical decision making, the problems of a purely empiric science and medical terminology.

Development of the system

We postulated, that a radiological diagnosis is made up of only few points:

1. First we have to perform an appropriate examination including the choice on the appropriate technique.

2. The resulting document or image is marked out by the technique used, and we will proceed to describing alterations which can be found at specific anatomical sites.

3. Keeping in mind all other signs and symptoms that we know from a certain patient, we will be able to summarize all features in the form of a diagnosis.

Each of these four elements: document, technique, anatomy and signs, can be treated independently and has its own relation to the diagnois. For example, the relation between a technique and a diagnosis lies in its potential to show it or not, an anatomic region may be altered in respect to some illness or not. The most significant relation exists between radiological signs that we recognize and a diagnosis. Then next time we have to do with similar diagnostic problems, we will remember all earlier information and compare how often similar anatomical, technical and qualitative or quantitative findings exist. If there is coincidence, we will add this case with the same diagnosis to our collection or memory, if there is partial or no coincidence, we will add new or other information and a new diagnosis.

This description resembles the way a radiologist does his work and gathers experience. At the beginning, his knowledge is limited. In learning and repeating the process described above again and again he will become experienced.

The system described here works in exactly the same manner. But there are two fundamental differences between our computer system and a medical doctor in this respect:

Our system is a simple tool and completely dependent on input:
If the person that enters the data lacks experience the quality of information will be poor.

On the other hand, as this system will grow by large amounts of relevant information it can be helpful as an active tool in remembering earlier decisions and compare all elements of information in it optionally. Unlike an expert system, the model works without rules or statistics and is simply based on the quantity and quality of entered data.

System specifications

The system runs on any PC, minicomputer or mainframe with a hard disk and 640k of memory. The program was built using a fourth generation language (Progress Software Corporation) which supplies all advanced features of a modern relational database management system such as data security, data protection, automatic recovery of data, networking and so on.

Retrieval and sorting of text and image documents

An arbitrary collection of radiological images may enclose several thousands of pictures. All these documents should be readily available and therefore the contents of the data base must be structured or "indexed". Indexing can be done in several ways: by anatomical site,

by techniques, by diagnosis or by authors. Several indices can be combined. If a document is entered in the system, indexing is done automatically; we ourselves use sorting by the anatomy code.

Supply of consistent nomenclature

The next very important demand is that the card file system uses a
consistent nomenclature. Otherwise we would have problems in retrieval
and data comparison; for example, we would never be sure that a complete research has been done. We solved this problem by implementing
common international catalogues for anatomy and diagnoses and created
our own catalogues for techniques and radiological and clinical signs.
The internal structure of all catalogue systems is open to individual
adoption and expansion but if the program is used for interindividual
data exchange, supervision of the catalogues will be inevitable.

Transparency

Data comparison and data valididation in medicine, as elsewhere, depends on the question:

Where do the data come from; are they reliable; who has found specific
results?

Therefore each data input in our system must be labelled by its
source, i.e. the doctor or institution or the source of literature.
This source can be protected resulting in "silent data", but if it is
removed, the data is removed as well. We postulate, that data is only
relevant when the source is known.

Administration of literature

If we use a catalogue system, it should not only be capable of ad-
ministrating our pictorial documents but also provide order in our
collection of literature. The combination of literature and individual data collection makes sense, as most of our knowledge is derived
from literature, and literature provides the substantiation. On the
other hand, in the literature we find collections of patients with
groups of signs which can be entered in the same way as individual
cases. Input of common literature, statistics and exceptional case
reports is possible and helps to establish a basic knowledge base.

"Intelligence"

We developed some "intelligent" features to accommodate data input
that allows not only the saving of data but also of the underlying
decisions leading to a diagnosis by building a knowledge base for
further diagnostic support.

All "intelligent" features of the system are based on the calculation
of the number of connections between selected attributes like anatomical, technical, radiological, clinical or diagnostic descriptions and
the final diagnosis. These connections are labelled by the name or the
grammalogue of the entering person and by the degree of reliability
which can be modified during data entry and data query. The advantage
of this technique lies in its high degree of transparency, as the user
is completely free in making decisions derived from the whole database, from his own experience or from specified data subgroups of
any source.

Time saving

An information system which is "better" than our traditional way of
collecting the results of our work should at least provide a minimum
of convenience and save time. It is evident that the handling of data
is much better, and the exchange of data with other systems is very
easy, if the systems are compatible, and that sorting and searching
are facilitated.

The question remains, whether entering data is really enhanced as
long as the user or his secretary is not yet familiar with this instrument. Reporting can be done as well, but again the question arises, if the normal habit of typing individual texts can be overcome
by computer generated reports.

Data input

Data input in our system is performed in two steps. The input of a
general data reflecting all common data like age, name, sex and so
on, can be done by a technician or secretary.

The second part of data input is done by the radiologist himself. He
has to choose a document and describe it by aid of the catalogue system (see Fig.1). Beginning with the technique used, he takes a term
from the catalogue in the inner shell into his description. He has

to continue with the description of the document, the anatomical site and finally with a description of signs. Starting from the technique used, the system will automatically propose a weighted list of possible terms for every next step from which he can select. With each new entry the system compares all previous constellations of signs in the system's memory and proposes a possible diagnosis. The user is completely free to accept it or to take a different one out of the catalogue of all possible terms or diagnoses. This way the user can "play" with different solutions and check the degree of probability of each constellation. The final diagnosis, however, is up to himself. He can accept the system's proposal substantiated by earlier decisions or make a new one.

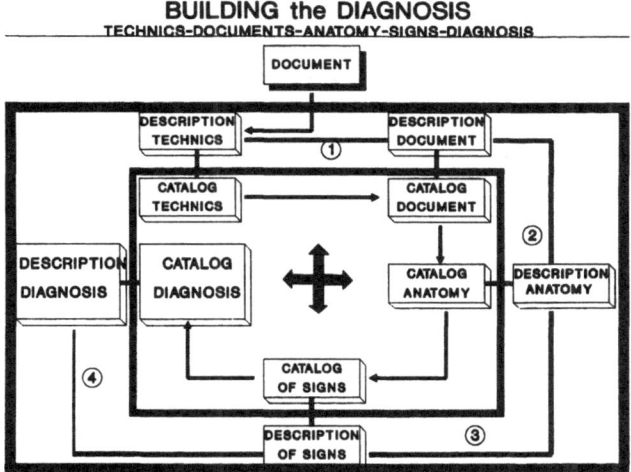

Fig.1. Schematic representation of the inner and outer shell of the diagnostic system. Each document is described in 4 steps, transferring terms from the catalogues to the descriptions

Final remarks

In its way of gathering experience the system described resembles the normal technique of radiological decision making. The use of a consistent nomenclature will provide the possibility of aggregating arbitrary amounts of data that can be exchanged with others. The system introduced here completely lives on real data and depends on the quality of these data. It is no expert system but has the potential to validate systems built on rules or algorithms. As the potential of the model lies in its amount of transparent data, it will prove its strength only if many of us use it and are willing to share common data.

MRI Multicenter Study – Clinical Evaluation

S. Bockenheimer, M. Meves, and A. Oberstein (Frankfurt/M., FRG)

The German Bundesministerium für Forschung und Technologie sponsors a multicenter study to evaluate both the clinical and the economic status of MRI in West Germany. The design of the study as regards clinical evaluation was outlined by us at the XIVth congress of this society last year in Udine. We will now present the results of the first analysis.

Twenty-three institutions using MR participated in the study. Over a 6-month period data were collected on more than 21 000 MRI examinations. We also collected the available information gained by other imaging procedures like ultrasound, CT and angiography. We gathered the MR diagnoses and in the follow-up, wherever possible, the final diagnosis as proven by surgery, histology and/or pathological anatomy, or any other definite outcome.

The amount of data allows us to judge the relative specificity and sensitivity of MRI in current diagnostic procedures, even for less common diseases.

Neurenteric Cyst of Bronchogenic Origin

B. Appel, E. Moens, I. Neetens, and A. Lowenthal (Antwerp, Belgium)

A 40-year-old woman was admitted after a sudden aggravation of a paraparesis and cauda equina syndrome, existing since the age of 12. From childhood she developed a progressive scoliosis, underwent several orthopedic interventions, and went through episodes of osteomyelitis.

X-ray of the spine showed an important scoliosis and abnormal lumbar vertebrae. There was no dysraphism. NMR demonstrated a large extramedullary, intradural, slightly inhomogeneous lesion invading the conus. CT scan confirmed the size and extent of the lesion. No myelography was performed.

Age of onset, the relapsing course and the erosion of the vertebrae suggested a developmental lesion such as a dermoid, lipoma or teratoma. A neurenteric cyst seemed less likely, since no clear congenital abnormality of the vertebrae existed.

At surgery a cystic lesion was found, containing a white gelatinous fluid, and beneath the cyst a fibrous string with calcifications. Histopathology revealed bronchial tissue. The fibrous string was partially ossified and lined by cylindrical epithelium. This lesion most probably results from an error very early in the embryological development and corresponds to a neurenteric cyst of bronchogenic origin, with a rather unusual localisation.

MR of Brain Metastases

G. Krol, N. Imam, J. Kim, and G. Sze

INTRODUCTION

Since its introduction, MR proved to be an effective method of diagnosis of intracranial tumors. Its sensitivity in the detection of intraaxial neoplasm, particularly low grade glioma, is now considered to be superior to that of CT scan. Generally accepted mode of MR evaluation of intracranial neoplasms is a spin-echo sequence with short and also prolonged TR/TE intervals. MR presentation of metastatic intraaxial lesions on T1 and T2 weighted sequences, as correlated with histological diagnosis is the subject of this investigation.

MATERIALS AND METHODS

Seventy-four patients with histologically proven systemic neoplasms and CT scans of the head revealing contrast enhancing parenchymal lesions, consistent with metastases were evaluated by MR, using routine T1 and T2 weighted spin echo sequences (axial plane, TR/TE 600/20, 2000/80/40 msec). Intensity patterns of the lesions, proceeding from the center to the periphery were evaluated on T1 and both first and second echo images of T2 weighted sequences. Traditional components of the neoplasm, including central tumor (without or with necrotic center), peripheral ring and edema were evaluated.

RESULTS

T1 weighted sequences: No abnormalities were observed in three patients, central hypointensity in 55, hyperintensity in 12 and mixed intensity in one. The tumor tissue appeared isointense to the brain tissue in three patients. The peripheral aspect of the tumor was well defined in the majority of patients (43). The formation of the identifiable ring along the periphery was noted in 34 patients. In the majority, the ring was hypointense (16). Isointense, hyperintense and mixed intensity of the ring was noted 9, 8 and 1 case, respectively. The periphery of the ring was well defined in 23 cases. Coarse configuration of the border was noted in two, and ill-defined in nine cases. There was no ring formation in 40 patients. No edema was identified surrounding the tumor on T1 image in 45 patients. In 25, hypointense area was identified consistent with edema. In four patients, the periphery was slightly hyperintense.

T2 weighted sequences ;

The center remained hypointense, became isointense, hyperintense or assumed mixed intensity (in 13,24,28 and 9 cases, respectively). Peri-tumoral ring was identified in 31 cases. In 20 the ring was hypointense. On the second echo there was further shift towards hyperintensity with 15 lesions remaining hypointense, 10 becoming isointense, 41 - hyperintense and 8 displaying mixed intensity. The ring formation was observed in slightly larger number of lesions, as compared to the first echo (38 as compared to 31).

Lesion visualization:

Demonstration of the various components of the tumor was superior on T2 weighted sequences. The tumor edema separation was not readily appreciated on T1 sequences in 25 lesions, not well defined in four and well defined in 16. By contrast, the separation was considered relatively well defined on long echo sequences combined in 50 patients. Hemorrhagic component, identified on short echo sequences as hyperintense, was seen in 22 lesions.

DISCUSSION

The subject of MR recognition of intraaxial neoplasms has been discussed by several investigators (1,2,3). Metastatic lesions were mentioned as a part of a larger series of primary brain tumors or lesions of non-neoplastic nature. Spin echo sequences with short and long TR/TE intervals constitute an accepted method of imaging of brain neoplasms. In general, the neoplastic process appears as an area of hypointensity on T1 and hyperintensity on T2 weighted images. Hemorrhage into pre-existing tumor may occur and is recognized as an area of hyperintensity on short echo sequences. The tendency to hemorrhage is recognized in metastatic lesions originating from melanoma and, less commonly from other neoplams such as renal, thyroid and bronchogenic carcinomas (4,5). Our study of the pattern of presentation of parenchymal metastases from common systemic neoplasms also indicates that the hemorrhagic component is most commonly encountered in melanomas and less commonly observed in other metastases. The tumor tissue is usually hypointense on T1 weighted sequences. When hyperintensity is identified, it is more likely to be located along the peripheral aspect of the tumor tissue. The majority of the lesions become iso- or hyperintense on T2 weighted sequences. Metastases from kidney carcinoma and sarcoma appear hyperintense on both first and second echos. Although the center is hyperintense, the peripheral ring, if identified, remains hypointense in the majority of cases. Occasionally, the tumor tissue cannot be identified. In our series, the diagnosis was made on the basis of detection of edematous area only in 6 patients, 5 of them with lung carcinoma.

SUMMARY

The MR appearance of intracranial metastases from common primary systemic neoplasms is variable. Typical ring configuration of enhancing lesion observed by CT is identified in less than 50% of patients. Short echo sequences are less informative with regard to assessment of the peritumoral edema as compared to T2 weighted sequences. Tumor-edema separation is usually unclear on T1 but better discernible on T2 weighted images. Hemorrhagic tendency, manisfested as hyperintensity on T1 image is observed in metastatic melanomas but less commonly in other metastases (breast, lung).

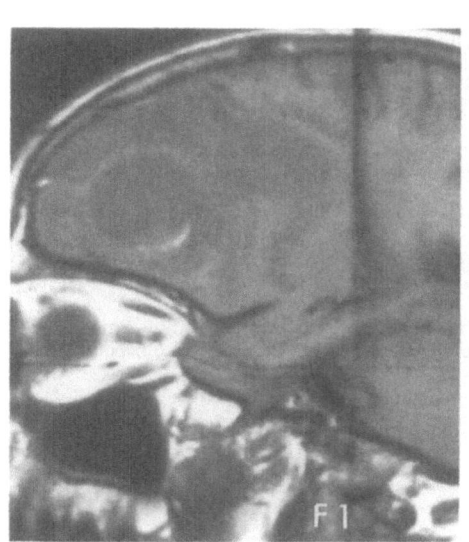

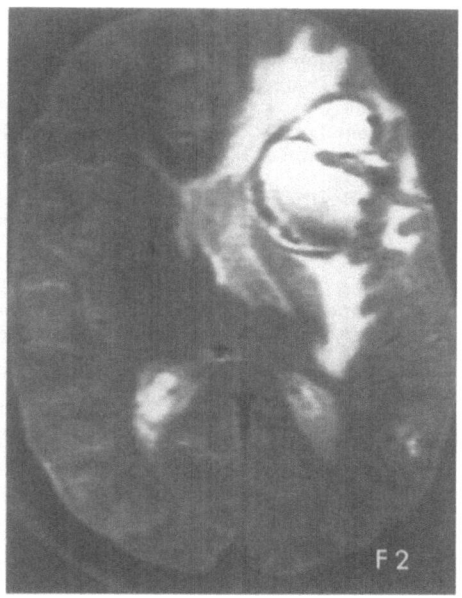

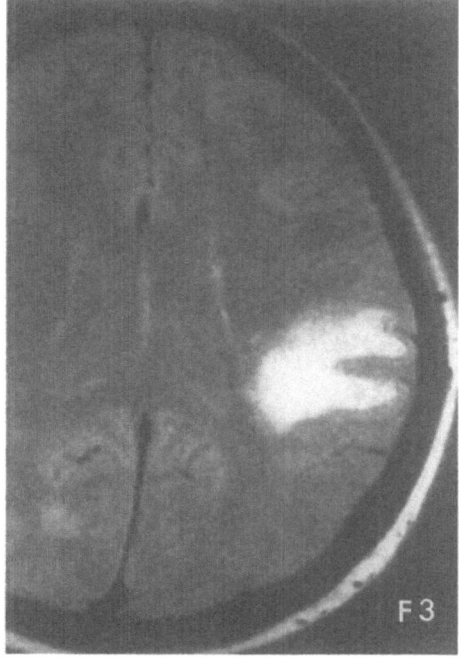

Fig. I. Hemorrhagic metastasis, melanoma. T I weighted sequence, sagittal view. Increased intensity is located along the periphery.

Fig. 2. Left frontal metastases, lung carcinoma. First echo, 2000/40. The central aspect of the lesion is hyperintense and ring hypointense.

Fig. 3. Left frontal metastases, lung carcinoma. T2 weighted sequence, E I, 2000/40. An area of edema is noted, no tumor tissue could be identified.

REFERENCES

1. Lee BCP, Kneeland JB, Cahill PT, Deck MDF. MR recognition of supratentorial tumors. AJNR, 1985;6:871-878.

2. Bilaniuk LT, Zimmerman RA, Wehrli RW, et al. Cerebral magnetic resonance: comparison of high and low field strength imaging. Radiology 1984;153:409-414.

3. Bradley WG Jr, Waluch V, Yadley RA, Wycoff RR. Comparison of CT and MR in 400 patients with suspected disease of the brain and cervical spinal cord. Radiology 1984;152:695-702.

4. Atlas SW, Grossman RI, Gormor JM, Guerry D, Hackney DB, Goldberg HI, Zimmerman RA, Bilaniuk LT. MR imaging of intracranial metastatic melanoma. Journal of Computer Assisted tomography, 577-582.

5. Atlas SC, Grossman RI, Gomori JM, Hackney DB, Goldberg HI, Zimmerman RA, Bilaniuk LT. Hemorrhagic intracranial malignant neoplasms: Spin-echo MR imaging. Radiology 1987;164:71-77.

MRI of Intrapetrous Bone Tumors (Except Acoustic Neuromas)

N. Martin, O. Sterkers, and H. Nahum

Introduction

In petrous bone all the tumors are located near to or are surrounded by bony structures; accurate detection and assessment extension is crucial in planning surgical approaches, but this may be difficult by CT due to interference by bone. Related to the absence of bone artifacts and its multiplanar display, MR is now a well-known diagnostic modality of choice for depicting posterior fossa diseases such as acoustic neuromas or paragangliomas. We retrospectively reviewed 30 petrous bone tumors and compared the abilities of CT and MR to detect, localize, and characterize these lesions.

Patients and Methods

A total of 30 patients were studied with MRI. Based on the anatomical locations of the lesions, they were divided into three groups: (a) middle ear: four had cholesteatomas, four cholesterol granulomas, three facial neuromas, and one brain hernia; (b) jugular foramen: three paragangliomas, one melanoma, one fibroinflammatory tumor, and one metastatic tumor; (c) petrous apex: meningiomas in six cases, nasopharyngeal carcinomas in four, one pailloma, and one cholesteatoma. MR examinations were performed with a 0.5-T unit (Magniscan, CGR). Multislice, spin-echo T1- and T2-weighted sequences were performed in all cases, and MR images were obtained in at least two planes. Thin sections (3-4 mm) were used for examinations of the middle ear lesions, with a 256 × 256 matrix. CT scans and pathologic or angiographic confirmation were available in all cases.

Results

All the lesions seen on CT were clearly demonstrated by MR.

Middle Ear Lesions. Cholesteatomas, cholesterol granulomas, and brain hernia were detected on CT as abnormal soft-tissue masses in the middle ear cavities, with erosion of ossicular chain in three cases. On MR, all cholesteatomas appeared as T1 iso- or hyposignal intensity masses relative to the brain, with a high signal intensity on T2-weighted sequences. Cholesterol granulomas, instead, had major variations: in three cases, the tumor had a well-defined, markedly increased signal intensity on both T1- and T2-weighted sequences; in one case, however, a pathologically confirmed cholesterol cyst, which appeared as expansive, well-defined cystic lesions, exhibited medium T1 and long T2 relaxation times. Brain hernia was clearly shown by dehiscence of the tegmen, especially on sagittal sequences, as a continuous mass with the brain.

The extension of these lesions was in all cases depicted in the middle ear cavities with CT and MR; in two cholesteatomas, however, supracanalicular or temporal fossa invasion were better shown with MR.

Facial neuromas involved the third segment in two cases and the geniculate ganglion in one case. CT demonstrated intrapetrous soft-tissue masses and bone erosion along the facial nerve anatomy. On MR, they appeared predominantly as medium T1- and T2-weighted signal intensity tumors. Their extension was more clearly shown in relation to the lack of bone signal and in the petrous course than in the extracranial extension to the posterior parotid space close to the external carotid artery.

Jugular Foramen. The three paragangliomas were detected on CT as contrast-enhanced irregular masses, with enlargement of jugular foramen. All were detected on MR images as medium T1- and long T2-weighted signal intensity areas with punctuate areas of signal void. The more precise relationship of the tumors to the adjacent vessels was defined with MR due to both tumoral and vascular enhancement on postcontrast CT. Jugular veins were flow-free in all cases, with adherence in one case, while both jugular vein and carotid arteries were displaced by a voluminous intra- and extracranial paraganglioma.

Fibroinflammatory tumor appeared as a contrast-enhanced lesion on CT with bony irregular destruction. On T2-weighted images, the tumor exhibited a heterogeneous rim of hypersignal intensity with a large hypointense central area which strongly evoked fibrous components.

These aspects were quite different from these of malignant melanoma, where the jugular foramen was smoothly enlarged by non-contrast-enhanced tumor; on MR it appeared as a well-delineated irregular and homogeneous mass, isointense on both T1- and T2-weighted sequences.

Petrous Apex Lesions. The five CPA meningiomas were isointense on T1-
weighted images; on T2-weighted sequences, three tumors were hyperintense, whereas the two others were iso- or hypointense. Only one tumor was slightly heterogeneous on the T2-weighted images. Vascular rim
and displacement of adjacent vessels was better seen with MR; but in
one case, encasement of the superior cerebellar artery was not seen by
MR or CT even in retrospective study. Intracanalicular extent was detected in two cases by MR but not CT, appearing larger and more medial
than intracanalicular neuromas did. Lastly, the large cervical extension of a CPA meningioma-en-plaque was more precisely examined by MR
in the petrous ridge than in the infratemporal fossa.

Papilloma of the CPA gave an isointense signal on T1- and T2-weighted
sequences with a heterogeneous appearance. Like in one meningioma, invasion of the cavernous sinus was better shown by MR, with close relation to the intracavernous carotid artery, but was never missed by CT.

In the four cases of skull base invasion by nasopharyngeal carcinomas, CT precisely defined bone destruction. On MR, the well-delineated
tumors were isointense on both T1 and T2 studies. Extension was better
seen on MR images in the petrous apex and the sphenoid bone related to
the lack of bone artifact, and in the infratemporal fossa related to
the good contrast between the muscles and the tumor. Relationship to
the Eustachian tube was shown in all cases. Encasement of the carotid
artery was present in three cases, better shown by MR especially in
its intrapetrous and intracavernous course; the permeability of jugular vein was assessed in all cases.

Lastly, cholesteatoma of the petrous apex appeared as an expansive,
hypodense non-contrast-enhanced lesion. CT bone destruction was extensive. On MR, the tumor exhibited long T1 and T2 relaxation times
relative to the brain. Extension was well delineated until middle ear
cavities as well as the internal contact with the carotid artery.

Discussion

Preceding reports (Gentry et al. 1987; Olsen et al. 1986; Press and
Hesselink 1988) have emphasized the superior ability of MR over that
of CT for detection of CPA and jugular foramen lesions. Also in our
study, all lesions detected by CT were well seen with MR.

MR is, however, able to characterize tumors better than CT. In the
middle ear cavities, CT has not proven helpful in differentiating

cholesteatomas from other soft-tissue density processes; in another
manner, a bluish eardrum can be related nonspecifically to cholesterol cyst, paragangliomas, or brain hernia. Only few papers have reported about MR appearances, and almost exclusively in the petrous apex
(Griffin et al. 1987; Valvassori 1988; Gentry et al. 1987). Cholesterol granulomas give a high signal intensity on T1- and T2-weighted
sequences secondary to a paramagnetic effect of hemoglobin breakdown
products; this aspect was regarded as characteristic of this tumor.
In our study, they appear so opposite to the hypo or medium T1 and
high T2 signal intensity of all cholesteatomas. However one rare expansive, pathologically proven cholesterol cyst, exhibited only a T1
medium signal intensity relative to the brain. Further experience is
necessary to evaluate all the various aspects of these tumors.

The brain hernia can be specifically demonstrated with sagittal sections as a continuous mass from brain through the erosion of the tegmen. Moreover this sagittal projection has the advantage of following
the plane of surgical approach.

To our knowledge the only reported facial neuromas involved the intracanalicular segment (Daniels et al. 1987). In our three patients they
were characterized by their location along the geniculate and mastoid
segment where they gave a medium T1 and T2 signal intensity.

In the jugular foramen, MR detects the vascular nature of paragangliomas with their "salt and pepper" pattern due to their hypervascularity
(Olsen et al. 1986). In our study, MR could differentiate them from the
T2-weighted hyposignal intensity of a fibroinflammatory tumor. However
other tumors, such as melanoma or nasopharyngeal carcinomas, gave only nonspecific iso T1- and T2-weighted signals.

In accord with the report of Press and Hesselink (1988), the majority
of our apical meningiomas were hyperintense and homogeneous on T2-
weighted sequences. Mottled appearance, previously described in meningiomas (Spagnoli et al. 1986, Zimmerman et al. 1985), was never
seen in our cases and, as observed by Gentry and Press, this aspect
is encountered less frequently in infratentorial lesions. The large
size, the center of the tumor relative to porus acousticus, and/or
the shape can help to differentiate them from acoustic neuromas.

Due to the lack of bone artifact and its superior soft-tissue contrast resolution, the role of MR in determining tumor extension to
the skull base has recently been emphasized (Teresi et al. 1987;
Barloon et al. 1987). Our study confirms the superiority of MR over

CT for evaluating the infiltration of infratemporal fossa, posterior
retroparotid space, or extension of intra- and extracranial tumors
through jugular foramen.

Extension of facial neuromas was more clearly depicted through the
intrapetrous route. In the middle ear cavities the invasion of cholesteatomas to the middle fossa and to the cells of the petrous apex
was precisely delineated.

Additional information regarding the relationship of the tumor to the
surrounding vessels such as jugular vein and carotid artery was given
by MR, especially with CT contrast-enhanced tumors of jugular foramen
(Olsen et al. 1986; Teresi et al. 1987). Encasement of the petrous
portion of the carotid artery was well delineated and related to its
signal void, as in the involvement of the cavernous sinus.

Lastly, brainstem and vascular relations (basilar artery, PICA) with
meningiomas were clearly delineated, with, in two cases, an intracanalicular extension not seen on CT.

MR was more helpful than CT for detection, assessment of extension,
and characterization of petrous bone tumors. But MR also has limitations, and CT better demonstrates subtle osseous changes of the skull
base or the precise relationship of the tumor to the osseous middle
ear structures (ossicular chain or lateral semicircular canal). In
no case were they misinterpreted, however, by MR.

MR thus seems a replacement for CT in the initial evaluation of intrapetrous bone pathology. CT will be used in a complementary status.

References

[1] Barloon TJ, Yuh WTC, DeMarino DP, Maves MD, Godersky JC, Dolan KD
     (1987) Infratemporal fossa meningioma: CT and MR findings. J
     Comput Assist Tomogr 11: 1050-1053
[2] Daniels DL, Millen SJ, Meyer GA, Pojunas KW, Kilgore DP,
     Shaffer KA, Williams AL, Haughton VM (1987) MR detection of tumor
     in the internal auditory canal. AJNR 148: 1219-1222
[3] Gentry LR, Jacoby CG, Turski PA, Houston LW, Strother CM,
     Sackett JF (1987) Cerebellopontine angle-petromastoid mass
     lesions: comparative study of diagnosis with MR imaging and CT.
     Radiology 162: 513-520
[4] Griffin C, DeLaPaz R, Enzmann D (1987) MR and CR correlation of
     cholesterol cysts of the petrous bone. AJNR 8: 825-829
[5] Olsen WL, Dillon WP, Kelly WM, Norman D, Brant-Zawadzki M,
     Newton TH (1986) MR imaging of paragangliomas. AJNR 7: 1039-1042
[6] Press GA, Hesselink JR (1988) MR imaging of cerebellopontine
     angle and internal auditory canal lesions at 1.5 T. AJNR 9:
     241-251

[7]   Spagnoli MV, Goldberg HI, Grossman RI, Bilaniuk LT, Gomori JN,
      Hackney DB, Zimmerman RA (1986) Intracranial meningiomas: high-
      field MR imaging. Radiology 161: 369-375
[8]   Teresi LM, Lufkin RB, Vinuela F, Dietrich RB, Wilson GH,
      Bentson JR, Hanafee WN (1987) MR imaging of the nasopharynx and
      floor of the middle cranial fossa Part II. Malignant tumors.
      Radiology 164: 817-821
[9]   Valvassori GE (1988) Diagnosis of retrocochlear and central
      vestibular disease by magnetic resonance imaging. Ann Otol
      Rhinol Laryngol 97: 19-22
[10] Zimmerman RD, Fleming CA, Saint-Louis LA, Lee BCP, Manning JJ,
      Deck MDF (1985) Magnetic resonance imaging of meningiomas.
      AJNR 6: 149-157

Significance of Virchow Robin Spaces in Magnetic Resonance Images of the Brain

A. Muraki, H. Manz, J. Smirniotopoulus, M. Carvlin,
and D. Schellinger (Washington, DC, USA)

Small, multiple foci of increased signal intensity (T2 weighted
images) in the centrum semiovale and basal ganglia are frequently
observed on magnetic resonance images of the brain. Often, these
findings are of doubtful significance with respect to the patient's
clinical state. Several explanations for this phenomenon have been
advanced and much controversy surrounds this issue. We correlated
images of 5 fresh and fixed brains obtained at 1.5 T and 4.7 T and
of 10 fixed brains obtained at 1.5 T with pathologic analysis of
these brains and also with an evaluation of the perivascular spaces
in fixed brain specimens from the Yakovlev collection of the Armed
Forces Institute of Pathology (AFIP). These foci of hyperintensity
in part correlated with the location of the deep penetrating arteries and probably represent extracellular water in the perivascular
(Virchow-Robin) spaces. These spaces typically enlarge with aging
and with various systemic disorders such as hypertension. We then
retrospectively reviewed 100 MR scans of patients with various
clinical/pathologic conditions and found that these hyperintense
foci were frequent findings. It is our conclusion that many of the
hyperintense foci in the centrum semiovale and basal ganglia represent extracellular water in the Virchow-Robin spaces.

Comparison of MR and CT in Patients with Intracranial Aneurysm Clips

S. Holtås, M. Olsson, B. Romner, and E.-M. Larsson (Lund, Sweden)

CT and MR images of the brain were obtained without complications in 16 patients operated upon for ruptured aneurysms using nonferromagnetic Yasargil Phynox or Sugita Elgiloy clips. These clips were not magnetized and did not move when introduced into our scanner (0.3 T Fonar β-3000 M) in a previous study. The artifacts caused by the clips were smaller on MR than on CT and anatomical structures such as brain stem and temporal lobe were therefore better visualized on MR. Brain tissue lesions corresponding to the frontotemporal surgical approach were seen in seven patients with MR and in six with CT. In three patients temporal lobe lesions seen on MR were not visualized on CT because of beam hardening artifacts. Lesions unrelated to the region of surgery were seen in nine patients with MR and in five with CT. In conclusion, our study shows that patients with nonferromagnetic Yasargil and Sugita clips can safely be examined in a 0.3 T Fonar MR scanner. MR provides more information than CT because of less disturbance of the image by metal artifacts and superior soft tissue discrimination.

Tentorial Meningiomas: Neuroradiological Considerations

F. P. Bernini, A. Scuotto, I. Muras, and F. A. Cioffi

Introduction

Meningiomas represent 7-12% of all posterior fossa tumors (Yasargil, 1980) and about 30% of posterior fossa meningiomas arise from the tentorium (Castellano and Ruggiero, 1953). Mostly cranial nerve findings, the subjective impression of an unsteady gait or ataxia dominate the clinical picture. The very slow increase of uncharacteristic clinical signs at the beginning of the disease may delay the onset of diagnostic measures. High resolution computed tomography (CT) has clearly become the mainstay in the diagnosis of such lesions, but is not without deficiencies. Recently, magnetic resonance (MR) imaging has been employed to evaluate these tumors (Zimmerman et al. 1985), but only high field strength MR scanners seem to be best suited for this purpose (Spagnoli, 1986). Inserted as they are on the tentorium, meningiomas occupy a region where the dural branches of cerebral arterial systems meet. Then angiography may still be needed to evaluate the typical meningeal vessels of the tumor or assess venous sinus invasion (Bernasconi et al. 1956; Nadjmi et al. 1975; Theron et al. 1978; Muras et al. 1988). This stimulated us to undertake a retrospective evaluation of our own case material, with emphasis on a comparison between CT and angiography.

Materials and Methods

We reviewed 20 patients with CT diagnosis of tentorial meningioma evaluated also with a complete angiographic study between June 1975 and December 1987. In earlier cases, selective catheterization of the external carotid artery and its branches was not uniformly performed as done nowadays. Only in 4 cases a MRI was performed, with a 0.5 T superconducting imager. 75% of cases were female; the age of patients ranged from 30 to 65 years. All cases were operated and the diagnosis was confirmed by histological investigations.

618

Results

CT scans delineated a mass in all the patients studied. Tumor diameter
ranged from 4 to 10 cm, and the majority of lesions were larger than
5 cm. Supra- and infratentorial extension "on iceberg" was observed in
6 cases. Calcifications within the tumor were noted unfrequently, and
contrast enhancement, usually in a homogeneous pattern, was present
in all cases. In one patient CT scans seemed to show a meningioma of
the free margin of the tentorium developing into the quadrigemino-pi-
neal region. A full angiographic investigation, however did not reveal pathological circulation and vascular displacements argued more
for a mesencephalic space-occupying lesion, confirmed at surgery
(Greitz, 1972; Papo et al. 1974). In two other cases with CT diagnosis of tentorial meningioma "on iceberg", angiography showed the dural
attachment of the tumor at the level of the occipital bone. In each of
the remaining patients angiography demonstrated almost one of the typical meningeal vessels at the tumoral insertion on the tentorium.
These branches originated from various sources. Meningiomas arising
laterally, near the petrous or the occipital insertion of the tentorium, were supplied chiefly by: the petrous, squamopetrous or distal
branches of the middle meningeal artery (Fig.1); the jugular and hypoglossal branches of the ascending pharyngeal artery (Fig.2); the meningeal branches of the occipital artery (Fig.3).

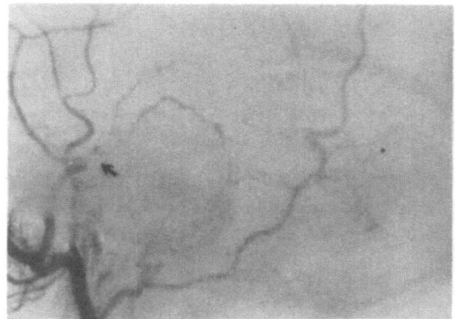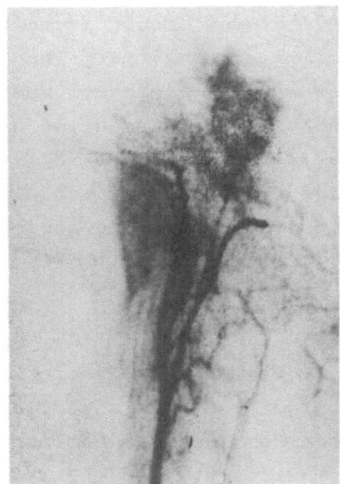

Fig.1. Meningioma of the lateral tentorial insertion receiving supply
from a posterior branch of the middle meningeal artery (arrow)

Fig.2. Meningioma of the petrous insertion of the tentorium. Opacification of the tumor from the ascending pharyngeal artery

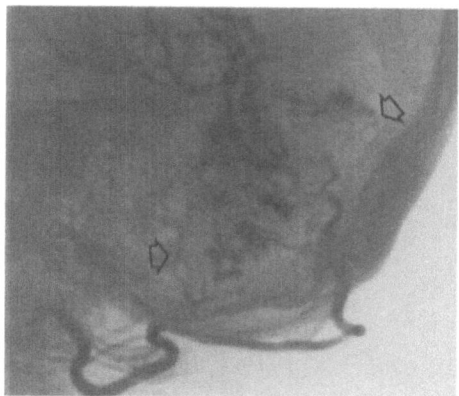

Fig.3. Meningioma "on iceberg" of the occipital insertion of the tentorium supplied by hypertrophied meningeal branches of the occipital
artery (arrows)

Meningiomas of the free tentorial edge or more posteriorly located in
the falco-tentorial region received meningeal branches coming from the
posterior group of intracavernous branches of the internal carotid artery (Fig.4); meningeal branches of the occipital artery; the posterior
meningeal artery (Fig.5). In two cases the meningioma was supplied by
hypertrophied tentorial artery arising from the carotid siphon and a
recurrent tentorial artery arising from the ophthalmic artery (Fig.6).
Angiography allowed also a better evaluation of the venous sinus invasion then was possible with CT.

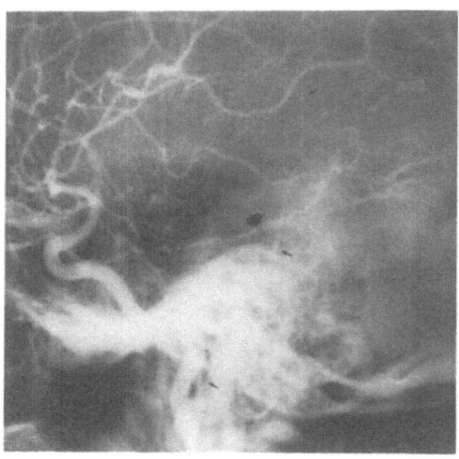
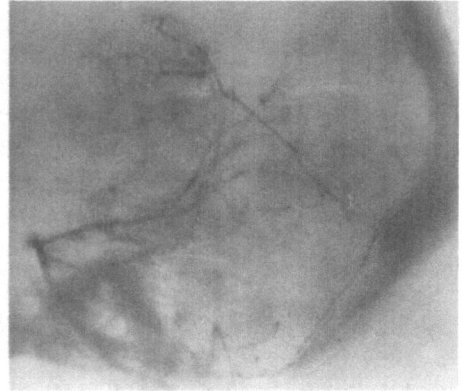

Fig.4.

Fig.5. Meningioma of free edge of the tentorium supplied by the posterior meningeal artery.

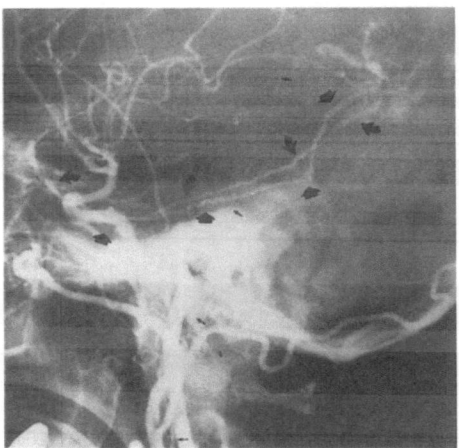

Fig.6. Falco-tentorial meningioma. Two hypertrophied tentorial arteries arise from the carotid siphon and the ophthalmic artery

On MRI all four meningiomas had local compressive effects on CSF spaces and neural structures, were practically isointense with the brain on T1-weighted images and demonstrated a moderate signal increase on T2-weighted images. Encroachment on the transverse sinus was seen once.

Discussion

High resolution CT usually affords easy recognition of the meningioma as a hyperdense, dural based tumor with smooth margins and dense, homogeneous contrast enhancement. There are only few deficiencies to this diagnostic modality such as the difficulty of obtaining good quality direct scans in more than one plane; the sometimes limited assessment of intraaxial, extraaxial, extradural or combined extension of the lesion. The parallel enhancement of blood vessels and meningiomas results also in a less convincing demonstration of vascular phenomena related to tumors, such as venous sinus invasion. In the experience of some AA. (Spagnoli et al. 1986) meningiomas are well demonstrated on highfield (1.5 T) MR images. Furthermore this diagnostic procedure is able to assess the vascularization of the tumor, its specific localization to the extraaxial compartment (visualized by means of various marginating characteristics) and to detect venous sinus invasion. We did not have the opportunity to study a more consistent number of our cases by MR. Although the diagnostic approach to tentorial meningiomas has been simplified by this technique, it is not likely to replace preoperative angiography in the demonstration of feeding pedicles

(Nadjmi et al. 1975; Theron et al. 1978; Muras et al. 1988). During development in several areas at the base of the skull, e.g. the tentorium, the primitive arterial supply regresses and a new arterial system takes over the blood supply. So the area is vascularized by two or more independent arterial systems, and when an arterial afferent becomes insufficient others enlarge to supply this area (Silvela and Zamarron, 1978). Thus only superselective and complete angiography allows each feeding vessel and the extent of the tumor blush to be defined. This permits also to evaluate the opportunity of a preoperative embolization of some dural pedicles.

Summary

We have discussed some aspects of the diagnosis of tentorial meningiomas, starting from a critical analysis of 20 personal cases observed from 1975 to 1987.

The extensive use of CT and MR has made possible a correct diagnosis and localization in almost any case. Angiography is an essential diagnostic procedure to guide the surgical approach. The necessity of an angiographic investigation as complete as possible is emphasized.

References

[1]   Bernasconi V, Cassinari V (1956) Un segno carotideo tipico di meningioma del tentorio. Chirurgia II: 586-588
[2]   Castellano F, Ruggiero G (1953) Meningiomas of posterior fossa. Acta Radiologica Suppl 104: 1-157
[3]   Greitz T (1972) Tumours of the quadrigeminal plate and adjacent structures. Acta Radiol Diagn 12: 513-538
[4]   Muras I, Cianciulli E, Scuotto A, Conforti R, Cioffi FA, Bernini FP (1988) Alcuni interessanti aspetti angiografici dei meningiomi intracranici. Atti VII Congr Naz Assoc Ital Neuroradiol Idelson-Napoli: 247-254
[5]   Nadjmi M, Ratzka M, Moissl G (1975) Angiographic aspects in meningiomas of the posterior cranial fossa. Advances in Neurosurgery 2: 250-252
[6]   Papo I, Salvolini U (1974) Meningiomas of the free margin of tentorium developing in the pineal region. Neuroradiology 7: 237-243
[7]   Silvela J, Zamarron MA (1978) Tentorial arteries arising from the external carotid artery. Neuroradiology 14: 267-269
[8]   Theron J, Bonafe A, Lasjaunias P, Clarisse J, Manelfe C (1978) Les mèningiomes de la tente du cervelet, J Neuroradiology 5: 69-81
[9]   Yasargil MG, Mortara RW, Curcic M (1980) Meningiomas of basal posterior cranial fossa. In: Krayenbhul H ed) Advances and Technical Standards in Neurosurgery, Vol 7, Chap. A. Springer-Verlag, Wien New York
[10] Zimmerman RD, Fleming CA, Saint Louis LA, Lee BC, Manning JJ, Deck MD (1985) Magnetic resonance imaging of meningiomas. AJNR 6: 149-157

Secondary High Flow Dural Arteriovenous Malformation (DAVMs) with Venous Drainage into a Venous Angioma After Neurosurgical Treatment of a Cavernous Angioma – A Case Presentation

S. Sielecki, J. P. Haas, H.-D. Langohr, and H.-P. Richter

INTRODUCTION

Dural arteriovenous malformations (DAVMs) represent abnormal shunts within the dura.The early case reports described the slow flow lesion. In 1964 van de Werf presented a case of spontaneous high flow dural arteriovenous malformations. Several authors have reported an association between DAVMs and other vascular malformation of the brain (Debrun and Chartres 1972; Djindjian and Merland 1978;Hieshima et al 1977).

CASE REPORT

A 21-year old man had a head injury after an epileptic episode.Plain CT scans disclosed fractures of the frontal bone (Fig.1) and a hyperdense lesion without mass effect in the left Sylvian region. In contrast enhanced CT there were a well circumscribed vascular abnormality in the basal ganglia and an area of irregular enhancement in the Sylvian region (Fig.3 and 4), both without mass effect. The ia-DSA of the left ICA showed a medusa-like network of numerous dilated medullar venules; they converged toward one transmedullar vein draining into the lateral sinus (Fig.2).CT signs and angiographic findings pointed to the diagnosis of venous malformation (venous angioma) and a cavernous angioma. After surgical treatment of the cavernous angioma there was a clinical detoriation with seizures and temporary neurologic deficits. CT scans 10 months after surgery showed nearly unchanged findings. The control angiography of the left ICA and ECA disclosed multiple dural arteriovenous fistulas from the territory of the ophthalmic, internal maxillary, middle meningeal and superficial temporal arteries with a high flow venous drainage resp. reflux into the previously demonstrated venous angioma (Fig.5 and 6).The venous phase in medullar veins resp. venous angioma was secondary disturbed.

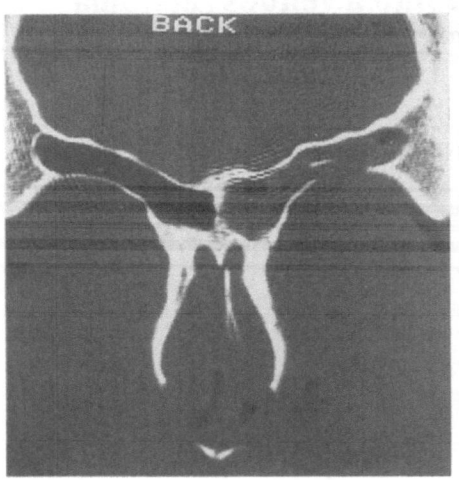

Fig. 1. High resolution CT, direct
coronal projection. Orbita roof
fracture with displaced fragment

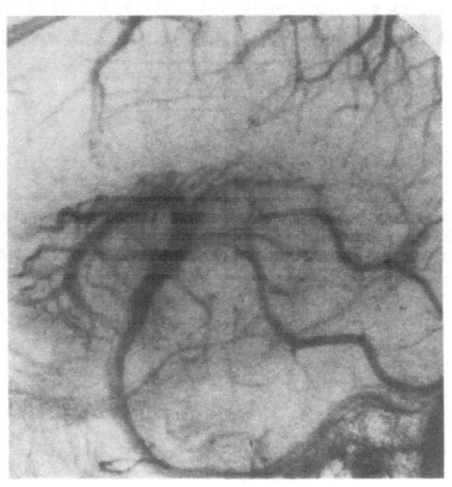

Fig. 2. Venous phase, left ICA
(ia-DSA). Large venous malformation in caudate and thalamus region; normal circulation time

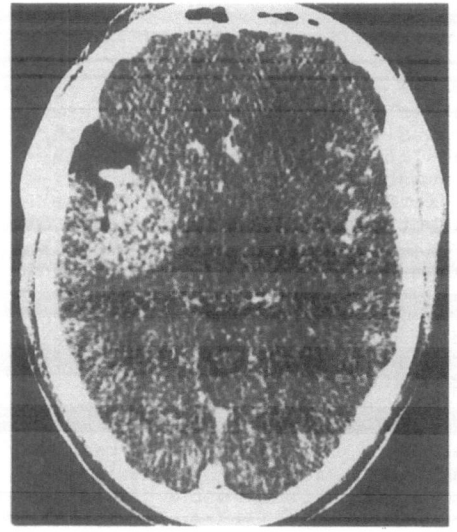

Fig. 3. Cavernous angioma. CT
after contrast infusion. In the
left Sylvian region an irregulary
shaped enhancing lesions is seen;
no mass effect

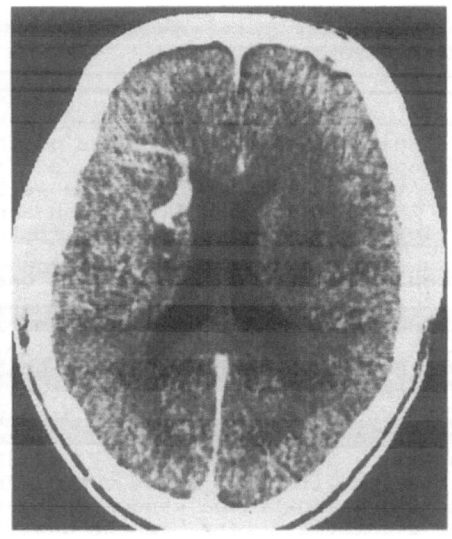

Fig. 4. Contrast enhanced CT.
A large vascular structure is
seen extending from caudate toward the region of insula

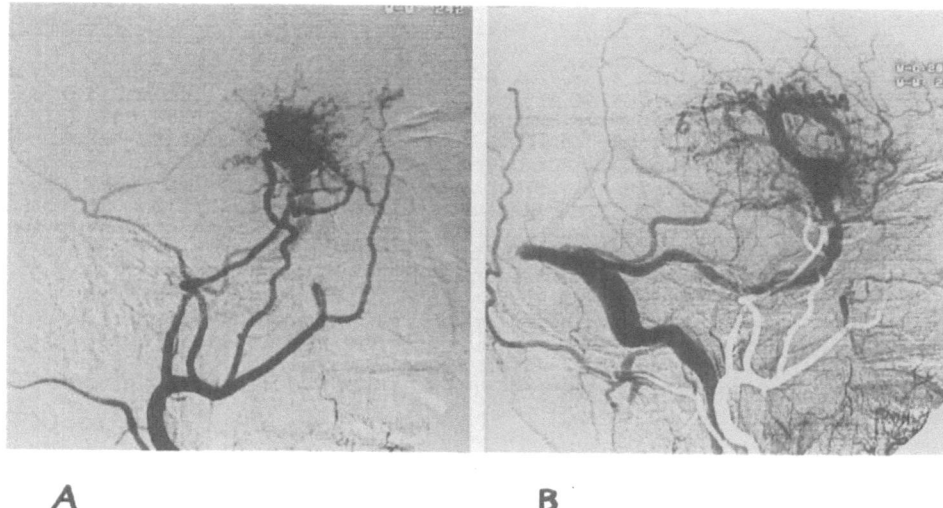

A   B

Fig. 5. Left external carotid angiography (ia-DSA), early (A) and late (B) arterial phase after the surgery demonstrates multiple dural AV-shunts with reflux into deep cerebral veins and a venous drainage mostly toward the lateral sinus

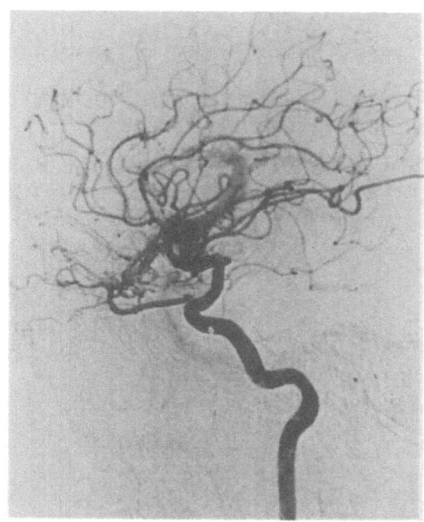

Fig. 6. Arterial phase of the left ICA)ia-DSA). There are several dural AV-fistulas in the territory of the posterior ethmoidal artery with reflux into the venous malformation

DISCUSSION

DAVMs are considered to be acquired lesions which develop secondary to venous obstruction due to a variety of causes e.g. trauma, infection or intracranial surgery (Aminoff 1973;Bitoh et al.1980;Djindjian et al.1973;Watanabe et al.1984). A combination of secondary developed multiple DAVMs, a venous and a cavernous angioma was in our opinion not described before. The presumable causative factors for DAVMs are very frequent but these malformations are relatively seldom in the population.These observations suggest that the pathogenesis of DSVMs is based on the preexistance of arteriovenous malformations connecting arterial meningeal branches and dural veins that are clinically quiescient but can be activated by a trigger factor (Clemens and Lodin 1968). The relatively rapid development of multiple AV-shunts in our patient after trauma and surgery support the hypothesis of preexistent changes of the dural vessels which premote formation of DAVMs.
The clinical detoriation was due probably to the disturbed hemodynamis of the venous phase.

REFERENCES

Arminoff MJ (1973) Vascular anomalies in the intracranial dura mater. Brain 96:601-612

Bitoh S, Hasegawa H, Fujuwara M, Nakata M (1980) Traumatic arteriovenous fistula between the middle meningeal artery and cortical vein. Surg Neurol 14:355-358

Clemens F, Lodin H (1968) Non-traumatic external carotid-cavernous sinus fistula. Clin Radiol 19:201-203

Debrun G, Chartres A (1972) Infra and supratentorial arteriovenous malformations: a general review about two cases of spontaneus supratentorial arteriovenous malformations of the dura. Neuroradiology 3:184-192

Djindjian R, Manelfe C, Picard L (1973a) Festules arterioveineuses carotide exterbe-sunus caverneux: étude angiographique á propos de 6 observations et revue de la littérature. Neurochirurgie 19:91-110

Djindjian R, Merland JJ (1987) Superselective arteriography of the external carotid artery. Springer, Berlin Heidelberg New York

Hieshima GB, Cahan LD, Berlin MS, Pribarm H (1971) Calvariel, orbital and dural vascular anomalies in herediatary hemorrhagic teleangiectasia. Surg Neurol 18:263-267

Van de Werf AJ (1964) Sur un cas d'avevrisme arterioveineux intradural bilateral de la fosse postéreure chez un enfant. Neurochirurgie 10:140-144

Watanabe A, Takahura Y, Ibuchi Y, Mizukami K (1984) Two cases of dural arteriovenous malformation occuring after intracranial sugery. Neuroraiology 26:375-380

Comparative Study of Ultrasound, MRI, CT, and Myopathological Findings in Generalized Neuromuscular Diseases

C. D. Reimers, M. Naegele, G. Fenzl, Th. N. Witt, K. Reimers, S. Wagner, D. Mautner, D. Hahn, and D. E. Pongratz

INTRODUCTION

Muscular imaging (ultrasound (US), computed tomography (CT), and magnetic resonance imaging (MRI)) is of increasing importance in the diagnosis of generalized neuromuscular disease (Reimers et al. 1988).

The purpose of this current study is to answer the following questions:
1. What is the morphological substrate of pathological sonographic and computed tomographic findings?
2. Is real-time sonography a sensitive method for the detection of fasciculations in spinal muscular atrophies and hereditary motor and sensory neuropathies?
3. Is there any contribution of muscular imaging to the differential diagnosis in degenerative myopathies?

PATIENTS AND METHODS

Up to now the myopathological findings of 136 muscle biopsies were compared to echo intensities of the same muscle. The samples were taken by open biopsy from tibialis anterior in 68, from biceps brachii in 31, from rectus femoris in 20, from vastus lateralis in 9, from deltoideus and gastrocnemius in 4 cases each. 38 of these specimen were correlated to densities in CT, too. Percentages of muscle parenchyma, interstitial fat and connective tissue were quantified by semiautomatic picture analysis (Leitz A.S.M.). Muscle US was performed in transversal and longitudinal sections using a linear array real-time scanner with a 3.75 MHz-transducer. Echo intensities were determined by computer assisted texture analysis. The region of interest extended from the superficial to the profound fascia of the muscle. The thickness of subcutaneous fat was measured by means of US investigation, too. A corresponding study concerning MRI has not yet been finished.

Fasciculations can be detected by means of real-time US in B- and M-mode technique in the form of short twitchings of muscle bundles. Their duration is about 0.2 to 0.5 seconds.

Between November 1986 and August 1988 we examined 31 adult patients (10 women, 21 men), aged 19 to 74 years, with non-hereditary spinal muscular atrophies and 16 adult patients (4 women, 12 men), aged 19 to 79 years, suffering from hereditary motor and sensory neuropathies. All patients were able to walk.

Furthermore 76 ambulatory patients, aged 14 to 79 years, suffering from degenerative myopathies (39x dystrophia myotonica, 18x facio-scapulohumeral, 10x X-linked, and 9x autosomal recessive limb girdle muscular dystrophy) have been investigated by US, 26 of them by MRI and 11 by CT, too. Up to 23 limb and trunk muscles have been examined sonographically on both sides.

RESULTS

The multiple correlation coefficients R between the echo intensities and densities in CT on one side and percentages of muscle parenchyma, interstitial fat and connective tissue on the other side are shown in table 1.

Table 1. US and CT compared to myopathological findings

	n	R
Ultrasound:		
Transverse scannings	125	0.622
Longitudinal scannings	93	0.654
Computed tomography	38	0.683

(n = number of muscle biopsies, R = multiple correlation coefficient).

The multiple correlation coefficients concerning US examinations increased by 0.08, if the thickness of the subcutaneous tissue was taken into account additionally. The multiple regression equation between echo intensities and muscle parenchyma, interstitial fat, and connective tissue proved that infiltration of the muscles by interstitial fat is considerably more echogenic than muscular fibrosis. Analogically an increase of interstitial fat markedly diminished muscle densities in CT, whereas muscular fibrosis results in slightly elevated densities.

In 25 of the 31 cases with spinal muscular atrophies (SMA) and 3 of the 16 patients with hereditary motor and sensory neuropathies (HMSN) fasciculations on the trunk and extremities were seen on neurological examination. Using real-time sonography fasciculations were found in 26 of the 31 patients with SMA and in 8 of the 16 patients with HMSN (table 2, fig. 1). They were most frequently localized in the quadriceps femoris, triceps surae, and the paraspinal muscles and only rarely seen in the forearm muscles, the rectus abdominis and tibialis anterior muscles. Fasciculations of profound muscles such as vastus intermedius, adductores femoris, and soleus were often visible by US only.

In general in advanced stages of myopathic diseases there was good agreement between sonographic, computed and magnetic resonance tomographic findings. Yet, in early stages MRI has been proved to be more sensitive than US and CT. Topic resolution was best in MRI and CT. Evaluation of echo intensities, CT densities, and signal intensities in MRI revealed typical distributions of mesenchymal alterations in many patients with degenerative myopathies. Some muscles were involved already in the beginning disease, whereas others were still normal and even hypertrophic in advanced stages. Table 3 presents a list of typical, but not pathognomonic distributions of the mesenchymal changes in degenerative myopathies.

Table 2. Detection of fasciculations by means of real-time sonography

	SMA fasciculations		HMSN fasciculations	
	+	-	+	-
Arms	17	12	0	4
Trunk	6	19	0	8
Legs	23	8	8	8
Total	26	5	8	8

(+ = patients with fasciculations in this region, - = patients without fasciculations in this region).

Table 3. Degenerative myopathies: Muscles affected in the beginning disease or in late stages only

	early affected muscles	lately affected muscles
Dystrophia myotonica	biceps brachii brachioradialis gastrocnemius, med. head	gastrocnemius, lat. head hamstrings deltoideus
facioscapulohumeral dystrophy	triceps brachii biceps brachii brachialis	supinator gastrocnemius vastus medialis
X-linked muscular dystrophy	rectus femoris vastus lateralis biceps brachii	sartorius gracilis supinator
limb girdle dystrophy	vastus intermedius vastus lateralis soleus	rectus abdominis deltoideus sartorius

COMMENT

Our results indicate that high echo intensities as well as low densities in CT are predominantly caused by an increase of interstitial fat. Similar to CT sonographic investigation gives a reliable impression of mesenchymal alterations in skeletal muscles. Yet, MRI is more sensitive (Naegele et al. 1988). In obese persons the thickness of subcutaneous fat layers must be considered to avoid false pathological assessments of echo intensities. The multiple correlation coefficients between echo intensities and CT densities on one hand and myopathological findings on the other hand were not quite satisfactory. We expect even higher correlation coefficients if further parameters were taken into account. These parameters could be the distribution of interstitial fat and connective tissue in the muscle biopsy specimen and of mesenchymal alterations in the whole muscle, the fibre size, and the muscle diameter.

Fasciculations are important differential diagnostic indicators of spinal muscular atrophies and sometimes of hereditary motor and sensory neuropathies, as they are only rarely found in aquired polyneuropathies. Our data prove higher sensitivity of real-time sonographic detection of fasciculations compared to clinical examination

630

only, especially in obese persons and fasciculations localized in
deep muscle layers.

Our results give further clues that evaluation of the distribution
and extent of mesenchymal alterations by means of muscular imaging
can contribute to differential diagnosis in degenerative myopathies.
This is of special interest in early stages, when typical clinical
features are still missing, or in late stages of the diseases, when
generalisation of the process blurs the characteristics.

REFERENCES

Naegele M, Karabensch F, Reimers CD, Hahn D (1988) Potential Use of
MRI for Skeletal Muscle in the Study of Neuromuscular Diseases: Cor-
relative Study CT, Ultrasound, EMG, Biopsy. Magn Reson Imaging 6
(Suppl. I): 72

Reimers CD, Naegele M, Fenzl G, Witt ThN, Müller W, Reimers K, Mautner D, Pongratz DE (1988) Bildgebende Verfahren (Sono-, Computer-
und Magnetresonanztomographie) an der Skelettmuskulatur bei gene-
ralisierten neuromuskulären Erkrankungen. Psycho 14: 665 - 679

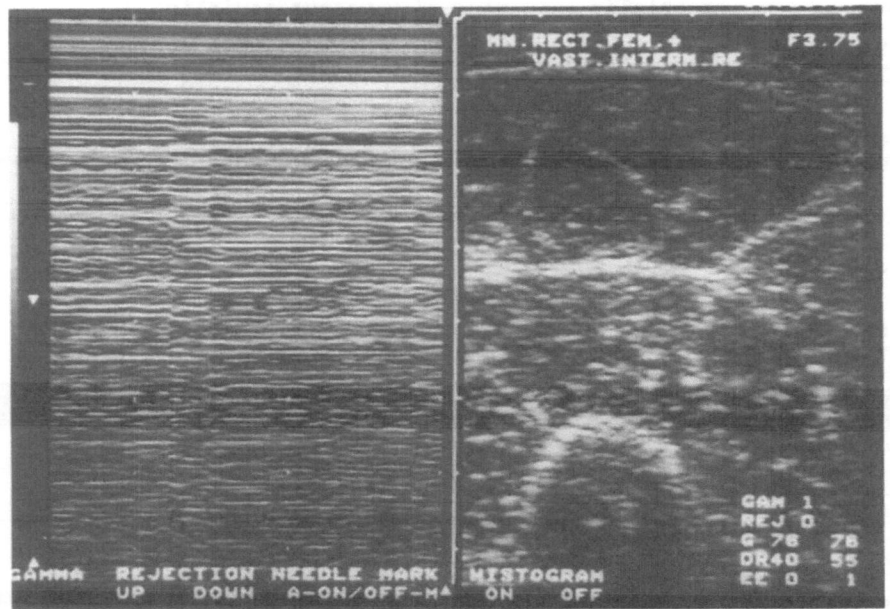

Fig. 1. 27-year-old man, hereditary motor and sensory neuropathy
type I, real-time-sonography of the right rectus femoris and vastus
intermedius muscles (transversal scanning). B-mode: Slightly increased echo intensities of the vastus intermedius muscle. M-mode:
Two fasciculations lasting for about 0.2 to 0.3 seconds.

CT Patterns of Recurrent Malignant Astrocytoma

K. Wallner, G. Krol, and M. Malkin

INTRODUCTION

Neoplasms arising from glial tissue are the most common primary intraaxial tumors of adulthood. Malignant forms of glioblastoma multiforme and anaplastic astrocytoma render generally poor prognosis with the majority of the patients surviving less than 1 year from the time of diagnosis. An attempt of complete resection of the lesion, followed by total brain irradiation constitutes an accepted mode of treatment of these tumors. The management of recurrence is not yet clearly outlined and repeat resection or limited irradiation may be employed. A definition of the spacial relationship of recurrent tumor with reference to the initial tumor bed is important for further surgical or radiotherapeutic management and is a subject of this investigation.

MATERIALS AND METHODS

Thirty-four patients with glioblastoma multiforme and anaplastic astrocytoma, treated by resection and followup whole brain radiation therapy had evidence of a recurrent disease on the CT scan. The initial resection of the tumor was considered total in twelve patients and partial in 16. In four patients only biopsy was performed. The recurrence was documented by followup CT's and occurred within two to 16 months after surgery (median: 6 months). Eighteen of these patients underwent a second operation. Evaluation of the configuration and spacial relationships between the recurrence and the primary tumor bed before surgery was done graphically. The largest initial and recurrent tumor areas were located on anatomically comparable CT slices. The CT images were then photographed and slides projected on each other, lifesize. The outline of the primary and recurrent tumors was drawn with exclusion of surrounding edema (Fig. 1A and B). The location of the recurrence was then related to the primary tumor bed (enhancement).

RESULTS

Seventy-eight per cent of tumors recurred within 2cm and 58% within 1 cm (Fig. 2 and 3) of the initial tumor margin. Large tumors were generally no more likely to recur further from the initial tumor margin than were the smaller tumors. No unifocal tumor recurred as the multifocal tumor. Only one tumor recurred in the contralateral hemisphere.

DISCUSSION

Initially, the investigators stressed the propensity for glioblastoma multiforme and anaplastic astrocytoma to infiltrate distant from the tumor bed areas of the brain (1). However, more recent work by Hochberg and Pruitt, investigating patterns of recurrence suggested that the majority of recurrent lesions occur in the proximity of the initial tumor bed (2). The present study, utilizing graphic method of superimposition of projected CT slides indicates that, indeed, recurrence after initial surgery occurs either within the tumor bed or close to its periphery.

The routine treatment of glioblastoma and anaplastic astrocytoma is resection followed by whole brain radiation therapy. The guidelines for management of recurrence are not definite. The spacial pattern of recurrence of the tumor observed in this study indicates that the majority recur at or at the close proximity of the initial tumor bed. Although no controls without RT treatment are available for comparison, the study suggests that local radiation therapy to the tumor bed with margin not smaller than 2-3 cm. from the periphery of enhancing component of the tumor may be sufficient. Recently introduced alternative treatment by seed implantation may be adequate, providing that the peritumoral tissue margin of minimum 2 cm. in thickness will receive an adequate irradiation dose.

SUMMARY

It is uncommon for glioblastoma and anaplastic astrocytoma to recur at the site distant from initial tumor bed. The majority of the recurrent lesions occur in close proximity of the initial margin of tumor enhancement. Focal radiation therapy and implantation with radioactive seeds may constitute and effective postoperative treatment, provided that an adequate tumor dose is delivered within 2 cm of the margin of the enhancing primary tumor.

REFERENCES

1. Concannon JP, Kramer S, Berry R: The extent of intracranial gliomata at autopsy and its relationship to techniques used in radiation therapy of brain tumors. Am J roent 84:99-107, 1960.

2. Hochberg FH, Pruitt A: Assumptions in the radiotherapy of glioblastoma. Neurology 30:907-911, 1980.

3. Salazar OM, Rubin P: The spread of glioblastoma multiforme as a determining factor in the radiation treated volume. Int J Radiation Oncol Biol Phys 1:627-637, 1976.

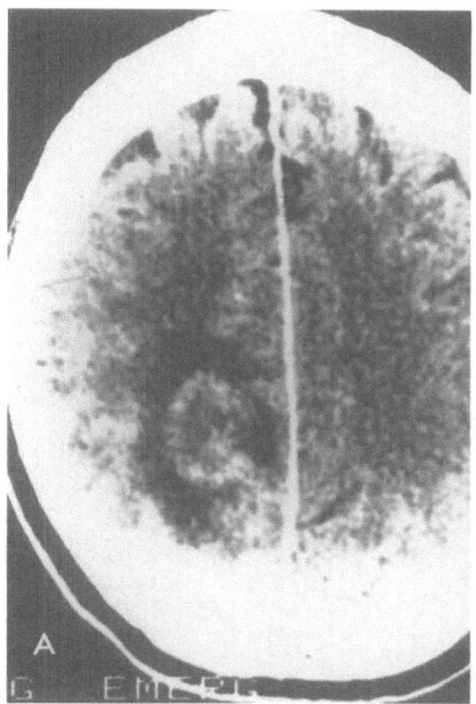

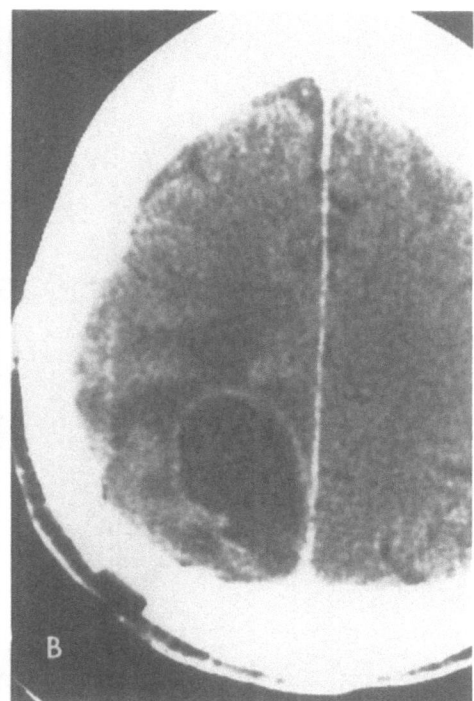

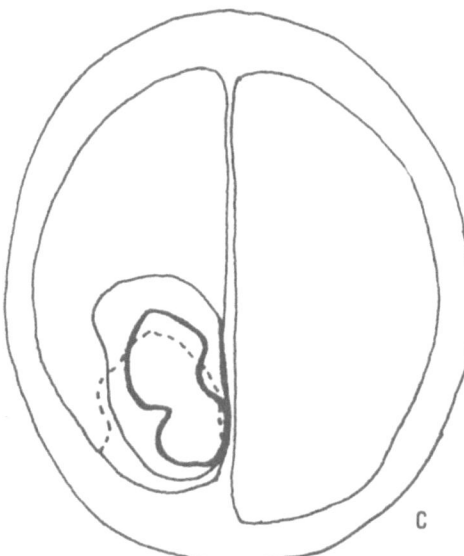

A. CT scan with contrast, preoperative study.

B. Followup CT scan with contrast. Abnormal enhancement is noted along the periphery, consistent with recurrent tumor.

C. Method. Contrast enhancing component of the tumor was traced manually on preoperative examination and the followup scan, showing recurrence. They were then photographed and projected on each other, taking into account the magnification corrections.

Continuous thick line – outline of the original tumor, interrupted line – outline of the recurrent tumor, continuous thin line – outline of the edema.

Arterial Circulation in the Posterior Fossa – A Comparative Radioanatomy and Doppler Ultrasound Study

M. Mull, A. Aulich, and M. Hennerici

INTRODUCTION

Since the development of a high-energy ultrasound pulsed-wave Doppler system operating at low emission frequencies (1-2 MHz) by Aaslid et al. in 1982, this method has been increasingly used for a non-invasive assessment of the major intracranial basal vessels from temporal and orbital ultrasonic windows (Hennerici et al. 1987 a, 1987 b). In contrast to the investigation of the anterior circle of Willis, identification of the vertebral (VA) and basilar (BA) arteries by transcranial Doppler (TCD) is difficult because of more frequent anatomical variations in the posterior circulation which limit the continuous tracing of particular vessels (Büdingen and Staudacher 1987).

PATIENTS and METHODS

To test the validity of TCD for the examination within the posterior fossa we compared TCD results with corresponding radioanatomic morphometrics in 58 patients. 37 patients suffered from cerebrovascular diseases which involved the vertebro-basilar system in 21 cases. 8 patients underwent the diagnostic studies because of brain tumors. 13 patients were evaluated because of various other reasons.
Angiograms of the vertebro-basilar system were performed by retrograde injections into the right or left brachial artery (n=36) or simultaneously into both brachial arteries (n=22). The nuchal position of the Doppler probe was indicated in the midline by an X-ray opaque marker. A micro-processor-controlled directional pulsed-wave Doppler device (EME Überlingen) was used. From a suboccipital nuchal approach Doppler signals were taken in 5 mm steps ranging from 30 to 125 mm insonation depth (Hennerici et al. 1987 a). According to the angiographical findings the nuchal probe position was adapted to obtain the optimal Doppler signal.

RESULTS

The radioanatomic data referring to vascular and bony reference points (Fig. 1) revealed a considerable interindividual variability known from the literature (Busch 1966, Krayenbühl and Yasargil 1957).

DISTANCE PROBE	n	MEAN DISTANCE [cm]	RANGE [cm]
- TUBERCULUM POSTERIOR OF THE ATLAS (a)	58	3.9	2.6 - 6.6
- VERTEBRAL ARTERY GROOVE OF THE ATLAS (b)	57	5.2	4.1 - 7.9
- BEGINNING OF THE BASILAR ARTERY (c)	35	8.7	7.0 - 10.6
- SUPERIOR BIFURCATION OF THE BASILAR ARTERY (d)	50	11.5	9.6 - 14.5
- DORSUM SELLAE (e)	58	11.7	10.0 - 15.4

Fig. 1. Schematic lateral view of the skull illustrating the suboccipital position of the transcranial Doppler (TCD) probe in relation to osseous and vascular reference points (a-e); note the thickness of nuchal soft tissue. The table shows our findings of radio-angiographic distances.

When comparing the angiographic point of commencement of the BA with the maximal depth of the Doppler signals, the total length of the BA could only exceptionally be traced (9%). Even its proximal part was missed in 30%. Identification of the beginning of the BA is limited on the basis of hemodynamic parameters as revealed by the analysis of flow velocities in different segments of the VAs and BAs in patients with normal angiographical findings and norm variants.
TCD findings of 3 patients had to be excluded because of technical reasons. Normal angiographic findings were confirmed by the TCD recordings in 25 patients. However, the non-invasive method failed to detect physiological and morphological variants in 15 patients (hypoplasia (n=10), kinkings or coilings (n=4), primitive trigeminal artery (n=1)).

15 patients showed pathological findings of the intracranial vertebro-basilar system revealed by angiography (5 affecting the VAs, 10 the BAs). 10 of the pathological conditions were confirmed by TCD. The TCD analysis provided reliable results in moderate stenosis (n=1, Fig.2), in hemodynamic alterations (subclavian steal phenomenon (n=2), VA-occlusion (n=1)).
Moreover, in 2 of 6 patients with angiographically occluded BA TCD demonstrated in addition reversal of flow in the seemingly occluded part of the BA (Fig. 3); in the other 4 patients no TCD signal could be found in the corresponding depth of the BA. TCD failed to detect angiographically circumscript stenosis of the VA (n=2) and to discriminate dilative arteriopathy (n=3) from other conditions with low flow phenomena.
In contrast to a normal angiogram, TCD examination revealed abnormal Doppler signals in 2 patients indicating a vascular lesion in the VA and/or posterior inferior cerebellar artery.

Thus the combined use of both methods added further information in 7 of 17 patients.

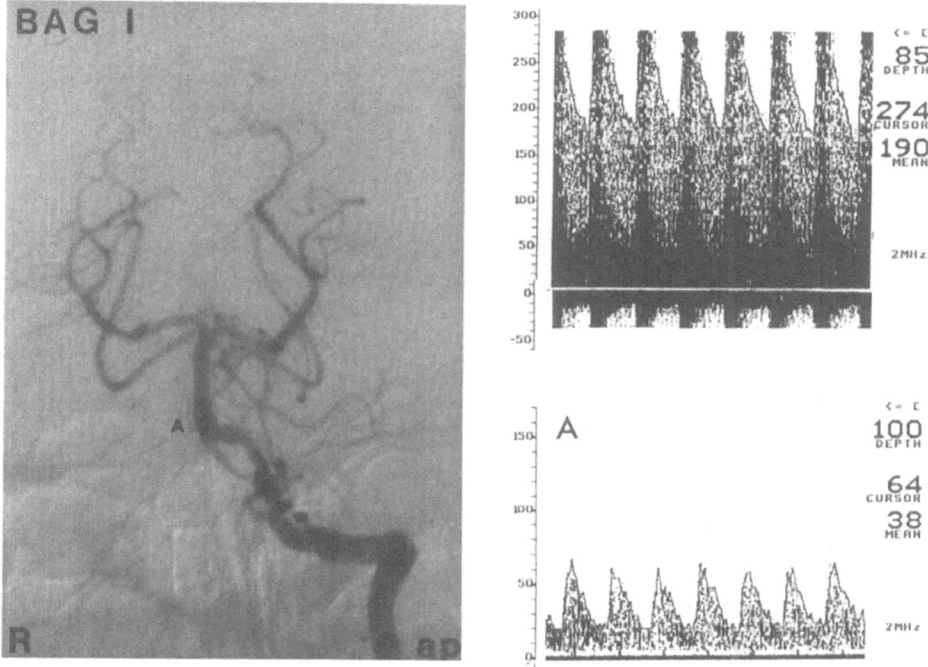

Fig. 2. Angiogram and TCD recordings of a 67-year-old man with bilateral
partial infarction in the posterior cerebral artery
territitory. Typical signs of moderate stenosis (below 100 mm depth = A)
correspond with the angiographically confirmed extended stenosis of the
left VA.
Abbreviations: BAG 1.= left retrograde brachial angiogram, R.= right;
ap. = anteriorposterior view.

CONCLUSIONS

TCD examination of the vertebro-basilar system is a supplementary method
to cerebral angiography. With regard to the numerous anatomical
variations and to the limitations in obtaining intracranial Doppler
signals especially in the depth of the BA, the assessment of the
posterior circulation should critically reflect the amount of
misdiagnoses from hemodynamic studies alone. However, the combination of
both methods may enhance their diagnostic validity.

638

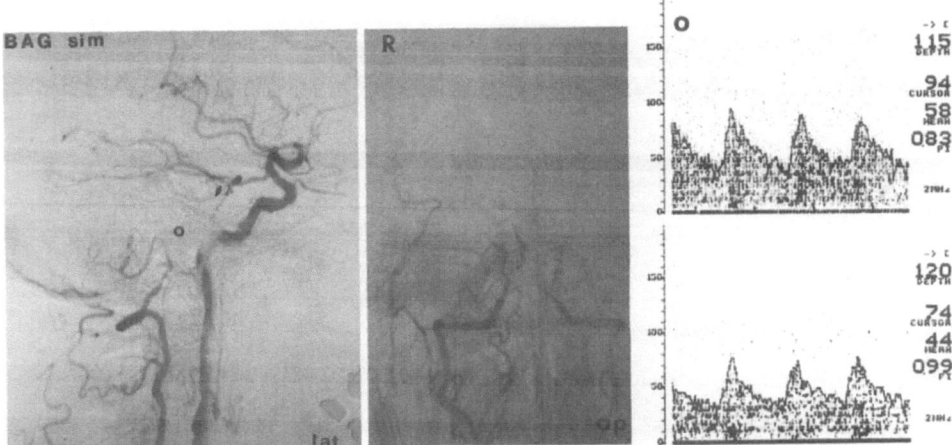

Fig.3 Angiogram and TCD spectra of a 60-year-old man with brain stem
infarction and TIAs in the vertebro-basilar territory.
Whereas the bilateral retrograde brachial arteriogram suggests filling of
the distal BA only via the posterior communicating artery (   ), TCD
spectra show reversal of flow reaching the proximal BA (O).
Abbreviations: BAG sim.= simultanous (injection in both arteries)
retrograde brachial arteriorgram; Lat.= lateral view.

REFERENCES

Aaslid R, Markwalder T-M, Nornes H (1982) Non-invasive transcranial
   Doppler ultrasound recording of flow veloty in basal cerebral
   arteries. J Neurosurg 57:769-774
Büdingen HJ, Staudacher T (1987) Die Identifizierung der Arteria
   basilaris mit der transcraniellen Doppler-Sonographie. Ultraschall 8:
   95-101
Busch W (1966) Beitrag zur Morphologie und Pathologie der Arteria
   basilaris (Untersuchungsergebnisse bei 1000 Gehirnen). Arch Psychiatr
   Nervenkr 208: 326-344.
Hennerici M, Rautenberg W, Sitzer G, Schwartz A (1987a) Transcranial
   Doppler ultrasound for the assessment of intracranial arterial flow
   velocity - part 1. Examination technique and normal values.
   Surg Neurol 27: 439-448
Hennerici M, Rautenberg W, Schwartz A (1987b) Transcranial Doppler
   ultrasound for the assessment of intracranial arterial flow velocity -
   part 2. Evaluation of intracranial disease. Surg Neurol 27: 523-532.
Krayenbühl H, Yasargil M G (1957) Die vaskulären Erkrankungen im Gebiet
   der Arteria vertebralis und Arteria basilaris. Thieme, Stuttgart, 1-170

Radiological Manifestations of Aneurysmatic Subarachnoid Hemorrhage After Acute Operation and Nimodipin Therapy

H. Traupe and K. Ritter

Introduction

Therapy of acute subarachnoidal aneurysmatic bleedings has changed.
Acute operation and therapy with calcium antagonists play a central
role in neurosurgical treatment. The object of our study was to
evaluate the influence of today's treatment on radiological features.
The following questions were answered:
1. Did the spectrum of complications seen in radiology change after
acute operation and/or nimodipin therapy,
2. Is there a change in frequency of functional changes of blood
vessels after acute operation and nimodipin therapy,
3. How often does hydrocephalus occur and is it of prognostic value,
4. Does early operation influence the development of ischemic
lesions visible in CT,
5. Does therapy with calcium antagonists demonstrate an effect on
the development of infarcts?

Patients/Methods

Distribution of age and sex in 90 patients studied lies within the
normal range found in literature.
All patients were evaluated angiographically and by CT. 136
angiographies and a total of 231 CT's before and after treatment
were studied.

Results

Cerebral vessels demonstrating aneurysms.

In 90 patients 108 aneurysms were diagnosed. The distribution of the
cerebral vessels demonstrating aneurysms was as follows:
The middle cerebral artery was most often involved (29%), followed
by the internal cerebral artery (23%) the anterior communicating
artery (25%) the anterior c.a. 7.4%, ramus comm. post. 3.7%, basilar
a. 5.8%, vert.a. 2.8% a.c.inf.post. 1.8% and one aneurysm of the a.
auditiva.

Amount of bleeding

In 86 patients blood within the subarachnoidal space was found. In
71% the CT localisation of the bleeding pointed to the site of the
aneurysm, in 29% CT did not indicate the site of the aneurysm.
The amount of subarachnoid blood was graduated according to Fisher
et al. 1980 and is included in brackets:
F1: no blood detected (10%), F2: diffuse layers of blood (19%), F3:
localized clots of blood (37%), F4: diffuse or no blood but
intracerebral or intraventricular clots (33%).

Functional changes of vessel diameter, spasm and vasodilatation.

76% of our patients demonstrated changes of vessel diameter. In Fig.1 a,b the frequency of functional changes of the blood vessels is shown during the first 2 weeks after acute hemorrhage (a) and from the 3. to the 14th week after bleeding (b). At day of admission 17 of 27, the second day 15 out of 18 and the third day 5 out of 10 patients demonstrated spasm or vasodilatation. Spasms dominated with 81% over vasodilatation (34%). Spasms were found in 48% unilaterally, in 26% bilaterally. There was no correlation between the amount of blood seen in CT and the frequency of spasms.

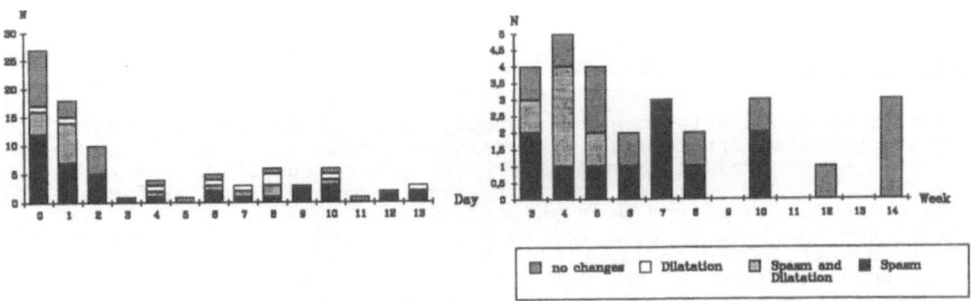

Fig. 1 a: Angiographic findings during the first two weeks after acute hemorrhage. The incidence of functional vessel disturbances is high during the first 2 days and declines significantly after the second day. Vasodilatation alone was only found during the first 10 days after bleeding.
Fig. 2 b: Spasms were observed up to the 10th week, the combination of spasms and vasodilatation was seen up to the 5th week.

Posthemorrhagic hydrocephalus

39 out of 90 patients showed dilatation of the ventricular spaces. At admission (first day) 7 out of 35 (20%), during the first week 17 out of 92, the second week 10 out of 30 (33%). The occurrence of ventricular dilatation (12 cases with severe hydrocephalus) was found in 66% of cases during the first 2 weeks. A significant correlation between the amount of blood seen in CT and development of hydrocephalus was only observed after intraventricular hemorrhage (77%).

Ischemic lesions

In 25 out of 46 patients who underwent early operation a complete follow-up study of CT examinations was available. In 9 of these cases (36%) ischemic lesions were observed in CT. In all of these cases functional alterations of the cerebral vessels were seen angiographically. Cases with spasms alone showed lesions in 17%, with spasms and vasodilatation the finding was observed in 66%. Patients with hydrocephalus demonstrated significant less lesions than with hydrocephalus.
Patients operated after 24 hours were followed up in 35 of 44 cases. 20 patients (57%) developed ischemic lesions.
In all cases where local edema was observed before operation,

demarcated lesions were seen in later CT studies. The findings of
ischemic lesions are summarized in Fig. 2 a,b..

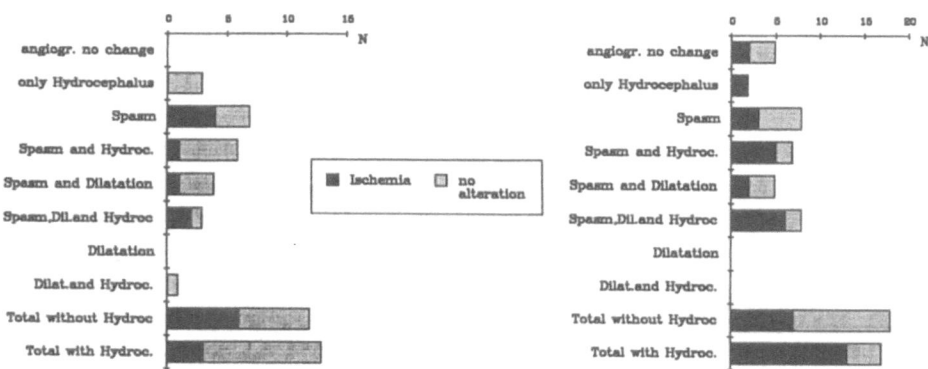

Fig. 2 a: Relation between radiological findings and the occurrence of
ischemic lesions in patients treated by acute operation.
Angiographic proven changes of the vessel diameter in a high degree
lead to ischemic lesions, whereas hydrocephalus has no influence or
even a "beneficial" effect on development of infarcts.
2b: In the group of late operated patients, the incidence of
ischemic lesions is higher, patients with hydrocephalus show
infarcts to a higher degree than without.

Therapy with calcium antagonists

28 out of 90 patients were treated with calcium antagonists, follow
up studies were available in 21 patients after nimodipin treatment
and in 47 cases without nimodipin therapy. In all patients who
underwent early operation as well as in patients with late operation
results after treatment with nimodipin were better than without.
Best results were seen in the group of late operated patients:
Ischemic lesions were seen in 75% without nimodipin therapy and in
31% with nimodipin therapy. The relation in early operated patients
was 61% without nimodipin to 44% with nimodipin Fig. 3 a,b..
Discussion

Spasms
Compared to common literature frequency and manifestation of cerebral
vasospasm in this study is found to a higher degree and earlier. If
the timing of angiography is taken into account, our results with a
frequency of 81% over all and 64% of spasms during the first 3 days
show poor correlation to elder literature and are comparable only to
those of Fisher et al. 1980 who found a frequency of 70% of spasms
in a group of 47 patients examined within the first 5 days.
As shown in our study, the frequency of spasms is not dependent on
the finding of subarachnoidal blood in CT. All patients without
evidence of subarachnoidal blood had spasms.
28% of our patients demonstrated manifest hydrocephalus, ventricular
dilatation was seen in 43%. Hydrocephalus was observed in 17 out of
90 patients within the first 5 days, which is in accordance to other
CT studies.

642

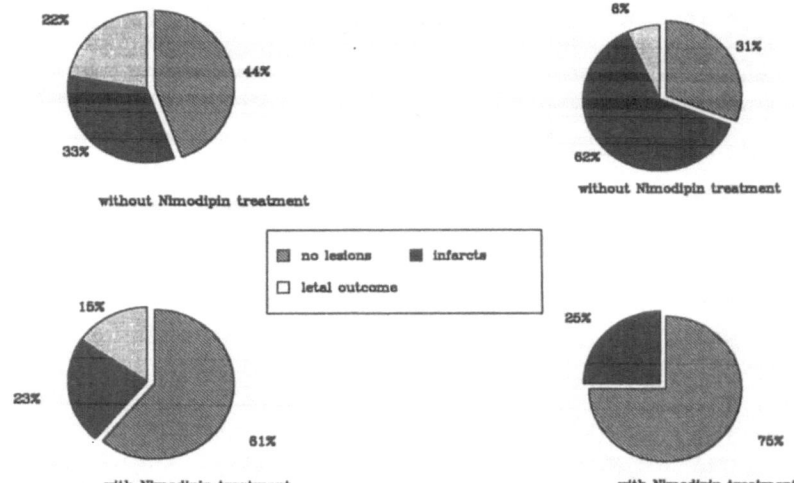

Fig. 3 a,b: Incidence of infarcts or letal outcome in patients
treated with/without calcium antagonists after acute operation,(a) and
late operation. In both groups the beneficial effect of nimodipin
therapy is evident.

The incidence of cerebral infarcts is remarkably lowered by acute
operation (36%) against late operated patients (57%).
The effect of treatment with calcium antagonists shows significant
ischemic lesions (20% less in the group of early operated patients
and 44% less in the group of late operated patients).
Our results show a considerable change in the radiological pattern
of posthemorrhagic angiographic and computertomographic findings and
are in good accordance with corresponding clinical studies (Auer
1984, Adams et al. 1983, Hunger et al. 1986, Allen et al. 1983, Koos
et al. 1985).

REFERENCES

Adams HP et al.(1983) CT and clinical correlations in recent
   aneurysmal sdbarachnoid hemorrhage:A preliminary report of the
   Cooperative Aneurysma Study.
   Neurology 33:981-88.
Allen G.S. et al.(1983) Cerebral arterial spasm - a controlled trial
   of nimodipine patients with subarachnoid hemorrhage.
   The New England Journal Of Medicine 308 No 11:619-24.
Auer LM, (1984) Acute operation and preventive nimodipine improve
   outcome in patients with ruptured cerebral aneurysms
   Neurosurgery 15 No1:57-66.
Fisher C.M. et al.(1980) Relation of cerebral vasospasm to
   subarachnoid hemorrhage visualized by computerized
   tomographic scanning. Neurosurgery 6:
Hunger J. et al. (1986) Spontane intrakranielle Blutung:
   Spätkomplikationen und Spätergebnisse. Nervenheilkunde 4:140-142
Koos W.T. et al.(1985) Nimodipine treatment of ischemicneurological
   Vasospasm to subarachnoid hemorrhage visualized by computerized
   tomographic scanning. Neurosurgery 6 No. 1.

Passage of Ultrasound Contrast Medium (Gas Bubbles) into the Cerebral Circulation

Th. Staudacher, P. Stoeter, and K. Berwing (Ravensburg, Bad Nauheim, FRG)

Ultrasound contrast medium containing microbubbles now is usually used for cardiologic examinations. After intravenous injection, the gas bubbles reach the right ventricle and a small portion of them after passage of the lung also reach the left ventricle and the aorta. To determine the amount of gas bubbles passing the cerebral arteries after i.v. injection of ultrasound contrast medium, we examined 10 patients during echocardiographic examinations with transcranial Doppler sonography of the middle cerebral artery. The amount of echoes depended on the dose of contrast medium administered and varied between different individuals, probably because of av shunts in the lung. In patients with septal defects, however, tremedous showers of ultrasound-reflecting gas bubbles can be demonstrated in the cerebral arteries. By now, even in these patients no side effects or complications were observed apart from transient sensations of taste. Therefore, it may be possible to inject this type of ultra-sound contrast medium without greater risk into the arterial system and even into cerebral arteries.

Diagnostic Value of Paramagnetic Contrast Media in the MR Evaluation of Intracranial Extraaxial Tumors

P. M. Parizel, J. Van Goethem, D. Balériaux, H. R. Degryse,
G. Rodesch, and A. M. De Schepper

INTRODUCTION

Many extraaxial tumors present MR signal intensities that are similar to normal brain tissue and are thus difficult to identify. In particular, meningiomas can pose a specific problem, because they are often isosignal to the adjacent brain parenchyma [Bydder et al. 1985, Bradac et al. 1987, Lee and Deck 1985, Sartor et al. 1987]. Anatomic distortion is the key to the MR diagnosis, but unenhanced MR images have been reported to be less accurate than CT in the diagnosis of benign extraaxial tumors [Haughton et al. 1986]. Since these tumors lack a blood-brain barrier and are usually richly vascularized, they are ideally suited for examination with paramagnetic contrast agents.

The present study was designed to evaluate the *comparative diagnostic accuracy* of non-contrast and contrast-enhanced MR in the diagnosis of benign extraaxial tumors and to assess the advantages of contrast-enhanced MR examinations in the presurgical work-up in these lesions. The MR contrast agents used were the paramagnetic gadolinium chelates *Gd-DTPA* (Schering AG, Berlin) and *Gd-DOTA* (Laboratoire Guerbet, Aulnay-sous-Bois).

MATERIAL AND METHODS

We have compared the precontrast T1 and T2 weighted images (T1 and T2 WI) and the postcontrast T1 WI in 63 patients with suspected extraaxial tumors of the central nervous system.

All subjects were examined on a superconducting MR unit operating at 0.5 T (Siemens Magnetom; Universitair Ziekenhuis Antwerpen, University of Antwerp) or on a superconducting 1.5 T system (Philips Gyroscan S15; Hôpital Erasme, Université Libre de Bruxelles).

The paramagnetic contrast media used were Gd-DTPA (30 patients) and Gd-DOTA (33 patients). The contrast agents were administered intravenously in a dosage of 0.1 mmol/kg body weight. Postcontrast T1 WI were obtained between 5 and 40 minutes of gadolinium injection, using at least two imaging planes.

RESULTS

In a series of 63 gadolinium-enhanced MR examinations in subjects with suspected intracranial extraaxial lesions, tumors were discovered in 45 patients. This group included patients with meningioma (n=26), acoustic schwannoma (n=8), trigeminal schwannoma (n=1), hemangiopericytoma (n=1), pituitary adenoma (n=6), craniopharyngioma (n=2), chordoma (n=1). In the remaining 18 patients, the MR studies were negative. This group included 8 patients in whom the MR examination was performed because of the suspicion of an acoustic schwannoma, and 10 patients suspected of a pituitary adenoma.

Our results are summarized in Table 1.

Table 1. Histologic diagnoses in 63 patients

Diagnosis	N (DTPA+DOTA)	n_1 (Gd-DTPA)	n_2 (Gd-DOTA)	Enhancement
MENINGIOMA	26	15	11	++
ACOUSTIC SCHWANNOMA	8	6	2	++
TRIGEMINAL SCHWANNOMA	1	0	1	++
PITUITARY ADENOMA	6	0	6	+
HEMANGIOPERICYTOMA	1	0	1	++
CRANIOPHARYNGIOMA	2	2	0	+
CHORDOMA	1	1	0	+
SUBTOTALS (EXTRAAXIAL TUMORS)	*45*	*24*	*21*	
NEG. SEARCH FOR ACOUSTIC NEUROMA	8	2	6	-
NEG. SEARCH FOR PITUITARY ADENOMA (INCLUDING 3 PATIENTS WITH EMPTY SELLA)	10	4	6	-
SUBTOTALS (NEGATIVE EXAMINATIONS)	*18*	*6*	*12*	
TOTALS (ALL PATIENTS)	*63*	*30*	*33*	

On T1 weighted spin echo sequences, high levels of contrast enhancement (i.e. T1 shortening) were observed in most extraaxial tumors, as indicated in Table 1. The use of Gd-DTPA or Gd-DOTA increased lesion conspicuity and improved the contrast resolution of the examination. The enhancement was most pronounced in meningiomas and schwannomas, which showed immediate, intense and sharply marginated contrast uptake. This strong enhancement enabled us to correctly diagnose several lesions that were missed initially on the precontrast images.

There were no significant differences in the level of contrast enhancement between the Gd-DTPA and Gd-DOTA groups. Both were safe and effective contrast media. The contrast injection was well tolerated in all patients. There were no adverse reactions either during the MR examination or in the next 24–48 hours.

DISCUSSION

The use of a paramagnetic contrast agent proved valuable in the identification of extraaxial lesions, improving overall tumor visibility, border definition, visualization of necrotic foci or areas of cystic degeneration, tumor versus edema separation, distinction between tumor and CSF loculations, evaluation of residual tumor or tumor recurrence in the postoperative patient. These advantages were especially helpful in the diagnosis of small lesions without mass effect or perilesionsal edema.

In *meningiomas*, the multiplanar enhanced MR examination allows the extent of the tumor mass to be delineated more completely and enables internal and peripheral vascularity, arterial encasement, and invasion of the dural venous sinuses to be visualized [Spagnoli et al. 1986]. In most meningiomas, there was enhancement of the tumor as well as of the adjacent dura, indicating tumor spread along the meninges. This finding is difficult if not impossible to demonstrate with CT.

In *acoustic schwannomas*, the postcontrast T1 WI were especially valuable in demonstrating small, intracanalar lesions, which may be easily overlooked on the precontrast MR study. In medium-sized and large acoustic schwannomas, the enhanced study improved tumor versus edema differentiation. However, in 2 patients with very large acoustic schwannomas surrounded by loculated CSF filled arachnoid cysts, the postcontrast MR examination did not provide additional information: these lesions were clearly outlined by the surrounding CSF, especially on the precontrast long TR images.

In *pituitary adenomas*, the relative enhancement was less pronounced. Paramagnetic gadolinium chelates have a limited role in macroadenomas but may be useful in demonstrating microadenomas that were not seen on the precontrast study.

CONCLUSIONS

In benign extraaxial tumors, which are approximately isointense with respect to adjacent cerebral structures, paramagnetic contrast agents improve contrast and lesion conspicuity, thus increasing the sensitivity of the MR examination [Breger et al. 1987, Haughton et al. 1988].

Both Gd-DTPA and Gd-DOTA were effective and safe paramagnetic contrast agents and there were no significant differences in the level of enhancement between the two groups.

Our experience suggests that Gd-DTPA or Gd-DOTA enhanced MR with multiplanar imaging is the method of choice in the preoperative evaluation of intracranial extraaxial tumors.

REFERENCES

Bydder GM, Kingsley DPE, Brown J, Niendorf HP, Young IR (1985) MR imaging of meningiomas including studies with and without Gadolinium-DTPA. J Comput Assist Tomogr 9: 690-697

Bradac GB, Riva A, Schörner W, Stura G (1987) Cavernous sinus meningiomas: an MRI study. Neuroradiology 29: 578-581.

Breger RK, Papke RA, Pojunas KW, Haughton VM, Williams AL, Daniels DL (1987) Benign extraaxial tumors: contrast enhancement with Gd-DTPA. Radiology 163: 427-429

Haughton VM, Rimm A, Sobocinski K, Papke RA, Daniels DL, Williams AL, Lynch R, Levine R (1986) Blinded clinical comparison of MR proton imaging and CT in neuroradiology. Radiology 160: 751-755.

Haughton VM, Rimm AA, Czervionke LF, Breger RK, Fisher ME, Papke RA, Hendrix LE, Strother CM, Turski PA, Williams AL, Daniels DL (1988) Sensitivity of Gd-DTPA-enhanced MR imaging of benign extraaxial tumors. Radiology 166: 829-833.

Lee BCP, Deck MDF (1985) Sellar and juxtasellar detection with MR. Radiology 157: 143-147.

Sartor K, Karnaze MG, Winthrop JD, Gado M, Hodges FJ (1987) MR imaging in infra-, para- and retrocerebellar lesions. Neuroradiolgy 29: 19

Spagnoli MV, Goldberg HI, Grossman RI, Bilaniuk LT, Gomori JM, Hackney DB, Zimmerman RA (1986) Intracranial meningiomas: high-field MR imaging. Radiology 161: 369-375.

Pulse-Synchronous Alterations of Contrast Density During Carotid Angiography

P. Stoeter and N. Prey

During the arterial phase of angiography pulse-synchronous changes of contrast density (CD) were recorded by cinematography (Heuck et al. 1969) and digital subtraction angiography (DSA) (Bürsch et al. 1981, Hall and Volz, 1986). The origin of these "pulsations" of CD and their relation to the arterial blood flow are examined in this study.

Model studies

A rubber tube of a diameter of 5,5 mm is injected mechanically with diluted (1:4) and heparinized blood at a rate of 2,5 (lo.5), 5 (21) and lo (42) ml/sec (cm/sec) (Fig.1). Pulsatile changes of flow are created by repeated short-lasting manual compressions of the tube. The velocity of flow is recorded by Doppler sonography. A 5-F-catheter is inserted into the tube, and 2 ml of contrast medium (CM) are injected at rates of o,5 - 2 ml/sec by a second injector. DSA images are acquired at high frequency (25/sec) on the 512 matrix of a Picker 211 DSA unit. Time-density curves are generated from regions of interest (ROI) in various distances from the site of injection. The amplitude of background density is subtracted.

In a distance of 2 cm from the tip of the catheter, the maximal amplitude of CD can be registrated at the end of the Doppler sonographic phase of acceleration of blood flow after a preceeding depression (Fig.1). Observation of consecutive DSA images shows that during a phase of reduced flow a pool of CM accumulates around the tip of the catheter and is moved foreward by the accelerated flow of the following ("early systolic") phase to the site of registration (ROI). Afterwards, the persisting blood flow dilutes the injected CM until the blood flow is interrupted again.

There is a close time relation between the alterations of blood flow and CD. The latency between the Doppler-sonographic begin of flow acceleration and the densographic maximum of CD is increased by a larger distance between the site of injection and ROI and reduced by an increased velocity of blood flow (Fig.2).

The maximal amplitude of CD and the index of density variation (amplitude of density "pulse": amplitude of maximal CD) are variable and depend mainly on the actual experimental set-up. In identical conditions and consecutive registrations, both parameters are reduced by an increasing distance between the site of injection and ROI. The maximal amplitude of CD is reduced, the index slightly increased by an augmentation of blood flow. A changing rate of injection of CM has no obvious influence on the latencies and other parameters mentioned above.

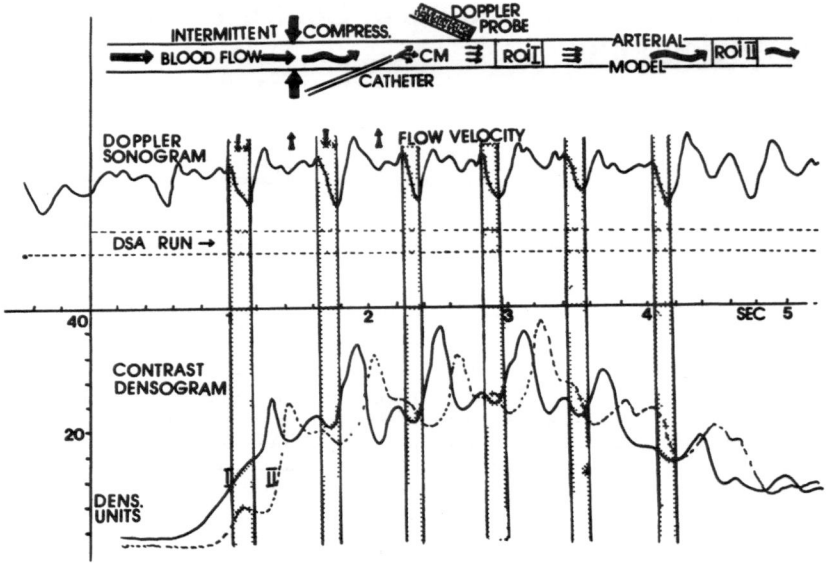

Fig.1. Arterial model and simultanously recorded Doppler sonogram and densogram of ROI I and II. Blood flow 2o cm/sec, CM 2 ml, rate of injection o,5 ml/sec.

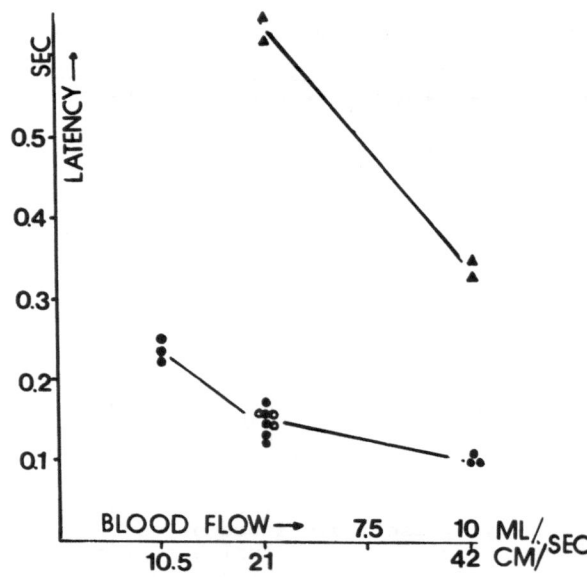

Fig.2. Latency between Doppler-sonographic begin of flow acceleration (=end of grey bar in Fig.1) and maximum of CD decreases with increasing rate of blood flow. Registration in a distance of 2 cm (●) and 2o cm (▲) from tip of catheter.

Clinical examinations:

In 8 patients with otherwise normal carotid angiograms, densograms
are generated from ROIs of the proximal and distal parts of the
internal carotid artery and the Ml/Al segments of the middle and
anterior cerebral arteries during the injection of 6 ml of iopamidole
(Solutrast, Byk-Gulden) (15o mgJ/ml) into the common or internal carotid
artery at a rate of 2 ml/sec. ECG und Doppler sonograms from the proximal
internal carotid (5 cases) or middle cerebral (3 cases) artery are
recorded simultaneously.

Pulse-synchronous changes of CD are observed in all cases (Fig.3)
except from 2 ROIs of the anterior cerebral artery. The maximal
amplitude of CD and the index of density variation decrease from
the proximal to the distal carotid and cerebral artery ROIs. As
in the model studies, the latency between the Doppler-sonographic
acceleration of flow and the maximum of CD increases with increasing
distance from the site of injection from o,o5 - o,1 sec in the
proximal part of the internal carotid artery to o,5 - o,7 sec in the
middle cerebral artery. This means that the velocity of propagation
of the flow wave (maximum of flow) is higher than the actual movement
of the particles (maximum of CD).

In one case of an occlusion of the internal carotid artery, the siphon
is opacified via the external carotid and ophthalmic artery after a
marked delay of 2 sec and CD is low but shows faint pulse-synchronous
alterations. The maximal CD within the proximal internal carotid stump
is higher and is reached earlier but without pulsations. (Fig.4, case 11)

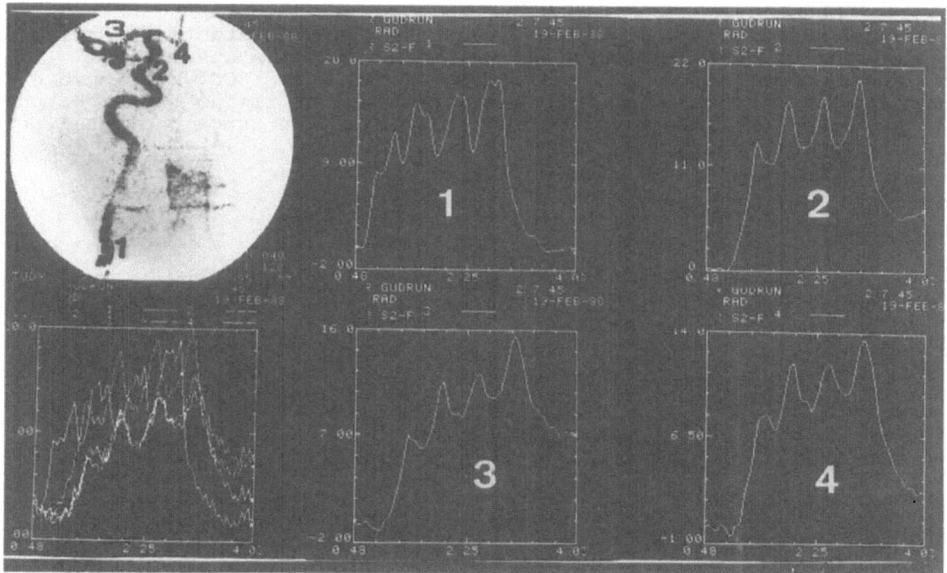

Fig. 3. High frequency DSA with ROIs within the proximal (1)
and distal (2) part of the internal carotid and the middle (3)
and anterior (4) cerebral artery and resulting densograms.

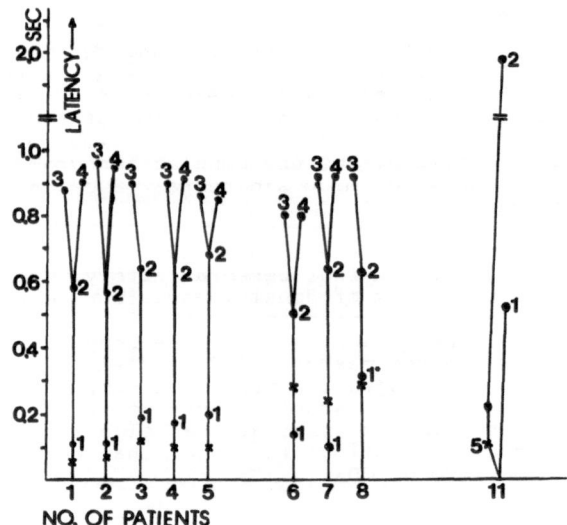

Fig. 4. Latency of Doppler-sonographic early systolic acceleration of flow (✖) and densographic maxima of CD (●) to R-wave of ECG (base line). Doppler sonogram of the proximal internal carotid (No. 1 - 5) and middle cerebral (no. 6 - 8) artery. ROIs as in Fig. 3. ROI 1* of case 8 is placed more distal than usual. No. 11: Internal carotid occlusion, Doppler sonogram and ROI 5 from external carotid artery (see text).

Summary and conclusions:

Pulse-synchronous changes of CD during carotid angiography are caused by the pulsating blood flow and have a close and constant time relation to the cardiac cycle. A summation of DSA images of a special ROI triggered according to its local delay of CD to the ECG, may improve image quality. In addition, the evaluation of the timing and amplitude of the pulse-like changes of CD may lead to a more functional analysis of arteriograms.

REFERENCES

Bürsch JH, Hahn HJ, Brennecke R, Grönemeier D, Heintzen PH (1981) Assessment of arterial blood flow measurements by digital angio-graphy. Radiology 14: 39 - 47
Hall A., Volz DJ (1986): Anwendungsmöglichkeiten der digitalen Subtraktionsangiographie in der Neuroradiologie. In: Nadjmi M (ed.): Digitale Subtraktionsangiographie in der Neuroradiologie. Thieme, Stuttgart
Heuck F, Piepgras U, Vanselow K (1969) Densitometrische Messungen des Blutstromvolumens der Arteria carotis. Radiologe 12: 443 - 448

Ultrasound Contrast Phenomena During the Injection of Contrast Medium into the Carotid Arteries

Th. Staudacher, P. Stoeter, N. Prey, and W. Sonntag (Ravensburg, FRG)

Injection of contrast medium into the carotid arteries induced numerous echoes of high intensity in the B scan and Doppler image of the
blood flow in the carotid and middle cerebral arteries. In order to
determine the case of this phenomenon we performed several in vitro
examinations.

1. There are only mild ultrasound effects if the injected and the
accepting fluids are of the same kind, i.e. injection of contrast
medium into contrast medium or blood into blood at a moderate velocity. This may be caused by turbulence of flow.

2. Injection of contrast medium into water or into a contrast medium
of a different kind induces typical Doppler and B scan reflections
due to interface effects.

3. Similar echoes are recorded if freshly aspirated contrast medium
containing some gas bubbles is injected into contrast medium or freshly aspirated blood into blood. Echoes also can be produced by injection of degassed contrast medium into contrast medium at high velocities above 1500 cm/sec. In these cases the echoes are probably
caused by gas bubbles which are either already present within the in-
jectate or are produced by cavitation. During carotid angiography the
ultrasound phenomena probably are due to a combination of turbulence
interfaces and gas bubbles.

List of Contributors

Abitbol M., Dept. of Neuroradiology, University Hospital, Besançon, France

Adelmann M.H., Dept. of Neurology, University of Frankfurt, FRG

Agnoli A.L., Dept. of Neuroradiology, University Hospital, Giessen, FRG

Aichner F., Dept. of Neurology, University of Innsbruck, Austria

Alesch F., Institute of Neuroradiology, Saarland University Homburg, FRG

Amicarelli I., Dept. of Radiology, Collemaggio Hospital, University of L'Aquila, Italy

Andreula C.F., Dept. of Neuroradiology, Policlinic, University of Bari, Italy

Arrué P., Dept. of Neuroradiology, CHU Purpan, Toulouse, France

Aschoff A., Dept. of Neurosurgery, University of Heidelberg, FRG

Aulich, A., Dept. of Neurology/Neuroradiology, University of Düsseldorf, FRG

Avni E.F., Dept. of Radiology, Erasme Hospital, University of Brussels, Belgium

Bakke S.J., Dept. of Neuroradiology and Neurosurgery, Rikshospitalet, University of Oslo, Norway

Bakker-Niezen S.H.,Dept. of Neurosurgery, Institute of Diagnostic Radiology,University Hospital, Nijmegen, The Netherlands

Balériaux D., Dept. of Radiology, Erasme Hospital, University of Brussels, Belgium

Bassi P., Dept. of Neuroradiology, U.S.L., Parma, Italy

Bavinzski G., Dept. of Neurosurgery, University of Vienna, Austria

Beck A., Dept. of Diagnostic Radiology, University of Freiburg, FRG

Becker H., Dept. of Diagnostic Radiology, MHH, Hannover, FRG

Beigelman C., Dept. of Radiology, Central Hospital, Strasbourg, France

Beltramello A., Dept. of Neuroradiology, University Hospital, Verona, Italy

Benati A., Dept. of Neuroradiology, University Hospital, Verona, Italy

Beomonte Zobel B., Dept. of Radiology, Collemaggio Hospital, University of L'Aquila, Italy

Bergström K., Dept. of Diagnostic Radiology and Neurology, University Hospital and Organic Chemistry, Uppsala, Sweden

Bergström M., Dept. of Diagnostic Radiology and Neurology, University Hospital and Organic Chemistry, Uppsala, Sweden

Berkefeld J, Dept. of Neuroradiology, University Hospital, Frankfurt, FRG

Berky M., Dept. of Radiology, Central Military Hospital, Budapest, Hungary

Bernini F.P., Dept. of Neuroradiology, C.T.O. Hospital, Naples, Italy

Berry I., Dept. of Neuroradiology, CHU Purpan, Toulouse, France

Bertalanaffy H., Dept. of Diagnostic Radiology, University of Freiburg, FRG

Bettag M., Dept. of Neurosurgery, University of Düsseldorf, FRG

Betz H., Dept. of Neurology, University of Heidelberg, FRG

Bock W.J., Dept. of Neurosurgery, University Hospital, Düsseldorf, FRG

Bonafé A., Dept. of Neuroradiology, CHU Purpan, Toulouse, France

Bonneville J.F., Dept. of Neuroradiology, University Hospital, Besançon, France

Bouchareb M., Dept. of Neuroradiology, University Hospital, Besançon, France

Bouguet D., Dept. of Neuroradiology, "La Pitie" Hospital, Paris, France

Boukobza M., Dept. of Neuroradiology, "La Pitie" Hospital, Paris, France

Bozzao A., Dept. of Radiology, Collemaggio Hospital, University of L'Aquila, Italy

Bradley W.G., Huntington Medical Research Institutes, Pasadena, CA 91105, USA

Brainin M., Dept. of Neurology, NO Landeskrankenhaus, Klosterneuburg, Austria

Brassel F., Dept. of Neuroradiology, MHH, Hannover, FRG

Brückmann H., Neuroradiology, Dept. of Neurology, RWTH Aachen, FRG

Bunke J., Dept. of Radiology, University of Cologne, FRG

Carella A., Dept. of Neuroradiology, Polyclinic, University of Bari, Italy

Castagna A., Dept. of Pediatrics, L. Sacco Hospital, University of Milan, Italy

Castaings L., Dept. of Anesthesiology, Fondation A. de Rothschild, Paris, France

Cattin F., Dept. of Neuroradiology, University Hospital, Besançon, France

Cavka K., Central Institute for Tumors, Zagreb, Yugoslavia

Cioffi F.A., Dept. of Neuroradiology, C.T.O. Hospital, Naples, Italy

Citrin C.M., Washington Imaging Center, Chevy Chase, MD; Uniformed Services University of the Health Sciences, Bethesda; George Washington University, Washington, DC, USA

Colombari R., Institute of Pathology, University Hospital, Verona, Italy

Conroy G., Dept. of Anatomy, Washington University, St. Louis, MO, USA

Cordes M., Radiological Clinic and Policlinic, Klinikum Rudolf Virchow, Standort Charlottenburg, Free University of Berlin, FRG

Corsico N., Research Dept., Bracco Industria Chimica, Milano, Italy

Cusmano F., Dept. of Neuroradiology, U.S.L., Parma, Italy

Da Pian R., Dept. of Neurosurgery, University Hospital, Verona, Italy

D'Aprile P., Dept. of Neuroradiology, Poyclinic, University of Bari, Italy

De La Porte C., Depts. of Radiology, Neurology, Neurosurgery and E.N.T., Universitair Ziekenhuis Antwerpen, Edegem, Belgium

De Schepper A.M., Depts. of Radiology, Neurology, Neurosurgery and E.N.T., Universitair Ziekenhuis Antwerpen, Edegem, Belgium

De Silva D., Dept. of Neuroradiology, Alfried Krupp Hospital, Essen, FRG

Deecke L., Neurological University Clinic, Vienna, Austria

Degryse H.R., Depts. of Radiology, Neurology, Neurosurgery and E.N.T., Universitair Ziekenhuis Antwerpen, Edegem, Belgium

Dekel D., Neuroradiological Section, Ch. Sheba Medical Center, Tel Aviv University for Advanced Technology, Elscint-Haifa, Israel

Derôme P., Dept. of Neurosurgery, Hôpital Foch, Suresnes, France

Dettmers Ch., Neurological Hospital, University of Bonn, FRG

Di Cesare E., Dept. of Radiology, Collemaggio Hospital, University of L'Aquila, Italy

Dicuonzo F., Dept. of Neuroradiology, Policlinic, University of Bari, Italy

Dietemann J.L., Dept. of Radiology, Central Hospital, Strasbourg, France

Dietrich B., Institute of Neuroradiology, Saarland University Homburg, FRG

Dietz H., Neurosurgical Hospital, MHH, Hannover, FRG

Dietz R., Elisabethen Hospital, Ravensburg, FRG

Döhring W., Dept. of Diagostic Radiology, MHH, Hannover, FRG

Drews U., Dept. of Anatomy, University of Tuebingen, FRG

Eberhard K. Dept. of Neuroradiology, University of Würzburg, FRG

Ehrmann D., Dept. of Neuroradiology, Elisabethen Hospital, Ravensburg, FRG

Eichstädt H., Radiological Clinic and Policlinic, Klinikum Rudolf Virchow, Standort Charlottenburg, Free University of Berlin, FRG

Eisenstadter A., Dept. of Neurology, NO Landeskrankenhaus, Klosterneuburg, Austria

Eldevik P., Dept. of Radiology, University of Wisconsin Hospital and Clinics, Madison, WI, USA

Eldridge R., National Institutes of Health, Bethesda, MD, USA

Elovaara I., Dept. of Neurology, University of Helsinki, Finland

Enzensberger W., Dept. of Neuroradiology, University of Frankfurt, FRG

Ethier R., Dept. of Radiology, Neurological Hospital and Institute, McGill University, Montreal, Canada

Fáiss J.H., Dept. of Neuroradiology, University of Tuebingen, FRG

Farchi G., Dept. of Neuroradiology, Polyclinic, University of Bari, Italy

Faubert C., Dept. of Radiology, Hospice Civil, Strasbourg, France

Feinendegen L.E., Dept. of Nuclear Medicine, University Hospital, Düsseldorf and Institute of Medicine, Nuclear Research Center, Jülich, FRG

Feivel M., Neuroradiological Section, Ch. Sheba Medical Center, Tel Aviv University for Advanced Technology, Elscint-Haifa, Israel

Felber S., Dept. of Neurology and Institute of Magnetic Resonance, University of Innsbruck, Austria

Feldges A., Neurosurgical Clinic, University Medical Center, Essen, FRG

Feliciani M., Dept. of Neurosciences, University "La Sapienza", Rome, Italy

Felix R., Radiological Clinic and Policlinic, Klinikum Rudolf Virchow,Standort Charlottenburg, Berlin, FRG

Fenzl G., Friedrich Baur-Institute, University of Munich, FRG

Ferri M., Dept. of Neurosurgery, U.S.L., Parma, Italy

Freitag J, Clinic of Neurology and Psychiatry, Med. Akademie Magdeburg, GDR

Friedburg H., Dept. of Diagnostic Radiology, University of Freiburg, FRG

Friedmann G., Dept. of Radiology, University of Cologne, FRG

Fritz P., Dept. of Radiology, University of Heidelberg, FRG

Góraj B., Dept. of Diagnostic Imaging, Institute of Radiology, Medical Academy, Lódź, Poland

Gaab M., Neurosurgical Hospital, MHH, Hannover, FRG

Gado M., Mallinckrodt Institute of Radiology, Washington University, St. Louis, MO, USA

Gallucci M., Dept. of Radiology, Collemaggio Hospital, University of L'Aquila, Italy

Gangarosa R., Clinical Science Center, Picker International, Ohio, USA

Gentile M.A., Dept. of Neuroradiology, Policlinic, University of Bari, Italy

Gerhard L., Institute of Neuropathology, University Medical Center, Essen, FRG

Gheuens J., Depts. of Radiology, Neurology, Neurosurgery and E.N.T., Universitair Ziekenhuis Antwerpen, Edegem, Belgium

Ginsberg L., Memorial Sloan-Kettering Cancer Center, New York, NY, USA

Goede G., Dept. of Diagnostic Radiology and Nuclear Medicine and Dept. of Physical Medicine and Medical Rehabilitation, Municipal Hospital München-Bogenhausen, FRG

Goldenberg G., Neurological Clinic, University of Vienna, Austria

Graves V., Dept. of Radiology, University of Wisconsin Hospital and Clinics, Madison, WI, USA

Grebmeier J., Interdisciplinary Dept. for MR-Tomography, University of Erlangen-Nürnberg, FRG

Grönlund G., Töölö Hospital, University of Helsinki, Finland

Grodd W., Dept. of Neuroradiology, University of Tuebingen, FRG

Gross-Fengels W., Institute for Radiology, University of Cologne, FRG

Grote E.H., Dept. of Neurosurgery, University of Tuebingen, FRG

Guglielmi G., Dept. of Neurosciences, University "La Sapienza", Rome, Italy

Guidetti G., Dept. of Neurosciences, University "La Sapienza", Rome, Italy

Haas J.P., Institute of Radiology, Municipal Hospital, Fulda, FRG

Hacker H., Dept. of Neuroradiology, University Hospital, Frankfurt, FRG

Hahn D., Friedrich Baur-Institute, University of Munich, FRG

Halbsguth A., Dept. of Radiology, University Hospital, Frankfurt/Main, FRG

Hald J., Dept. of Neuroradiology and Neurosurgery, Rikshospitalet, University of Oslo, Norway

Harilainen A., Töölö Hospital, University of Helsinki, Finland

Harth P., Dept. of Neuroradiology, University of Frankfurt, FRG

Hartmann A., Neurological Hospital, University of Bonn, FRG

Hassler W., Dept. of Neurosurgery, University of Tuebingen, FRG

Haubitz B., Dept. of Neuroradiology, MHH, Hannover, FRG

Hauss C., Elisabethen Hospital, Ravensburg, FRG

Hawnaur J.M., Dept. of Diagnostic Radiology, University of Manchester, England

Hedde J.P., Dept. of Radiology, Klinikum Rudolf Virchow, Standort Charlottenburg, Free University of Berlin, FRG

Heindel W.,Dept. of Radiology, University of Cologne, FRG

Heinrich P., Clinic of Neurology and Psychiatry, Med. Akademie Magdeburg, GDR

Heiss W.D., Max Planck Society for Neurological Research and Dept. of Neurology, University of Cologne, FRG

Henkes H., Radiological Clinic and Policlinic, Klinikum Rudolf Virchow, Standort Charlottenburg, Free University of Berlin, FRG

Hennerici, M., Dept. of Neurology/Neuroradiology, University of Düsseldorf, FRG

Henning J., Dept. of Radiology, University of Freiburg, FRG

Herholz K., Max Planck Society for Neurological Research and Dept. of Neurology, University of Cologne, FRG

Herzog H., Institute of Medicine, Nuclear Research Center, Jülich, FRG

Heun R., Max-Planck-Society, Clinical Research Unit for MS, Würzburg, FRG

Hofmann E., Dept. of Diagnostic Radiology, University of Freiburg, FRG

Holl K., Neurosurgical Hospital, MHH, Hannover, FRG

Holland I.M, Dept. of Neuroradiology, University Hospital, Nottingham, UK

Hosten N., Radiological Clinic and Policlinic, Klinikum Rudolf Virchow, Standort Charlottenburg, Free University of Berlin, FRG

Huber G., Institute of Neuroradiology, Saarland-University, Homburg, FRG

Huk W.J., Dept. of Neuroradiology, Neurosurgical Clinic, University of Erlangen-Nürnberg, FRG

Imam N., Memorial Sloan-Kettering Cancer Center, New York, USA

Imberti M., Dept. of Neuroradiology, U.S.L., Parma, Italy

Isherwood I., Dept. of Diagnostic Radiology, University of Manchester, England

Jagodziński Z., Dept. of Neurotraumatology, Medical Academy, Łódź, Poland

Jaspan T., Dept. of Neuroradiology, University Hospital, Nottingham, UK

Jenkins J. Dept. of Diagnostic Radiology, University of Manchester, England

Jeung M.Y., Dept. of Radiology, Central Hospital, Strasbourg, France

Jimenez J.L., Dept. of Radiology, Paris XI University, Kremlin Biçetre, France

Jinkins J.R., Huntington Medical Research Institutes, Pasadena, CA, USA

Jusić A., Central Institute for Tumors, Zagreb, Yugoslavia

Kahn T., Institute of Diagnostic Radiology, University Hospital, Düsseldorf, FRG

Kaiser-Kupfer M., National Institutes of Health Bethesda, MD, USA

Kamler A., Dept. of Neuroradiology and Neurosurgery, Clinical Hospital Center Rebro, University of Zagreb, Yugoslavia

Kamman R. L., Dept. of Magnetic Resonance, University Hospital, Groningen, The Netherlands

Kappos L., Max-Planck-Society, Clinical Research Unit for MS, Würzburg, FRG

Kaufmann H.J., Dept. of Pediatric Radiology, Klinikum Rudolf Virchow, Standort Charlottenburg, Free University of Berlin, FRG

Keil W., Practicing Radiologist, Würzburg, FRG

Köhler D., Dept. of Radiology, Klinikum Rudolf Virchow, Standort Charlottenburg, University of Berlin, FRG

Kühne D., Dept. of Neuroradiology, Alfried Krupp Hospital, Essen, FRG

Kikuchi Y., Dept. of Radiology, University of Wisconsin Hospital and Clinics, Madison, WI, USA

Kim J., Memorial Sloan-Kettering Cancer Center, New York, NY, USA

Kiwit J. C.W., Dept. of Neurosurgery, University Hospital Düsseldorf, FRG

Klose U., Dept. of Neuroradiology, University of Tuebingen, FRG

König E., Dept. of Neuroradiology, University of Tuebingen, FRG

Knosp E., Dept. of Neurosurgery, University of Vienna, Austria

Koch R.D., Clinic of Neurology and Psychiatry, Med. Akademie Magdeburg, GDR

Kollmann F., Dept. of Radiology, University Hospital, Frankfurt-Main, FRG

Kopits S.E., Washington Imaging Center, Chevy Chase, MD, USA

Kopytek M., Dept. of Diagnostic Imaging, Institute of Radiology, Medical Academy, Łódź, Poland

Koulousakis A., Neurosurgical Hospital, University of Cologne, FRG

Krol G., Memorial Sloan-Kettering Cancer Center, New York, NY, USA

Kubina G., Dept. of Neurology, Elisabethen Hospital, Ravensburg, FRG

Kutluk K., Dept. of Radiology, Section of Neuroradiology, University of Freiburg, FRG

Kuwert T., Institute of Medicine, Nuclear Research Center, Jülich, FRG

Laasonen E.M., Töölö Hospital, University of Helsinki, Finland

Lanfermann H., Institute of Radiology, University of Cologne, FRG

Lang S., Dept. of Neurology, Landeskrankenhaus Klosterneuburg, Austria

Langen K.-J., Dept. of Nuclear Medicine, University Hospital, Düsseldorf, FRG

Langer M., Radiological Clinic and Policlinic, Klinikum Rudolf Virchow, Standort Charlottenburg, Berlin, FRG

Langohr H.-D., Institute of Neurology and Neurophysiology, Municipal Hospital, Fulda, FRG

Langström B., Dept. of Diagnostic Radiology and Neurology, University Hospital and Organic Chemistry, Uppsala, Sweden

Lasjaunias P., Dept. of Radiology, Paris XI University, Kremlin Bicetre, France

Laub G., Siemens Medical Systems, Erlangen, FRG

Laun A., Dept. of Neurosurgery, University Hospital
Giessen, FRG

Lazzarin A., Dept. of Pediatrics, L. Sacco Hospital,
University of Milan, Italy

Lefebre C., Radiological Clinic and Policlinic, Klinikum Rudolf Virchow, Standort Charlottenburg, Free University of Berlin, FRG

Lepoire J., Dept. of Neurosurgery, Hôpital St. Julien,
Nancy, France

Lilius G., Töölö Hospital, University of Helsinki, Finland

Lilja A., Neuroradiology, Dept. of Diagnostic Radiology, Akademiska Hospital, Uppsala, Sweden

Lindegaard K.-F., Dept. of Neuroradiology and Neurosurgery, Rikshospitalet, University of Oslo, Norway

Lins E., Dept. of Neurosurgery, University of Düsseldorf, FRG

Livian S., Dept. of Neuroradiology, Scientific Institute, San Raffaele Hospital, Milan, Italy

Löffler W., Siemens Medical Systems, Erlangen, FRG

Löhlein A., Dept. of Orthopedic Surgery, University
of Heidelberg, FRG

Lorey C., Dept. of Radiology, University Hospital,
Frankfurt-Main, FRG

Lorusso A., Dept. of Neuroradiology, Policlinic, University of Bari, Italy

Lundberg P.O., Dept. of Diagnostic Radiology and Neurology, University Hospital and Organic Chemistry, Uppsala, Sweden

Lundin P., Dept. of Diagnostic Radiology and Neurology,
University Hospital and Organic Chemistry, Uppsala,
Sweden

Maida E., Neurological University Clinic, Vienna, Austria

Majno M., Dept. of Neuroradiology, San Raffaele Hospital, University of Milan, Italy

Malenica B.,Central Institute for Tumors, Yugoslavia

Malkin M., Memorial Sloan-Kettering Cancer Center, New
York, NY, USA

Mandić A., Central Institue for Tumors, Zagreb, Yugoslavia

Manelfe C.,Dept. of Neuroradiology, CHU Purpan, Toulouse,
France

Martin J.J., Depts. of Radiology, Neurology, Neurosurgery and E.N.T., Universitair Ziekenhuis Antwerpen, Edegem, Belgium

Martin N., Neuroradiology, Dept. of Radiology, Beaujon Hospital, Clichy, France

Maschio A., Dept. of Neuroradiology, University Hospital, Verona, Italy

Masciocchi C., Dept. of Radiology, Collemaggio Hospital, University of L`Aquila, Italy

Mayer T.E., Dept. of Radiology, University Hospital, Frankfurt-Main, FRG

Melanson D., Dept. of Radiology, Neurological Hospital and Institute, McGill University, Montreal, Canada

Mende U., Dept. of Radiotherapy, University of Heidelberg, FRG

Menichelli F., Dept. of Neuroradiology, General Regional Hospital, Ancona, Italy

Menozzi R., Dept. of Neuroradiology, U.S.L., Parma, Italy

Merland J.J., Lariboisière Hospital, Paris, France

Merx J.L., Dept. of Neuroradiology, Institute of Diagnostic Radiology, University Hospital Nijmegen, The Netherlands

Metzger M., Dept. of Neuroradiology, "La Pitie" Hospital, Paris, France

Michael T., Dept. of Pediatrics, Klinikum Rudolf Virchow, Standort Charlottenburg, Free University of Berlin, FRG

Müller D., Clinic of Neurology and Psychiatry, Med. Akademie Magdeburg, GDR

Müller-Forell W., Dept. of Neuroradiology, University Hospital Mainz, FRG

Mooyaart E.L., Dept. of Magnetic Resonance, University Hospital, Groningen, The Netherlands

Moret J., Dept. of Interventional Neuroradiology, Fondation Rothschild, Paris, France

Muessig M., Dept. of Neurology, Saarland University, Homburg-Saar, FRG

Muhr C., Dept. of Diagnostic Radiology and Neurology, University Hospital and Organic Chemistry, Uppsala, Sweden

Mull, M., Dept. of Neurology/Neuroradiology, University of Düsseldorf, FRG

Muras I., Dept. of Neuroradiology, C.T.O. Hospital, Naples, Italy

Myllynen P., Töölö Hospital, University of Helsinki, Finland

Nadjmi M., Dept. of Neuroradiology, University of Würzburg, FRG

Naegele M., Friedrich Baur-Institute, University of Munich, FRG

Nahser H.C., Dept. of Neuroradiology, Alfried Krupp Hospital, Essen, FRG

Nahum H., Neuroradiology, Dept. of Radiology, Beaujon Hospital, Clichy, France

Nakstad P., Dept. of Neuroradiology and Neurosurgery, Rikshospitalet, University of Oslo, Norway

Nemath M.-N., Neurosurgical Hospital, MHH, Hannover, FRG

Neuhold A., Dept. of Neurosurgery, University of Vienna and Institute for Diagnostic Imaging, Hospital Rudolfiner-haus, Vienna, Austria

Nierhaus A., Neurological Hospital, University of Bonn, FRG

Nomblot C., Dept. of Neuroradiology, CHU Purpan, Toulouse, France

Nouy I., Dept. of Neuroradiology, University Hospital, Besançon, France

Özturk E., Dept. of Neurosurgery, University of Vienna, Austria

Ott D., Dept. of Neuroradiology, University of Freiburg, FRG

Paladini R., Dept. of Neuroradiology, Policlinic, University of Bari, Italy

Palmbach M., Dept. of Neuroradiology and Neurosurgery, University of Tuebingen, FRG

Parizel P.M., Depts. of Radiology, Neurology, Neurosur-gery and E.N.T., Universitair Ziekenhuis Antwerpen, Edegem, Belgium

Parry D.M., National Institutes of Health, Bethesda, MD, USA

Partington C., Dept. of Radiology, University of Wis-consin Hospital and Clinics, Madison, WI, USA

Pasqualin A., Dept. of Neurosurgery, University Hospi-tal, Verona, Italy

Pasquini U., Dept. of Neuroradiology, General Regional Hospital, Ancona, Italy

Passariello R., Dept. of Radiology, Collemaggio Hospital, University of L'Aquila, Italy

Patay Z., Dept. of Radiology, Central Military Hospital, Budapest, Hungary

Pavone P., Dept. of Radiology, Collemaggio Hospital, University of L'Aquila, Italy

Pawlik G., Max Planck Society for Neurological Research and Dept. of Neurology, University of Cologne, FRG

Perini S., Dept. of Neuroradiology, University Hospital, Verona, Italy

Pesce Delfino V., Dept. of Anthropology, Institute of Zoology and Comparative Anatomy, University of Bari, Italy

Piazza P., Dept. of Neuroradiology, U.S.L., Parma, Italy

Picard L., Dept. of Neuroradiology, Hôpital St. Julien, Nancy, France

Piepgras C., Institute of Neuroradiology, Saarland-University, Homburg, FRG

Pieralli S., Dept. of Neuroradiology, San Raffaele Hospital, University of Milan, Italy

Pikus A., National Institutes of Health Bethesda, MD, USA

Piovani E., Dept. of Neuroradiology, University Hospital, Verona,Italy

Pongratz D.E., Friedrich Baur-Institute, University of Munich, FRG

Posner J., Memorial Sloan-Kettering Cancer Center, New York, USA

Poutiainen E., Dept. of Neurology, University of Helsinki, Finland

Prère J., Dept. of Neuroradiology, CHU Purpan, Toulouse, France

Prevo R.L., Dept. of Radiology, Ziekenhuis "De Stadsmaten", Enschede, The Netherlands

Prey N., Dept. of Neuroradiology, Elisabethen Hospital, Ravensburg, FRG

Purgold S., Dept. of Neuroradiology, University Hospital, Hamburg Eppendorf, FRG

Raininko R., Dept. of Diagnostic Radiology, University of Helsinki, Finland

Ratzka M., Dept. of Neuroradiology, University of Würzburg, FRG

Reifenberger G., Dept. of Neuropathology, University of Düsseldorf, FRG

Reimers K., Friedrich Baur-Institute, University of Munich, FRG

Reisner T., Neurological University Clinic, Vienna, Austria

Resta M., Dept. of Neuroradiology, Policlinic, University of Bari, Italy

Richling B., Dept. of Neurosurgery, University of Vienna, Austria

Richter H.-P., Institute of Neurosurgery, Municipal Hospital, Fulda, FRG

Righi C., Dept. of Neuroradiology, Scientific Institute, San Raffaele Hospital, Milan, Italy

Ringelstein E.B., Neuroradiology, Dept. of Neurology, RWTH Aachen, FRG

Ritter K., Dept. of Neuroradiology, University Hospital, Hamburg Eppendorf, FRG

Rodesch C., Dept. of Radiology, Paris XI University, Kremlin Biçetre, France

Rodesch G., Dept. of Radiology, Erasmus Hospital, Free University of Brussels, Belgium

Rodiek S.O., Dept. of Diagnostic Radiology and Nuclear Medicine and Dept. of Physical Medicine and Medical Rehabilitation, Municipal Hospital München Bogenhausen, FRG

Rohrbach E., Max-Planck-Society, Clinical Research Unit for MS, Würzburg, FRG

Rolfes H., Dept. of Neuroradiology, University Hospital, Frankfurt, FRG

Roosen N., Dept. of Neurosurgery, University Hospital, Düsseldorf, FRG

Rossi R., Dept. of Radiology, I.N.R.C.A., Ancona, Italy

Rosta L., Dept. of Neuroradiology, University Hospital, Verona, Italy

Rota E., Institute of Medicine, Nuclear Research Center, Jülich, FRG

Rothwell C.I., Dept. of Neuroradiology, University Hospital, Nottingham, UK

Roy-Camille R., Dept. of Neuroradiology, "La Pitie" Hospital, Paris, France

Ruggieri P., Siemens Medical Systems, Erlangen, FRG

Rumbach L., Dept. of Radiology, Central Hospital, Strasbourg, France

Salvolini U., Dept. of Neuroradiology, General Regional Hospital, Ancona, Italy

Sauter R., Siemens Medical Systems, Erlangen, FRG

Scarpa, Institute of Pathology, University Hospital, Verona, Italy

Schimrigk K., Dept. of Neurology, Saarland University, Homburg-Saar, FRG

Schindler E., Dept. of Neurosurgery, University of Vienna, Austria

Schlote W., Dept. of Neuroradiology, University of Frankfurt, FRG

Schober R., Dept. of Neuropathology, University of Düsseldorf, FRG

Schroth G., Dept. of Neuroradiology, University Hospital Mainz and Dept. of Neuroradiology, University of Tuebingen, FRG

Schuhknecht B., Dept. of Neuroradiology, University of Würzburg, FRG

Schuierer G., Dept. of Neuroradiology, Neurosurgical Clinic, University of Nürnberg-Erlangen, FRG

Schumacher M., Dept. of Neuroradiology, University of Freiburg, FRG

Scienza R., Dept. of Neurosurgery, University Hospital, Verona, Italy

Scotti G., Dept. of Neuroradiology, San Raffaele Hospital, University of Milan, Italy

Scuotto A., Dept. of Neuroradiology, C.T.O. Hospital, Naples, Italy

Söder R., Dept. of Neuroradiology, University of Frankfurt, FRG

Selosse P., Depts. of Radiology, Neurology, Neurosurgery and E.N.T., Universitair Ziekenhuis Antwerpren, Edegem, Belgium

Sherman J.L., Washington Imaging Center, Chevy Chase, MD 20815; Uniformed Services University of the Health Sciences, Bethesda, MD; George Washington University Medical Center, Washington, DC, USA

Sick H., Dept. of Anatomy, Inst. Louis-Pasteur Strasbourg, France

Sielecki S., Institute of Radiology, Municipal Hospital, Fulda, FRG

Silipo P., Dept. of Neurosciences, University "La Sapienza", Rome, Italy

Simuni S., Central Institute for Tumors, Yugoslavia

Skalpe I.O., Dept. of Neuroradiology and Neurosurgery, Rikshospitalet, University of Oslo, Norway

Solymosi L., Dept. of Neuroradiology, Neurosurgical Hospital, Universiy of Bonn

Sonntag W., Elisabethen Hospital, Ravensburg, FRG

Sostarko M., Central Institute for Tumors, Zagreb, Yugoslavia

Sorteberg W., Dept. of Neuroradiology and Neurosurgery, Rikshospitalet, University of Oslo, Norway

Splendiani A., Dept. of Radiology, Collemaggio Hospital, University of L'Aquila, Italy

Sörensen N., Dept. of Neuroradology, University of Würzburg, FRG

Staudacher T. Dept. of Neurology, Elisabethen Hospital, Ravensburg, FRG

Städt D., Max-Planck-Society, Clinical Research Unit for MS, Würzburg and Dept. of Neuroradiology, University of Würzburg, FRG

Steinbrich W., Institute of Radiology, University of Cologne, FRG

Steinmetz H., Dept. of Neuroradiology and Neurosurgery, University of Tuebingen, FRG

Sterkers O., Neuroradiology, Dept. of Radiology,Beaujon Hospital, Clichy, France

Stiglbauer R., Dept. of Neurosurgery, University of Vienna, Austria

Stoeter P., Dept. of Neuroradiology, Elisabethen Hospital, Ravensburg, FRG

Stojanović J., Dept. of Neuroradiology and Neurosurgery, Clinical Hospital Center Rebro, University of Zagreb, Yugoslavia

Strother C., Dept. of Radiology, University of Wisconsin Hospital and Clinics, Madison, WI, USA

Strutz J., Dept. of Radiology, Section of Neuroradiology, University of Freiburg, FRG

Sze G., Memorial Sloan-Kettering Cancer Center, New York, NY, USA

Szelies B., Max Planck Society for Neurological Research and Dept. of Neurology, University of Cologne, FRG

Tadmor R., Neuroradiological Section, Ch. Sheba Medical Center, Tel Aviv University for Advanced Technology, Elscint-Haifa, Israel

Tajahmady T., Dept. of Radiology, Central Hospital, Strasbourg, France

Tampieri D., Dept. of Radiology, Neurological Hospital and Institute, McGill University, Montreal, Canada

Tang Y.S., Dept. of Neuroradiology, University Hospital, Besançon, France

Terbrugge K., Dept. of Radiology, Paris XI University, Kremlin Biçetre, France

Thaller N., Central Institute for Tumors, Zagreb, Yugoslavia

Thijssen H.O.M., Dept. of Neuroradiology, Institute of Diagnostic Radiology, University Hospital Nijmegen, The Netherlands

Thijssen M.A.O., Dept. of Physics, Institute of Diagnostic Radiology, University Hospital Nijmegen, The Netherlands

Thron A., Dept. of Neurology, University of Aachen, FRG

Thun F., Radiological Institute, University of Cologne, FRG

Tirone P., Research Dept., Bracco Industria Chimica, Milano, Italy

Tjan T.G., Dept. of Radiology, St. Elizabeth Hospital, Tilburg, The Netherlands

Trabert W., Dept. of Neurology, Saarland University, Homburg-Saar, FRG

Traupe H., Dept. of Neuroradiology, University Hospital, Hamburg Eppendorf, FRG

Treisch J., Dept. of Radiology, Klinikum Rudolf Virchow, Standort Charlottenburg, Free University of Berlin, FRG

Triulzi F., Dept. of Neuroradiology, San Raffaele Hospital, University of Milan, Italy

Turi M., Dept. of Neuroradiology and Neurosurgery, Clinical Hospital Center Rebro, University of Zagreb, Yugoslavia

Ulrich F., Dept. of Neurosurgery, University of Düsseldorf, FRG

Unusic J., Dept. of Neuroradiology and Neurosurgery, Clinical Hospital Center Rebro, University of Zagreb, Yugoslavia

Valanne L., Dept. of Radiology, Kivelä Hospital, Helsinki, Finland

Van de Heyning P., Depts. of Radiology, Neurology, Neurosurgery and E.N.T., Universitair Ziekenhuis Antwerpen, Edegem, Belgium

Van der Velde E.A., Dept. of Radiology, Ziekenhuis "De Stadsmaten", Enschede, The Netherlands

Van Goethem J., Dept. of Radiology, Universitair Ziekenhuis, University of Antwerp, Edegem, Belgium

Van Vyve M., Depts. of Radiology, Neurology, Neurosurgery and E.N.T., Universitair Ziekenhuis Antwerp,
Edegem, Belgium

Van Woensel M.P.L.M., Department of Physics, Institute
of Diagnostic Radiology, University Hospital Nijmegen,
The Netherlands

Vannier M., Mallinckrodt Institute of Radiology, Washington
University, St. Louis, MO, USA

Viars P., Dept. of Neuroradiology, "La Pitie" Hospital,
Paris, France

Vidovi M.,Central Institute for Tumors, Yugoslavia

Vielvoye G.J., Dept. of Radiology, Ziekenhuis "De
Stadsmaten", Enschede, The Netherlands

Virta A., Dept. of Radiology, Kivelä Hospital, Helsinki,
Finland

Visciani A., Dept. of Neuroradiology, Scientific Institute, San Raffaele Hospital, Milan, Italy

Vogl G., Dept. of Neuroradiology, University of Tuebingen,
FRG

Volle E., Dept. of Radiology, Klinikum Rudolf Virchow,
Standort Charlottenburg, Free University of Berlin, FRG

Vouge M., Dept. of Radiology, Hospice Civil, Strasbourg,
France

Wackenheim A., Dept. of Radiology, Hospice Civil,
Strasbourg, France

Wagner S., Friedrich Baur-Institute, University of
Munich, FRG

Wallner K., Memorial Sloan-Kettering Cancer Center, New
York, NY USA

Werner G.T., Dept. of Diagnostic Radiology and Nuclear
Medicine and Dept. of Physical Medicine and Medical Re-
habilitation, Municipal Hospital München-Bogenhausen,
FRG

Wessel K., Dept. of Neuroradiology, University Hospital
Mainz, FRG

Whittemore A.R., Huntington Medical Research Institutes, Pasadena, CA, USA

Wicke L,. Institute for Diagnostic Imaging, Hospital
Rudolfinerhaus, Vienna, Austria

Wienhard K., Max Planck Society for Neurological Research
and Dept. of Neurology, University of Cologne, FRG

Will B., Dept. of Neuroradiology, University of Tuebingen, FRG

Wilmink J.T., Dept. of Diagnostic Radiology, Section of Neuroradiology, University Hospital, Groningen, The Netherlands

Wilson A.R.M., Queen's Medical Centre, University Hospital, Nottingham, England

Winkels G., Philips Medical System, Best, The Netherlands

Witt T.N., Friedrich Baur-Institute, University of Munich, FRG

Woelki U., Dept. of Neuroradiology, University of Frankfurt, FRG

Worthington B.S., Queen's Medical Centre, University Hospital, Nottingham, England

Yeh S., Memorial Sloan-Kettering Cancer Center, New York, NY, USA

Zamboni G., Institute of Pathology, University Hospital, Verona, Italy

Zanella F.E., Institute of Radiology, University of Cologne, FRG

Zeilstra D.J., Dept. of Neurosurgery, University Hospital, Groningen, The Netherlands

Zeumer H., Dept. of Neuroradiology, University Hospital, Hamburg Eppendorf, FRG

The most precise diagnosis of CNS diseases

W. J. Huk, University of Erlangen-Nürnberg;
G. F. Gademann, University of Heidelberg;
G. Friedmann, Cologne

Magnetic Resonance Imaging of Central Nervous System Diseases

Functional Anatomy – Imaging – Neurological Symptoms – Pathology

With contributions by numerous experts

1989. 635 figures in 765 separate illustrations.
Approx. 530 pages. Hard cover.
ISBN 3-540-17641-1

This book provides an outstanding description of diseases of the central nervous system (CNS) and their presentation by magnetic resonance imaging (MRI). Stress is layed upon neuropathological peculiarities of the diseases, knowledge of which is of great importance for the correct evaluation of their impact on signal intensity and for the choice of adequate imaging parameters. The clinical section is preceded by a list of leading neurological symptoms and their topical correlations which serves to obtain accuracy not only in formulating diagnostic questions, but also in performing the examination.

The excellent detailed presentation of the anatomy of the CNS in the MR image allows a more profound study of the relationship between the site of the lesion and its effects on function and, with it, the symptoms, than has ever been the case in existing radiological books.

Springer-Verlag Berlin
Heidelberg New York London
Paris Tokyo Hong Kong

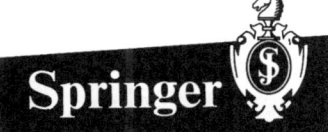

Springer

E. Kazner, S. Wende, T. Grumme, O. Stochdorph,
R. Felix, C. Claussen (Eds.)

Computed Tomography and Magnetic Resonance Tomography of Intracranial Tumors

A Clinical Perspective

2nd fully revised and expanded edition.
1989. 738 figures in 2993 separate illustrations.
Approx. 720 pages. Hard cover
ISBN 3-540-50576-8

This internationally recognized standard work on cerebral computer tomography has been completely revised and expanded to include magnetic resonance imaging.

It systematically presents the clinical diagnosis and differential diagnosis of virtually all cerebral tumors. Cranial base and orbital lesions are also included.

The authors' vast experience with CT and MRI in almost 10,000 cases of verified space-occupying lesions and orbital diseases lays a solid foundation for this second edition. The comprehensive illustrations include not just the typical, but also the rare tumors and atypical sites. The new WHO classification was used for the tumor categorization. The section on differential diagnosis offers complete coverage of all non-neoplastic, space-occupying intracranial lesions: inflammatory diseases, AIDS related diseases, acute demyelinization, granulomas, cysts, parasites, hemorrhages, vascular anomalies and brain infarctions.

Springer-Verlag Berlin
Heidelberg New York London
Paris Tokyo Hong Kong

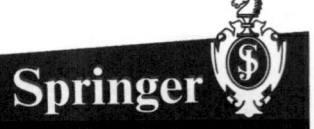